EVOLUTION OF MICROBIAL PATHOGENS

DISCARDED

EVOLUTION OF MICROBIAL PATHOGENS

EDITED BY

H. STEVEN SEIFERT
Department of Microbiology-Immunology
Feinberg School of Medicine
Northwestern University
Chicago, Illinois

AND

VICTOR J. DiRITA
Unit for Laboratory Animal Medicine and
Department of Microbiology and Immunology
University of Michigan
Ann Arbor, Michigan

ASM PRESS

Washington, D.C.

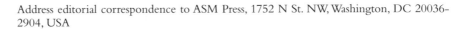

Address editorial correspondence to ASM Press, 1752 N St. NW, Washington, DC 20036-2904, USA

Send orders to ASM Press, P.O. Box 605, Herndon, VA 20172, USA
Phone: (800) 546-2416 or (703) 661-1593
Fax: (703) 661-1501
E-mail: books@asmusa.org
Online: estore.asm.org

Library of Congress Cataloging-in-Publication Data

Evolution of microbial pathogens / edited by H. Steven Seifert and Victor J. DiRita.
    p. ; cm.
  Includes bibliographical references and index.
  ISBN-13: 978-1-55581-300-0 (hardcover)
  ISBN-10: 1-55581-300-3 (hardcover)
  1. Pathogenic bacteria—Evolution. 2. Bacterial genetics. I. Seifert, H. Steven. II. DiRita, Victor J.
  [DNLM: 1. Bacteria—genetics. 2. Bacteria—pathogenicity. 3. Evolution, Molecular. 4. Fungi—genetics. 5. Fungi—pathogenicity.
QW 50 E93 2006]
QR201.B34E76 2006
579.3'165—dc22   2005032862

10 9 8 7 6 5 4 3 2 1

Cover design by Meral Dabcovich, VisPer

Cover photo: Scanning electron micrograph of enteropathogenic *Escherichia coli* adhering to cultured HeLa cells. Courtesy of Jorge Giron, University of Arizona.

CONTENTS

CONTRIBUTORS

Stephen B. Beres
Department of Pathology, Baylor College of Medicine, One Baylor Plaza, Houston, TX 77030

A. Casadevall
Departments of Microbiology and Immunology and of Medicine, Albert Einstein College of Medicine, Bronx, NY 10461

Vaughn S. Cooper
Department of Microbiology, 212 Rudman Hall, University of New Hampshire, Durham, NH 03824

William A. Day
Bacteriology Division, U.S. Army Medical Research Institute of Infectious Diseases, Fort Detrick, MD 21702

Rob DeSalle
Molecular Biology Laboratory, American Museum of Natural History, Molecular Laboratories, Central Park West at 79th St., New York, NY 10024

Ulrich Dobrindt
Institut für Molekulare Infektionsbiologie, Universität Würzburg, D-97070 Würzburg, Germany

David H. Figurski
Department of Microbiology, College of Physicians and Surgeons, Columbia University, 701 West 168th St., New York, NY 10032

J. Ross Fitzgerald
Centre for Infectious Diseases, Medical Microbiology, University of Edinburgh Medical School, Teviot Place, Edinburgh, Scotland, United Kingdom

Jeffrey I. Gordon
Center for Genome Sciences, Washington University School of Medicine, St. Louis, MO 63108

Nicole M. Green
Department of Pathology, Baylor College of Medicine, One Baylor Plaza, Houston, TX 77030

Jörg Hacker
Institut für Molekulare Infektionsbiologie, Universität Würzburg, D-97070 Würzburg, Germany

Bianca Hochhut
Institut für Molekulare Infektionsbiologie, Universität Würzburg, D-97070 Würzburg, Germany

Deborah A. Hogan
Department of Microbiology and Immunology, Dartmouth Medical School, Hanover, NH 03755

James B. Kaper
Center for Vaccine Development, Department of Microbiology and Immunology, University of Maryland School of Medicine, Baltimore, MD 21201

Roberto Kolter
Department of Microbiology and Molecular Genetics, Harvard Medical School, Boston, MA 02115

Ruiting Lan
School of Biotechnology and Biomolecular Sciences, University of New South Wales, Sydney, New South Wales 2052, Australia

Jeffrey G. Lawrence
Pittsburgh Bacteriophage Institute and Department of Biological Sciences, University of Pittsburgh, Pittsburgh, PA 15260

Martin C. J. Maiden
The Peter Medawar Building for Pathogen Research and Department of Zoology, University of Oxford, South Parks Road, Oxford OX1 3SY, United Kingdom

Anthony T. Maurelli
Department of Microbiology and Immunology, F. Edward Hébert School of Medicine, Uniformed Services University of the Health Sciences, Bethesda, MD 20814-4799

Didier Mazel
Unité Plasticité du Génome Bactérien, Institut Pasteur, 25 rue du Dr. Roux, 75724 Paris cedex 15, France

Margaret J. McFall-Ngai
Department of Medical Microbiology and Immunology, University of Wisconsin, Madison, WI 53706

John J. Mekalanos
Department of Microbiology and Molecular Genetics, Harvard Medical School, Building D1, Room 421, 200 Longwood Ave., Boston, MA 02115

Rachel Muir
Departments of Genetics and of Microbiology and Immunology, Stanford University School of Medicine, Stanford, CA 94305

James M. Musser
Department of Pathology, Baylor College of Medicine, One Baylor Plaza, Houston, TX 77030

James P. Nataro
Department of Pediatrics, Department of Medicine, Department of Microbiology and Immunology, and Center for Vaccine Development, University of Maryland School of Medicine, Baltimore, MD 21201

Paul J. Planet
Molecular Biology Laboratory, American Museum of Natural History, Molecular Laboratories, Central Park West at 79th St., New York, NY 10024

Alexander S. Pym
Medical Research Council of South Africa, 491 Ridge Road, P.O. Box 70380, Overport 4067, Durban, South Africa

Sean D. Reid
Department of Microbiology and Immunology, Wake Forest University School of Medicine, Winston-Salem, NC 27157

Peter R. Reeves
School of Molecular and Microbial Biosciences, University of Sydney, Sydney, New South Wales 2006, Australia

Dean Rowe-Magnus
Department of Microbiology, Clinical Integrative Biology Division. Sunnybrook & Women's College Health Sciences Centre, 2075 Bayview Ave., S1–26A, Toronto, Ontario, Canada M4N 3N5

Peter M. Small
Global Health Program, P.O. Box 23350, Seattle, WA 98102

Judith N. Steenbergen
Department of Microbiology and Immunology, Albert Einstein College of Medicine, Bronx, NY 10461

O. Colin Stine
Department of Epidemiology and Preventive Medicine and Department of Pediatrics, University of Maryland School of Medicine, Baltimore, MD 21201

Man-Wah Tan
Departments of Genetics and of Microbiology and Immunology, Stanford University School of Medicine, Stanford, CA 94305

Rachel Urwin
The Peter Medawar Building for Pathogen Research and Department of Zoology, University of Oxford, South Parks Road, Oxford OX1 3SY, United Kingdom

INTRODUCTION

The 1976 edition of the classic textbook *The Microbial World* by Stanier, Adelberg, and Ingraham (3) relegated the topics "Microbial Pathogenicity" and "Microbial Diseases of Man" to chapters 29 and 30 of a 31-chapter book. Such was the appreciation of microbial pathogenesis in the field of microbiology in the 1970s. More detailed coverage of microbial pathogens is found in the 1978 edition of *Bailey and Scott's Diagnostic Microbiology* (1), but that book is also a time capsule of the breadth and depth of knowledge in pathogenic microbiology at that time—before the genetics and genomics revolutions of the last 30 years. The sole reference to Legionnaires' disease makes no mention of *Legionella pneumophila*, which had yet to be discovered. Likewise, although enteropathogenic and enteroxigenic *Escherichia coli* are covered, enterohemorrhagic *E. coli* was not mentioned at all. And of course in 1978 there was no appreciation at all that a microbe, *Helicobacter pylori*, causes human ulcers.

Any active field of study will accumulate new information after nearly 30 years, but in the area of pathogenic microbiology the fruits of research since the 1970s have been quite extraordinary. Not only have new microbial diseases been uncovered, but appreciation about the diversity of mechanisms underlying the way that microbes and hosts interact has also grown. Microbes that have historically been challenging to study in the laboratory have yielded to the ingenuity of researchers who have brought an impressive toolbox of techniques and experimental models to bear on questions of microbial pathogenicity. The 1980s saw the development and application of genetic approaches for uncovering new virulence factors. The 1990s were a time of incredible advances in the study of how microbes exploit or disrupt host cell functions, and the field of "cellular microbiology" was born. Currently we are in the genomic era, with dozens of genomes from pathogenic microbes being mined for new virulence factors and therapeutic targets using bioinformatics and high-throughput approaches and new genome sequences appearing weekly. The quantum leap in knowledge from the field of genomics has also reinvigorated the study of microbial physiology, microbial metabolism, and microbial communities in a diverse range of environments. It is the amazing amount of data available from prokaryotic genome sequences which has fueled a renewed interest in the study of the evolution of microbes, and in parallel the study of the evolution of microbial pathogens. It is at this point that we considered the suggestion of assembling a book that could provide central concepts about evolution to the microbiological community in the context of pathogenesis. Given our interest in the subject, as well as the fact that sufficient knowledge to allow a thoughtful approach to it is now available, we decided to take on the project.

Most biologists like to speculate about the evolution of their particular area of focus, but to discuss evolution intelligently requires familiarity with the basic concepts about the subject. Evolutionary biologists have much to teach general physiologists, biochemists, geneticists, and infectious disease specialists, but the concepts and language of this area of study have become sufficiently specialized that there are barriers to a microbiologist who wants to learn more about evolution. This leads to a scenario where microbiologists sometimes make evolutionary arguments that are not well supported by the accepted theories of evolution.

It is often assumed that traits associated with pathogenicity were acquired as a way to improve the fitness of those microbes living in an otherwise hostile host environment. This is a simplistic view of a complicated relationship between microbes and the many environments they encounter. We undoubtedly place too much emphasis on the host and disease in trying to understand selection forces operating on microbes that live in a wide range of environments. Environmental reservoirs, where pathogens spend so much more time relative to that spent in a susceptible host who then becomes sick, may be better places to look for answers to questions of how pathogenicity traits have become fixed in microbial populations.

In this context, disease may simply be a consequence of specific microbial mechanism acting on a host that does not have a long natural history of coevolution with the microbe. A theme that has emerged from recent work on pathogenic microbes challenges even the basic notion of what a pathogen is. Microbes that cause disease in some hosts may be perfectly harmless in others. In turn, mechanisms that have evolved to enable microbes to disrupt the host in a way that causes symptoms and disease can be used by other microbes or in other hosts to establish asymptomatic, long-term associations.

The genomic era has provided new knowledge regarding the evolution of specific pathogenic species, in which some of the common themes, such as pathogenicity islands, are seen in action. Valuable information can be obtained by determining the genome sequence of pathogenic microbes as well as closely related non-pathogenic strains. This has enabled investigators to focus on unique sequences in the pathogenic strains both as a way to design new control strategies, and as a way to better understand the forces that govern evolution of pathogenicity. Why, for example, are some serogroups of a particular species pathogenic whereas others are not? What traits have evolved along with serogroup specificity that contribute to this segregation of specific antigenic types with virulence traits?

As we assembled this book, the topic of bacterial genetics kept cropping up in the majority of the chapters. To understand the process of evolution in bacteria without thinking about the horizontal transmission of genetic material within and between species is like trying to understand a baseball box score without thinking about hits, runs or errors. Rather than offer a basic primer for bacterial genetics (or baseball), we refer readers who are not familiar with the details of genetic processes to the textbook *Molecular Genetics of Bacteria* by Snyder and Champness (2) or any of the wonderful texts that also describe the mechanisms of gene exchange such as transformation, transduction, and conjugation.

Our goal with this book is to offer a current understanding of virulence evolution with the microbiologist in mind. The content is offered from three different perspectives. In the first section, our emphasis is on broad themes and the business of how evolution is studied. Principles that relate not only to pathogenesis, but to evolution in general, are covered in some detail by looking at specific cases. The second section offers examples of how problems common to a number of pathogens have been solved in evolutionary terms. This section also discusses the question of how microbial ecology has played a role in the evolution of pathogenicity. These first two sections discuss model systems that have provided new knowledge relevant to study of many other microbes. In the third section, we focus on a few well-studied classes of pathogens to learn how they may have evolved their disease-causing mechanisms. In this section we see some more specific examples of the themes developed in the first two sections, but the points are more finely drawn. In all chapters we are fortunate to have as collaborators outstanding authors who have made important contributions to the literature regarding their topics. Each section is also introduced and put into broader perspective by an eminent investigator whose own work relates to that section. We have learned a lot about both evolution in general, the evolution of pathogenic systems, and examples from specific microbial pathogens while assembling this book. We hope it will be useful to many who are learning about or studying pathogenic microbes and set the stage for further research into this important area of biology.

HANK S. SEIFERT
VICTOR J. DiRITA

REFERENCES

1. **Finegold, S. M., W. J. Martin, and E. G. Scott.** 1978. *Bailey and Scott's Diagnostic Microbiology,* 5th ed. C.V. Mosby Company, St. Louis, Mo.
2. **Snyder, L., and W. Champness.** 2003. *Molecular Genetics of Bacteria,* 2nd ed. ASM Press, Washington, D.C.
3. **Stanier, R. Y., E. A. Adelberg, and J. L. Ingraham.** 1976. *The Microbial World,* 4th ed. Prentice-Hall, Englewood Cliffs, N.J.

GENERAL CONCEPTS OF MICROBIAL EVOLUTION

I

PART I OVERVIEW

John J. Mekalanos

I

The field of microbial pathogenesis spans a century of research effort. Over the last few decades, the study of microbial pathogens has focused on pragmatic topics such as vaccine development and the identification of virulence factors and their molecular effects on the host. This work leaves a legacy that is a storehouse of knowledge on many important pathogens, as well as a template for studying newly identified pathogens. How evolution shaped the traits of pathogenic microbes has been an interesting and important question, but less research has been devoted to it than to other topics related to pathogens. Investigators interested in evolution per se have traditionally devoted their attention to tractable model systems, and some important pathogens certainly do not easily fall into this category.

But the introduction of large-scale genome sequencing projects has led to great interest in understanding the evolution of microbes, and of microbial pathogens in particular. Indeed, the paper describing the first complete genome sequence of a free-living organism, that of *Haemophilus influenzae,* compared the attenuated Rd laboratory strain with the sequences of

virulence genes (e.g., genes encoding capsular polysaccharides, fimbriae, and iron uptake systems) previously cloned from more pathogenic clinical isolates (10). This sort of comparative analysis can lead to insights about how particular bacterial pathogens have evolved and has accelerated as more and more genomic sequences have been deposited in open databases. Comparative genomics has matured as a field and will contribute importantly to our understanding of horizontal gene transfer and genetic variations linked to virulence and pathogen emergence. Jeffrey Lawrence provides a thorough description of how the availability of genome sequence data has influenced the study of evolution and the types of genetic variation that are apparently linked to alterations in the virulence of pathogenic bacterial species. He points out that some questions about evolution of pathogens are now approachable for really the first time because of genome sequence data mining. Lawrence also reminds us that significant variation takes place by point mutation as well as by the acquisition or loss of large gene clusters. Thus, genome sequence data can provide a deeper understanding of the mutational processes compared with what we could learn from low-resolution methods that were routinely used in the pregenomic era. New methods such as microarray

John J. Mekalanos, Department of Microbiology and Molecular Genetics, Harvard Medical School, Building D1, Room 421, 200 Longwood Ave., Boston, MA 02115.

Evolution of Microbial Pathogens, Edited by H. S. Seifert and V. J. DiRita, © 2006 ASM Press, Washington, D.C.

analysis of gene content have been used to identify genome variation among closely related strains. For example, microarray-based studies have identified patterns of horizontal gene acquisition that correlate with the emergence of pathogenic clones of *Vibrio cholerae* (6) and *Pseudomonas aeruginosa* (24) from environmental strains of relatively lower virulence potential. Microarray analysis has been applied to gene loss as well as acquisition. Using this approach, for example, Israel et al. isolated *Helicobacter pylori* isolates that arose in one individual 6 years after the original sequenced isolate J99 was isolated from that person (11). The study demonstrated considerable genetic diversity among the newer isolates compared with the reference isolate, showing that "microevolution," as the authors termed it, is occurring continuously in the specialized niche in which *H. pylori* is found.

An analysis like this was not impossible before the genome sequence revolution. Other methods using protein isoforms or restriction fragment length polymorphisms might have hinted at such variation, but, as Lawrence points out, genome analysis empowers biological approaches to understand the driving forces and consequences of variation. One of the more interesting of these is the analysis of so-called contingency loci. We have understood for some time that genes may be activated or silenced by random changes that occur in runs of repetitive nucleotides, through the process of slipped-strand mispairing during DNA replication. But the complete genome sequences of some pathogens have made clear that this mechanism represents a major, and perhaps predominant, force in generating diversity within a strain or indeed a bacterial species (18, 19).

Vaughn Cooper provides a wonderful overview of how bacterial evolution may be studied in the laboratory. He highlights, among other model systems, experiments from the laboratory of Richard Lenski using lines of *Escherichia coli* that were established in 1988 and have evolved over 20,000 generations by now. This rich resource has enabled Lenski and his colleagues to address several basic questions

important to evolutionary biologists, including the conditions under which it is advantageous for a population to evolve a greater mutation rate. Pathogenic strains of some species have mutator phenotypes, suggesting the obvious conclusion that higher mutation rates must be particularly beneficial to pathogens that exist in highly selective host environments where adaptation equates to survival. But experimental work has shown that the advantage of the mutator phenotype is only transient, and Cooper points out that evolution of high mutation rates is in fact not unique to pathogenic bacteria, as several of the Lenski long-term domesticated *E. coli* populations evolved to high-mutator phenotypes.

Cooper goes on to discuss the important confluence of evolution research and vaccine development. In a sense, the early development of live vaccines by repeated passage of viruses or bacteria under in vitro conditions to derive mutants that were no longer fit for efficient in vivo replication represents a form of accelerated experimental evolution from pathogen to non-pathogen. The ideal vaccine strain frequently emerged that was easy to grow in the laboratory but that could only transiently infect the host and thus caused no overt symptoms of infection. The mutations driving this attenuation are not simply the result of replication cycles per se because attenuation by this method fails completely if serial passage through animals is used in place of in vitro culture on laboratory media or cell lines. Indeed, the latter method generally selects for more virulent strains rather than less virulent strains. Cooper points out that this may be due to the artificial nature of the transmission between hosts in serial passage experiments. When there is a virtual certainty that a pathogen will become transmitted to a new host, as is the case in serial passage experiments, selection for overall more virulent isolates occurs because these do not have to accommodate the negative effects on transmission of host morbidity or, worse, rapid host lethality. Successful natural pathogens must balance pathogenicity (which usually correlates with rapid replication and host morbidity) with transmission efficiency (which may be optimal only if the host remains active while infected). The role that natural transmission plays in the evolution of virulence is thus an interesting question, and perhaps even more challenging than the analysis of virulence mechanisms. Interesting observations have been made along this line. For example, the regulatory system controlling expression of *Bordetella bronchiseptica* virulence may control transmission by down-regulating virulence and up-regulating environmental survival genes (1, 23). In another example, *V. cholerae* cells present in the stools of cholera victims appear to be more readily able to infect experimental animals than cells of the same strain grown in laboratory media to stationary phase (16).

A confounding issue in the study of transmission, of course, is that natural routes of transmission of many pathogens are not easy to duplicate in the laboratory on a scale large enough to generate statistically significant data. Transmission may also be influenced in the natural environment by factors that are not integrated into experimental models designed to explore this aspect of pathogen biology. For example, predation by bacteriophage correlates dramatically with the dynamics of cholera epidemics in Bangladesh (8, 9). Thus, factors that modulate phage predation would likely have a profound effect on the evolution of this pathogen and could explain the emergence of new *V. cholerae* serogroups and biotypes over the last century.

Questions of transmission necessarily raise the issue of the host populations available to the microbe, and how microbial populations can most efficiently exploit the host populations in order to be maintained. Not all members of a host population are the same, and issues of susceptibility influenced by innate or acquired immune status, age, or genetic background come into play. This is further elaborated by Martin Maiden and Rachel Urwin, who introduce the population biology term "R_0," which describes the number of offspring that a microbe must produce in order to be maintained within a susceptible population. Clearly

any value for R_0 that is greater than 1 means that the microbe will persist over the long term within the host population. The term is dependent on the availability of susceptible hosts, which, in turn, can be dictated by the pathogenicity of the microbe. If the host is eliminated too easily, the microbe loses its niche and then R_0 can fall below 1. This is not a concern for microbes that have environmental niches outside of hosts, but for obligate pathogens this balance is critical and is likely what leads to chronic persistent states that characterize the pathogenicity of microbes such as *Mycobacterium tuberculosis.*

As population biologists, Maiden and Urwin naturally concern themselves with how well represented is the genome diversity within pathogenic isolates that are studied around the world. Although the microbiologist may select a single, pure colony as his or her starting point for studying pathogenicity, the population biologist is more aware of how this methodology sacrifices the diversity that is the engine of evolution. This is of most concern where populations are known to be diverse and the concept of a "type" strain that might serve as an exemplar for the species is questionable at best. Nevertheless, the clonal nature of many pathogens—characterized by low levels of genetic diversity—is by now well accepted. In some cases it is easy to understand the lack of diversity, particularly in the case of obligate pathogens in which the opportunity for genetic exchange is very limited. But even in cases in which genetic exchange and horizontal gene acquisition are known to take place, there is a clonality to population structures that is difficult to understand. Perhaps amplification within the host represents the rate-limiting bottleneck in evolution of some pathogens because it is so tightly linked to transmission. In such a case, the stochastic first clone "though the door" so enables itself for further host amplification and transmission that local epidemics and global pandemics emerge without further selection needed. Clearly there are also selection pressures operating that influence the clonality of some pathogen population structures. The population dynamics and structures of disease-causing microbes are of more than simply academic interest, as Maiden and Urwin point out, because a full understanding of them is essential for developing effective vaccine strategies.

Much of evolution takes place by mutation and selection, which are relatively slow processes, but rapid acquisition of virulence traits has occurred with the introduction of pathogenicity islands in many species. This is the subject of the chapter by Hochhut, Dobrindt, and Hacker. These large regions of the genome are generally present in pathogenic strains and absent in closely related but non-pathogenic strains of the same species. As pointed out by Hochhut and colleagues, pathogenicity islands may encode myriad traits, from secretion systems and toxins to adherence organelles and iron acquisition systems. One of the benefits of the genome era in the study of microbial pathogens is the ability to rapidly identify potential pathogenicity islands by their location in the chromosome and their G+C content relative to the rest of the chromosome.

Where do pathogenicity islands come from? That they arose from a source outside of the microbe in which they reside is an unavoidable hypothesis, but a potential source is really not known for any island. With their apparent site preferences for genome integration—often within genes that encode small RNA molecules such as tRNAs—and the phage-like integrases they can encode, they certainly seem as if they borrowed their integration mechanisms from phages. Some pathogenicity islands may parasitize helper phages for their transmission, as has been dramatically demonstrated by the island encoding the toxic shock toxin of *Staphylococcus aureus* (15, 21). This mechanism is analogous to the coliphage P2/P4 cycle in its overall mechanics (14). The steps in the transmission of other islands are only beginning to be revealed. Pathogenicity island excision in *Yersinia* (12) and in *V. cholerae* (20) proceeds through a site-specific excision and circulization mechanism that is analogous to prophage chromosomal excision. In the case of *Yersinia*,

horizontal transmission after excision has been observed experimentally (13), but this has not been demonstrated for the *Vibrio* island.

Phages also encode numerous virulence factors that depend on the function of unlinked bacterial genes present on chromosomal islands. For example, the CTX phage encodes cholera toxin which is extracellularly secreted by type II secretion pathways (4), whereas some prophages encode effectors that are secreted by type III secretion systems encoded on pathogenicity islands (3, 7). Clearly the coevolution of phages with pathogenicity islands may extend beyond such linked biological function into areas such as transmission, exclusion, restriction/modification, and lysogenic immunity. A balance between the role of phages in transmission of islands and the deleterious effect that phages have on host cell viability may lead to paradoxical antagonism between these genetic elements. This is reminiscent of the balance that must be reached between host transmission and virulence for the bacterial pathogen as discussed above.

While dramatic changes in the pathogenicity of bacterial clones have been linked to the acquisition of plasmids, phages, transposons, and islands, in contrast, chromosomal recombinational events have been less frequently linked to such evolutionary leaps in pathobiological fitness. One clear example is the conversion of a *V. cholerae* El Tor O1 biotype strain into the O139 serogroup through replacement of the gene cluster encoding the O1 antigen by genes encoding the O139 antigen and capsule. Strains of the O139 serogroup caused a huge epidemic in South Asia in 1992–1993 despite the fact that the emergent O139 strain encoded exactly the same virulence factors as the earlier endemic O1 El Tor strain. Microarray analysis confirm earlier data that the seventh-pandemic El Tor O1 strains and the emergent O139 strains are virtually the same clone albeit with different lipopolysaccharide gene clusters. Since 1993, the O139 and O1 seventh-pandemic El Tor strains have coexisted in South Asia as stably endemic causes of cholera. Initially, the O139 serogroup was predicted to displace the resident

O1 strain simply because immunity to *V. cholerae* is largely dependent on anti-O antigen humoral responses. The huge O1-resistant population would understandably "select" for the dominence of the O139 strains. However, the balance has shifted back and forth through the following decade, suggesting that host susceptibility may be only one factor in predicting the evolutionary fitness of the two serogroups. Phage susceptibility may also play a role and could have been the driving factor in the emergence of the novel serogroup to begin with, given that phages have a profound effect on environmental persistence and thus transmission of *V. cholerae* (8, 9).

How recombinational events assembled the O139 gene cluster remains a mystery. A mobile element, IS*1358*, is found in both the O1 and O139 gene clusters and may have provided homology for recombination (2). Two other unrelated serogroups, O69 and O141, also carry genes that are found in the O139 locus, suggesting they may have donated portions of the O139 gene ensemble (2, 17). How the multiple gene transfers required to assemble a functional O139 antigen biosynthetic cluster occurred without selection and amplification of the individual steps remains unclear. Nonetheless, the emergence of *V. cholerae* O139 provides an exceptionally strong example that multiple rare horizontal gene acquisitions and recombinational events do occur and can then can be selected by a combination of factors that probably include host susceptibility (e.g., preexisting immunity), compatibility with virulence factor function (e.g., pilus assembly and toxin secretion), and transmission efficiency in the environment (e.g., phage resistance or ecological fitness).

It is easy to see how acquisition of new traits may advance the evolution toward virulence. Less obvious, although predicted by evolutionary theory, is when loss of traits leads to enhanced virulence. The principle of antagonistic pleiotrophy, discussed in Cooper's chapter as well as in that of Day and Maurelli, holds that traits beneficial for one niche may be harmful in another. For a pathogen that may have evolved from a free-living saprophyte or even from a commensal, traits that once served well may be detrimental when trying to grow within a host. The term "pathoadaptive mutation" has been coined for mutations that inactivate genes whose products are detrimental for survival in hosts. The so-called antivirulence genes subject to such loss fall into different categories. Among other examples, Day and Maurelli describe the intriguing story of lysine decarboxylase (*cadA*) gene loss in pathogenic *Shigella* as compared with the closely related nonpathogenic *E. coli*. The product of lysine decarboxylase is cadaverine, which serves to inhibit some of the virulence functions of *Shigella*. This mutation (the loss of *cadA*) is a feature of the *Shigella* genus that occurred at least four times before in the evolutionary history of *Shigella* compared with that of *E. coli*.

Day and Maurelli restrict their discussion to gene loss that clearly occurs as an evolutionary event, leading to new lineages. If one considers pathoadaptive mutation perhaps more broadly, it is clear that gene loss is a widespread mechanism in bacterial pathogenesis (22). For example, strains of *P. aeruginosa* associated with cystic fibrosis accumulate mutations in the complex regulatory circuit that controls alginate production, leading to high-level alginate synthesis in these isolates (5). Antigenic or phase variation processes might themselves be considered examples of pathoadaptive mutations. Perhaps these examples do not necessarily lead to the evolutionary "black holes" described by Day and Maurelli, wherein one species lacks a specific gene expressed by its ancestors, but these examples nonetheless make clear that adaptation in pathogenesis can occur by phenotypic loss as well as by phenotypic gain.

Evolutionary studies of microbial pathogens will continue to reveal numerous surprises. If loss of function can drive pathogenic fitness as well as gain of function, then it would indeed be quite difficult to interpret raw genetic content of pathogens without studies aimed at quantifying the effects of every variation in the context of every other variation. This is a daunting task for sure but now possible with availability of complete genomic sequences of pathogenic and nonpathogenic bacterial strains and species. It is also quite clear that these studies will continue to rely on genetic approaches that target the identification of virulence genes and experimental animal models that reveal the function of these genes within the host.

REFERENCES

1. **Akerley, B. J., P. A. Cotter, and J. F. Miller.** 1995. Ectopic expression of the flagellar regulon alters development of the Bordetella-host interaction. *Cell* **80:**611–620.
2. **Bik, E. M., A. E. Bunschoten, R. D. Gouw, and F. R. Mooi.** 1995. Genesis of the novel epidemic Vibrio cholerae O139 strain: evidence for horizontal transfer of genes involved in polysaccharide synthesis. *EMBO J.* **14:**209–216.
3. **Campellone, K. G., D. Robbins, and J. M. Leong.** 2004. EspFU is a translocated EHEC effector that interacts with Tir and N-WASP and promotes Nck-independent actin assembly. *Dev. Cell.* **7:**217–228.
4. **Davis, B. M., E. H. Lawson, M. Sandkvist, A. Ali, S. Sozhamannan, and M. K. Waldor.** 2000. Convergence of the secretory pathways for cholera toxin and the filamentous phage, CTXphi. *Science* **288:**333–335.
5. **Deretic, V., M. J. Schurr, and H. Yu.** 1995. Pseudomonas aeruginosa, mucoidy and the chronic infection phenotype in cystic fibrosis. *Trends Microbiol.* **3:**351–356.
6. **Dziejman, M., E. Balon, D. Boyd, C. M. Fraser, J. F. Heidelberg, and J. J. Mekalanos.** 2002. Comparative genomic analysis of Vibrio cholerae: genes that correlate with cholera endemic and pandemic disease. *Proc. Natl. Acad. Sci. USA* **99:**1556–1561.
7. **Ehrbar, K., and W. D. Hardt.** 2005. Bacteriophage-encoded type III effectors in Salmonella enterica subspecies 1 serovar Typhimurium. *Infect. Genet. Evol.* **5:**1–9.
8. **Faruque, S. M., M. J. Islam, Q. S. Ahmad, A. S. Faruque, D. A. Sack, G. B. Nair, and J. J. Mekalanos.** 2005. Self-limiting nature of seasonal cholera epidemics: role of host-mediated amplification of phage. *Proc. Natl. Acad. Sci. USA* **102:**6119–6124.
9. **Faruque, S. M., I. B. Naser, M. J. Islam, A. S. Faruque, A. N. Ghosh, G. B. Nair, D. A. Sack, and J. J. Mekalanos.** 2005. Seasonal epidemics of cholera inversely correlate with the prevalence of environmental cholera phages. *Proc. Natl. Acad. Sci. USA* **102:**1702–1707.
10. **Fleischmann, R. D., M. D. Adams, O. White,** R. A. Clayton, E. F. Kirkness, A. R. Kerlavage, C. J. Bult, J. F. Tomb, B. A. Dougherty, J. M. Merrick, et al. 1995. Whole-genome random sequencing and assembly of Haemophilus influenzae Rd. *Science* **269:**496–512.
11. **Israel, D. A., N. Salama, U. Krishna, U. M. Rieger, J. C. Atherton, S. Falkow, and R. M. Peek, Jr.** 2001. Helicobacter pylori genetic diversity within the gastric niche of a single human host. *Proc. Natl. Acad. Sci. USA* **98:**14625–14630.
12. **Lesic, B., S. Bach, J. M. Ghigo, U. Dobrindt, J. Hacker, and E. Carniel.** 2004. Excision of the high-pathogenicity island of Yersinia pseudotuberculosis requires the combined actions of its cognate integrase and Hef, a new recombination directionality factor. *Mol. Microbiol.* **52:**1337–1348.
13. **Lesic, B., and E. Carniel.** 2005. Horizontal transfer of the high-pathogenicity island of *Yersinia pseudotuberculosis. J. Bacteriol.* **187:**3352–3358.
14. **Lindqvist, B. H., G. Deho, and R. Calendar.** 1993. Mechanisms of genome propagation and helper exploitation by satellite phage P4. *Microbiol. Rev.* **57:**683–702.
15. **Lindsay, J. A., A. Ruzin, H. F. Ross, N. Kurepina, and R. P. Novick.** 1998. The gene for toxic shock toxin is carried by a family of mobile pathogenicity islands in Staphylococcus aureus. *Mol. Microbiol.* **29:**527–543.
16. **Merrell, D. S., S. M. Butler, F. Qadri, N. A. Dolganov, A. Alam, M. B. Cohen, S. B. Calderwood, G. K. Schoolnik, and A. Camilli.** 2002. Host-induced epidemic spread of the cholera bacterium. *Nature* **417:**642–645.
17. **Mooi, F. R., and E. M. Bik.** 1997. The evolution of epidemic Vibrio cholerae strains. *Trends Microbiol.* **5:**161–165.
18. **Moxon, E. R., P. B. Rainey, M. A. Nowak, and R. E. Lenski.** 1994. Adaptive evolution of highly mutable loci in pathogenic bacteria. *Curr. Biol.* **4:**24–33.
19. **Parkhill, J., B. W. Wren, K. Mungall, J. M. Ketley, C. Churcher, D. Basham, T. Chillingworth, R. M. Davies, T. Feltwell, S. Holroyd, K. Jagels, A. V. Karlyshev, S. Moule, M. J. Pallen, C. W. Penn, M. A. Quail, M. A. Rajandream, K. M. Rutherford, A. H. van Vliet, S. Whitehead, and B. G. Barrell.** 2000. The genome sequence of the food-borne pathogen Campylobacter jejuni reveals hypervariable sequences. *Nature* **403:**665–668.
20. **Rajanna, C., J. Wang, D. Zhang, Z. Xu, A. Ali, Y. M. Hou, and D. K. Karaolis.** 2003. The vibrio pathogenicity island of epidemic Vibrio cholerae forms precise extrachromosomal circular excision products. *J. Bacteriol.* **185:**6893–6901.
21. **Ruzin, A., J. Lindsay, and R. P. Novick.** 2001. Molecular genetics of SaPI1—a mobile patho-

genicity island in Staphylococcus aureus. *Mol. Microbiol.* **41:**365–377.

22. **Sokurenko, E. V., D. L. Hasty, and D. E. Dykhuizen.** 1999. Pathoadaptive mutations: gene loss and variation in bacterial pathogens. *Trends Microbiol.* **7:**191–195.

23. **Vergara-Irigaray, N., A. Chavarri-Martinez, J. Rodriguez-Cuesta, J. F. Miller, P. A. Cotter, and G. Martinez de Tejada.** 2005. Evaluation of the role of the Bvg intermediate phase in Bordetella pertussis during experimental respiratory infection. *Infect. Immun.* **73:**748–760.

24. **Wolfgang, M. C., B. R. Kulasekara, X. Liang, D. Boyd, K. Wu, Q. Yang, C. G. Miyada, and S. Lory.** 2003. Conservation of genome content and virulence determinants among clinical and environmental isolates of Pseudomonas aeruginosa. *Proc. Natl. Acad. Sci. USA* **100:**8484–8489.

STUDYING EVOLUTION USING GENOME SEQUENCE DATA

Jeffrey G. Lawrence

2

The appearance of the first complete genome sequence from a free-living microorganism in 1995, that of the γ-proteobacterium *Haemophilus influenzae* (58), revolutionized the way molecular evolutionary biologists could examine the patterns reflecting—and thereby infer the processes driving—the evolution of microbes. Until that time, microbial molecular evolution was explored using sequences of individual genes obtained from disparate taxa. Many of the sequences available for inspection were determined by researchers working on their genes of interest, resulting in very little systematic or representative sampling either of gene sequences or of taxa; one used what sequences one could find and carefully chose which sequences to obtain directly, to augment the publicly available data. Initially, the features of genes were examined independently (a necessity for the first few sequences determined in the 1970s), but even then important evolutionary patterns were recognized, such as the nonrandom usage of synonymous codons that varied greatly for genes between organisms, but far less for genes within organisms (65–67). Individual gene sequences were also compared

to presumed homologues from conspecific strains, or from distantly related organisms, to examine properties of bacterial populations as well as to examine relationships among populations and species by use of molecular phylogenetics (45, 47, 48, 76, 79, 111, 147). Theories pertaining to microbial evolution could be devised and tested using the data available (e.g., see references 47, 123, and 124), and the field advanced to offer a somewhat cohesive view of microbial evolutionary processes. Yet questions that demanded more data to be addressed (136) in a satisfactory manner always arose.

The accumulation of well-annotated, complete genome sequences now offers an unprecedented view into the biology of microorganisms, including powerful and practical applications such as the inference of metabolic pathways and lifestyle choices without any experimental evidence. These data could be gleaned from careful analysis of the presence and absence of genes with homologues with known (or, more likely, inferred) functions in other organisms. For example, the spirochete *Borrelia burgdorferi* is notoriously recalcitrant to easy growth and manipulation in the laboratory; but its genome sequences offered an unobstructed view into its metabolic capabilities, including the lack of biosynthetic capabilities but increased capacities for both transport of

Jeffrey G. Lawrence, Pittsburgh Bacteriophage Institute and Department of Biological Sciences, University of Pittsburgh, Pittsburgh, PA 15260.

Evolution of Microbial Pathogens, Edited by H. S. Seifert and V. J. DiRita, © 2006 ASM Press, Washington, D.C.

nutrients and chemotaxis (20, 21, 59). Similarly, analyses of the genome of the endosymbiont *Buchnera aphidicola* (which lives within specialized organs of its hosts, the sap-feeding aphids) demonstrated the retention of biosynthetic pathways for amino acids lacking from plant phloem, but the loss of biosynthetic pathways (assuming a prototrophic ancestor) for amino acids found in adequate supplies (11, 12, 169, 181, 196, 211, 212). Such introspective analyses (those that focused on the properties of a single genome) were soon joined by comparisons between genome sequences—allowing the investigation of even larger scale questions, such as the gain and loss of genes (117, 119, 121, 157, 159) or the dynamics of genomic rearrangements (50, 129, 130, 141)—as additional genome sequences allowed for the assessment of differences between genomes with a high degree of accuracy. Finally, the availability of large numbers of genome sequences opened up opportunities for addressing new sets of evolutionary questions that could not be previously answered, or even asked.

Crafting a chapter detailing how genome sequences can be used to examine microbial evolution is a daunting task, since entire books could be written on the topic. Herein I will not discuss any one topic in depth, as many will be given appropriate coverage in other sections of this book. Rather, I will review briefly the many ways genomes can change over time, how these processes are inferred by analysis of extant sequences, and how these data sets can be employed to address broad-scale evolutionary questions.

MECHANISMS OF GENOMIC CHANGE

Nucleotide Substitutions

Genes certainly change by point mutation, and it is primarily this sort of variation among genomes that has been under scrutiny since the dawn of microbial population biology in the 1970s (22, 146, 151, 190, 191, 213). Such mutations were analyzed by way of the resulting variant isoforms of proteins (termed "allozymes") that were distinguished by gel electrophoresis and appropriate enzyme assays; this methodology eventually gave way to more direct assays of genome variability, including the identification of restriction fragment length polymorphisms and finally direct determination of the DNA sequence itself.

Although organisms certainly can adapt by the acquisition of novel sequences (as will be discussed below), genetic variability is ultimately generated by mutational processes; therefore, understanding the dynamics of mutational processes forms the critical cornerstone in any model for bacterial genome evolution. In the "pregenomic" era, one could examine evolution by point mutational processes by performing surveys of gene sequences from numerous naturally occurring organisms, which offered a view into which mutations had been tolerated by natural selection, and hence were still observed in the population (33, 45, 47, 80, 142, 147, 202). Alternatively, one could examine evolution in laboratory environments; here, one typically focused on a particular gene or pathway, since methods were not readily available to identify important mutational changes that could have occurred at any location in the genome (14, 31, 32, 38, 39, 46, 78, 122, 160, 172, 177, 206). What have complete genome sequences brought to the table that has changed how these processes are examined? Three benefits that are notable.

First, novel mutational changes (e.g., suppressors) have been examined for decades by cloning the genes in question; this was a long and sometimes complex process (e.g., if false "suppressors" arose via expression from high-copy-number plasmids), and often required the laborious sequencing of large segments of DNA. But the availability of complete genome sequences for most model organisms has reduced the previously tedious task of gene identification and characterization to the sequencing of a few dozen bases, thereby localizing the mutation in question quite rapidly. Second, the availability of multiple genomic sequences has the potential for improving the gene annotation of all genomes, thus providing a wealth of information on a gene of interest, even if it had not been characterized in the organism under study. For example, the functions of genes in the cobalamin biosynthetic pathway in *Salmonella enterica* were inferred by homology of these genes to the cognate genes in *Pseudomonas denitrificans* (180), in which extensive biochemical characterization of the encoded proteins had been performed (10). These comparisons now allow for more distantly related proteins involved in cobalamin biosynthesis to be identified with a high degree of confidence in other genome sequences.

Last, and perhaps most exciting, is the use of microarray technology to examine how patterns of gene expression have changed, whether between naturally occurring organisms or artificially evolved populations. Microarrays contain segments of DNA representing all of the genes in a genome, and they can be used as hybridization templates to DNA or mRNA isolated from other organisms. Pioneering work by Rosenzweig using the yeast *Saccharomyces cerevisiae* showed how overall patterns of gene expression changed in response to adaptation to new laboratory environments (54). While these studies showed global patterns of adaptation, and gave a more comprehensive view of global metabolic change than earlier work in *Escherichia coli* (179), they provided only fruits for endless (albeit thought-provoking) speculation on the underlying causes of the evolutionary changes. A superb and more complete example of this approach is the work of Lenski and colleagues (30), who employed comparative analyses of parallel alterations in microarray-inferred gene expression patterns to infer where critical point mutations had occurred during evolution in a glucose-limited environment. Here, mutations in the *spoT* gene were inferred, and the changes in the gene were verified by direct sequencing.

Microarrays (and, to a lesser extent, multilocus sequence typing [see chapter 3]) can also be used to identify some of the variation among strains closely related to an isolate with a complete genome sequence available. In microarrays, the probe is DNA from strains of bacteria closely related to the organism used to construct the microarray, which, when hybridized to the microarray, show which genes are absent from these strains (56). For example, this approach clearly demonstrated that the genomes of pathogenic strains of *E. coli* (157), *Streptococcus* (176), *Helicobacter pylori* (90, 182), and *Staphylococcus aureus* (51) are quite diverse. In contrast, the genomes of *Mycobacterium tuberculosis* isolates show little diversity (99), in agreement with previous data using more limited data sets (150). This last point is important, as some pathogens can be quite diverse at some loci and not at others (e.g., the *Salmonella rfb* locus encoding the O-antigen is hypervariable in gene content [219], which could be overlooked in multilocus sequence typing surveys). While this does not shed light on point mutational processes, it does demonstrate how new technologies can be brought to bear to address rapidly questions once thought to be unanswerable (in this case, how widely distributed, or how variable, particular genes are within a bacterial "species").

Recombination

As bacteria reproduce by binary fission, homologous recombination between genes found among closely related strains was once thought to be rare, with periodic selection of rare advantageous mutations being a popular and fairly well-supported view (123). This perspective began to shift in the 1990s when it was shown that genes in *E. coli* did not have congruent phylogenies (47, 76, 77). More striking examples were found in *Neisseria* and *Streptococcus*, and it was soon recognized that exchange of DNA among closely related strains was a potent evolutionary force (34, 52, 53, 136, 199, 200). Yet these were hard-won data, derived from experiments in which the DNA sequences of homologous regions of DNA were obtained from numerous strains. How can individual whole-genome sequences be used to examine the significance of this process in bacterial diversification, or in the cohesion of lineages? The answer is clear: they cannot. But the first wave of experimentation showing the importance of recombination opened up additional questions that are readily addressed via the examination of genome sequences: What is the distribution of fragment sizes participating in recombinational events? How are these events distributed across the chromosome? Is recombination equally likely across all regions of the chromosome among all strains with similar overall relatedness? These questions require whole-genome sequences to be addressed, and some data are available to begin to answer these questions. For example, several genomes of the pathogen *S. enterica* are publicly available (40, 140, 141, 161, 163), and several more are being completed. Similarly, there are numerous genomes of *E. coli* and the related pathogenic taxon *Shigella* (16, 93, 167, 209, 210). The aim of these projects may be to discern which genes allow each serovar of this species to be pathogenic in different host organisms (49), but the data set may also be used to delineate domains of free recombination, calculate the size of fragments mobilized by recombination mechanisms, and so forth. While the relative significance of recombination, gene transfer, and mutational processes will vary among lineages, complete genome sequences provide much-needed data to begin resolving these thorny issues.

Indeed, these data may prove useful as powerful correlates to the original aims of the projects: strain-specific genes allowing certain patterns of pathogenicity should show a lower probability of recombination among other salmonellae, potentially leading to "speciation" events (108), which could create evolutionarily distinct lineages. While the concept of microbial species is still hotly debated (26, 27, 107, 108, 132, 133, 208), both the identification of niche-specific genes and an understanding of how reproductive isolation is established (a hallmark of most species concepts [137, 139, 207]) are central to constructing a framework for understanding lineage diversification, regardless of how "species" are defined.

Confounding this issue is the problem that it is not clear how a bacterial species is effectively delineated, either on theoretical grounds or in practice (28). The eukaryote-centric idea that species share a common genome pool (137, 138) derived from obligate recombination accompanying reproduction, a biological oddity that does not constrain any prokaryotic lineage. The acquisition of niche-specific genes, coupled with the mechanisms of bacterial recombination that exchange only segments of genomes, would lead to some regions of bacterial chromosomes experiencing reproductive isolation with cognate regions in a sister lineage, while other regions do not. These bacteria would be considered species at some loci, but not at others (108). A more pragmatic view that members of species share a common ecologic niche is comfortable from a theoretic standpoint but difficult to implement by examination of strains, and can only be arbitrarily predicted from sequence data. For example, genetic differences arise every few generations in an average bacterium; which differences are of ecological importance and which are "ecologically neutral"? The only concept that is certain in this arena is that a bacterial species concept adopted in the 21st century, one that recognizes the scope of lifestyle variation among microbial lineages, will have little in common with what Haeckel, and certainly Linnaeus, once posited.

Replication Slippage

One class of point mutational change is the gain or loss of small numbers of bases by replication slippage events (Fig. 1). This mechanism is employed as a reversible way of activating or deactivating genes in many pathogens in several ways, including (i) changing the spacing between promoter recognition sites, thus altering a gene's expression level (187), or (ii) silencing genes by including a "slippery" sequence within a protein-coding region that is not a multiple of 3 (thereby shifting the downstream sequence in or out of frame) (92). Such "contingency loci" are often, but not always, found to encode antigenic determinants, and thus allow these organisms to change their outward appearance rapidly and at random. Whole-

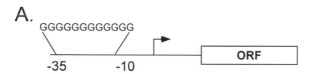

A.

GGGGGGGGGGGG

-35   -10

ORF

B. *3 Repeats : In Frame*

ATG GAT CAG ATC AGA TCA TTG ACC GGG ...

4 Repeats : Out of Frame

ATG GAT CAG ATC AGA TCA GAT CAT TGA CCG GG ...
                                     ***

FIGURE 1   Replication slippage events. (A) Slippage at polynucleotide repeats can affect promoter regions, thereby altering expression at downstream loci. Here, replication slippage in the polyguanosine region can alter the separation and relative orientation of sites required for σ-factor recognition of the gene's promoter. (B) Slippage within open reading frames can stochastically move downstream regions in and out of frame. Here, addition of a pentameric repeat to a region found in-frame will cause the downstream region of the gene to be translated out-of-frame, resulting in a useless protein or premature translation termination.

genome sequences have been used to identify putative contingency loci by finding simple sequence repeats (83), then assessing their variation among closely related strains of bacteria (either naturally occurring or generated in the laboratory).

Inversion

Aside from point mutational changes, larger DNA rearrangements may also occur within genomes. Inversions have attracted attention since the 1980s, when Roth and colleagues showed that inversions of some regions of the *Salmonella* chromosome appeared to be "permissive," or readily obtained, while others were not (131, 145, 188, 189). These data, when combined with the striking similarity between the genetic maps of *Salmonella* and its sister taxon *E. coli* (15, 186) (aside from the known terminus–centric inversion [184]), implied that there were global factors at work constraining the rearrangement of bacterial chromosomes. The finding that strongly host-adapted strains of *Salmonella* showed extensive evidence for genome rearrangements

(126, 128, 130, 153, 185) was unexpected, and raised questions as to what factors are important in constraining chromosome structure, and how and when these constraints may be released.

Since that time, two lines of research have employed whole-genome sequences to address this tantalizing proposal. First, comparison of gene synteny among closely related bacteria (how gene order is conserved) showed that inversions were common only when they were symmetrical with respect to the origin or terminus of replication (50). Second, work initially presented by Louarn and others identified oligomeric sequences that were present only on leading strands of replication and showed nonuniform distributions: they were more abundant near the replication terminus (19, 166). The implication from these data was that these sequences may be involved in replication termination, and inversion of sequences that were asymmetrical with respect to the terminus of replication would be counterselected. An example of one such octomeric sequence in the genome of the α-proteobacterium *Mesorhizo-*

bium loti (96) is shown in Figure 2 (81a, 113, 114). Here, the sequence is found primarily on the leading strand of replication, and increases markedly in abundance near the terminus of replication. This sequence is distributed in a similar manner among many members of the α-proteobacteria, although its position in each genome is not conserved (114); moreover, such distributions are not the result of mutational biases that could occur as replication ends (such as deoxynucleoside triphosphate pool depletion), and are not found at other locations around the genome. These data strongly support the hypothesis that such sequences play important roles in genome biology, and may constrain inversion that are not symmetrical with respect to the origin or terminus of replication, or limit the acquisition of foreign DNA from organisms with such sequences abundant on both strands. Such global constraints on genome evolution cannot be uncovered without whole-genome sequences as primary data sets.

Insertions and Deletions

In addition to the alteration of existing DNA, genomes may change by the gain of novel genetic information from outside sources (9, 159). Much has been made of horizontal gene transfer (HGT) and its ability to introduce novel traits into organisms, altering their adaptive potential and evolutionary trajectory (41, 43, 104, 106). Yet many ways of identifying genes acquired by HGT—such as an unusually high level of similarity to genes found in an otherwise unrelated taxon—do not rely upon whole-genome sequences. For example, numerous transfer events involving genes encoding aminoacyl-tRNA synthetases were elucidated from fine-scale phylogenetic analyses, although complete genome sequences did serve to expand the data set (215). The bacterial origin of genes responsible for fungal invasion of ruminant intestinal tracts was also evident without genome sequences (61).

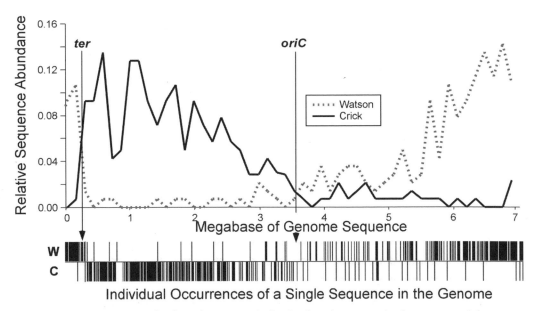

FIGURE 2 Occurrences of a skewed, asymmetrically distributed sequence in the genome of the α-proteobacterium *Mesorhizobium loti*. The lower panel depicts each sequence on either the Watson (top) or Crick (bottom) strand as a hash mark. The abundance of this sequence on each strand is tabulated in the graph above; the origin and terminus of replication can be inferred from analyses of G+C skew (183) as well as the distribution of the octomer depicted here. Data are from H. Hendrickson and J. G. Lawrence (81a). The origin was distinguished from the terminus by (i) the position of the *dnaA* gene (typically origin-proximal), and (ii) the orientation of *rrn* operons encoding rRNAs (typically transcribed away from the origin of replication).

Yet there are ways of detecting DNA insertions that become possible only after whole-genome sequences are available. The most straightforward method entails the comparison of genomes of relatively closely related organisms. Here, genes present in only one genome are apparent; the difference could have arisen by either deletion of genes in one strain or insertion in the other. There are two ways of distinguishing between these possibilities. The first method is again phylogenetic, wherein one observes either a gene's conservation among, or absence from, closely related taxa. The second method for distinguishing between insertions and deletions relies upon the whole-genome sequences, and also serves as a primary method for detecting insertion events without phylogenetic data. With this method, one can devise numerous parametric measures of the mutational biases peculiar to any one lineage, such as nucleotide composition (116, 117), dinucleotide and trinucleotide frequencies (97), codon usage biases (73, 98, 144, 148), nucleotide skew, or patterns inferred from Markov chain analyses (81). These measures allow for quantitative description of genes native to any one genome, independent of phylogenetic comparisons. Genes falling outside the distribution of one or more parameters can be described as "atypical" for that genome. One example is the apparent insertion of foreign genes into the *nuo* operon of *Neisseria meningi-*

tidis (Fig. 3); here, atypical genes as measured by several parameters are dispersing genes otherwise found clustered in other bacterial genomes (e.g., in *E. coli*). Such operon disruption is not unusual; although the structure of certain operons may be conserved among distantly related genomes (36, 109), most operons have a short evolutionary lifespan (36).

A gene may appear atypical for numerous reasons: (i) the sequence is short, and lacks the information required for accurate measurement; (ii) the sequence is atypical because natural selection acts on this gene in a different fashion than the majority of genes in the genome (e.g., some genes encoding ribosomal proteins in *E. coli* are highly AT rich, primarily due to their unusually high lysine content, encoded by the preferred AAA codon); and (iii) the gene evolved in a different genome, and parameters measuring the mutational biases it experienced reflect those of the donor genome, not the genome in which the gene currently resides. Therefore, this gene may be considered an insertion. However, careful consideration of these data is paramount, since one may easily overlook the effects of gene size or unusual selection in making a conclusion that an atypical gene was introduced by gene transfer (118).

Like the phylogenetic approaches, these parametric approaches have been successful in identifying genes introduced into a genome (116, 158, 159). Unlike phylogenetic approa-

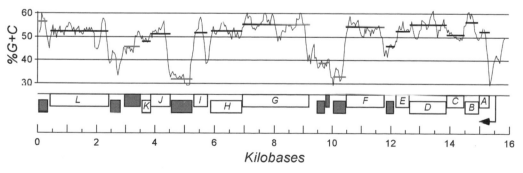

FIGURE 3 A portion of the *Neisseria meningitidis* Z2491 genome (162) containing the *nuo* operon (encoding an NADH dehydrogenase). The genes depicted in gray have been inserted into this genome, likely by horizontal gene transfer, dispersing the *nuo* genes. The plot above shows the overall G+C content over a 200-bp sliding window; non-*nuo* genes show atypical G+C content, as well as other unusual properties. The average G+C content for each gene is shown as a horizontal bar on the plot.

ches, however, parametric approaches are limited to their detection of genes recently inserted into a genome; as time passes, these genes will be subject to the mutational biases of their new genomic context—imparted by the mutational proclivities of the DNA polymerases found in the new genome; the composition of the deoxynucleoside triphosphate pools; the number, nature, and efficiency of the error correction systems; the identities and abundances of the tRNAs (leading to codon usage bias); and other factors. This amelioration of the gene sequence limits the detection of inserted DNA to those genes recently acquired. Phylogenetic approaches can detect ancient transfer events, but application of these methods relies upon the depth and breadth of the sequence database, the efficacy of phylogenetic methodologies, and the ability to reject alternative hypotheses, and can be confounded by the proliferation of gene families and the failure of the investigator to distinguish between orthologous and paralogous genes (170, 171). A combination of these approaches may be necessary to identify, in a clear and robust fashion, genes that have been introduced by horizontal transfer (118). Insertion of foreign DNA has been identified as a major force shaping the evolution of pathogenic organisms (9, 34, 69–72, 156). Perhaps the most striking case involves the comparison of the 5.5-Mb genome of enterohemorrhagic *E. coli* O157:H7 (167) with the 4.7-Mb genome of the nonpathogenic laboratory strain *E. coli* K-12 (16); about 1.5 Mb of DNA is unique to one or the other genome, illustrating the vast impact of newly acquired DNA in the diversification of organisms once believed to be highly similar but for the pathogenicity aspect of the O157 strain.

In addition, the deletion of DNA sequences may also play important adaptive roles (37). For example, the deletion of the *cadA* gene from the *Shigella* genome is one of the factors contributing to the pathogenicity of this organism (135); similar data implicate the selective advantage of the deletion of the *ompT* gene from the same organism (152). Unless remnants of a pseudogene are left behind (as they are in some taxa for long periods [203]) clearly indicating that a deletion has taken place, then deletions can be distinguished from insertions using the methods detailed above, where insertions often, but not always, bear unusual compositional patterns. Among sets of closely related genomes, insertions may be distinguished from deletions by phylogenetics comparisons, where the loss of a gene is the most parsimonious explanation for differences in gene content.

Deletions can be a major driving force during genome reduction, whereby large portions—perhaps even the majority—of the genetic material of an organism are lost over time, with little gain of new genes (see chapter 6). This process occurs primarily among obligate pathogens, parasites, and endosymbionts. *Mycoplasma genitalium*, *Rickettsia prowazekii*, and *B. aphidicola* represent examples of taxa whose genomes are highly reduced in gene content. The causative agent of leprosy, *Mycobacterium leprae*, has also lost a great many genes, but their remnant pseudogenes still remain in the genome (29). These pseudogenes likely indicate that the process of genome reduction has proceeded to a lesser degree than in the taxa noted above (115). The process of genome reduction is driven by the small effective population size and little recombination among strains of these lineages, and is tolerated since many of the genes lost encode biosynthetic and degradative pathways, which are not under strong selection for retention in environments where nutrients are in constant supply and composition (3–6).

Lessons from Bacteriophages

No chapter on prokaryotic genome evolution would be complete without consideration of the bacteriophage. Phage genomes provide powerful model systems for bacterial genome analysis. They provide a test ground for gene identification, having in many cases well-recognized facets to their overall gene organization. Phage genomes evolve by mutation, recombination, and gene insertion and deletion and contain numerous genes of unknown function that push PSI-BLAST annotation to its limits (18). Moreover, each phage genome is related to numerous other genomes, both bacteriophage and bacterial, in complex ways

(112). In addition, phage genomes are often found embedded in bacterial genomes as prophages (115), necessitating their identification, and coevolve with the genomes of their bacterial hosts as they play an active role in recombination and gene exchange processes. The complexities of the relationships among phage genomes (112, 178) exacerbate the problems of taxonomy and phylogeny in these groups since (i) DNA transfer events involve much large fractions of the total genome size, and (ii) there is no stable "core" of genes—analogous to rRNA genes or genes encoding the transcription and translation machinery—to rely upon when constructing phylogenies.

Yet some of the lessons learned by comparative phage genomics provide important insights into bacterial genome evolution. First is the importance of gene loss and acquisition in their evolution, evident not only among the double-stranded DNA phages (82, 94), but in single-stranded DNA phages as well (112). Phage genomes are constrained in their ability to acquire genes, since only a certain amount can be packaged efficiently into the capsid; this constraint mimics the constraint on bacterial genome size, wherein only a finite amount of information can be maintained under selection, preventing runaway growth in genome size (107, 121). Moreover, analysis of the recombination events introducing genes into phage genomes makes it clear that only genes increasing the fitness of the phage are retained; some "junk DNA" appears to be retained in some genomes only to satisfy the requirements for proper genome size. Similarly, bacterial genomes discard enormous amounts of introduced DNA that is not under selection for function (116, 117, 120, 121). One lesson here is simple: introduction of a novel gene certainly does not guarantee its retention over evolutionary time.

Lastly, more recent analyses of numerous mycobacteriophage genomes has demonstrated two salient points (165). First, bacteriophage genomes and bacterial genomes share a common gene pool. This is not merely to say that prophages are found in bacteria; rather, genes that increase the fitness of bacteria may also increase the fitness of phages (e.g., genes encoding tRNA, subunits of DNA polymerases, restriction/modification systems). Second, a remarkable number of novel genomes are still being discovered in bacteriophage (and bacterial) genomes, representing a vast reservoir of genetic information. The intimate relationships between phages and their bacterial hosts makes the quantitation and characterization of this gene pool of critical importance for the understanding of all prokaryotic genomes, phage and host alike.

INFERENCE OF PHYLOGENY AND ORGANISMAL EVOLUTION

Whole Genomes and a New Era

In 1965, Zuckerkandl and Pauling proposed the use of molecules as tools to infer the evolutionary history of organisms bearing those molecules (221, 222), arguing that the history of substitutions (amino acid substitutions at that time) provided a record of changes that occurred along the evolutionary paths of these organisms. Decades have been devoted to devising clever and robust methods of untangling the signal from the noise in these substitutional patterns to provide a plausible view of evolutionary history, especially when much time has passed and the signal/noise ratio has become very small. This method opened the door to the classification of microorganisms—which otherwise had few reliable characters available from which taxonomy or phylogeny could be inferred—especially utilizing the sequence of universally distributed rRNAs.

For 30 years, phylogenies have been constructed from rRNA gene sequences (or, early on, the shared distributions of fragments generated by nuclease digestion), which were used as templates for the evolutionary histories of the organisms containing these genes. Sometimes these studies yielded dramatic results, such as uncovering the *Archaea* as a separate domain of life (214). Yet the advent of complete genome sequences in the mid-1990s reinforced an idea that had been festering on the back burners of evolutionary thought for some time: the existence of significant amounts of HGT, involving more than transposons or genes conferring antibiotic resistance, meant that the phylogeny of a gene could no longer be trivially associated with the phylogeny of an organism. At its most extreme interpretation, Doolittle argued that perhaps there could be no such concept as "organismal" phylogeny among organisms that exchange genes with such ease (41–44). At the other extreme, one may consider HGT to be a source of "noise" in the phylogenetic signal that must be corrected and accounted for like any other (103). The truth undoubtedly lies somewhere between these extremes, and its pursuit has led to novel approaches to addressing this particular evolutionary issue, one that certainly captures the imagination of many microbiologists.

Supergene Trees

One way to circumvent the limitations of constructing organismal phylogenies from protein-coding genes is to use multiple genes, thereby increasing the size of the data set. If one assumed that horizontal transfer was rare, then mutational "noise" could be overcome by amplifying the remnant signals found in multiple genes, thus allowing organismal phylogeny to be deduced. At this point, if some genes provided "signal" that was in dramatic disagreement with the overall single phylogeny obtained from this concatenated set of protein sequences (often referred to as a "supergene"), then they could be discarded. This approach has been used and, not surprisingly, the results reinforced the delineation of major clades of organisms inferred from rRNA gene cladograms (17). Whole-genome sequences offered the availability of (presumably) orthologous sequences from a number of genomes, enabling this analysis to be performed on a previously unattainable scale.

"Gene Content" Phylogenies

In contrast to "supergene" trees, gene content phylogenies could only be constructed after complete genome sequences became available in large numbers; therefore, like microarray studies of gene expression, this methodology represents an approach to a scientific question that arose in the so-called postgenomic era. While many investigators implemented variants of this method, the central idea remained the same: one would use the presence or absence of a gene as a character in constructing an organismal phylogeny (57, 201, 205). These methods had the advantage that alignment of sequences was no longer required, eliminating a well-known error-prone, but highly crucial, step in the phylogenetic process. Yet like all other approaches to this question, this one has its drawbacks, including the "convergence" of organisms having undergone genome reduction, misidentification of paralogous genes as orthologous genes, and the ever-present confounding effect of HGT.

"Signature Genes" and Deep Phylogeny

Some investigators have approached organismal phylogeny from a different philosophical standpoint. Rather than attempting to use complete genome sequences to deduce the relationships among all extant life forms, these same sequences could be analyzed for other features that provided insight into "deep" phylogenetic relationships. One approach has been to identify sequences (genes, or even oligonucleotide patterns) that are shared among members of a group (1, 64, 74, 75, 216). Here the question being addressed is not "What are the exact relationships among a set of organisms?" but rather "Which organisms belong to a particular group?" One could ask, then, if all methanogens fell into a single group (which is not predicted by rRNA gene phylogenies, which place *Methanopyrus kandleri* at the base of the archaeal lineage [198]), and other broad evolutionary questions. Signature sequences—such as insertion/deletion events in conserved proteins—can be used to define groups, and even identify genes that have experienced gene transfer or other evolutionary processes (68). Genomic signatures can also be used on a finer scale. For example, the polarity of a gene transfer event between the pathogens *Haemophilus* and *Neisseria* (i.e., which was the donor and which was the recipient) was determined by the presence of the "signature" *Haemophilus* uptake sequence at the transferred locus in *Neisseria*, indicating that *Haemophilus* was the likely donor (102).

The Utility of Such a "Tree of Life"

Although complete genome sequences have offered unprecedented abilities to examine the tree of life, its meaning is hotly debated among microbiologists (63). Perhaps even the most conservative microbiologist would agree that there is no gene that has not experienced horizontal transfer at some point, somewhere among extant lineages. More dramatically, many may agree that perhaps extant genomes contain no genes that have been passed down by vertical inheritance from mother cell to daughter cell; that is, every gene has been subject to transfer at some point in its history. At this point opinions diverge, and the "Ship of Theseus" analogy for genome evolution [first heard by the author from Ford Doolittle, adapting the argument made by Plutarch [*Vita Thesei*, p. 22 23]] has been argued from both sides. That is, it one replaces all of the planks of the mythical ship over time, is it the same ship? If not, what has it changed into? By analogy, is it meaningful to even think about an "organismal" phylogeny if what one could follow (when provided with an omniscient microscope examining all cell divisions since the origin of life) was the history of cytoplasm, independent of genetic material? Here some would argue that organismal phylogeny is meaningless, since it does not reflect the multitude of histories of the heritable genetic material in that organism; the "tree of life" would be more accurately represented as a "web of life." Others would argue that genes may come and go, but the organism remains (as does the Ship of Theseus); after all, the molecules in our bodies are turned over regularly, and even this author would argue that he remains himself during the turnover of his constituent parts (though perhaps becoming a bit more forgetful and a bit grumpier during the process). It is unlikely that further genome sequences will ever resolve this issue, since it is a philosophical matter and not a biological one, and the fastest computers and best data sets are poor tools for the dissection of metaphysical problems. Perhaps the best that can be accomplished is to recognize that the history of an organism cannot be equated with the diverse histories of the genes that define that organism.

NEW BIOLOGICAL APPROACHES ENABLED BY COMPLETE GENOME SEQUENCES

Gene Identification: Small Open Reading Frames

Clearly genes were identified robustly prior to complete genome sequences, even in the absence of genetic or biochemical evidence of predicted gene function. Indeed, most of the tools taking advantage of complete genome sequences (such as the identification of genes by virtue of homologues in other taxa, or the assignment of protein coding sequences based on patterns of nucleotide composition, dinucleotide frequencies, codon usage bias, etc.) were employed using sequences available from the sequence database. Yet one approach relies on the comparison of complete genomes to identify genes; here, very small protein-coding regions are identified by examining sequence conservation between related taxa (110, 155). For protein-coding genes, synonymous substitutions (those that do not alter amino acid identity) outnumber nonsynonymous substitution (those that do change amino acid identity) since nonsynonymous substitutions are more likely to be eliminated by purifying selection. What makes this approach unique is that the complete genome sequences provide the necessary values for the mean and variance of these substitution rates. Utilizing these values, one can identify small annotated open reading frames that lie outside these parameters, allowing one to place a confidence value on whether a segment of DNA is protein-coding or not. This method allows genome annotation to evolve beyond "a gene or not a gene, that is the question" and provide quantitative values behind the prediction of the most difficult protein-coding regions to predict. Small RNAs offer even more challenges; rates of evolution of their sequence are highly dependent upon secondary structure as well as function, and global patterns of constraint—such as those imposed by the genetic code—are not available for interpretation of observed variation.

Gene Identification: Contingency Loci et Alia

Some pathogenic organisms use clever molecular tricks to turn genes on and off at random. Examples include the switching of flagellar types by site-specific recombination in *S. enterica* (197, 220), alteration of host-recognition tail-fiber proteins in bacteriophages Mu and P1 by similar mechanisms (89, 95), the switching of host cell recognition in a *Bordetella* phage via error-prone reverse transcription (127), and the stochastic inactivation of genes presenting surface antigens by recombination in *Bacteroides* (101, 164) or replication slippage in *H. influenzae* (92). The use of replication slippage as a mechanism for the stochastic inactivation of genes provides a sequence signature. For example, long stretches of single nucleotides in promoter regions, such as that controlling expression of Opc proteins in *Neisseria* (187), allow replication slippage to randomly control the strength of a promoter by varying the spacing between the −10 and −35 binding sites for RNA polymerase. Similarly, polynucleotide repeats within coding regions (where N mod 3 ≠ 0) can randomly shift regions downstream of these repeats in or out of their proper reading frame, depending on the number of repeats (92). As mentioned above, scanning complete genome sequences for such repeated sequences allows for the identification of putative contingency loci from genomic sequences without prior genetic or biochemical evidence (85).

Here, data gleaned from careful analyses of genes of interest have allowed for the development of computer algorithms for the detection of genes that may employ similar mechanisms for their expression. Similar computational methods have been applied to identify genes possibly involved in ribosomal frameshifting (13, 195), or genes that may be translated

by incorporating selenocysteine into UGA codons (8). In this case, the genomic approach results in reciprocal benefits: the genome sequence allows for the identification of novel genes encoding selenocysteine-bearing proteins, and the identification of these proteins allows for better annotation of the genome, since the selenocysteine UGA codon would likely be interpreted as a stop codon by automated genome annotation programs.

Minimal Genome Size

How small can the genome of a free-living organism be? This concept has been much speculated upon prior to the acquisition of complete genome sequences (105, 134, 168). The publication of the genome sequence for *M. genitalium* (60, 83) provided access to several new approaches to address this issue. First, one may use this "smallest" of genomes to determine which genes have homologues in most or all other genomes (7, 149, 175); this analysis provides an initial estimate of the number of "universally required" gene products, minus those undetectable because of nonorthologous replacement and other confounding processes. In this case the number turns out to be about 250 genes, or a bit more than half of the gene complement of *M. genitalium*. A second approach is to use the *M. genitalium* genome as a starting point and eliminate genes, one by one, to determine if they are essential for this organism (86); analogous projects are being performed in yeast (62, 154) and other organisms. Using this approach, about 300 genes were found to be essential for life. Interestingly, some of the "universal" genes found in comparative analyses could be eliminated experimentally without effect (100), and others were not found in the closely related taxon *Mycoplasma pulmonis* (23).

In this way, one may directly assess what a minimal genome size is for a particular organism and its corresponding lifestyle. Such projects provide insight into the possible nature of the most recent common ancestor of all known life, and were not conceivable prior to the acquisition of complete genome sequences, necessary for providing both the substrates for the analyses and the perspective to interpret the results. Yet strong caveats accompany such extrapolative studies, since the label "required for life" in an experimental setting depends entirely upon growth conditions. After all, the *lac* operon is essential for growth of *E. coli* on minimal lactose medium.

Evolution of Metabolic Pathways

As is clear, whole-genome sequences allow for the identification of metabolic pathways in organisms even when they cannot be grown in pure culture, as was the case for the identification of pathways for amino acid biosynthesis in the endosymbiont *B. aphidicola* (196). In addition, genomic sequences can "jump-start" genetic and biochemical analysis by allowing the inference of genes (by homology) involved in metabolic pathways, which can be used to direct experimentation; this was the case for characterization of genes involved in lipopolysaccharide biosynthesis in *Haemophilus* (84). This analysis can be extended to examine the distribution of metabolic pathways among organisms, allowing inferences regarding the evolution of metabolic pathways. For example, the origins of the tricarboxylic acid cycle as a separate biosynthetic pathway for amino acid metabolism become clear upon the inspection of even a small number of genomes and their complements of the genes involved (87). Similarly, the remarkable plasticity in the once-presumed "universal" glycolytic pathway became evident only after comparison of the constituent genes among completely sequenced genomes (35). The involvement of HGT in the evolution of methylotrophy in some bacterial lineages—whereby genes for enzymes and the synthesis of required cofactors were obtained from methanogenic *Archaea*—is robustly supported by the whole-genome sequences of methanogens (24). Similarly, the role of HGT in the evolution of photosynthetic organisms, involving the transfer of core components of the complex photosynthetic apparatus, was made possible only through the availability of whole-genome sequences (173,

174). These examples demonstrate how the elucidation of the way in which metabolism has evolved over the course of organismal diversification, a hard-fought pursuit without genome sequences (e.g., the evolution of aromatic amino acid metabolism [2]) is made possible to a degree hitherto unimagined in the pregenomic era.

Evolution of Genomes

Lastly, we can use genome sequences to examine genomes themselves as entities, and examine processes that occur at genomic scales. For example, in 1997 Wolfe and Shields proposed that hemiascomycete yeasts (those related to the laboratory workhorse *S. cerevisiae*) may have evolved through whole-genome duplication (217). The idea was intriguing, and had both merit and some support by the available data. Like any proposal making plausible but not conclusive extrapolations, this hypothesis attracted its fair share of skepticism, which was laid to rest with the subsequent exquisite analysis of partial genome sequences from multiple species of yeasts (218). Whole-genome duplications have been proposed at several junctures in the evolution of extant eukaryotes (e.g., see reference 143), and complete genome sequences from multicellular eukaryotes will allow similar rigorous analyses to confirm this route of organismal evolution. Similarly, rates of chromosomal rearrangements can be assessed among various taxa (25, 88, 192–194), and the growth of genomes by tandem duplications (55) and their association with potential *cis*-acting regulatory sequences (125, 204) can be assessed, all providing insight into how dynamic genomes change over time.

CHAPTER SUMMARY

- Genomes evolve by gene modification, gene loss, and gene gain.
- Variant genes may arise by mutation or by recombination.
- In some lineages, gene gain can be a profound influence, allowing adaptation by providing new functions.
- Gene loss can be a potent evolutionary

force, both removing unused functions and preventing the expression of potentially problematic genes.

- Different genes have different susceptibilities to gene gain and loss.
- Reconstruction of the tree of life must account for both vertical and horizontal inheritance.

ACKNOWLEDGMENTS

I thank H. Hendrickson for helpful discussions and for sharing unpublished data, and E. Presley for helpful comments on the manuscript.

This work was supported by grant MCB-0217278 from the National Science Foundation.

REFERENCES

1. Abe, T., S. Kanaya, M. Kinouchi, Y. Ichiba, T. Kozuki, and T. Ikemura. 2003. Informatics for unveiling hidden genome signatures. *Genome Res.* 13:693–702.
2. Ahmad, S., W. G. Weisburg, and R. A. Jensen. 1990. Evolution of aromatic amino acid biosynthesis and application to the fine-tuned phylogenetic positioning of enteric bacteria. *J. Bacteriol.* 172:1051–1061.
3. Andersson, J. O. 2000. Evolutionary genomics: is *Buchnera* a bacterium or an organelle? *Curr. Biol.* 10:R866–R868.
4. Andersson, J. O., and S. G. Andersson. 1999. Genome degradation is an ongoing process in *Rickettsia. Mol. Biol. Evol.* 16:1178–1191.
5. Andersson, J. O., and S. G. Andersson. 1999. Insights into the evolutionary process of genome degradation. *Curr. Opin. Genet. Dev.* 9:664–671.
6. Andersson, S. G., A. Zomorodipour, J. O. Andersson, T. Sicheritz-Ponten, U. C. Alsmark, R. M. Podowski, A. K. Naslund, A. S. Eriksson, H. H. Winkler, and C. G. Kurland. 1998. The genome sequence of *Rickettsia prowazekii* and the origin of mitochondria. *Nature* 396:133–140.
7. Arigoni, F., F. Talabot, M. Peitsch, M. D. Edgerton, E. Meldrum, E. Allet, R. Fish, T. Jamotte, M. L. Curchod, and H. Loferer. 1998. A genome-based approach for the identification of essential bacterial genes. *Nat. Biotechnol.* 16:851–856.
8. Backofen, R., N. S. Narayanaswamy, and F. Swidan. 2002. Protein similarity search under mRNA structural constraints: application to targeted selenocysteine insertion. *In Silico Biol.* 2:275–290.
9. Barinaga, M. 1996. A shared strategy for virulencey. *Science* 272:1261–1263.

10. Battersby, A. R. 1994. How nature builds the pigments of life: the conquest of vitamin B_{12}. *Science* 264:1551–1557.
11. Baumann, L., P. Baumann, and N. A. Moran. 1998. The endosymbiont (*Buchnera*) of the aphid *Diuraphis noxia* contains all the genes of the tryptophan biosynthetic pathway. *Curr. Microbiol.* 37:58–59.
12. Baumann, L., P. Baumann, N. A. Moran, J. Sandstrom, and M. L. Thao. 1999. Genetic characterization of plasmids containing genes encoding enzymes of leucine biosynthesis in endosymbionts (*Buchnera*) of aphids. *J. Mol. Evol.* 48:77–85.
13. Bekaert, M., L. Bidou, A. Denise, G. Duchateau-Nguyen, J. P. Forest, C. Froidevaux, I. Hatin, J. P. Rousset, and M. Termier. 2003. Towards a computational model for −1 eukaryotic frameshifting sites. *Bioinformatics* 19:327–335.
14. Bennett, A. F., K. M. Dao, and R. E. Lenski. 1990. Rapid evolution in response to high-temperature selection. *Nature* 346:79–81.
15. Berlyn, M. K. 1998. Linkage map of *Escherichia coli* K-12, edition 10: the traditional map. *Microbiol. Mol. Biol. Rev.* 62:814–984.
16. Blattner, F. R., G. R. Plunkett, C. A. Bloch, N. T. Perna, V. Burland, M. Riley, J. Collado-Vides, J. D. Glasner, C. K. Rode, G. F. Mayhew, J. Gregor, N. W. Davis, H. A. Kirkpatrick, M. A. Goeden, D. J. Rose, B. Mau, and Y. Shao. 1997. The complete genome sequence of *Escherichia coli* K-12. *Science* 277:1453–1474.
17. Brown, J. R., C. J. Douady, M. J. Italia, W. E. Marshall, and M. J. Stanhope. 2001. Universal trees based on large combined protein sequence data sets. *Nat. Genet.* 28:281–285.
18. Brussow, H., C. Canchaya, and W. D. Hardt. 2004. Phages and the evolution of bacterial pathogens: from genomic rearrangements to lysogenic conversion. *Microbiol. Mol. Biol. Rev.* 68:560–602.
19. Capiaux, H., F. Cornet, J. Corre, M. Guijo, K. Perals, J. E. Rebollo, and J. Louarn. 2001. Polarization of the *Escherichia coli* chromosome. A view from the terminus. *Biochimie* 83:161–170.
20. Casjens, S., and W. M. Huang. 1993. Linear chromosomal physical and genetic map of *Borrelia burgdorferi*, the Lyme disease agent. *Mol. Microbiol.* 8:967–980.
21. Casjens, S., N. Palmer, R. van Vugt, W. M. Huang, B. Stevenson, P. Rosa, R. Lathigra, G. Sutton, J. Peterson, R. J. Dodson, D. Haft, E. Hickey, M. Gwinn, O. White, and C. M. Fraser. 2000. A bacterial genome in flux: the twelve linear and nine circular extrachromosomal DNAs in an infectious isolate of the Lyme disease spirochete *Borrelia burgdorferi. Mol. Microbiol.* 35:490–516.

22. **Caugant, D. A., L. F. Mocca, C. E. Frasch, O. Froholm, W. D. Zollinger, and R. K. Selander.** 1987. Genetic structure of *Neisseria meningitidis* populations in relation to serogroup, serotype, and outer membrane protein pattern. *J. Bacteriol.* **169:**2781–2792.

23. **Chambaud, I., R. Heilig, S. Ferris, V. Barbe, D. Samson, F. Galisson, I. Moszer, K. Dybvig, H. Wroblewski, A. Viari, E. P. Rocha, and A. Blanchard.** 2001. The complete genome sequence of the murine respiratory pathogen *Mycoplasma pulmonis*. *Nucleic Acids Res.* **29:** 2145–2153.

24. **Chistoserdova, L., J. A. Vorholt, R. K. Thauer, and M. E. Lidstrom.** 1998. C1 transfer enzymes and coenzymes linking methylotrophic bacteria and methanogenic Archaea. *Science* **281:**99–102.

25. **Coghlan, A., and K. H. Wolfe.** 2002. Fourfold faster rate of genome rearrangement in nematodes than in *Drosophila*. *Genome Res.* **12:**857–867.

26. **Cohan, F. M.** 1994. Genetic exchange and evolutionary divergence in prokaryotes. *Trends Ecol. Evol.* **9:**175–180.

27. **Cohan, F. M.** 2001. Bacterial species and speciation. *Syst. Biol.* **50:**513–524.

28. **Cohan, F. M.** 2002. What are bacterial species? *Annu. Rev. Microbiol.* **56:**457–487.

29. **Cole, S. T., K. Eiglmeier, J. Parkhill, K. D. James, N. R. Thomson, P. R. Wheeler, N. Honore, T. Garnier, C. Churcher, D. Harris, K. Mungall, D. Basham, D. Brown, T. Chillingworth, R. Connor, R. M. Davies, K. Devlin, S. Duthoy, T. Feltwell, A. Fraser, N. Hamlin, S. Holroyd, T. Hornsby, K. Jagels, C. Lacroix, J. Maclean, S. Moule, L. Murphy, K. Oliver, M. A. Quail, M. A. Rajandream, K. M. Rutherford, S. Rutter, K. Seeger, S. Simon, M. Simmonds, J. Skelton, R. Squares, S. Squares, K. Stevens, K. Taylor, S. Whitehead, J. R. Woodward, and B. G. Barrell.** 2001. Massive gene decay in the leprosy bacillus. *Nature* **409:**1007–1011.

30. **Cooper, T. F., D. E. Rozen, and R. E. Lenski.** 2003. Parallel changes in gene expression after 20,000 generations of evolution in *Escherichia coli*. *Proc. Natl. Acad. Sci. USA* **100:**1072–1077.

31. **Cooper, V. S., A. F. Bennett, and R. E. Lenski.** 2001. Evolution of thermal dependence of growth rate of *Escherichia coli* populations during 20,000 generations in a constant environment. *Int. J. Org. Evol.* **55:**889–896.

32. **Cooper, V. S., D. Schneider, M. Blot, and R. E. Lenski.** 2001. Mechanisms causing rapid and parallel losses of ribose catabolism in evolving populations of *Escherichia coli* B. *J. Bacteriol.* **183:** 2834–2841.

33. **Crawford, I. P., and R. Milkman.** 1991. Orthologous and paralogous divergence, reticulate evolution, and lateral gene transfer in bacterial *trp* genes, p. 77–95. *In* R. K. Selander, A. G. Clark, and T. S. Whittam (ed.), *Evolution at the Molecular Level*. Sinauer Associates, Sunderland, Mass.

34. **Crook, D. W., and B. G. Spratt.** 1998. Multiple antibiotic resistance in *Streptococcus pneumoniae*. *Br. Med. Bull.* **54:**595–610.

35. **Dandekar, T., S. Schuster, B. Snel, M. Huynen, and P. Bork.** 1999. Pathway alignment: application to the comparative analysis of glycolytic enzymes. *Biochem. J.* **343:**115–124.

36. **Dandekar, T., B. Snel, M. Huynen, and P. Bork.** 1998. Conservation of gene order: a fingerprint of proteins that physically interact. *Trends Biochem. Sci.* **23:**324–328.

37. **Day, W. A., Jr., R. E. Fernandez, and A. T. Maurelli.** 2001. Pathoadaptive mutations that enhance virulence: genetic organization of the *cadA* regions of *Shigella* spp. *Infect. Immun.* **69:** 7471–7480.

38. **Dean, A. M., D. E. Dykhuizen, and D. L. Hartl.** 1986. Fitness as a function of beta-galactosidase activity in *Escherichia coli*. *Genet. Res.* **48:**1–8.

39. **Dean, A. M., D. E. Dykhuizen, and D. L. Hartl.** 1988. Fitness effects of amino acid replacements in the beta-galactosidase of *Escherichia coli*. *Mol. Biol. Evol.* **5:**469–485.

40. **Deng, W., S. R. Liou, G. Plunkett III, G. F. Mayhew, D. J. Rose, V. Burland, V. Kodoyianni, D. C. Schwartz, and F. R. Blattner.** 2003. Comparative genomics of *Salmonella enterica* serovar Typhi strains Ty2 and CT18. *J. Bacteriol.* **185:**2330–2337.

41. **Doolittle, W. F.** 1999. Lateral genomics. *Trends Cell Biol.* **9:**M5–M8.

42. **Doolittle, W. F.** 1999. Phylogenetic classification and the universal tree. *Science* **284:**2124–2129.

43. **Doolittle, W. F.** 2000. The nature of the universal ancestor and the evolution of the proteome. *Curr. Opin. Struct. Biol.* **10:**355–358.

44. **Doolittle, W. F.** 2000. Uprooting the tree of life. *Sci. Am.* **282:**90–95.

45. **DuBose, R. F., D. E. Dykhuizen, and D. L. Hartl.** 1988. Genetic exchange among natural isolates of bacteria: recombination within the *phoA* gene of *Escherichia coli*. *Proc. Natl. Acad. Sci. USA* **85:**7036–7040.

46. **Dykhuizen, D. E., A. M. Dean, and D. L. Hartl.** 1987. Metabolic flux and fitness. *Genetics* **115:**25–31.

47. **Dykhuizen, D. E., and L. Green.** 1991. Recombination in *Escherichia coli* and the definition of biological species. *J. Bacteriol.* **173:**7257–7268.

48. **Dykhuizen, D. E., S. A. Sawyer, L. Green, R. D. Miller, and D. L. Hartl.** 1985. Joint distribution of insertion elements IS*4* and IS*5* in natural isolates of *Escherichia coli*. *Genetics* **111:**219–231.

49. **Edwards, R. A., G. J. Olsen, and S. R. Maloy.**

2002. Comparative genomics of closely related Salmonellae. *Trends Microbiol.* **10:**94–99.

50. Eisen, J. A., J. F. Heidelberg, O. White, and S. L. Salzberg. 2000. Evidence for symmetric chromosomal inversions around the replication origin in bacteria. *Genome Biol.* **1:**1–11.

51. Enright, M. C., N. P. Day, C. E. Davies, S. J. Peacock, and B. G. Spratt. 2000. Multilocus sequence typing for characterization of methicillin-resistant and methicillin-susceptible clones of *Staphylococcus aureus. J. Clin. Microbiol.* **38:** 1008–1015.

52. Feil, E. J., E. C. Holmes, D. E. Bessen, M. S. Chan, N. P. Day, M. C. Enright, R. Goldstein, D. W. Hood, A. Kalia, C. E. Moore, J. Zhou, and B. G. Spratt. 2001. Recombination within natural populations of pathogenic bacteria: short-term empirical estimates and long-term phylogenetic consequences. *Proc. Natl. Acad. Sci. USA* **98:**182–187.

53. Feil, E. J., J. M. Smith, M. C. Enright, and B. G. Spratt. 2000. Estimating recombinational parameters in *Streptococcus pneumoniae* from multilocus sequence typing data. *Genetics* **154:**1439–1450.

54. Ferea, T. L., D. Botstein, P. O. Brown, and R. F. Rosenzweig. 1999. Systematic changes in gene expression patterns following adaptive evolution in yeast. *Proc. Natl. Acad. Sci. U.S.A.* **96:** 9721–9726.

55. Ferrier, D. E., and P. W. Holland. 2001. Ancient origin of the Hox gene cluster. *Nat. Rev. Genet.* **2:**33–38.

56. Fitzgerald, J. R., and J. M. Musser. 2001. Evolutionary genomics of pathogenic bacteria. *Trends Microbiol.* **9:**547–553.

57. Fitz-Gibbon, S. T., and C. H. House. 1999. Whole genome-based phylogenetic analysis of free-living microorganisms. *Nucleic Acids Res.* **27:**4218–4222.

58. Fleischmann, R. D., M. D. Adams, O. White, R. A. Clayton, E. F. Kirkness, A. R. Kerlavage, C. J. Bult, J.-F. Tomb, B. A. Dougherty, J. M. Merrick, K. McKenney, G. G. Sutton, W. FitzHugh, C. A. Fields, J. D. Gocayne, J. D. Scott, R. Shirley, L. I. Liu, A. Glodek, J. M. Kelley, J. F. Weidman, C. A. Phillips, T. Spriggs, E. Hedblom, M. D. Cotton, T. Utterback, M. C. Hanna, D. T. Nguyen, D. M. Saudek, R. C. Brandon, L. D. Fine, J. L. Fritchman, J. L. Fuhrmann, N. S. Geoghagen, C. L. Gnehm, L. A. McDonald, K. V. Small, C. M. Fraser, H. O. Smith, and J. C. Venter. 1995. Whole-genome random sequencing and assembly of *Haemophilus influenzae* Rd. *Science* **269:**496–512.

59. Fraser, C. M., S. Casjens, W. M. Huang, G. G. Sutton, R. Clayton, R. Lathigra, O. White, K. A. Ketchum, R. Dodson, E. K. Hickey, M. Gwinn, B. Dougherty, J. F. Tomb, R. D. Fleischmann, D. Richardson, J. Peterson, A. R. Kerlavage, J. Quackenbush, S. Salzberg, M. Hanson, R. van Vugt, N. Palmer, M. D. Adams, J. Gocayne, J. C. Venter, et al. 1997. Genomic sequence of a Lyme disease spirochaete, *Borrelia burgdorferi. Nature* **390:**580–586.

60. Fraser, C. M., J. D. Gocayne, O. White, M. D. Adams, R. A. Clayton, R. D. Fleischmann, C. J. Bult, A. R. Kerlavage, G. Sutton, J. M. Kelley, J. L. Fritchman, J. F. Weidman, K. V. Small, M. Sandusky, J. L. Fuhrmann, D. T. Nguyen, T. R. Utterback, D. M. Saudek, C. A. Phillips, J. M. Merrick, J.-F. Tomb, B. A. Dougherty, K. F. Bott, P.-C. Hu, T. S. Lucier, S. N. Peterson, H. O. Smith, C. A. I. Hutchison, and J. C. Venter. 1995. The minimal gene complement of *Mycoplasma genitalium. Science* **270:**397–403.

61. Garcia-Vallve, S., A. Romeu, and J. Palau. 2000. Horizontal gene transfer of glycosyl hydrolases of the rumen fungi. *Mol. Biol. Evol.* **17:** 352–361.

62. Giaever, G., A. M. Chu, L. Ni, C. Connelly, L. Riles, S. Veronneau, S. Dow, A. Lucau-Danila, K. Anderson, B. Andre, A. P. Arkin, A. Astromoff, M. El-Bakkoury, R. Bangham, R. Benito, S. Brachat, S. Campanaro, M. Curtiss, K. Davis, A. Deutschbauer, K. D. Entian, P. Flaherty, F. Foury, D. J. Garfinkel, J. H. Gerstein, D. Gotte, U. Guldener, J. H. Hegemann, S. Hempel, Z. Herman, D. F. Jaramillo, D. E. Kelly, S. L. Kelly, P. Kotter, D. LaBonte, D. C. Lamb, N. Lan, H. Liang, H. Liao, L. Liu, C. Luo, M. Lussier, R. Mao, P. Menard, S. L. Ooi, J. L. Revuelta, C. J. Roberts, M. Rose, P. Ross-Macdonald, B. Scherens, G. Schimmack, B. Shafer, D. D. Shoemaker, S. Sookhai-Mahadeo, R. K. Storms, J. N. Strathern, G. Valle, M. Voet, G. Volckaert, C. Y. Wang, T. R. Ward, J. Wilhelmy, E. A. Winzeler, Y. Yang, G. Yen, E. Youngman, K. Yu, H. Bussey, J. D. Boeke, M. Snyder, P. Philippsen, R. W. Davis, and M. Johnston. 2002. Functional profiling of the *Saccharomyces cerevisiae* genome. *Nature* **418:**387–391.

63. Gogarten, J. P., W. F. Doolittle, and J. G. Lawrence. 2002. Prokaryotic evolution in light of gene transfer. *Mol. Biol. Evol.* **19:**2226–2238.

64. Graham, D. E., R. Overbeek, G. J. Olsen, and C. R. Woese. 2000. An Archaeal genomic signature. *Proc. Natl. Acad. Sci. USA* **97:**3304–3308.

65. Grantham, R., C. Gautier, and M. Gouy. 1980. Codon frequencies in 119 individual genes confirm consistent choices of degenerate bases according to genome type. *Nucleic Acids Res.* **8:**1893–1912.

66. Grantham, R., C. Gautier, M. Gouy, M. Jacobzone, and R. Mercier. 1981. Codon cata-

log usage is a genome strategy modulated for gene expressivity. *Nucleic Acids Res.* **9**:43–74.

67. **Grantham, R., C. Gautier, M. Gouy, R. Mercier, and A. Pave.** 1980. Codon catalog usage and the genome hypothesis. *Nucleic Acids Res.* **8**:r49–r62.

68. **Griffiths, E., and R. S. Gupta.** 2002. Protein signatures distinctive of chlamydial species: horizontal transfers of cell wall biosynthesis genes *glmU* from Archaea to chlamydiae and *murA* between chlamydiae and *Streptomyces. Microbiology* **148**:2541–2549.

69. **Groisman, E. A., and H. Ochman.** 1993. Cognate gene clusters govern invasion of host epithelial cells by *Salmonella typhimurium* and *Shigella flexneri. EMBO J.* **12**:3779–3787.

70. **Groisman, E. A., and H. Ochman.** 1994. How to become a pathogen. *Trends Microbiol.* **2**:289–294.

71. **Groisman, E. A., and H. Ochman.** 1996. Pathogenicity islands: bacterial evolution in quantum leaps. *Cell* **87**:791–794.

72. **Groisman, E. A., and H. Ochman.** 1997. How *Salmonella* became a pathogen. *Trends Microbiol.* **5**:343–349.

73. **Guerdoux-Jamet, P., A. Hénaut, P. Nitschké, J. L. Risler, and A. Danchin.** 1997. Using codon usage to predict genes origin: is the *Escherichia coli* outer membrane a patchwork of products from different genomes? *DNA Res.* **4**:257–265.

74. **Gupta, R. S.** 2001. The branching order and phylogenetic placement of species from completed bacterial genomes, based on conserved indels found in various proteins. *Int. Microbiol.* **4**:187–202.

75. **Gupta, R. S., and E. Griffiths.** 2002. Critical issues in bacterial phylogeny. *Theor. Popul. Biol.* **61**:423–434.

76. **Guttman, D. S., and D. E. Dykhuizen.** 1994. Clonal divergence in *Escherichia coli* as a result of recombination, not mutation. *Science* **266**:1380–1383.

77. **Guttman, D. S., and D. E. Dykhuizen.** 1994. Detecting selective sweeps in naturally occurring *Escherichia coli. Genetics* **138**:993–1003.

78. **Hall, B. G.** 1998. Activation of the *bgl* operon by adaptive mutation. *Mol. Biol. Evol.* **15**:1–5.

79. **Hartl, D. L., and D. E. Dykhuizen.** 1984. The population genetics of *Escherichia coli. Annu. Rev. Genet.* **18**:31–68.

80. **Hartl, D. L., M. Medhora, L. Green, and D. E. Dykhuizen.** 1986. The evolution of DNA sequences in *Escherichia coli. Philos. Trans. R. Soc. Lond. B* **312**:191–204.

81. **Hayes, W. S., and M. Borodovsky.** 1998. How to interpret an anonymous bacterial genome: machine learning approach to gene identification. *Genome Res.* **8**:1154–1171.

81a. **Hendrickson, H., and J.G. Lawrence.** 2006. Selection for chromosome architecture in bacteria. *J. Mol. Evol.*, in press.

82. **Hendrix, R. W., M. C. M. Smith, R. N. Burns, M. E. Ford, and G. F. Hatfull.** 1999. Evolutionary relationships among diverse bacteriophages and prophages: all the world's a phage. *Proc. Natl. Acad. Sci. USA* **96**:2192–2197.

83. **Himmelreich, R., H. Plagens, H. Hilbert, B. Reiner, and R. Herrmann.** 1996. Comparative analysis of the genomes of the bacteria *Mycoplasma pneumoniae* and *Mycoplasma genitalium. Nucleic Acids Res.* **25**:701–712.

84. **Hood, D. W., M. E. Deadman, T. Allen, H. Masoud, A. Martin, J. R. Brisson, R. D. Fleischmann, J. C. Venter, J. C. Richards, and E. R. Moxon.** 1996. Use of the complete genome sequence information of *Haemophilus influenzae* strain Rd to investigate lipopolysaccharide biosynthesis. *Mol. Microbiol.* **22**:951–965.

85. **Hood, D. W., M. E. Deadman, M. P. Jennings, M. Bisercic, R. D. Fleischmann, J. C. Venter, and E. R. Moxon.** 1996. DNA repeats identify novel virulence genes in *Haemophilus influenzae. Proc. Natl. Acad. Sci. USA* **93**:11121–11125.

86. **Hutchison, C. A., S. N. Peterson, S. R. Gill, R. T. Cline, O. White, C. M. Fraser, H. O. Smith, and J. C. Venter.** 1999. Global transposon mutagenesis and a minimal *Mycoplasma* genome. *Science* **286**:2165–2169.

87. **Huynen, M. A., T. Dandekar, and P. Bork.** 1999. Variation and evolution of the citric-acid cycle: a genomic perspective. *Trends Microbiol.* **7**:281–291.

88. **Huynen, M. A., B. Snel, and P. Bork.** 2001. Inversions and the dynamics of eukaryotic gene order. *Trends Genet.* **17**:304–306.

89. **Iino, T., and K. Kutsukake.** 1981. *Trans*-acting genes of bacteriophages P1 and Mu mediate inversion of a specific DNA segment involved in flagellar phase variation of *Salmonella. Cold Spring Harbor Symp. Quant. Biol.* **45**:11–16.

90. **Israel, D. A., N. Salama, C. N. Arnold, S. F. Moss, T. Ando, H. P. Wirth, K. T. Tham, M. Camorlinga, M. J. Blaser, S. Falkow, and R. M. Peek, Jr.** 2001. *Helicobacter pylori* strain-specific differences in genetic content, identified by microarray, influence host inflammatory responses. *J. Clin. Investig.* **107**:611–620.

91. **Itoh, T., K. Takemoto, H. Mori, and T. Gojobori.** 1999. Evolutionary instability of operon structures disclosed by sequence comparisons of complete microbial genomes. *Mol. Biol. Evol.* **16**:332–346.

92. **Jennings, M. P., D. W. Hood, I. R. A. Peak,**

M. Virji, and E. R. Moxon. 1995. Molecular analysis of a locus for the biosynthesis and phase-variable expression of the lacto-N-neotetraose terminal lipopolysaccharide structure in *Neisseria meningitidis. Mol. Microbiol.* **18:**729–740.

93. Jin, Q., Z. Yuan, J. Xu, Y. Wang, Y. Shen, W. Lu, J. Wang, H. Liu, J. Yang, F. Yang, X. Zhang, J. Zhang, G. Yang, H. Wu, D. Qu, J. Dong, L. Sun, Y. Xue, A. Zhao, Y. Gao, J. Zhu, B. Kan, K. Ding, S. Chen, H. Cheng, Z. Yao, B. He, R. Chen, D. Ma, B. Qiang, Y. Wen, Y. Hou, and J. Yu. 2002. Genome sequence of *Shigella flexneri* 2a: insights into pathogenicity through comparison with genomes of *Escherichia coli* K12 and O157. *Nucleic Acids Res.* **30:**4432–4441.

94. Juhala, R. J., M. E. Ford, R. L. Duda, A. Youlton, G. F. Hatfull, and R. W. Hendrix. 2000. Genomic sequences of bacteriophages HK97 and HK022: pervasive genetic mosaicism in the lambdoid bacteriophages. *J. Mol. Biol.* **299:**27–51.

95. Kamp, D., and R. Kahmann. 1981. The relationship of two invertible segments in bacteriophage Mu and *Salmonella typhimurium* DNA. *Mol. Gen. Genet.* **184:**564–566.

96. Kaneko, T., Y. Nakamura, S. Sato, E. Asamizu, T. Kato, S. Sasamoto, A. Watanabe, K. Idesawa, A. Ishikawa, K. Kawashima, T. Kimura, Y. Kishida, C. Kiyokawa, M. Kohara, M. Matsumoto, A. Matsuno, Y. Mochizuki, S. Nakayama, N. Nakazaki, S. Shimpo, M. Sugimoto, C. Takeuchi, M. Yamada, and S. Tabata. 2000. Complete genome structure of the nitrogen-fixing symbiotic bacterium *Mesorhizobium loti. DNA Res.* **7:**331–338.

97. Karlin, S., and C. Burge. 1995. Dinucleotide relative abundance extremes: a genomic signature. *Trends Genet.* **11:**283–290.

98. Karlin, S., J. Mrazek, and A. M. Campbell. 1998. Codon usages in different gene classes of the *Escherichia coli* genome. *Mol. Microbiol.* **29:**1341–1355.

99. Kato-Maeda, M., J. T. Rhee, T. R. Gingeras, H. Salamon, J. Drenkow, N. Smittipat, and P. M. Small. 2001. Comparing genomes within the species *Mycobacterium tuberculosis. Genome Res.* **11:**547–554.

100. Koonin, E. V. 2000. How many genes can make a cell: the minimal-gene-set concept. *Annu. Rev. Genomics Hum. Genet.* **1:**99–116.

101. Krinos, C. M., M. J. Coyne, K. G. Weinacht, A. O. Tzianabos, D. L. Kasper, and L. E. Comstock. 2001. Extensive surface diversity of a commensal microorganism by multiple DNA inversions. *Nature* **414:**555–558.

102. Kroll, J. S., K. E. Wilks, J. L. Farrant, and P. R. Langford. 1998. Natural genetic exchange between *Haemophilus* and *Neisseria:* intergeneric transfer of chromosomal genes between major human pathogens. *Proc. Natl. Acad. Sci. USA* **95:**12381–12385.

103. Kurland, C. G. 2000. Something for everyone. *EMBO Rep.* **1:**92–95.

104. Lawrence, J. G. 1997. Selfish operons and speciation by gene transfer. *Trends Microbiol.* **5:**355–359.

105. Lawrence, J. G. 1999. Gene transfer and minimal genome size, p. 32–38. *In* A. Knoll, M. J. Osborn, J. Baross, H. Berg, N. R. Pace, and M. Sogin (ed.), *Size Limits of Very Small Organisms.* National Research Council, Washington, D.C.

106. Lawrence, J. G. 1999. Gene transfer, speciation, and the evolution of bacterial genomes. *Curr. Opin. Microbiol.* **2:**519–523.

107. Lawrence, J. G. 2001. Catalyzing bacterial speciation: correlating lateral transfer with genetic headroom. *Syst. Biol.* **50:**479–496.

108. Lawrence, J. G. 2002. Gene transfer in bacteria: speciation without species? *Theor. Popul. Biol.* **61:**449–460.

109. Lawrence, J. G. 2002. Shared strategies in gene organization among prokaryotes and eukaryotes. *Cell* **110:**407–413.

110. Lawrence, J. G. 2003. When ELFs are ORFs, but don't act like them. *Trends Genet.* **19:**131–132.

111. Lawrence, J. G., D. E. Dykhuizen, R. F. DuBose, and D. L. Hartl. 1989. Phylogenetic analysis using insertion sequence fingerprinting in *Escherichia coli. Mol. Biol. Evol.* **6:**1–14.

112. Lawrence, J. G., G. F. Hatfull, and R. W. Hendrix. 2002. Imbroglios of viral taxonomy: genetic exchange and failings of phenetic approaches. *J. Bacteriol.* **184:**4891–4905.

113. Lawrence, J. G., and H. Hendrickson. 2003. Lateral gene transfer: when will adolescence end? *Mol. Microbiol.* **50:**739–749.

114. Lawrence, J. G., and H. Hendrickson. 2004. Chromosome structure and constraints on lateral gene transfer. *Dynam. Genet.* **50:**319–336.

115. Lawrence, J. G., R. W. Hendrix, and S. Casjens. 2001. Where are the pseudogenes in bacterial genomes? *Trends Microbiol.* **9:**535–540.

116. Lawrence, J. G., and H. Ochman. 1997. Amelioration of bacterial genomes: rates of change and exchange. *J. Mol. Evol.* **44:**383–397.

117. Lawrence, J. G., and H. Ochman. 1998. Molecular archaeology of the *Escherichia coli* genome. *Proc. Natl. Acad. Sci. USA* **95:**9413–9417.

118. Lawrence, J. G., and H. Ochman. 2002. Reconciling the many faces of gene transfer. *Trends Microbiol.* **10:**1–4.

119. Lawrence, J. G., and J. R. Roth. 1996. Selfish operons: Horizontal transfer may drive the evolution of gene clusters. *Genetics* **143:**1843–1860.

120. **Lawrence, J. G., and J. R. Roth.** 1998. Roles of horizontal transfer in bacterial evolution, p. 208–225. *In* M. Syvanen and C. I. Kado (ed.), *Horizontal Transfer.* Chapman and Hall, London, United Kingdom.

121. **Lawrence, J. G., and J. R. Roth.** 1999. Genomic flux: genome evolution by gene loss and acquisition, p. 263–289. *In* R. L. Charlebois (ed.), *Organization of the Prokaryotic Genome.* ASM Press, Washington, D.C.

122. **Lenski, R. E., M. Slatkin, and F. J. Ayala.** 1989. Mutation and selection in bacterial populations: alternatives to the hypothesis of directed mutation. *Proc. Natl. Acad. Sci. USA* **86:**2775–2778.

123. **Levin, B.** 1981. Periodic selection, infectious gene exchange, and the genetic structure of *E. coli* populations. *Genetics* **99:**1–23.

124. **Levin, B. R.** 1988. Frequency-dependent selection in bacterial populations. *Philos. Trans. R. Soc. Lond. B* **319:**459–472.

125. **Levings, P. P., and J. Bungert.** 2002. The human β-globin locus control region: a center of attraction. *Eur. J. Biochem.* **269:**1589–1599.

126. **Liu, G. R., A. Rahn, W. Q. Liu, K. E. Sanderson, R. N. Johnston, and S. L. Liu.** 2002. The evolving genome of *Salmonella enterica* serovar Pullorum. *J. Bacteriol.* **184:**2626–2633.

127. **Liu, M., R. Deora, S. R. Doulatov, M. Gingery, F. A. Eiserling, A. Preston, D. J. Maskell, R. W. Simons, P. A. Cotter, J. Parkhill, and J. F. Miller.** 2002. Reverse transcriptase-mediated tropism switching in *Bordetella* bacteriophage. *Science* **295:**2091–2094.

128. **Liu, S. L., and K. E. Sanderson.** 1995. The chromosome of *Salmonella paratyphi* A is inverted by recombination between *rrnH* and *rrnG. J. Bacteriol.* **177:**6585–6592.

129. **Liu, S. L., and K. E. Sanderson.** 1995. Rearrangements in the genome of the bacterium *Salmonella typhi. Proc. Natl. Acad. Sci. USA* **92:**1018–1022.

130. **Liu, S. L., and K. E. Sanderson.** 1996. Highly plastic chromosomal organization in *Salmonella typhi. Proc. Natl. Acad. Sci. USA* **93:**10303–10308.

131. **Mahan, M. J., and J. R. Roth.** 1991. Ability of a bacterial chromosome segment to invert is dictated by included material rather than flanking sequence. *Genetics* **129:**1021–1032.

132. **Majewski, J., and F. M. Cohan.** 1999. DNA sequence similarity requirements for interspecific recombination in *Bacillus. Genetics* **153:**1525–1533.

133. **Majewski, J., P. Zawadzki, P. Pickerill, F. M. Cohan, and C. G. Dowson.** 2000. Barriers to genetic exchange between bacterial species: *Streptococcus pneumoniae* transformation. *J. Bacteriol.* **182:**1016–1023.

134. **Maniloff, J.** 1996. The minimal cell genome: "On being the right size". *Proc. Natl. Acad. Sci. USA* **93:**10004–10006.

135. **Maurelli, A. T., R. E. Fernández, C. A. Bloch, C. K. Rode, and A. Fasano.** 1998. "Black holes" and bacterial pathogenicity: a large genomic deletion that enhances the virulence of *Shigella* spp. and enteroinvasive *Escherichia coli. Proc. Natl. Acad. Sci. USA* **95:**3943–3948.

136. **Maynard Smith, J., N. H. Smith, M. O'Rourke, and B. G. Spratt.** 1993. How clonal are bacteria? *Proc. Natl. Acad. Sci. USA* **90:**4384–4388.

137. **Mayr, E.** 1942. *Systematics and the Origin of Species.* Columbia University Press, New York, N.Y.

138. **Mayr, E.** 1954. Change of genetic environment and evolution, p. 156–180. *In* J. S. Huxley, A. C. Hardy, and E. B. Ford (ed.), *Evolution as a Process.* Allen and Unwin, London, United Kingdom.

139. **Mayr, E.** 1963. *Animal Species and Evolution.* Harvard University Press, Cambridge, Mass.

140. **McClelland, M., L. Florea, K. Sanderson, S. W. Clifton, J. Parkhill, C. Churcher, G. Dougan, R. K. Wilson, and W. Miller.** 2000. Comparison of the *Escherichia coli* K-12 genome with sampled genomes of a *Klebsiella pneumoniae* and three *Salmonella enterica* serovars, Typhimurium, Typhi and Paratyphi. *Nucleic Acids Res.* **28:**4974–4986.

141. **McClelland, M., K. E. Sanderson, J. Spieth, S. W. Clifton, P. Latreille, L. Courtney, S. Porwollik, J. Ali, M. Dante, F. Du, S. Hou, D. Layman, S. Leonard, C. Nguyen, K. Scott, A. Holmes, N. Grewal, E. Mulvaney, E. Ryan, H. Sun, L. Florea, W. Miller, T. Stoneking, M. Nhan, R. Waterston, and R. K. Wilson.** 2001. Complete genome sequence of *Salmonella enterica* serovar Typhimurium LT2. *Nature* **413:**852–856.

142. **McKane, M., and R. Milkman.** 1995. Transduction, restriction and recombination patterns in *Escherichia coli. Genetics* **139:**35–43.

143. **McLysaght, A., K. Hokamp, and K. H. Wolfe.** 2002. Extensive genomic duplication during early chordate evolution. *Nat. Genet.* **31:**200–204.

144. **Médigue, C., T. Rouxel, P. Vigier, A. Hénaut, and A. Danchin.** 1991. Evidence of horizontal gene transfer in *Escherichia coli* speciation. *J. Mol. Biol.* **222:**851–856.

145. **Miesel, L., A. Segall, and J. R. Roth.** 1994. Construction of chromosomal rearrangements in *Salmonella* by transduction: inversions of nonpermissive segments are not lethal. *Genetics* **137:**919–932.

146. **Milkman, R.** 1973. Electrophoretic variation in *Escherichia coli* from natural sources. *Science* **182:**1024–1026.

147. **Milkman, R., and I. P. Crawford.** 1983. Clustered third-base substitutions among wild strains of *Escherichia coli*. *Science* **221:**378–379.

148. **Moszer, I., E. P. Rocha, and A. Danchin.** 1999. Codon usage and lateral gene transfer in *Bacillus subtilis*. *Curr. Opin. Microbiol.* **2:**524–528.

149. **Mushegian, A. R., and E. V. Koonin.** 1996. A minimal gene set for cellular life derived by comparison of complete bacterial genomes. *Proc. Natl. Acad. Sci. USA* **93:**10268–10273.

150. **Musser, J. M., A. Amin, and S. Ramaswamy.** 2000. Negligible genetic diversity of *Mycobacterium tuberculosis* host immune system protein targets: evidence of limited selective pressure. *Genetics* **155:**7–16.

151. **Musser, J. M., D. A. Bemis, H. Ishikawa, and R. K. Selander.** 1987. Clonal diversity and host distribution in *Bordetella bronchiseptica*. *J. Bacteriol.* **169:**2793–2803.

152. **Nakata, N., T. Tobe, I. Fukuda, T. Suzuki, K. Komatsu, M. Yoshikawa, and C. Sasakawa.** 1993. The absence of a surface protease, OmpT, determines the intercellular spreading ability of *Shigella:* the relationship between the *ompT* and *kcpA* loci. *Mol. Microbiol.* **9:**459–468.

153. **Ng, I., S.-L. Liu, and K. Sanderson.** 1999. Role of genomic rearrangements in producing new ribotypes of *Salmonella typhi*. *J. Bacteriol.* **181:**3536–3541.

154. **Niedenthal, R., L. Riles, U. Guldener, S. Klein, M. Johnston, and J. H. Hegemann.** 1999. Systematic analysis of *S. cerevisiae* chromosome VIII genes. *Yeast* **15:**1775–1796.

155. **Ochman, H.** 2002. Distinguishing the ORFs from the ELFs: short bacterial genes and the annotation of genomes. *Trends Genet.* **18:**335–337.

156. **Ochman, H., and E. A. Groisman.** 1995. The evolution of invasion in enteric bacteria. *Can. J. Microbiol.* **41:**555–561.

157. **Ochman, H., and I. B. Jones.** 2000. Evolutionary dynamics of full genome content in *Escherichia coli*. *EMBO J.* **19:**6637–6643.

158. **Ochman, H., and J. G. Lawrence.** 1996. Phylogenetics and the amelioration of bacterial genomes, p. 2627–2637. *In* F. C. Neidhardt, R. Curtiss III, J. L. Ingraham, E. C. C. Lin, K. B. Low, B. Magasanik, W. S. Reznikoff, M. Riley, M. Schaechter, and H. E. Umbarger (ed.), *Escherichia coli and Salmonella typhimurium: Cellular and molecular biology,* 2nd ed. American Society for Microbiology, Washington, D.C.

159. **Ochman, H., J. G. Lawrence, and E. Groisman.** 2000. Lateral gene transfer and the nature of bacterial innovation. *Nature* **405:**299–304.

160. **Papadopoulos, D., D. Schneider, J. Meier-Eiss, W. Arber, R. E. Lenski, and M. Blot.** 1999. Genomic evolution during a 10,000-generation experiment with bacteria. *Proc. Natl. Acad. Sci. USA* **96:**3807–3812.

161. **Parkhill, J.** 2002. The importance of complete genome sequences. *Trends Microbiol.* **10:**219–220.

162. **Parkhill, J., M. Achtman, K. D. James, S. D. Bentley, C. Churcher, S. R. Klee, G. Morelli, D. Basham, D. Brown, T. Chillingworth, R. M. Davies, P. Davis, K. Devlin, T. Feltwell, N. Hamlin, S. Holroyd, K. Jagels, S. Leather, S. Moule, K. Mungall, M. A. Quail, M. A. Rajandream, K. M. Rutherford, M. Simmonds, J. Skelton, S. Whitehead, B. G. Spratt, and B. G. Barrell.** 2000. Complete DNA sequence of a serogroup A strain of *Neisseria menigitidis* Z2491. *Nature* **404:**502–506.

163. **Parkhill, J., G. Dougan, K. D. James, N. R. Thomson, D. Pickard, J. Wain, C. Churcher, K. L. Mungall, S. D. Bentley, M. T. Holden, M. Sebaihia, S. Baker, D. Basham, K. Brooks, T. Chillingworth, P. Connerton, A. Cronin, P. Davis, R. M. Davies, L. Dowd, N. White, J. Farrar, T. Feltwell, N. Hamlin, A. Haque, T. T. Hien, S. Holroyd, K. Jagels, A. Krogh, T. S. Larsen, S. Leather, S. Moule, P. O'Gaora, C. Parry, M. Quail, K. Rutherford, M. Simmonds, J. Skelton, K. Stevens, S. Whitehead, and B. G. Barrell.** 2001. Complete genome sequence of a multiple drug resistant *Salmonella enterica* serovar Typhi CT18. *Nature* **413:**848–852.

164. **Patrick, S., J. Parkhill, L. J. McCoy, N. Lennard, M. J. Larkin, M. Collins, M. Sczaniecka, and G. Blakely.** 2003. Multiple inverted DNA repeats of *Bacteroides fragilis* that control polysaccharide antigenic variation are similar to the *hin* region inverted repeats of *Salmonella typhimurium*. *Microbiology* **149:**915–924.

165. **Pedulla, M. L., M. E. Ford, J. M. Houtz, T. Karthikeyan, C. Wadsworth, J. A. Lewis, D. Jacobs-Sera, J. Falbo, J. Gross, N. R. Pannunzio, W. Brucker, V. Kumar, J. Kandasamy, L. Keenan, S. Bardarov, J. Kriakov, J. G. Lawrence, W. R. Jacobs, R. W. Hendrix, and G. F. Hatfull.** 2003. Origins of highly mosaic mycobacteriophage genomes. *Cell* **113:**171–182.

166. **Perals, K., F. Cornet, Y. Merlet, I. Delon, and J. M. Louarn.** 2000. Functional polarization of the *Escherichia coli* chromosome terminus: the *dif* site acts in chromosome dimer resolution only when located between long stretches of opposite polarity. *Mol. Microbiol.* **36:**33–43.

167. **Perna, N. T., G. Plunkett, V. Burland, B. Mau, J. D. Glasner, D. J. Rose, G. F. Mayhew, P. S. Evans, J. Gregor, H. A. Kirkpatrick, G.**

Posfai, J. Hackett, S. Klink, A. Boutin, Y. Shao, L. Miller, E. J. Grotbeck, N. W. Davis, A. Lim, E. T. Dimalanta, K. D. Potamousis, J. Apodaca, T. S. Anantharaman, J. Lin, G. Yen, D. C. Schwartz, R. A. Welch, and F. R. Blattner. 2001. Genome sequence of entero-haemorrhagic *Escherichia coli* O157:H7. *Nature* **409:**529–533.

168. **Pirie, N. W.** 1973. "On being the right size". *Annu. Rev. Microbiol.* **27:**119–132.

169. **Plague, G. R., C. Dale, and N. A. Moran.** 2003. Low and homogeneous copy number of plasmid-borne symbiont genes affecting host nutrition in *Buchnera aphidicola* of the aphid *Uroleucon ambrosiae. Mol. Ecol.* **12:**1095–1100.

170. **Ragan, M. A.** 2001. Detection of lateral gene transfer among microbial genomes. *Curr. Opin. Genet. Dev.* **11:**620–626.

171. **Ragan, M. A.** 2001. On surrogate methods for detecting lateral gene transfer. *FEMS Microbiol. Lett.* **201:**187–191.

172. **Rainey, P. B., and M. Travisano.** 1998. Adaptive radiation in a heterogeneous environment. *Nature* **394:**69–72.

173. **Raymond, J., O. Zhaxybayeva, J. P. Gogarten, and R. E. Blankenship.** 2003. Evolution of photosynthetic prokaryotes: a maximum-likelihood mapping approach. *Philos. Trans. R. Soc. Lond. B* **358:**223–230.

174. **Raymond, J., O. Zhaxybayeva, J. P. Gogarten, S. Y. Gerdes, and R. E. Blankenship.** 2002. Whole-genome analysis of photosynthetic prokaryotes. *Science* **298:**1616–1620.

175. **Razin, S.** 1997. The minimal cellular genome of *Mycoplasma. Indian J. Biochem. Biophys.* **34:**124–130.

176. **Reid, S. D., N. M. Green, J. K. Buss, B. Lei, and J. M. Musser.** 2001. Multilocus analysis of extracellular putative virulence proteins made by group A *Streptococcus*: population genetics, human serologic response, and gene transcription. *Proc. Natl. Acad. Sci. USA* **98:**7552–7557.

177. **Riley, M. S., V. S. Cooper, R. E. Lenski, L. J. Forney, and T. L. Marsh.** 2001. Rapid phenotypic change and diversification of a soil bacterium during 1000 generations of experimental evolution. *Microbiology* **147:**995–1006.

178. **Rohwer, F., and R. Edwards.** 2002. The Phage Proteomic Tree: a genome-based taxonomy for phage. *J. Bacteriol.* **184:**4529–4535.

179. **Rosenzweig, R. F., R. R. Sharp, D. S. Treves, and J. Adams.** 1994. Microbial evolution in a simple unstructured environment: genetic differentiation in *Escherichia coli. Genetics* **137:**903–917.

180. **Roth, J. R., J. G. Lawrence, M. Rubenfield, S. Kieffer-Higgins, and G. M. Church.** 1993. Characterization of the cobalamin (vitamin B$_{12}$) biosynthetic genes of *Salmonella typhimurium. J. Bacteriol.* **175:**3303–3316.

181. **Rouhbakhsh, D., C. Y. Lai, C. D. von Dohlen, M. A. Clark, L. Baumann, P. Baumann, N. A. Moran, and D. J. Voegtlin.** 1996. The tryptophan biosynthetic pathway of aphid endosymbionts (*Buchnera*): genetics and evolution of plasmid-associated anthranilate synthase (*trpEG*) within the aphididae. *J. Mol. Evol.* **42:**414–421.

182. **Salama, N., K. Guillemin, T. K. McDaniel, G. Sherlock, L. Tompkins, and S. Falkow.** 2000. A whole-genome microarray reveals genetic diversity among *Helicobacter pylori* strains. *Proc. Natl. Acad. Sci. USA* **97:**14668–14673.

183. **Salzberg, S. L., A. J. Salzberg, A. R. Kerlavage, and J. F. Tomb.** 1998. Skewed oligomers and origins of replication. *Gene* **217:**57–67.

184. **Sanderson, K. E., and C. A. Hall.** 1970. F-prime factors of *Salmonella typhimurium* and an inversion between *S. typhimurium* and *Escherichia coli. Genetics* **64:**215–228.

185. **Sanderson, K. E., and S. L. Liu.** 1998. Chromosomal rearrangements in enteric bacteria. *Electrophoresis* **19:**569–572.

186. **Sanderson, K. E., and J. R. Roth.** 1988. Linkage map of *Salmonella typhimurium*, edition 7. *Microbiol. Rev.* **52:**485–532.

187. **Sarkari, J., N. Pandit, E. R. Moxon, and M. Achtman.** 1994. Variable expression of the Opc outer membrane protein in *Neisseria meningitidis* is caused by size variation of a promoter containing poly-cytidine. *Mol. Microbiol.* **13:**207–217.

188. **Segall, A., M. J. Mahan, and J. R. Roth.** 1988. Rearrangement of the bacterial chromosome: forbidden inversions. *Science* **241:**1314–1318.

189. **Segall, A. M., and J. R. Roth.** 1989. Recombination between homologies in direct and inverse orientation in the chromosome of *Salmonella*: intervals which are nonpermissive for inversion formation. *Genetics* **122:**737–747.

190. **Selander, R. K., and B. R. Levin.** 1980. Genetic diversity and structure in *Escherichia coli* populations. *Science* **210:**545–547.

191. **Selander, R. K., R. M. McKinney, T. S. Whittam, W. F. Bibb, D. J. Brenner, F. S. Nolte, and P. E. Pattison.** 1985. Genetic structure of populations of *Legionella pneumophila. J. Bacteriol.* **163:**1021–1037.

192. **Semple, C., and K. H. Wolfe.** 1999. Gene duplication and gene conversion in the *Caenorhabditis elegans* genome. *J. Mol. Evol.* **48:**555–564.

193. **Seoighe, C., N. Federspiel, T. Jones, N. Hansen, V. Bivolarovic, R. Surzycki, R. Tamse, C. Komp, L. Huizar, R. W. Davis, S.**

Scherer, E. Tait, D. J. Shaw, D. Harris, L. Murphy, K. Oliver, K. Taylor, M. A. Rajandream, B. G. Barrell, and K. H. Wolfe. 2000. Prevalence of small inversions in yeast gene order evolution. *Proc. Natl. Acad. Sci. USA* **97**:14433–14437.

194. Seoighe, C., and K. H. Wolfe. 1998. Extent of genomic rearrangement after genome duplication in yeast. *Proc. Natl. Acad. Sci. USA* **95**:4447–4452.

195. Shah, A. A., M. C. Giddings, J. B. Parvaz, R. F. Gesteland, J. F. Atkins, and I. P. Ivanov. 2002. Computational identification of putative programmed translational frameshift sites. *Bioinformatics* **18**:1046–1053.

196. Shigenobu, S., H. Watanabe, M. Hattori, Y. Sakaki, and H. Ishikawa. 2000. Genome sequence of the endocellular bacterial symbiont of aphids *Buchnera* sp. APS. *Nature* **407**:81–86.

197. Silverman, M., J. Zieg, M. Hilmen, and M. Simon. 1979. Phase variation in *Salmonella*: genetic analysis of a recombinational switch. *Proc. Natl. Acad. Sci. USA* **76**:391–395.

198. Slesarev, A. I., K. V. Mezhevaya, K. S. Makarova, N. N. Polushin, O. V. Shcherbinina, V. V. Shakhova, G. I. Belova, L. Aravind, D. A. Natale, I. B. Rogozin, R. L. Tatusov, Y. I. Wolf, K. O. Stetter, A. G. Malykh, E. V. Koonin, and S. A. Kozyavkin. 2002. The complete genome of hyperthermophile *Methanopyrus kandleri* AV19 and monophyly of Archaeal methanogens. *Proc. Natl. Acad. Sci. USA* **99**:4644–4649.

199. Smith, J. M., C. G. Dowson, and B. G. Spratt. 1991. Localized sex in bacteria. *Nature* **349**:29–31.

200. Smith, N. H., E. C. Holmes, G. M. Donovan, G. A. Carpenter, and B. G. Spratt. 1999. Networks and groups within the genus *Neisseria*: Analysis of *argF*, *recA*, *rho*, and 16S rRNA sequences from human *Neisseria* species. *Mol. Biol. Evol.* **16**:773–783.

201. Snel, B., P. Bork, and M. Huynen. 1999. Genome phylogeny based on gene content. *Nat. Genet.* **21**:108–110.

202. Stoltzfus, A., J. F. Leslie, and R. Milkman. 1988. Molecular evolution of the *Escherichia coli* chromosome. I. Analysis of structure and natural variation in a previously uncharacterized region between *trp* and *tonB*. *Genetics* **120**:345–358.

203. Tamas, I., L. Klasson, B. Canbäck, A. K. Näslund, A. S. Eriksson, J. J. Wernegreen, J. P. Sandström, N. A. Moran, and S. G. Andersson. 2002. 50 million years of genomic stasis in endosymbiotic bacteria. *Science* **296**:2376–2379.

204. Tanimoto, K., Q. Liu, J. Bungert, and J. D. Engert. 1999. Effects of altered gene order or orientation of the locus control region on human β-globin gene expression in mice. *Nature* **398**:344–348.

205. Tekaia, F., A. Lazcano, and B. Dujon. 1999. The genomic tree as revealed from whole proteome comparisons. *Genome Res.* **9**:550–557.

206. Treves, D. S., S. Manning, and J. Adams. 1998. Repeated evolution of an acetate-crossfeeding polymorphism in long-term populations of *Escherichia coli*. *Mol. Biol. Evol.* **15**:789–797.

207. Vrba, E. S. (ed.). 1985. *Species and Speciation*. Transvaal Museum, Pretoria, South Africa.

208. Ward, D. M. 1998. A natural species concept for prokaryotes. *Curr. Opin. Microbiol.* **1**:271–277.

209. Wei, J., M. B. Goldberg, V. Burland, M. M. Venkatesan, W. Deng, G. Fournier, G. F. Mayhew, G. Plunkett III, D. J. Rose, A. Darling, B. Mau, N. T. Perna, S. M. Payne, L. J. Runyen-Janecky, S. Zhou, D. C. Schwartz, and F. R. Blattner. 2003. Complete genome sequence and comparative genomics of *Shigella flexneri* serotype 2a strain 2457T. *Infect. Immun.* **71**:2775–2786.

210. Welch, R. A., V. Burland, G. Plunkett III, P. Redford, P. Roesch, D. Rasko, E. L. Buckles, S. R. Liou, A. Boutin, J. Hackett, D. Stroud, G. F. Mayhew, D. J. Rose, S. Zhou, D. C. Schwartz, N. T. Perna, H. L. Mobley, M. S. Donnenberg, and F. R. Blattner. 2002. Extensive mosaic structure revealed by the complete genome sequence of uropathogenic *Escherichia coli*. *Proc. Natl. Acad. Sci. USA* **99**:17020–17024.

211. Wernegreen, J. J., and N. A. Moran. 2000. Decay of mutualistic potential in aphid endosymbionts through silencing of biosynthetic loci: *Buchnera* of *Diuraphis*. *Proc. R. Soc. Lond. B* **267**:1423–1431.

212. Wernegreen, J. J., A. O. Richardson, and N. A. Moran. 2001. Parallel acceleration of evolutionary rates in symbiont genes underlying host nutrition. *Mol. Phylogenet. Evol.* **19**:479–485.

213. Whittam, T. S., H. Ochman, and R. K. Selander. 1983. Multilocus genetic structure in natural populations of *Escherichia coli*. *Proc. Natl. Acad. Sci. USA* **80**:1751–1755.

214. Woese, C. R., and G. E. Fox. 1977. Phylogenetic structure of the prokaryotic domain: the primary kingdoms. *Proc. Natl. Acad. Sci. USA* **74**:5088–5090.

215. Woese, C. R., G. J. Olsen, M. Ibba, and D. Soll. 2000. Aminoacyl-tRNA synthetases, the genetic code, and the evolutionary process. *Microbiol. Mol. Biol. Rev.* **64**:202–236.

216. **Woese, C. R., E. Stackebrandt, T. J. Macke, and G. E. Fox.** 1985. A phylogenetic definition of the major eubacterial taxa. *Syst. Appl. Microbiol.* **6:**143–151.

217. **Wolfe, K. H., and D. C. Shields.** 1997. Molecular evidence for an ancient duplication of the entire yeast genome. *Nature* **387:**708–713.

218. **Wong, S., G. Butler, and K. H. Wolfe.** 2002. Gene order evolution and paleopolyploidy in hemiascomycete yeasts. *Proc. Natl. Acad. Sci. USA* **99:**9272–9277.

219. **Xiang, S. H., A. M. Haase, and P. R. Reeves.** 1993. Variation of the *rfb* gene clusters in *Salmonella enterica. J. Bacteriol.* **175:**4877–4884.

220. **Zieg, J., M. Silverman, M. Hilmen, and M. Simon.** 1977. Recombinational switch for gene expression. *Science* **196:**170–172.

221. **Zuckerkandl, E.** 1965. The evolution of hemoglobin. *Sci. Am.* **212:**110–118.

222. **Zuckerkandl, E., and L. Pauling.** 1965. Molecules as documents of evolutionary history. *J. Theor. Biol.* **8:**357–366.

POPULATION DYNAMICS OF BACTERIAL PATHOGENS

Martin C. J. Maiden and Rachel Urwin

3

Bacterial infectious disease is a dynamic process: individual hosts of bacterial pathogens are well, become ill, and recover or die, and host populations experience successive periods of high and low disease incidence. The incidence of distinct pathogen types rises and falls, often for reasons that are not readily apparent. Different bacterial diseases exhibit diversity in the geographical and chronological time scales over which they occur: some diseases are endemic, persisting in human populations over many years or decades, and others occur in epidemic outbreaks of varying duration and size, ranging from localized increases in disease incidence lasting a short duration to large-scale global pandemics lasting for months or years. Some diseases affect a particular subset of the human population, while others attack all members of a population indiscriminately. These epidemiological differences reflect variation in the natural history of bacterial pathogens, and defining this variation is important not only for improving our understanding of bacterial pathogens and pathogenesis, but also for designing improved public health measures. This is a multidisciplinary endeavor that combines inferences from medical microbiology with epidemiological, evolutionary, and population-based techniques and concepts.

Bacterial pathogens can be considered to be ideal subjects for population studies. In practical terms, it is relatively easy to handle large numbers of bacterial isolates, and the small genome sizes and rapid growth rates typical of the prokaryotes are an additional advantage. From a public health perspective, the significance of bacterial populations in the spread of human disease provides a powerful motivation, and population studies have a major role to play in understanding both functional and evolutionary aspects of pathogenesis. Although studies of pathogen populations have been relatively underexploited to date, there has been a recent increase in interest that has been stimulated by the advent of cost-effective high-resolution isolate characterization techniques, especially those based on high-throughput nucleotide sequence determination, and the concomitant availability of complete genome sequences for many pathogens. While studies have confirmed many of the paradigms of bacterial population biology, they are also providing novel and unexpected insights into pathogen, and indeed human, evolution.

Martin C. J. Maiden and Rachel Urwin, The Peter Medawar Building for Pathogen Research and Department of Zoology, University of Oxford, South Parks Road, Oxford OX1 3SY, United Kingdom.

Evolution of Microbial Pathogens, Edited by H. S. Seifert and V. J. DiRita, © 2006 ASM Press, Washington, D.C.

BACTERIAL PATHOGENS: AN OVERVIEW

Human bacterial pathogens reflect the great diversity of the prokaryotic world, and it is intriguing that there are examples of genetically unrelated bacteria that have adopted similar ways of exploiting humans as an ecological niche. For example, the gram-positive organism *Streptococcus pneumoniae* and the gram-negative organisms *Haemophilus influenzae* and *Neisseria meningitidis* are distant from each other in evolutionary terms, yet all three inhabit the upper respiratory tract of humans, are spread by aerosols, have capsules composed of polysaccharide, and can cause meningitis (9, 67, 112). Most of the intimate associations that bacteria establish with humans can be categorized as either commensal or pathogenic: there are few well-documented examples of true symbiotic bacteria in humans, although colonization by various commensal organisms may have beneficial effects—for example, by limiting the growth of more harmful flora or providing a nutritional benefit (56). Commensal organisms infect their hosts without causing an overt pathology, whereas infection with a pathogen results in a disease syndrome that is damaging to the host. Bacterial pathogens can be further defined by subdivision into three categories: obligate, opportunistic, and "accidental." In common with other biological classifications, the boundaries between these groupings can be blurred, and the relationships of bacteria with their hosts are probably better regarded as a continuum rather than strict categories, but useful working definitions can be made.

Obligate pathogens have no environmental reservoir in the form of an active population outside the host or hosts; in addition, they rely on the induction of a disease syndrome for host-to-host transmission. Examples include bacteria as genetically different as the acid-fast organism *Mycobacterium tuberculosis,* the causative agent of tuberculosis (13, 127, 146); the treponeme *Treponema pallidum,* which causes syphilis (45, 120, 126); the gram-positive sporulating bacterium *Bacillus anthracis* (60, 74);

and the gram-negative enteric pathogen *Salmonella enterica* serovar Typhi (103).

Opportunistic pathogens do not rely on causing a disease pathology for their growth and spread; however, when these organisms cause disease in a host, this can promote spread to other hosts or in the environment. A wide range of bacteria fall into this class, including zoonotic pathogens, some human commensal organisms that occasionally cause disease, and a number of environmental bacteria. *Yersinia pestis,* which causes bubonic plague in humans, is naturally a pathogen of rodents, transmitted by an insect vector, the flea (137). It can be transmitted to humans by flea bites, and once in the human population can develop into pneumonic plague, which is spread from person to person by aerosol transmission, no longer requiring the original host or vector (102). *Vibrio cholerae,* the causative agent of cholera, is a naturally occurring environmental organism, commonly found in water courses throughout the world (91, 98). However, when this organism adopts the pathogenic habit, the very large quantities of vibrios released into the environment in the stools of cholera victims provide a source of infection for dissemination in the environment generally (91).

Accidental pathogens occasionally cause a pathology in the human host that does not promote the spread of the bacterium to other hosts or to the environment (70, 78). Therefore, the pathology is not an "opportunity" for the microbe, and the disease may indeed be inimical to further spread. An example is *Legionella pneumophila,* an environmental organism that infects humans only when it is introduced into the lungs by aerosols generated by water-handling systems such as air-conditioning units (46, 119). It does not spread among humans, who are a "dead end" host. This is also the case for the food-borne pathogen *Listeria monocytogenes,* which is an environmental contaminant of certain human foodstuffs, specifically non-pasteurized milk (122). Although both organisms are responsible for disease outbreaks, these are caused by a single point of contamination and are not transmitted among infected individuals.

Many accidental pathogens are part of the commensal flora of humans, and the diseases they cause can be considered to be the result of a failed or dysfunctional relationship between the bacterium and its host. A striking example is meningitis and septicemia caused by *N. meningitidis*. This meningococcus is widely regarded as a highly aggressive pathogen (52, 93, 143); however, this organism is a commensal inhabitant of the human nasopharynx found in all human populations analyzed to date, with carriage rates as high as 40% of individuals (18, 19). The great majority of infected individuals do not develop meningococcal disease, which, although individually devastating, is uncommon.

Within-Host Dynamics

After successful infection, the microbe-host relationship may be either acute or chronic. Chronic infectious diseases such as tuberculosis and syphilis may persist for many years or even decades, while some acute infections may last only periods of hours— meningococcal meningitis and septicemia providing two of the more extreme examples. In cases of infection by *M. tuberculosis* and *T. pallidum,* the chronic state is not infectious to other hosts, with activation of an acute infection providing opportunities for host-to-host transmission. Both of these organisms are widely disseminated; it has been estimated that one-third to one-half of the human population is infected with *M. tuberculosis* (13), and high incidences of infection with *T. pallidium* been reported in the absence of treatment (126). A rather different strategy is employed by *S. enterica* serovar Typhi: in this case, a small number of chronic, asymptomatic carriers can act as a focus of infection for many individuals who develop acute infections over periods spanning many years.

Pathogens that cause an acute disease include both accidental pathogens, such as the meningococcus, and some obligate pathogens, such as *B. anthracis. B. anthracis* causes a fatal dissemi-

nated infection in infected hosts, usually large ungulates, and exploits its ability to produce durable endospores by infecting its target population by ingestion (49). By producing large quantities of spores that can lie dormant in the soil for many years or decades, this organism may have alleviated or averted the problems associated with killing too many of the host population in a single disease outbreak, as endospores will survive in the soil for long periods of time, until the host population has recovered (30–32, 74). Acute infections may be accompanied by rapid within-host evolution of the pathogen as it adapts to growth in the host; however, in the majority of cases this is another example of dead-end evolution that has no long-term significance to the bacterium (70).

Mechanisms of Spread among Hosts

The population dynamics of obligate bacterial pathogens and commensals in humans are greatly influenced by the mechanisms by which the bacteria spread among hosts as, to persist in a given host population, such organisms must transmit effectively. In practical terms, in order for a pathogen to become successfully established in a host population, every infected host must give rise to the infection of at least one further susceptible host. The basic reproductive number (R_0) is essentially the average number of offspring that a bacterium produces, which must equal or exceed unity if the organism is to persist in the host population. This concept is central to any theoretical modeling of the population biology of bacterial pathogens (5). If obligate pathogens are too efficient at causing disease and a consequent host response, their spread can be self-limiting as susceptible hosts are removed by death or the development of immunity, and there may be a minimum host population size that can sustain a particular pathogen (5). If the susceptible host population drops below this minimum size, the pathogen dies out. A chronic infection state can overcome this problem by extending the transmission interval to one that enables new susceptible hosts to arise by population growth.

Obligate pathogens can exploit a wide range of transmission mechanisms, which are usually promoted by the disease syndrome caused. Pulmonary tuberculosis, for example, is a highly infectious condition with the violent coughing of the diseased individual efficiently spreading *M. tuberculosis* to other hosts (13, 127), and the lesions caused by *T. pallidum* on the sexual organs are highly infectious (126). Typhoid fever is associated with the release of large quantities of bacteria in the stools of diseased humans, promoting the spread of the pathogen by the fecal-oral route (65).

As opportunistic pathogens can survive in the absence of the host, dramatic effects on the human population will not affect the population of the microbe as a whole. Indeed, the proportion of the population that causes disease in humans may be insignificant in terms of the population biology of the bacterium: this is the case for both *L. pneumophila* and *L. monocytogenes*. Accidental pathogens that are also commensals must persist in the face of the negative impact on host-to-host transmission caused by the death or incapacitation of a proportion of infected hosts (133). Meningococcal disease, for example, is caused by septicemic growth of the bacterium (111, 136), and once in the bloodstream, the bacterium cannot spread to other hosts with the possible exception of the laboratory-acquired infection (15).

EXPLOITING PATHOGEN DIVERSITY IN THE STUDY OF PATHOGENS

Population Diversity

Populations of certain bacterial pathogens are genetically highly diverse (e.g., *N. meningitidis* [61, 76] and the enteric pathogen *Campylobacter jejuni* [28]), while others, such as *M. tuberculosis* and *Bordetella pertussis,* are remarkably uniform (51, 131, 142, 144). In each case, the level of diversity and the degree to which it is structured are likely to be due, at least in part, to the selective pressures imposed by the pathogen-host relationship and can therefore be interpreted to provide insights into the biology of the pathogen. Population genetic studies are founded on the premise that evolutionary forces acting on individuals in the population generate and maintain genetic diversity and determine its structure. Analyses of genetic diversity that reveal the evolutionary processes acting on the population therefore provide insights into the biology of the organism in question. These processes include mutation, genetic exchange, selection, demographic processes, and stochastic events.

Mutation is used here to describe the various processes whereby novel genetic variants arise within a population by events such as base substitution, deletion, and insertion (141) (Fig. 1). Once it has arisen by mutation, genetic variation can be reassorted into novel genotypes by the various mechanisms that mediate genetic exchange between organisms (62). As bacteria are asexual organisms, the sharing of genetic material among cells that do not share a common mother cell is confined to the mobilization of genetic material by parasexual processes such as genetic transformation, conjugation, and phage-mediated transduction (62, 68, 132, 148). These processes mobilize small fragments of the genome at any one time, and are known collectively as horizontal genetic exchange, or more colorfully as "localized sex"—the latter emphasizing the limited extent of the genetic transfer when compared with fully sexual processes (85). The term "lateral gene transfer" is employed here to indicate the subset of horizontal genetic exchange events that result in the transfer of complete genes among organisms. Horizontal genetic exchange also describes the transfer of gene fragments of homologous genes, resulting in mosaic gene structures (79, 82, 100).

The mechanisms and relative frequencies of mutation and genetic exchange have attracted much interest as dominant influences in generating genetic variants in bacteria (38, 41, 42, 128), but possibly the most important influence on the structure and diversity of bacterial populations is the evolutionary process of natural selection, which acts on genetic variants once they have arisen (141) (Fig. 2). Selection can promote the spread of novel variants, a process known as positive or diversifying selection, or

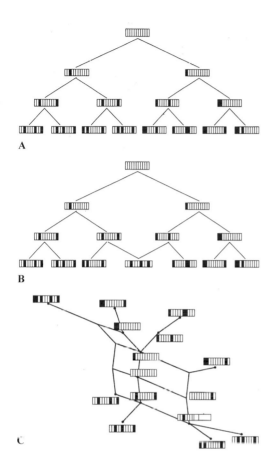

A

B

C

FIGURE 1 The evolution of bacterial populations. Simulated nucleotide sequence data sets are used to illustrate the phylogenetic processes that influence the structure of microbial populations. (A) A strictly clonal population, where new alleles appear as a result of mutations that accumulate by vertical transmission of genetic material. (B) Illustration of how a bifurcating phylogeny can be disrupted by the exchange of genetic material between distantly related strains. (C) Frequent recombination among members of a population can lead to a blurring of phylogenetic relationships, with multiple possible evolutionary pathways between strains (58).

prevent their spread, which is conversely known as negative or stabilizing selection (12, 149). Some variations may be neither selected for nor selected against; such variations are said to be neutral. The genetic variation present at chromosomal sites subject to these different selection pressures is characteristic and can be identified and quantified in population studies, especially those that collect and analyze nucleotide sequence data (12, 99, 149). The structure of the genetic variation present in populations is also influenced by what can be termed "demographic processes," such as rapid population growth or contraction, or "geographical" structuring, which results in isolated subpopulations (39, 96). Finally, a population may be importantly influenced by stochastic events, such as a subset of a population evolving the capacity to exploit a novel niche (44, 66, 72, 117), or spreading from one geographical location to another. This type of process may have been important in the emergence of a number of bacterial pathogens (131). For a bacterium, "geography" may operate on a number of scales: in addition to referring to the country-to-country spread of a pathogen, it can also refer to the isolation of a subset of organisms in a different host in the same geographical area, or even in a different location within the same host.

The selective and demographic processes that act on pathogen populations are of interest as they will, to at least some extent, reflect host-microbe interactions: studies of the genetic diversity of pathogens therefore provide insights into these processes that may be difficult or impossible to obtain by other means. The population approach entails the assembly of collections of isolates of known provenance through structured sampling; measuring the variation present in the population, preferably by nucleotide sequence determination; and the interpretation of this variation with model-based (parametric) theoretical frameworks.

The extent to which population studies reveal pathogen biology depends on the quality and quantity of the data available, set against the diversity of the population and the availability of suitable data analysis techniques. Recent technical advances permit the rapid and accurate collection of data describing genetic variation, especially by nucleotide sequence determination, which accurately and definitively identifies genetic variation (22, 78) (see chapter 2). In combination with complete

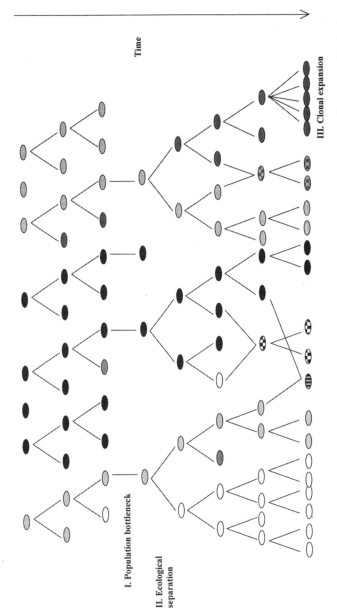

FIGURE 2 Selective and demographic effects on bacterial population structure. Novel genetic variants (represented in the figure by different shading) arise in a population as a result of mutation. Mechanisms that facilitate genetic exchange between organisms lead to reassortment of this variation into new genotypes. (I) Stochastic events such as population bottlenecks or periodic selection can lead to a reduction in the population diversity that is often accompanied by a decline in population size. (II) Reproductive isolation may result from ecological separation of a subpopulation (e.g., following adaptation to a new niche). (III) An increase in frequency in the population of a highly successful clone results in an "epidemic" population structure.

genome sequences, which are now available for many bacterial pathogens (14, 24, 45, 47, 53, 59, 104, 106, 107, 125, 135), this technology permits the cost-effective collection of large volumes of high-quality data from any part of the genome. These data are amenable to a range of analytical approaches (35, 40, 41, 51, 55, 62, 75, 101, 147). Consequently, population studies are now more likely to be limited by the quality and extent of the population samples available. There are two aspects to this sampling: obtaining isolates of pathogen populations and sampling the genetic variation within the genomes of the isolates obtained.

Population Sampling

Axenic technique is the defining methodology of microbiology, and its introduction was crucial to the development of the scientific investigation of bacterial disease; however, the isolation of bacteria into pure cultures necessarily removes population diversity that may exist within a single host. Population diversity is represented, at least to some degree, in the collections of pure cultures that are available for many bacterial pathogens, some of which span many decades and large geographical areas. Few of these collections, however, have been assembled within the context of representatively sampling the genetic diversity of a defined population (Fig. 3) (50, 78). This is an important considera-

tion, as the sampling rationale used for assembling isolate collections affects the inferences that can be drawn from them (61, 90, 94). For several aspects of pathogen population biology, there is a need for well-designed population sampling for many, and perhaps all, bacterial pathogens.

A number of factors influence the design of sampling strategies for population studies, including the natural history of the organism, the extent of variation present in the population, and practical issues of sample size and isolation procedure (90). The first consideration in the design of a sampling strategy is the identification of the target population. In many cases this will be what might be termed the "natural population" of the pathogen in question, that is to say, the population that is subject to the evolutionary forces that the population genetic analyses seek to investigate.

The simplest case is a bacterium that is solely or principally found in humans and that necessarily causes a disease syndrome as its primary mode of transmission among hosts (121, 126, 127). In such cases, a collection of disease isolates may represent the natural population quite well. However, many bacteria that cause disease in humans are commensal, environmental, or animal-associated organisms whose association with humans is incidental or even accidental (93, 122, 137): sampling the genetic diversity of

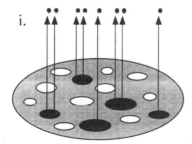 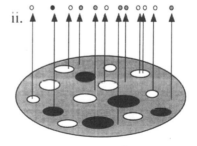

FIGURE 3 Sampling bacterial pathogen populations. Some bacterial pathogen populations are highly diverse, with only a subset of extant genotypes associated with disease. In this case, a collection of disease isolates will be unrepresentative of the diversity present in the whole population (i). A sampling strategy designed to target the whole population can help redress biased strain collections and provide insights into the mechanisms of pathogenicity (ii).

natural population of such organisms is more challenging and requires the microbiologist to leave the confines of the purely clinical laboratory. The level of diversity of the population under investigation is also important—the more diverse the population, the more extensive the sampling required, although this will also depend on the extent to which population diversity is structured (23, 94). Consequently, there is no "one size fits all" strategy for population sampling, and for each population, multiple studies may be necessary, with earlier studies informing the design of later studies.

The nature of the question or questions to be addressed is also central to study design. Investigations of the effects of vaccine introduction at the population level will have to sample the bacterial population under selection and include an analysis of the loci that encode the vaccine antigen (27, 87, 140). Studies of virulence may require an emphasis on isolates obtained from disease and an investigation of the biology of virulence determinants (88, 144). Framing questions on the basis of precollected samples is possible, but such analyses will be constrained by the context in which the isolate collection was assembled. Unfortunately, the majority of pre-existing bacterial isolate collections are not useful to address many important questions: it is, for example, unfortunate that we do not have population samples of many pathogens, or indeed commensals, from the pre-antibiotic era.

Within-Genome Diversity

Once an appropriate collection of isolates is available, it is necessary to choose the genetic loci to be examined and the methods to be used to measure the variation present. Prior to the widespread availability of molecular techniques, genetic variation had to be inferred from phenotypic characters. This approach can be successful if there is a close association between genotype and phenotype, as is the case with the Kaufmann-White serotyping scheme for *S. enterica* (108). Much of the success of this scheme as an epidemiological tool is due to the targeted antigen being a good surrogate for

genetic lineage. Agreement between a serological characteristic and genotype does not occur in all other bacteria, and can be obscured by factors that are spurious from a population genetic point of view, such as the expression levels of a given antigen.

A major advance in the study of bacterial populations was the application of multilocus enzyme electrophoresis (MLEE) (123). Of the phenotypic isolate characterization techniques employed on a large scale, this is the most closely related to genotype and has the advantage that it can be applied to a wide range of organisms (10, 11, 89, 97). The technique infers genetic variation by measuring the mobility differences during starch gel electrophoresis of variants of metabolic enzymes (electromorphs) (123). The application of biochemical staining techniques permits many different enzymes to be resolved from a single crude cell lysate. However, in addition to the limitation imposed by reliance on a specific stain for each of the enzymes analyzed, the technique only resolves protein variants that have different electrostatic charges, thus indexing a minority of the genetic variation present (80). Widespread adoption of the technique was also hampered by perceived difficulties in the technique, poor portability of the data among laboratories, and difficulties in comparing the results between different studies.

The advances in molecular and bioinformatics technologies has provided additional opportunities. Contiguous nucleotide sequences are the data of choice for population and evolutionary studies as they definitively measure variation, they are easily portable and their quality is assured, and there is a wealth of information present in nucleotide sequence data that can be interpreted by a range of population genetic and phylogenetic analysis techniques. A particular advantage is that nucleotide sequences provide information on both the extent and nature of the genetic diversity present in the population. A plethora of other techniques are available for measuring genetic variation in the bacteria (62, 141), but in no case are these as informative or readily interpreted as nucleotide sequence variation, and these approaches shall not be discussed in more detail here.

The availability of complete pathogen genome sequences, combined with PCR-based direct nucleotide sequence determination techniques, enables the genetic variation of virtually any locus of a pathogen to be measured. Consequently, the loci to be included in a study can be driven by the questions to be addressed rather than by practical considerations such as which variation is most easily measured. Many studies of pathogens concern those parts of the microbe that interact with the human host either directly (e.g., surface antigens) or indirectly (e.g., antibiotic targets). These genes, or more specifically certain parts of them, are likely to be under positive selection, and will be characterized by a ratio of nonsynonymous to synonymous substitutions (d_N/d_S) of greater than unity (83, 109, 139, 149). This indicates that, for a given gene or part of a gene, most of the base substitutions change the amino acid sequence of the protein encoded by the gene and are therefore likely to have a phenotypic effect. Determining the strength of selection at given loci, and even nucleotide residues, is valuable in studies of pathogenesis; however, these genes are unlikely to reflect the variation present in the genome as a whole, as positive selection can promote the spread of a given variant in the population (34, 92, 113, 129, 141).

Many of the models employed in population genetic analyses make use of the concept of neutral genetic variation, which in terms of nucleotide sequences is characterized by $d_N/d_S = 1$, but as discussed above, such variation is rare in the compact genomes of most prokaryotes. As in MLEE, nucleotide sequence variation in housekeeping genes that encode enzymes of central metabolism is frequently employed to investigate the population structure of bacterial pathogens (80). These genes are under stabilizing selection for conserved metabolic function (i.e., are expected to exhibit d_N/d_S ratios <1) (29). In other words, most of the base substitutions observed in the gene are

silent, in that they do not change the amino acid sequence of the encoded protein and are therefore unlikely to have a phenotypic effect. As many of the base substitutions within these relatively slowly evolving genes are synonymous, this variation is often regarded as a surrogate for neutral variation: at the very least, such variation provides a benchmark for comparisons with genes under positive selection. The use of variation in fragments of several housekeeping loci distributed around the chromosome for the typing of bacteria has been termed "multilocus sequence typing" (MLST) (80). Additional diversity, which is frequently indexed in bacterial characterization techniques, includes that found in noncoding regions, intergenic regions, or episomal elements or phage (43, 57, 73, 134). In practice, these types of variation, which are very popular in molecular typing schemes, are difficult to interpret in population genetic models, as they may be generated and maintained by a variety of selective forces that are not representative of the genome as a whole (48).

The number of loci to be used in a population study will depend on the diversity of the organism and the questions to be addressed (3, 38, 65, 77). The concept of analyzing complete genome sequences is attractive, and may be possible in the near future in purely technical terms; however, the analytical techniques and computational power required for the interpretation of this quantity of information for more than a very few isolates (54) are unlikely to be available for some time. In practice, multiple loci distributed around the chromosome have been examined; these loci often number between 6 and 20, which has enabled many of the basic models of bacterial population structure to be investigated (36–41, 55, 61, 128).

MODELS OF BACTERIAL POPULATION STRUCTURE

The clonal population structure is the basic paradigm for prokaryotes, established on the basis of the haploid asexual nature of bacteria (124). Bacterial population growth takes place by cell division that results in two daughter cells, both genetically identical to their mother cell (50). An important consequence of this process is that all genetic information is transmitted vertically from one generation to the succeeding generation. When combined with diversity reduction events resulting from selective (periodic selection) (69) or stochastic (bottlenecking) (1) processes, this inevitably leads to a clonal population structure comprising genetically distinct lineages. These lineages are characterized by linkage equilibrium of genetic variation at loci distributed around the chromosome (86). Analyzing the evolutionary history and structure of strictly clonal populations is relatively straightforward as they will be accurately modeled by conventional bifurcating phylogenetic trees (16, 33, 84).

Population data from several obligate bacterial pathogens are consistent with the clonal model, including *M. tuberculosis* (4, 8, 51), *Y. pestis* (3), *B. anthracis* (21, 59, 110), and *S. enterica* serovar Typhi (16, 65). Each of these pathogens exhibits relatively low levels of population diversity, which is consistent with the idea that they arose relatively recently from a single clone or lineage of a saprophytic or commensal organism. Concurrent with developing a pathogenic life cycle, these organisms have become reproductively isolated from their ancestral populations (4, 21, 47, 59, 64, 105). In *M. tuberculosis,* for example, reproductive isolation might be a consequence of its intracellular location (63), which limits contact with exogenous prokaryotic DNA. The fact that resistance to antimicrobial compounds in *M. tuberculosis* is invariably due to the accumulation of point mutations in the drug targets (114, 115, 118), rather than to the acquisition of drug resistance by horizontal genetic exchange, is consistent with this bacterium being reproductively isolated.

Comparisons between the genomes of *M. tuberculosis* and its relative *M. leprae,* which is also an obligate intracellular pathogen, indicate another possible consequence of the low genetic diversity, clonality, and reproductive isolation. The genomes of these related pathogens are of a similar size; however, that of *M. leprae* shows extensive evidence for gene decay when compared to the *M. tuberculosis* genome (25). Only 50% of the *M. leprae* genome is protein encoding, compared to 91% of *M. tuberculosis,* and the genome contains in excess of 1,000 pseudogenes, compared to the 6 found in *M. tuberculosis* (106, 112, 125). This type of gene loss is consistent with Müller's ratchet (141), a process whereby small asexual populations inevitably lose genetic material (6) (see chapter 6). Similar scenarios have been seen in other intracellular parasites, including the typhus agent *Rickettsia prowazekii* (7).

Intracellular location cannot explain the apparent reproductive isolation of *Y. pestis, B. anthracis,* or *S. enterica* serovar Typhi. However, it is possible that *Y. pestis* and *B. anthracis* are reproductively isolated from their parental populations as a consequence of their pathogenic lifestyle and specialized transmission mechanisms (49, 137). This explanation is less plausible for *S. enterica* serovar Typhi, which, although it has a specialized site in the human host (the spleen), is also an enteric organism that frequently travels through the environment (65). Furthermore, clonality appears to be a feature of subvariants of *S. enterica,* which as a group represent a diverse organism with an apparently clonal population structure (65). This clonal structure is apparently maintained in the face of horizontal genetic exchange, as there is evidence for lateral gene transfer at some antigen-encoding loci of these organism, demonstrating that they are not reproductively isolated (71). In this case, it is possible that clonality is maintained by a different mechanism such as niche adaptation or epistasic effects (116).

In the absence of selective effects, clonal population structures will not persist when horizontal genetic exchange is prevalent, as genetic variation will be reassorted over time, leading to a nonclonal (sometimes referred to as panmictic) population structure (86). In such a population, genetic variation is at linkage equilibrium typified by random association of alleles around the chromosome. Two predominantly nonclonal pathogens have been described to date: *Helicobacter pylori* and *Neisseria gonorrhoeae,* both of which are naturally competent for transformation and have been associated with mixed infections following the colonization of a single host with two or more unrelated strains (81). *H. pylori* is genetically very diverse, and estimates of recombination rate, relative to mutation, and of recombination fragment size are consistent with recombination driving this diversity (38). Recombination is at least as likely to occur as mutation, and the average recombination fragment size is around 400 bp, less than one-half of the average coding sequence length for this organism, which is estimated at 945 bp (138). Consequently, many of the recombination events occurring in *H. pylori* are intragenic, generating novel alleles. This observation is reflected in the data deposited in the *H. pylori* MLST database (http://helicobacter. mlst.net/): from a total of 380 isolates, there are a 370 unique sequence types (or haplotypes) based on the sequences obtained from the seven housekeeping genes examined, with the number of unique alleles at each locus ranging from 303 to 340.

H. pylori apparently has an ancient association with humans, most of the time colonizing the stomach asymptomatically, and its genetic variation at a global scale has been used to investigate human migration patterns (39). In contrast to *H. pylori*, *N. gonorrheoae* is highly uniform at housekeeping loci despite evidence of frequent genetic recombination and reassortment of this low-level diversity (145).

Many of the pathogenic bacterial populations examined to date are neither fully clonal nor completely nonclonal and have population structures that are intermediate between fully clonal and nonclonal (29, 55, 86, 130). When the populations of such organisms are examined, many genotypes are recovered that are not linked by robust phylogenetic relationships; nevertheless, groups of related genotypes are repeatedly recovered from diverse geographically and chronologically separated sources (41, 55). The meningococcus is one of the best studied examples of such organisms. Initial examination of MLEE data sets suggested that this organism exhibited a clonal population

structure (20), but subsequent analysis showed that this was a consequence of the over-representation of certain genotypes in isolate collections, a problem exacerbated by the fact that certain meningococci are more likely to cause disease than others (86). A number of subsequent analyses have demonstrated that the meningococcus has a fundamentally nonclonal population structure, comprising clonal complexes that do not share a treelike phylogeny with each other (55).

Members of clonal complexes are diverse but share sufficient genetic similarity to indicate that they share a common ancestor. The epidemic clone, or "clone dominance," model was invoked to explain the apparent presence of clones in nonclonal populations (86). This concept envisages that, in a recombining population, variants arise from time to time that have a fitness advantage over the rest of the population for host-to-host transmission. These fit variants will spread to transitorily dominate the population, diversifying by recombination. While providing a possible explanation for the presence of clonal complexes, this idea does not explain the observation that certain genotypes persist despite high levels of recombination. It is possible that selection for fitness stabilizes clonal complexes in the population, with fit, parental types persisting during spread (150). A further, as yet unresolved, problem is the association of certain meningococcal clonal complexes with virulence; as the meningococcus is an accidental pathogen, it is unclear how clonal complexes with increased virulence ("hyperinvasive lineages") compete successfully with clonal complexes that do not cause disease.

The epidemic clone model has been applied successfully to several other bacteria, including *C. jejuni*, in which clonal complexes may correspond to particular host organism preferences (28); *Streptococcus pneumoniae*, in which capsular type and virulence are associated with clonal complex (17); and *Staphylococcus aureus*, in which certain clonal complexes are associated with antibiotic resistance (26, 40). In summary, the data available so far from a range of diverse organisms suggest that, although based on housekeeping genes, clonal complexes are associated with phenotypic qualities that may be subject to selection. At present, a number of heuristic approaches have been proposed for examining clonal complex population structure, but to date no parametric quantitative methods for defining and exploring this population structure have been developed. Such methods will be essential to further understanding the population biology of the many "semiclonal" pathogenic bacteria and establishing the relationship of this structure to phenotypic characters of readvance to disease.

CONCLUSIONS AND PROSPECTS

Bacterial infectious diseases, major causes of human morbidity and mortality worldwide, remain imperfectly controlled. There are, for example, no effective vaccines against any pathogen that exhibits more than a few antigenic variants, and the prophylactic use of broad-spectrum antimicrobial agents is often ineffective and can lead to resistance. Where the biology of host-to-host transmission is understood at the population level, public health measures can be effective, and the importance of population data in both fundamental research and public health is increasingly recognized (95). Despite recent advances (2, 38, 150), however, there remains a paucity of the parametric descriptions of bacterial population structure, evolution, and epidemiology that are necessary to make the robust predictions required for both fundamental research and the design and implementation of intervention strategies. It is in these areas where the next developments in the analysis of bacterial pathogen populations are most urgently needed, and, as many of the tools for this work are now available, the prospects of developments in this area are especially exciting.

CHAPTER SUMMARY

- Bacterial populations are both dynamic and highly diverse, with recombination modifying or erasing clonal population structure.

- Pathogens, like nonpathogenic bacteria, consequently exhibit a range of population structures, depending on the balance of mechanistic and chance factors with evolutionary forces imposed by host-pathogen interactions.
- The patterns of variation in pathogen populations, when interpreted in an evolutionary context, represent a source of inference on bacteria pathogenesis.
- This rich seam of novel information is now being mined by a combination of high-throughput genetics characterization with novel analysis techniques.

REFERENCES

1. **Achtman, M.** 1997. Microevolution and epidemic spread of serogroup A *Neisseria meningitidis*—a review. *Gene* **192:**135–140.
2. **Achtman, M.** 2001. Population structure of *Helicobacter pylori* and other pathogenic bacterial species, p. 311–321. *In* Helicobacter pylori: *Molecular and Cellular Biology.* Horizon Scientific Press, Wymondham, Norfolk, United Kingdom.
3. **Achtman, M., K. Zurth, G. Morelli, G. Torrea, A. Guiyoule, and E. Carniel.** 1999. *Yersinia pestis,* the cause of plague, is a recently emerged clone of *Yersinia pseudotuberculosis. Proc. Natl. Acad. Sci. USA* **96:**14043–14048.
4. **Alland, D., T. S. Whittam, M. B. Murray, M. D. Cave, M. H. Hazbon, K. Dix, M. Kokoris, A. Duesterhoeft, J. A. Eisen, C. M. Fraser, and R. D. Fleischmann.** 2003. Modeling bacterial evolution with comparative-genome-based marker systems: application to Mycobacterium tuberculosis evolution and pathogenesis. *J. Bacteriol.* **185:**3392–3399.
5. **Anderson, R. M., and R. M. May.** 1991. *Infectious Diseases of Humans.* Oxford University Press, Oxford, United Kingdom.
6. **Andersson, D. I., and D. Hughes.** 1996. Muller's ratchet decreases fitness of a DNA-based microbe. *Proc. Natl. Acad. Sci. USA* **93:**906–907.
7. **Andersson, J. O., and S. G. Andersson.** 1999. Genome degradation is an ongoing process in *Rickettsia. Mol. Biol. Evol.* **16:**1178–1191.
8. **Baker, L., T. Brown, M. C. Maiden, and F. Drobniewski.** 2004. Silent nucleotide polymorphisms and a phylogeny for *Mycobacterium tuberculosis. Emerg. Infect. Dis.* **10:**1568–1577.
9. **Bakir, M., A. Yagci, N. Ulger, C. Akbenlioglu, A. Ilki, and G. Soyletir.** 2001. Asymptomatic carriage of *Neisseria meningitidis* and *Neisseria lactamica* in relation to *Streptococcus pneumoniae* and *Haemophilus influenzae* colonization in healthy

children: apropos of 1400 children sampled. *Eur. J. Epidemiol.* **17**:1015–1018.

10. **Beltran, P., G. Delgado, A. Navarro, F. Trujillo, R. K. Selander, and A. Cravioto.** 1999. Genetic diversity and population structure of Vibrio cholerae. *J. Clin. Microbiol.* **37**:581–590.

11. **Beltran, P., S. A. Plock, N. H. Smith, T. S. Whittam, D. C. Old, and R. K. Selander.** 1991. Reference collection of strains of the Salmonella typhimurium complex from natural. *J. Gen. Microbiol.* **137**:601–606.

12. **Bielawski, J. P., and Z. Yang.** 2003. Maximum likelihood methods for detecting adaptive evolution after gene duplication. *J. Struct. Funct. Genomics* **3**:201–212.

13. **Bloom, B. R.** 1994. *Tuberculosis: Pathogenesis, Protection and Control.* ASM Press, Washington, D.C.

14. **Boucher, Y., C. L. Nesbo, and W. F. Doolittle.** 2001. Microbial genomes: dealing with diversity. *Curr. Opin. Microbiol.* **4**:285–289.

15. **Boutet, R., J. M. Stuart, E. B. Kaczmarski, S. J. Gray, D. M. Jones, and N. Andrews.** 2001. Risk of laboratory-acquired meningococcal disease. *J. Hosp. Infect.* **49**:282–284.

16. **Boyd, E. F., F. S. Wang, T. S. Whittam, and R. K. Selander.** 1996. Molecular genetic relationships of the salmonellae. *Appl. Environ. Microbiol.* **62**:804–808.

17. **Brueggemann, A. B., D. T. Griffiths, E. Meats, T. Peto, D. W. Crook, and B. G. Spratt.** 2003. Clonal relationships between invasive and carriage *Streptococcus pneumoniae* and serotype- and clone-specific differences in invasive disease potential. *J. Infect. Dis.* **187**:1424–1432.

18. **Cartwright, K. A. V., J. M. Stuart, D. M. Jones, and N. D. Noah.** 1987. The Stonehouse survey: nasopharyngeal carriage of meningococci and *Neisseria lactamica*. *Epidemiol. Infect.* **99**:591–601.

19. **Caugant, D. A., E. A. Høiby, P. Magnus, O. Scheel, T. Hoel, G. Bjune, E. Wedege, J. Eng, and L. O. Frøholm.** 1994. Asymptomatic carriage of *Neisseria meningitidis* in a randomly sampled population. *J. Clin. Microbiol.* **32**:323–330.

20. **Caugant, D. A., L. F. Mocca, C. E. Frasch, L. O. Frøholm, W. D. Zollinger, and R. K. Selander.** 1987. Genetic structure of *Neisseria meningitidis* populations in relation to serogroup, serotype, and outer membrane protein pattern. *J. Bacteriol.* **169**:2781–2792.

21. **Cherif, A., S. Borin, A. Rizzi, H. Ouzari, A. Boudabous, and D. Daffonchio.** 2003. Bacillus anthracis diverges from related clades of the Bacillus cereus group in 16S-23S ribosomal DNA intergenic transcribed spacers containing tRNA genes. *Appl. Environ. Microbiol.* **69**:33–40.

22. **Clarke, S. C.** 2002. Nucleotide sequence-based typing of bacteria and the impact of automation. *Bioessays* **24**:858–862.

23. **Clough, H. E., D. Clancy, P. D. O'Neill, and N. P. French.** 2003. Bayesian methods for estimating pathogen prevalence within groups of animals from faecal-pat sampling. *Prev. Vet. Med.* **58**:145–169.

24. **Cole, S. T., R. Brosch, J. Parkhill, T. Garnier, C. Churcher, D. Harris, S. V. Gordon, K. Eiglmeier, S. Gas, C. E. Barry III, F. Tekaia, K. Badcock, D. Basham, D. Brown, T. Chillingworth, R. Connor, R. Davies, K. Devlin, T. Feltwell, S. Gentles, N. Hamlin, S. Holroyd, T. Hornsby, K. Jagels, B. G. Barrell, et al.** 1998. Deciphering the biology of *Mycobacterium tuberculosis* from the complete genome sequence. *Nature* **393**:537–544.

25. **Cole, S. T., K. Eiglmeier, J. Parkhill, K. D. James, N. R. Thomson, P. R. Wheeler, N. Honore, T. Garnier, C. Churcher, D. Harris, K. Mungall, D. Basham, D. Brown, T. Chillingworth, R. Connor, R. M. Davies, K. Devlin, S. Duthoy, T. Feltwell, A. Fraser, N. Hamlin, S. Holroyd, T. Hornsby, K. Jagels, C. Lacroix, J. Maclean, S. Moule, L. Murphy, K. Oliver, M. A. Quail, M. A. Rajandream, K. M. Rutherford, S. Rutter, K. Seeger, S. Simon, M. Simmonds, J. Skelton, R. Squares, S. Squares, K. Stevens, K. Taylor, S. Whitehead, J. R. Woodward, and B. G. Barrell.** 2001. Massive gene decay in the leprosy bacillus. *Nature* **409**:1007–1011.

26. **Crisostomo, M. I., H. Westh, A. Tomasz, M. Chung, D. C. Oliveira, and H. de Lencastre.** 2001. The evolution of methicillin resistance in *Staphylococcus aureus*: similarity of genetic backgrounds in historically early methicillin-susceptible and -resistant isolates and contemporary epidemic clones. *Proc. Natl. Acad. Sci. USA* **98**:9865–9870.

27. **Dabernat, H., M. A. Plisson-Saune, C. Delmas, M. Seguy, G. Faucon, R. Pelissier, H. Carsenti, C. Pradier, M. Roussel-Delvallez, J. Leroy, M. J. Dupont, F. De Bels, and P. Dellamonica.** 2003. Haemophilus influenzae carriage in children attending French day care centers: a molecular epidemiological study. *J. Clin. Microbiol.* **41**:1664–1672.

28. **Dingle, K. E., F. M. Colles, R. Ure, J. Wagenaar, B. Duim, F. J. Bolton, A. J. Fox, D. R. A. Wareing, and M. C. J. Maiden.** 2002. Molecular characterisation of *Campylobacter jejuni* clones: a rational basis for epidemiological investigations. *Emerg. Infect. Dis.* **8**:949–955.

29. **Dingle, K. E., F. M. Colles, D. R. A. Wareing, R. Ure, A. J. Fox, F. J. Bolton, H. J. Bootsma, R. J. L. Willems, R. Urwin, and M. C. J. Maiden.** 2001. Multilocus sequence typing system for *Campylobacter jejuni*. *J. Clin. Microbiol.* **39**:14–23.

30. **Dragon, D. C., and R. P. Rennie.** 1995. The ecology of anthrax spores: tough but not invincible. *Can. Vet. J.* **36:**295–301.

31. **Dragon, D. C., and R. P. Rennie.** 2001. Evaluation of spore extraction and purification methods for selective recovery of viable Bacillus anthracis spores. *Lett. Appl. Microbiol.* **33:**100–105.

32. **Dragon, D. C., R. P. Rennie, and B. T. Elkin.** 2001. Detection of anthrax spores in endemic regions of northern Canada. *J. Appl. Microbiol.* **91:**435–441.

33. **Dykhuizen, D. E., D. S. Polin, J. J. Dunn, B. Wilske, V. Preac Mursic, R. J. Dattwyler, and B. J. Luft.** 1993. *Borrelia burgdorferi* is clonal: implications for taxonomy and vaccine development. *Proc. Natl. Acad. Sci. USA* **90:**10163–10167.

34. **Elena, S. F., V. S. Cooper, and R. E. Lenski.** 1996. Punctuated evolution caused by selection of rare beneficial mutations. *Science* **272:**1802–1804.

35. **Enright, M. C., D. A. Robinson, G. Randle, E. J. Feil, H. Grundmann, and B. G. Spratt.** 2002. The evolutionary history of methicillin-resistant *Staphylococcus aureus* (MRSA). *Proc. Natl. Acad. Sci. USA* **99:**7687–7692.

36. **Enright, M. C., and B. G. Spratt.** 1998. A multilocus sequence typing scheme for *Streptococcus pneumoniae:* identification of clones associated with serious invasive disease. *Microbiology* **144:**3049–3060.

37. **Enright, M. C., B. G. Spratt, A. Kalia, J. H. Cross, and D. E. Bessen.** 2001. Multilocus sequence typing of *Streptococcus pyogenes* and the relationships between emm type and clone. *Infect. Immun.* **69:**2416–2427.

38. **Falush, D., C. Kraft, N. S. Taylor, P. Correa, J. G. Fox, M. Achtman, and S. Suerbaum.** 2001. Recombination and mutation during long-term gastric colonization by *Helicobacter pylori:* estimates of clock rates, recombination size, and minimal age. *Proc. Natl. Acad. Sci. USA* **98:**15056–15061.

39. **Falush, D., T. Wirth, B. Linz, J. K. Pritchard, M. Stephens, M. Kidd, M. J. Blaser, D. Y. Graham, S. Vacher, G. I. Perez-Perez, Y. Yamaoka, F. Megraud, K. Otto, U. Reichard, E. Katzowitsch, X. Wang, M. Achtman, and S. Suerbaum.** 2003. Traces of human migrations in *Helicobacter pylori* populations. *Science* **299:**1582–1585.

40. **Feil, E. J., J. E. Cooper, H. Grundmann, D. A. Robinson, M. C. Enright, T. Berendt, S. J. Peacock, J. M. Smith, M. Murphy, B. G. Spratt, C. E. Moore, and N. P. Day.** 2003. How clonal is *Staphylococcus aureus? J. Bacteriol.* **185:**3307–3316.

41. **Feil, E. J., E. C. Holmes, D. E. Bessen, M. S. Chan, N. P. Day, M. C. Enright, R. Goldstein, D. W. Hood, A. Kalia, C. E. Moore, J. Zhou,** and **B. G. Spratt.** 2001. Recombination within natural populations of pathogenic bacteria: short-term empirical estimates and long-term phylogenetic consequences. *Proc. Natl. Acad. Sci. USA* **98:**182–187.

42. **Feil, E. J., M. C. J. Maiden, M. Achtman, and B. G. Spratt.** 1999. The relative contributions of recombination and mutation to the divergence of clones of *Neisseria meningitidis. Mol. Biol. Evol.* **16:**1496–1502.

43. **Fernandez, J., A. Fica, G. Ebensperger, H. Calfullan, S. Prat, A. Fernandez, M. Alexandre, and I. Heitmann.** 2003. Analysis of molecular epidemiology of Chilean Salmonella enterica serotype Enteritidis isolates by pulsed-field gel electrophoresis and bacteriophage typing. *J. Clin. Microbiol.* **41:**1617–1622.

44. **Fierer, J., and D. G. Guiney.** 2001. Diverse virulence traits underlying different clinical outcomes of Salmonella infection. *J. Clin. Investig.* **107:**775–780.

45. **Fraser, C. M., S. J. Norris, G. M. Weinstock, O. White, G. G. Sutton, R. Dodson, M. Gwinn, E. K. Hickey, R. Clayton, K. A. Ketchum, E. Sodergren, J. M. Hardham, M. P. McLeod, S. Salzberg, J. Peterson, H. Khalak, D. Richardson, J. K. Howell, M. Chidambaram, T. Utterback, L. McDonald, P. Artiach, C. Bowman, M. D. Cotton, J. C. Venter, et al.** 1998. Complete genome sequence of *Treponema pallidum*, the syphilis spirochete. *Science* **281:**375–388.

46. **Fraser, D. W., T. R. Tsai, W. Orenstein, W. E. Parkin, H. J. Beecham, R. G. Sharrar, J. Harris, G. F. Mallison, S. M. Martin, J. E. McDade, C. C. Shepard, and P. S. Brachman.** 1977. Legionnaires' disease: description of an epidemic of pneumonia. *N. Engl. J. Med.* **297:**1189–1197.

47. **Garnier, T., K. Eiglmeier, J. C. Camus, N. Medina, H. Mansoor, M. Pryor, S. Duthoy, S. Grondin, C. Lacroix, C. Monsempe, S. Simon, B. Harris, R. Atkin, J. Doggett, R. Mayes, L. Keating, P. R. Wheeler, J. Parkhill, B. G. Barrell, S. T. Cole, S. V. Gordon, and R. G. Hewinson.** 2003. The complete genome sequence of Mycobacterium bovis. *Proc. Natl. Acad. Sci. USA* **100:**7877–7882.

48. **Grundmann, H., S. Hori, M. C. Enright, C. Webster, A. Tami, E. J. Feil, and T. Pitt.** 2002. Determining the genetic structure of the natural population of Staphylococcus aureus: a comparison of multilocus sequence typing with pulsed-field gel electrophoresis, randomly amplified polymorphic DNA analysis, and phage typing. *J. Clin. Microbiol.* **40:**4544–4546.

49. **Guidi-Rontani, C., M. Weber-Levy, E.**

Labruyere, and M. Mock. 1999. Germination of Bacillus anthracis spores within alveolar macrophages. *Mol. Microbiol.* **31:**9–17.

50. **Gupta, S., and M. C. J. Maiden.** 2001. Exploring the evolution of diversity in pathogen populations. *Trends Microbiol.* **9:**147–192.

51. **Gutacker, M. M., J. C. Smoot, C. A. Migliaccio, S. M. Ricklefs, S. Hua, D. V. Cousins, E. A. Graviss, E. Shashkina, B. N. Kreiswirth, and J. M. Musser.** 2002. Genome-wide analysis of synonymous single nucleotide polymorphisms in Mycobacterium tuberculosis complex organisms: resolution of genetic relationships among closely related microbial strains. *Genetics* **162:**1533–43.

52. **Harrison, L. H., M. A. Pass, A. B. Mendelsohn, M. Egri, N. E. Rosenstein, A. Bustamante, J. Razeq, and J. C. Roche.** 2001. Invasive meningococcal disease in adolescents and young adults. *JAMA* **286:**694–699.

53. **Hinton, J. C.** 1997. The *Escherichia coli* genome sequence: the end of an era or the start of the FUN? *Mol. Microbiol.* **26:**417–422.

54. **Holden, M. T., E. J. Feil, J. A. Lindsay, S. J. Peacock, N. P. Day, M. C. Enright, T. J. Foster, C. E. Moore, L. Hurst, R. Atkin, A. Barron, N. Bason, S. D. Bentley, C. Chillingworth, T. Chillingworth, C. Churcher, L. Clark, C. Corton, A. Cronin, J. Doggett, L. Dowd, T. Feltwell, Z. Hance, B. Harris, H. Hauser, S. Holroyd, K. Jagels, K. D. James, N. Lennard, A. Line, R. Mayes, S. Moule, K. Mungall, D. Ormond, M. A. Quail, E. Rabbinowitsch, K. Rutherford, M. Sanders, S. Sharp, M. Simmonds, K. Stevens, S. Whitehead, B. G. Barrell, B. G. Spratt, and J. Parkhill.** 2004. Complete genomes of two clinical Staphylococcus aureus strains: evidence for the rapid evolution of virulence and drug resistance. *Proc. Natl. Acad. Sci. USA* **101:**9786–9791.

55. **Holmes, E. C., R. Urwin, and M. C. J. Maiden.** 1999. The influence of recombination on the population structure and evolution of the human pathogen *Neisseria meningitidis. Mol. Biol. Evol.* **16:**741–749.

56. **Hooper, L. V., T. Midtvedt, and J. I. Gordon.** 2002. How host-microbial interactions shape the nutrient environment of the mammalian intestine. *Annu. Rev. Nutr.* **22:**283–307.

57. **Huard, R. C., L. C. de Oliveira Lazzarini, W. R. Butler, D. van Soolingen, and J. L. Ho.** 2003. PCR-based method to differentiate the subspecies of the Mycobacterium tuberculosis complex on the basis of genomic deletions. *J. Clin. Microbiol.* **41:**1637–1650.

58. **Huson, D. H.** 1998. SplitsTree: analyzing and visualizing evolutionary data. *Bioinformatics* **14:**68–73.

59. **Ivanova, N., A. Sorokin, I. Anderson, N. Galleron, B. Candelon, V. Kapatral, A. Bhattacharyya, G. Reznik, N. Mikhailova, A. Lapidus, L. Chu, M. Mazur, E. Goltsman, N. Larsen, M. D'Souza, T. Walunas, Y. Grechkin, G. Pusch, R. Haselkorn, M. Fonstein, S. D. Ehrlich, R. Overbeek, and N. Kyrpides.** 2003. Genome sequence of Bacillus cereus and comparative analysis with Bacillus anthracis. *Nature* **423:**87–91.

60. **Jensen, G. B., B. M. Hansen, J. Eilenberg, and J. Mahillon.** 2003. The hidden lifestyles of Bacillus cereus and relatives. *Environ. Microbiol.* **5:**631–640.

61. **Jolley, K. A., J. Kalmusova, E. J. Feil, S. Gupta, M. Musilek, P. Kriz, and M. C. Maiden.** 2000. Carried meningococci in the Czech Republic: a diverse recombining population. *J. Clin. Microbiol.* **38:**4492–8.

62. **Joyce, E. A., K. Chan, N. R. Salama, and S. Falkow.** 2002. Redefining bacterial populations: a post-genomic reformation. *Nat. Rev. Genet.* **3:**462–473.

63. **Kaufmann, S. H.** 2001. How can immunology contribute to the control of tuberculosis? *Nat. Rev. Immunol.* **1:**20–30.

64. **Keim, P., and K. L. Smith.** 2002. Bacillus anthracis evolution and epidemiology. *Curr. Top. Microbiol. Immunol.* **271:**21–32.

65. **Kidgell, C., U. Reichard, J. Wain, B. Linz, M. Torpdahl, G. Dougan, and M. Achtman.** 2002. *Salmonella typhi*, the causative agent of typhoid fever, is approximately 50,000 years old. *Infect. Genet. Evol.* **2:**39–45.

66. **Kohler, S., S. Michaux-Charachon, F. Porte, M. Ramuz, and J. P. Liautard.** 2003. What is the nature of the replicative niche of a stealthy bug named Brucella? *Trends Microbiol.* **11:**215–219.

67. **Lehmann, D., W. Yeka, T. Rongap, A. Javati, G. Saleu, A. Clegg, A. Michael, T. Lupiwa, M. Omena, and M. P. Alpers.** 1999. Aetiology and clinical signs of bacterial meningitis in children admitted to Goroka Base Hospital, Papua New Guinea, 1989–1992. *Ann. Trop. Paediatr.* **19:**21–32.

68. **Levin, B. R.** 1988. The evolution of sex in bacteria, p. 194–211. *In* R. C. Michod and B. R. Levin (ed.), *The Evolution of Sex.* Sinauer Associates, Sunderland, Mass.

69. **Levin, B. R.** 1981. Periodic selection, infectious gene exchange and the genetic structure of *E. coli* populations. *Genetics* **99:**1–23.

70. **Levin, B. R., and J. J. Bull.** 1994. Short-sighted evolution and the virulence of pathogenic microorganisms. *Trends Microbiol.* **2:**76–81.

71. **Li, J., K. Nelson, A. C. McWhorter, T. S. Whittam, and R. K. Selander.** 1994. Recombinational basis of serovar diversity in *Salmonella enterica. Proc. Natl. Acad. Sci. USA* **91:**2552–2556.

72. **Li, J., H. Ochman, E. A. Groisman, E. F. Boyd, F. Solomon, K. Nelson, and R. K. Selander.** 1995. Relationship between evolutionary rate and cellular location among the Inv/Spa invasion proteins of *Salmonella enterica. Proc. Natl. Acad. Sci. USA* **92:**7252–7256.

73. **Liebana, E., L. Garcia-Migura, C. Clouting, F. A. Clifton-Hadley, E. Lindsay, E. J. Threlfall, S. W. McDowell, and R. H. Davies.** 2002. Multiple genetic typing of Salmonella enterica serotype typhimurium isolates of different phage types (DT104, U302, DT204b, and DT49) from animals and humans in England, Wales, and Northern Ireland. *J. Clin. Microbiol.* **40:**4450–4456.

74. **Little, K.** 2002. A brief guide to anthrax. *Nurs. Times* **98:**28–29.

75. **Liu, S. V., N. J. Saunders, A. Jeffries, and R. F. Rest.** 2002. Genome analysis and strain comparison of correia repeats and correia repeat-enclosed elements in pathogenic *Neisseria. J. Bacteriol.* **184:**6163–6173.

76. **Maiden, M. C.** 2002. Population structure of *Neisseria meningitidis,* p. 151–170. *In* C. Ferreirós, M. T. Criado, and J. Vázquez (ed.), *Emerging Strategies in the Fight against Meningitis: Molecular and Cellular Aspects.* Horizon Scientific Press, Wymondham, Norfolk, United Kingdom.

77. **Maiden, M. C. J.** 2000. Characterisation of bacterial isolates with molecular techniques: multi locus sequence typing, p. 183–197. *In* P. Andrew, P. Oyston, G. L. Smith, and D. E. Stewart-Tull (ed.), *Fighting Infection in the 21st Century.* Blackwell Science Publishers, Oxford, United Kingdom.

78. **Maiden, M. C. J.** 2000. High-throughput sequencing in the population analysis of bacterial pathogens. *Int. J. Med. Microbiol.* **290:**183–190.

79. **Maiden, M. C. J.** 1993. Population genetics of a transformable bacterium: the influence of horizontal genetical exchange on the biology of *Neisseria meningitidis. FEMS Microbiol. Lett.* **112:**243–250.

80. **Maiden, M. C. J., J. A. Bygraves, E. Feil, G. Morelli, J. E. Russell, R. Urwin, Q. Zhang, J. Zhou, K. Zurth, D. A. Caugant, I. M. Feavers, M. Achtman, and B. G. Spratt.** 1998. Multilocus sequence typing: a portable approach to the identification of clones within populations of pathogenic microorganisms. *Proc. Natl. Acad. Sci. USA* **95:**3140–3145.

81. **Martin, I. M., A. Ghani, G. Bell, G. Kinghorn, and C. A. Ison.** 2003. Persistence of two genotypes of *Neisseria gonorrhoeae* during transmission. *J. Clin. Microbiol.* **41:**5609–5614.

82. **Maynard Smith, J.** 1992. Analysing the mosaic structure of genes. *J. Mol. Evol.* **34:**126–129.

83. **Maynard Smith, J.** 1994. Estimating selection by comparing synonymous and substitutional changes. *J. Mol. Evol.* **39:**123–128.

84. **Maynard Smith, J.** 1989. Trees, bundles or nets. *Trends Ecol. Evol.* **4:**302–304.

85. **Maynard Smith, J., C. G. Dowson, and B. G. Spratt.** 1991. Localized sex in bacteria. *Nature* **349:**29–31.

86. **Maynard Smith, J., N. H. Smith, M. O'Rourke, and B. G. Spratt.** 1993. How clonal are bacteria? *Proc. Natl. Acad. Sci. USA* **90:**4384–4388.

87. **Mooi, F. R., Q. He, H. van Oirschot, and J. Mertsola.** 1999. Variation in the *Bordetella pertussis* virulence factors pertussis toxin and pertactin in vaccine strains and clinical isolates in Finland. *Infect. Immun.* **67:**3133–3134.

88. **Mooi, F. R., H. van Oirschot, K. Heuvelman, H. G. van der Heide, W. Gaastra, and R. J. Willems.** 1998. Polymorphism in the *Bordetella pertussis* virulence factors P.69/pertactin and pertussis toxin in The Netherlands: temporal trends and evidence for vaccine-driven evolution. *Infect. Immun.* **66:**670–675.

89. **Moore, P. S., M. W. Reeves, B. Schwartz, B. G. Gellin, and C. V. Broome.** 1989. Intercontinental spread of an epidemic group A *Neisseria meningitidis* strain. *Lancet* **ii:**260–262.

90. **Morris, C. E., M. Bardin, O. Berge, P. Frey-Klett, N. Fromin, H. Girardin, M. H. Guinebretiere, P. Lebaron, J. M. Thiery, and M. Troussellier.** 2002. Microbial biodiversity: approaches to experimental design and hypothesis testing in primary scientific literature from 1975 to 1999. *Microbiol. Mol. Biol. Rev.* **66:**592–616.

91. **Morris, J. G., Jr.** 2003. Cholera and other types of vibriosis: a story of human pandemics and oysters on the half shell. *Clin. Infect. Dis.* **37:**272–280.

92. **Moxon, E. R., P. B. Rainey, M. A. Nowak, and R. E. Lenski.** 1994. Adaptive evolution of highly mutable loci in pathogenic bacteria. *Curr. Biol.* **4:**24–32.

93. **Munro, R.** 2002. Meningococcal disease: treatable but still terrifying. *Intern. Med. J.* **32:**165–169.

94. **Murray, M.** 2002. Sampling bias in the molecular epidemiology of tuberculosis. *Emerg. Infect. Dis.* **8:**363–369.

95. **Musser, J. M.** 1996. Molecular population genetic analysis of emerged bacterial pathogens: selected insights. *Emerg. Infect. Dis.* **2:**1–17.

96. **Musser, J. M., J. S. Kroll, D. M. Granoff, E. R. Moxon, B. R. Brodeur, J. Campos, H. Dabernat, W. Frederiksen, J. Hamel, G. Hammond, et al.** 1990. Global genetic structure and molecular epidemiology of encapsulated *Haemophilus influenzae. Rev. Infect. Dis.* **12:**75–111.

97. **Musser, J. M., J. S. Kroll, E. R. Moxon, and R. K. Selander.** 1988. Clonal population structure of encapsulated *Haemophilus influenzae. Infect. Immun.* **56:**1837–1845.

98. **Naidoo, A., and K. Patric.** 2002. Cholera: a

continuous epidemic in Africa. *J. R. Soc. Health* **122**:89–94.

99. **Nei, M., and T. Gojobori.** 1986. Simple methods for estimating the numbers of synonymous and nonsynonymous nucleotide substitutions. *Mol. Biol. Evol.* **3**:418–426.

100. **Normark, B. H., and S. Normark.** 2002. Evolution and spread of antibiotic resistance. *J. Intern. Med.* **252**:91–106.

101. **Ochman, H., and S. R. Santos.** 2003. Eyeing bacterial genomes. *Curr. Opin. Microbiol.* **6**:109–113.

102. **Oyston, P.** 2001. Plague virulence. *J. Med. Microbiol.* **50**:1015–1017.

103. **Pang, T., M. M. Levine, B. Ivanoff, J. Wain, and B. B. Finlay.** 1998. Typhoid fever—important issues still remain. *Trends Microbiol.* **6**:131–133.

104. **Parkhill, J., M. Achtman, K. D. James, S. D. Bentley, C. Churcher, S. R. Klee, G. Morelli, D. Basham, D. Brown, T. Chillingworth, R. M. Davies, P. Davis, K. Devlin, T. Feltwell, N. Hamlin, S. Holroyd, K. Jagels, S. Leather, S. Moule, K. Mungall, M. A. Quail, M. A. Rajandream, K. M. Rutherford, M. Simmonds, J. Skelton, S. Whitehead, B. G. Spratt, and B. G. Barrell.** 2000. Complete DNA sequence of a serogroup A strain of *Neisseria meningitidis* Z2491. *Nature* **404**:502–506.

105. **Parkhill, J., and C. Berry.** 2003. Genomics: relative pathogenic values. *Nature* **423**:23–25.

106. **Parkhill, J., G. Dougan, K. D. James, N. R. Thomson, D. Pickard, J. Wain, C. Churcher, K. L. Mungall, S. D. Bentley, M. T. Holden, M. Sebaihia, S. Baker, D. Basham, K. Brooks, T. Chillingworth, P. Connerton, A. Cronin, P. Davis, R. M. Davies, L. Dowd, N. White, J. Farrar, T. Feltwell, N. Hamlin, A. Haque, T. T. Hien, S. Holroyd, K. Jagels, A. Krogh, T. S. Larsen, S. Leather, S. Moule, P. O'Gaora, C. Parry, M. Quail, K. Rutherford, M. Simmonds, J. Skelton, K. Stevens, S. Whitehead, and B. G. Barrell.** 2001. Complete genome sequence of a multiple drug resistant Salmonella enterica serovar Typhi CT18. *Nature* **413**:848–852.

107. **Parkhill, J., B. W. Wren, K. Mungall, J. M. Ketley, C. Churcher, D. Basham, T. Chillingworth, R. M. Davies, T. Feltwell, S. Holroyd, K. Jagels, A. V. Karlyshev, S. Moule, M. J. Pallen, C. W. Penn, M. A. Quail, M. A. Rajandream, K. M. Rutherford, A. H. van Vliet, S. Whitehead, and B. G. Barrell.** 2000. The genome sequence of the food-borne pathogen *Campylobacter jejuni* reveals hypervariable sequences. *Nature* **403**:665–668.

108. **Popoff, M. Y., J. Bockemuhl, and F. W. Brenner.** 1998. Supplement 1997 (no. 41) to the Kauffmann-White scheme. *Res. Microbiol.* **149**:601–604.

109. **Posada, D., K. A. Crandall, M. Nguyen, J. C. Demma, and R. P. Viscidi.** 2000. Population genetics of the *porB* gene of *Neisseria gonorrhoeae*: different dynamics in different homology groups. *Mol. Biol. Evol.* **17**:423–436.

110. **Priest, F. G., M. Baker, L. W. J. Baillie, E. C. Holmes, and M. C. J. Maiden.** 2004. Population structure and evolution of the *Bacillus cereus* group. *J. Bacteriol.* **186**:7959–7970.

111. **Quagliarello, V., and W. M. Scheld.** 1992. Bacterial meningitis: pathogenesis, pathophysiology, and progress. *N. Engl. J. Med.* **327**:864–872.

112. **Quagliarello, V. J., and W. M. Scheld.** 1993. New perspectives on bacterial meningitis. *Clin. Infect. Dis.* **17**:603–610.

113. **Rainey, P. B., and M. Travisano.** 1998. Adaptive radiation in a heterogeneous environment. *Nature* **394**:69–72.

114. **Ramaswamy, S., and J. M. Musser.** 1998. Molecular genetic basis of antimicrobial agent resistance in Mycobacterium tuberculosis: 1998 update. *Tuber. Lung Dis.* **79**:3–29.

115. **Ramaswamy, S. V., A. G. Amin, S. Goksel, C. E. Stager, S. J. Dou, H. El Sahly, S. L. Moghazeh, B. N. Kreiswirth, and J. M. Musser.** 2000. Molecular genetic analysis of nucleotide polymorphisms associated with ethambutol resistance in human isolates of Mycobacterium tuberculosis. *Antimicrob. Agents Chemother.* **44**:326–336.

116. **Reeves, P. R.** 1992. Variation in O-antigens, niche-specific selection and bacterial populations. *FEMS Microbiol. Lett.* **79**:509–516.

117. **Reid, S. D., C. J. Herbelin, A. C. Bumbaugh, R. K. Selander, and T. S. Whittam.** 2000. Parallel evolution of virulence in pathogenic *Escherichia coli*. *Nature* **406**:64–67.

118. **Riska, P. F., W. R. Jacobs, Jr., and D. Alland.** 2000. Molecular determinants of drug resistance in tuberculosis. *Int. J. Tuberc. Lung Dis.* **4**:S4–S10.

119. **Roig, J., M. Sabria, and M. L. Pedro-Botet.** 2003. Legionella spp.: community acquired and nosocomial infections. *Curr. Opin. Infect. Dis.* **16**:145–151.

120. **Salazar, J. C., K. R. Hazlett, and J. D. Radolf.** 2002. The immune response to infection with Treponema pallidum, the stealth pathogen. *Microbes Infect.* **4**:1133–1140.

121. **Sasaki, S., F. Takeshita, K. Okuda, and N. Ishii.** 2001. Mycobacterium leprae and leprosy: a compendium. *Microbiol. Immunol.* **45**:729–736.

122. **Schwarzkopf, A.** 1996. Listeria monocytogenes—aspects of pathogenicity. *Pathol. Biol. (Paris)* **44**:769–774.

123. **Selander, R. K., D. A. Caugant, H. Ochman, J. M. Musser, M. N. Gilmour, and T. S.**

Whittam. 1986. Methods of multilocus enzyme electrophoresis for bacterial population genetics and systematics. *Appl. Environ. Microbiol.* **51:** 837–884.

124. **Selander, R. K., and B. R. Levin.** 1980. Genetic diversity and structure in *Escherichia coli* populations. *Science* 210:545–547.

125. **Seshadri, R., I. T. Paulsen, J. A. Eisen, T. D. Read, K. E. Nelson, W. C. Nelson, N. L. Ward, H. Tettelin, T. M. Davidsen, M. J. Beanan, R. T. Deboy, S. C. Daugherty, L. M. Brinkac, R. Madupu, R. J. Dodson, H. M. Khouri, K. H. Lee, H. A. Carty, D. Scanlan, R. A. Heinzen, H. A. Thompson, J. E. Samuel, C. M. Fraser, and J. F. Heidelberg.** 2003. Complete genome sequence of the Q-fever pathogen Coxiella burnetii. *Proc. Natl. Acad. Sci. USA* **100:**5455–5460.

126. **Singh, A. E., and B. Romanowski.** 1999. Syphilis: review with emphasis on clinical, epidemiologic, and some biologic features. *Clin. Microbiol. Rev.* **12:**187–209.

127. **Smith, I.** 2003. Mycobacterium tuberculosis pathogenesis and molecular determinants of virulence. *Clin. Microbiol. Rev.* **16:**463–496.

128. **Smith, J. M., E. J. Feil, and N. H. Smith.** 2000. Population structure and evolutionary dynamics of pathogenic bacteria. *Bioessays* **22:**1115–1122.

129. **Spiers, A. J., S. G. Kahn, J. Bohannon, M. Travisano, and P. B. Rainey.** 2002. Adaptive divergence in experimental populations of Pseudomonas fluorescens. I. Genetic and phenotypic bases of wrinkly spreader fitness. *Genetics* **161:**33–46.

130. **Spratt, B. G., and M. C. J. Maiden.** 1999. Bacterial population genetics, evolution and epidemiology. *Proc. R. Soc. Lond. Ser. B* 354:701–710.

131. **Sreevatsan, S., X. Pan, K. E. Stockbauer, N. D. Connell, B. N. Kreiswirth, T. S. Whittam, and J. M. Musser.** 1997. Restricted structural gene polymorphism in the *Mycobacterium tuberculosis* complex indicates evolutionarily recent global dissemination. *Proc. Natl. Acad. Sci. USA* **94:**9869–9874.

132. **Stewart, G. J., and C. A. Carlson.** 1986. The biology of natural transformation. *Annu. Rev. Microbiol.* **40:**211–235.

133. **Stollenwerk, N., and V. A. Jansen.** 2003. Meningitis, pathogenicity near criticality: the epidemiology of meningococcal disease as a model for accidental pathogens. *J. Theor. Biol.* **222:**347–359.

134. **Takahashi, S., S. Detrick, A. A. Whiting, A. J. Blaschke-Bonkowksy, Y. Aoyagi, E. E. Adderson, and J. F. Bohnsack.** 2002. Correlation of phylogenetic lineages of group B

Streptococci, identified by analysis of restriction-digestion patterns of genomic DNA, with infB alleles and mobile genetic elements. *J. Infect. Dis.* **186:**1034–1038.

135. **Tettelin, H., N. J. Saunders, J. Heidelberg, A. C. Jeffries, K. E. Nelson, J. A. Eisen, K. A. Ketchum, D. W. Hood, J. F. Peden, R. J. Dodson, W. C. Nelson, M. L. Gwinn, R. DeBoy, J. D. Peterson, E. K. Hickey, D. H. Haft, S. L. Salzberg, O. White, R. D. Fleischmann, B. A. Dougherty, T. Mason, A. Ciecko, D. S. Parksey, E. Blair, H. Cittone, E. B. Clark, M. D. Cotton, T. R. Utterback, H. Khouri, H. Qin, J. Vamathevan, J. Gill, V. Scarlato, V. Masignani, M. Pizza, G. Grandi, L. Sun, H. O. Smith, C. M. Fraser, E. R. Moxon, R. Rappuoli, and J. C. Venter.** 2000. Complete genome sequence of *Neisseria meningitidis* serogroup B strain MC58. *Science* **287:** 1809–1815.

136. **Tinsley, C., and X. Nassif.** 2001. Meningococcal pathogenesis: at the boundary between the pre- and post-genomic eras. *Curr. Opin. Microbiol.* **4:**47–52.

137. **Titball, R. W., J. Hill, D. G. Lawton, and K. A. Brown.** 2003. Yersinia pestis and plague. *Biochem. Soc. Trans.* **31:**104–107.

138. **Tomb, J. F., O. White, A. R. Kerlavage, R. A. Clayton, G. G. Sutton, R. D. Fleischmann, K. A. Ketchum, H. P. Klenk, S. Gill, B. A. Dougherty, K. Nelson, J. Quackenbush, L. Zhou, E. F. Kirkness, S. Peterson, B. Loftus, D. Richardson, R. Dodson, H. G. Khalak, A. Glodek, K. McKenney, L. M. Fitzegerald, N. Lee, M. D. Adams, J. C. Venter, et al.** 1997. The complete genome sequence of the gastric pathogen Helicobacter pylori. *Nature* **388:**539–547.

139. **Urwin, R., E. C. Holmes, A. J. Fox, J. P. Derrick, and M. C. Maiden.** 2002. Phylogenetic evidence for frequent positive selection and recombination in the meningococcal surface antigen PorB. *Mol. Biol. Evol.* **19:**1686–1694.

140. **Urwin, R., J. E. Russell, E. A. Thompson, E. C. Holmes, I. M. Feavers, and M. C. Maiden.** 2004. Distribution of surface protein variants among hyperinvasive meningococci: implications for vaccine design. *Infect. Immun.* **72:** 5955–5962.

141. **van Belkum, A., M. Struelens, A. de Visser, H. Verbrugh, and M. Tibayrenc.** 2001. Role of genomic typing in taxonomy, evolutionary genetics, and microbial epidemiology. *J. Clin. Microbiol.* **14:**547–560.

142. **van der Zee, A., F. Mooi, J. Van Embden, and J. Musser.** 1997. Molecular evolution and host adaptation of *Bordetella* spp.: phylogenetic analysis

using multilocus enzyme electrophoresis and typing with three insertion sequences. *J. Bacteriol.* **179:**6609–6617.

143. **van Deuren, M., P. Brandtzaeg, and J. W. van der Meer.** 2000. Update on meningococcal disease with emphasis on pathogenesis and clinical management. *Clin. Microbiol. Rev.* **13:** 144–166.

144. **Van Loo, I. H., K. J. Heuvelman, A. J. King, and F. R. Mooi.** 2002. Multilocus sequence typing of *Bordetella pertussis* based on surface protein genes. *J. Clin. Microbiol.* **40:**1994–2001.

145. **Viscidi, R. P., and J. C. Demma.** 2003. Genetic diversity of Neisseria gonorrhoeae housekeeping genes. *J. Clin. Microbiol.* **41:**197–204.

146. **Weissler, J. C.** 1993. Tuberculosis—immunopathogenesis and therapy. *Am. J. Med. Sci.* **305:**52–65.

147. **Whittam, T. S., and A. C. Bumbaugh.** 2002. Inferences from whole-genome sequences of bacterial pathogens. *Curr. Opin. Genet. Dev.* **12:**719–725.

148. **Wilkins, B. M.** 1995. Gene transfer by bacterial conjugation: diversity of systems and functional specialisations, p. 32–59. *In* S. Baumberg, J. P. W. Young, E. M. H. Wellington, and J. R. Saunders (ed.), *Population Genetics of Bacteria.* Cambridge University Press, Cambridge, United Kingdom.

149. **Yang, Z., and J. P. Bielawski.** 2000. Statistical methods for detecting molecular adaptation. *Trends Ecol. Evol.* **15:**496–503.

150. **Zhu, P., A. van der Ende, D. Falush, N. Brieske, G. Morelli, B. Linz, T. Popovic, I. G. Schuurman, R. A. Adegbola, K. Zurth, S. Gagneux, A. E. Platonov, J. Y. Riou, D. A. Caugant, P. Nicolas, and M. Achtman.** 2001. Fit genotypes and escape variants of subgroup III *Neisseria meningitidis* during three pandemics of epidemic meningitis. *Proc. Natl. Acad. Sci. USA* **98:**5234–5239.

THE STUDY OF MICROBIAL ADAPTATION BY LONG-TERM EXPERIMENTAL EVOLUTION

Vaughn S. Cooper

4

The process of becoming a pathogen necessarily involves evolutionary adaptation to a novel host environment. The molecular mechanisms of virulence that differentiate pathogenic from commensal organisms—including secretion systems, toxins, adhesion and invasion strategies, and the like—are often expressed with exquisite precision, and seem to be obvious adaptations. But the evolutionary processes that gave rise to these traits are still poorly understood, largely because adaptation often involves much more than a few predictable mutations. For example, the candidate-gene approach is insufficient because of potentially substantial contributions of interactions among genes and historical contingencies that predisposed their assembly. Even quantifying adaptation may be difficult because fitness is not easily defined and measured precisely in the context of an evolving pathogen. Fitness is always dependent upon the environment, so subtle variations in environmental conditions may significantly affect the relative advantage of a genotype. In principle, a detailed temporal sequence of all the genetic and phenotypic changes leading to the emergence of a pathogen might overcome these challenges, but these data are rarely attainable in natural systems.

Experimental evolution, the research approach discussed in this chapter, permits study of the fundamental processes of adaptation that underlie microbial evolution under controlled laboratory conditions. Long-term evolution experiments with microbes have displayed numerous elements of the complexity of natural systems and have therefore permitted the study of fundamental questions in evolutionary biology, ecology, physiology, and genetics. This chapter focuses on a few long-term, open-ended studies as well as other relevant experiments that best illustrate specific problems. Despite many excellent studies using fungal and viral models (2, 11, 16, 18, 51, 80, 97, 122, 134, 135), this chapter is focused primarily on bacterial systems with occasional mention of viral systems. Specific topics under consideration include the dynamics of adaptation, the genetic and physiological bases of fitness, causes of specialization and functional losses, evolution of mutation rates, and models of the evolution of virulence. However, experimental evolution has not, to date, emphasized the evolution of pathogens, so there is much still to be done. At

Vaughn S. Cooper, Department of Microbiology, 212 Rudman Hall, University of New Hampshire, Durham, NH 03824.

Evolution of Microbial Pathogens, Edited by H. S. Seifert and V. J. DiRita, © 2006 ASM Press, Washington, D.C.

the end of the chapter I will address prospects for future experiments to study the evolution of pathogens.

To the evolutionary biologist or ecologist concerned with large-scale processes, microbial model systems have several distinct advantages. Bacteria and viruses are typically easy to grow and quantify, especially in comparison with higher eukaryotes. Hundreds of generations of reproduction can be observed in some bacteria during the time required for a single generation of fruit flies. Furthermore, many bacteria have easily accessible genetics and tools for manipulation, especially in the case of the most commonly used species, *Escherichia coli*. In the view of some, however, the simplicity of microbes somehow limits their utility or relevance for ecological and evolutionary studies. Their limited genetic exchange, uncomplicated laboratory environments, and simple behaviors form the basis of arguments that conclusions derived from microbial models cannot be extrapolated to higher systems.

These criticisms are debatable in general, and most are irrelevant for microbiologists concerned with properties unique to bacteria or viruses. Realizing the inherent interest in pathogens, microbiologists typically have not sought to extrapolate, but rather to dissect. Over the last several decades, countless mechanisms of survival, physiology, invasion, and pathogenesis have been described, as reviewed in other chapters in this volume. However, the evolutionary origin of these mechanisms and their contributions to reproductive fitness remain poorly described. As a result, the evolutionary success of the microbe as a complete reproductive unit cannot be predicted by reductionist methods.

Allowing well-studied microorganisms to evolve in defined laboratory environments represents a fusion of reductionism and the study of complex population biological processes. Using an arsenal of molecular genetic techniques, competing bacteria can be marked, engineered to perform certain functions, or reconstituted to an ancestral state after novel genotypes and phenotypes have evolved. Microbiologists using this approach do not perform the artificial selection of plant and animal breeders, who generally focus on a specific trait, because manipulating individual cells is difficult and, moreover, not a reasonable model of the evolution of populations in nature. Instead, a simple environment is constructed in the laboratory that acts alone as the agent of natural selection on the microbial population. Mutations naturally arise that improve the relative growth of certain genotypes, but even if the advantage is substantial, many cell generations and a patient investigator are required to observe evolutionary change. The open-ended nature of the selection (as opposed to schemes focusing on a specific trait) also raises a second problem: even in a highly specific environment, what traits exactly were under the influence of natural selection? The uncertainties surrounding the basic outcome of these experiments—the genetic and phenotypic targets of adaptation—highlight certain limitations and argue for further refinement of microbial selection experiments. I will begin by describing the general methods in greater detail.

CULTURE TECHNIQUES

The easiest method of propagating bacterial populations is serial batch culture in flasks or tubes. At the end of a defined period of time, an aliquot from an existing population is introduced into a new flask containing fresh media that permit further growth. In principle, these transfers could occur at any time during the growth phase of the bacterial population, but in practice, most transfers occur once the population has exhausted the resources in the media and entered stationary phase. As a result, the freshly diluted population begins each cycle in a semiquiescent state that results in a lag phase prior to resuming exponential growth. The population size and resource concentration also fluctuate during each cycle. Despite complex population dynamics, selection typically acts most strongly during the exponential growth phase and less strongly during lag phase or stationary phase in batch culture (36, 70, 124), although if the interval between transfers is very long, then selection to survive starvation can also be of considerable importance (44, 125).

A different form of selection occurs in continuous culture (37, 38, 56, 107), in which chemostats maintain the bacterial population size, growth rate, and nutrient concentration at a predetermined, constant level. In chemostats, the rate of input of fresh media and the rate of removal of exhausted media and living cells are equal. As a result, the culture neither ever reaches stationary phase nor grows maximally, resulting in selection for maximum competitive ability for substrates at low concentration. One challenge of continuous culture is contamination, because the constant influx of fresh media and efflux of exhausted media and bacteria opens the system to unwanted microbes. An additional complication (or benefit, depending on the interpretation) of chemostat experiments is the potential for environmental partitioning and subsequent divergence of bacterial subpopulations that grow on the surfaces of the vessels. Because batch culture discards the exhausted culture vessel at regular intervals, such "wall growth" is less of a problem under that regimen.

In unshaken liquid culture or on solid agar surfaces, genetically uniform populations may rapidly evolve heterogeneity (62, 63, 87, 101, 114, 119). One example involving *Pseudomonas fluorescens* is discussed in detail below. Because static or solid cultures have environmental structure and prevent mixing, adaptation to different microenvironments is possible. These mutants may occasionally be distinguished on the basis of colony morphology, and the spatial structure of distinct colonies may be preserved and propagated by replica plating. Unfortunately, enumerating the total population size and the relative proportion of various mutants still requires that all cells be resuspended in liquid, which destroys the spatial structure.

A growing trend is to replace flasks, chemostats, or petri dishes with laboratory plants or animals as the venue for selection (e.g., see reference 48). Even if the starting animal is a germfree mouse, however, these systems may prove far more complicated and less predictable than a chemostat. For all culture methods, and these host models in particular, the construction and use of clear, selectively neutral markers is essential to differentiate among competing genotypes and to identify contaminants. Truly neutral markers are surprisingly rare, so this first step is often limiting to the experimental design.

ESTIMATING FITNESS

The most important currency in the majority of these experiments is reproductive *fitness,* a property that is frequently discussed but rarely measured. Fitness is the measurement of an organism's ability to reproduce in a given environment, but it is also relative to the ability of different variants. Because fitness is always dependent upon environment, methods for its estimation vary, but generally depend on the relative growth rate of the competing genotypes. In batch culture, fitness can be estimated directly by inoculating separately marked genotypes in fresh medium and allowing them to compete for resources during one or more transfer periods. Relative fitness is simply the ratio of the growth rates of the two competitors, which can be inferred using plate counts at inoculation and at the end of the competition (see references 37 and 71 for details). This equation can be described as

$$W_{ij} = \frac{\ln [N_i(1) / N_i(0)]}{\ln [N_j(1)/N_j(0)]}$$

Here, the fitness of strain i relative to strain j, W_{ij}, is the ratio of the strain densities, N_i and N_j, at 0 and 1 days. A slightly different fitness measure, the *selection rate constant,* can be calculated for both batch and continuous cultures (37):

$$r_{ij} = \frac{\ln [N_i(t)/N_i(0)] - \ln [N_j(t)/N_j(0)]}{t}$$

Here, the selection rate constant, r, is the *difference* in the rates of growth (per unit time), whereas fitness is the corresponding *ratio*. The use of r rather than W to quantify fitness is preferable when the difference between competitors is especially great, as it is less sensitive to sampling error under these conditions (117).

Several fitness components can be used as surrogates of organismal fitness, if the experimental design prevents more absolute measures. Maximum growth rate during exponential phase, the duration of lag phase, death rate, estimates of nutrient affinity, total biomass, and other factors can each describe different elements of fitness. Nonetheless, let the experimenter beware: when fitness components are measured in isolated isogenic cultures and not in head-to-head competition, important differences in relative fitness may be undetected. Significant *relative* growth differences may be observed between strains that exhibit identical growth curves in isolation. These need not require direct antagonism between competitors, either; subtle reductions in the duration of lag or increased resource affinity can produce substantial relative advantages.

MECHANISMS OF ECOLOGICAL EXCLUSION

Many microbial population biology experiments have tested a small number of defined genotypes for competitive dominance in a particular environment, and some have identified the mechanisms responsible for the ecological superiority of the dominant genotype. Because these experiments focus more on the ecological *fate* of genetic and phenotypic variation, as opposed to its evolutionary *origin,* they are not the focus of this chapter. Nonetheless, several are worth mentioning as examples. Zamenhof and Eichhorn (133) demonstrated that tryptophan auxotrophic mutants of a parental prototrophic strain of *Bacillus subtilis* are competitively superior to the parent in chemostat environments containing tryptophan. Derepressed mutants that produced unneeded tryptophan constitutively were at a clear competitive disadvantage in supplemented media. When the authors added indole—a precursor that auxotrophic mutants could use to convert to tryptophan—to the growth medium, the relative advantage of tryptophan auxotrophy was reduced but not eliminated. From these results,

the authors concluded that the mechanism responsible for competitive exclusion was some form of energy conservation, which might eventually lead to the selective elimination of extraneous structural genes. Furthermore, they argued that the reduced advantage of mutants in the presence of indole was a product of the extra energy expended to convert indole to tryptophan.

Dykhuizen (35) refuted this energy conservation hypothesis in a series of competitions between various mutants in chemostats. The key assumption of this hypothesis is that the strength of selection against producers is equivalent to the amount of energy saved by mutants that eliminate unneeded processes. Dykhuizen estimated these quantities under conditions similar to those employed by Zamenhof and Eichhorn, but found that auxotrophs were favored at a rate 3 orders of magnitude greater than the theoretical percentage of the energy budget devoted to tryptophan production. Moreover, the discrepancy in the two estimates was consistent across growth phases, population size, and population density. The energy conservation hypothesis also predicts that polar nonsense mutants, which produce no transcript, should grow faster than missense mutants, which produce malfunctioning transcripts. However, this was not observed. Because all measurements suggested that the combined cost of peptide synthesis and the production of intermediate metabolites was vastly less than the observed advantage of auxotrophy, some other unknown selective advantage must have been favored. Thus, the "motive force" of regressive evolution, or the disabling and loss of unused coding sequence, may only rarely be energy conservation. Despite these clear findings, many evolutionary arguments still assume that natural selection acts frequently and powerfully to conserve energy expenditure. In fact, more subtle or complex interactions between genes and their products may favor gene silencing and deletion.

Ecological superiority may also result from active exclusion, best exemplified by the toxins produced by *E. coli* known as colicins (104,

105). Colicins pose a paradox, because the capacity to produce toxin usually slows cell growth and the actual production of toxin is lethal to the cell. How such a trait evolved is mysterious, because natural selection must have favored a trait lethal to individuals that manifested it. Yet another problem is that the benefits of killing one's competitors, such as increased access to nutrients, are accessible to all neighbors, and not just genetic relatives. However, when the environment is physically structured, colicin producers may kill sensitive neighbors and allow their slower growing relatives to reproduce without being overwhelmed by fast-growing sensitive competitors. Chao and Levin (17) studied this phenomenon in structured, soft-agar habitats and found that colicin producers indeed were at an advantage. Surprisingly, clones resistant to colicins did not subsequently evolve because of their especially slow growth. What is most interesting is that a stable balance of sensitive and producing cells was achieved, suggesting that the burdens of colicin production facilitate coexistence of both resistant and sensitive populations. These experiments explain one aspect of prokaryotic altruism (committing suicide for the benefit of genetic relatives) and also highlight the importance of environmental structure in determining evolutionary outcomes.

Another key series of experiments by Hartl et al. (54) investigated whether naturally occurring genetic variation in enzymes affects fitness or is selectively neutral. The authors isolated several alleles of the enzyme 6-phosphogluconate dehydrogenase (encoded by *gnd*) in *E. coli*. They placed each variant in a common genetic background, and concluded that each affected fitness of this strain by no more than 1%, the limit of experimental detection. However, when these alleles were placed in different genetic backgrounds, they interacted strongly with other loci and altered fitness much more significantly. So, while most variation may be selectively neutral in any single environment, certain alleles may have strong effects in other environments and may promote adaptation. Together, these studies emphasize

the potential for substantial interactions between genes (epistasis) for any given trait, and suggest that even genes obviously tied to the structure or function of an adaptive trait may not have been the most important object of natural selection.

EXPERIMENTAL DESIGN: OPEN-ENDED EVOLUTION

Laboratory microbial populations are typically founded from a single clone without any initial genetic variation. However, genetic and phenotypic homogeneity does not last long in most large microbial populations. With a typical per-genome, per-generation mutation rate among bacteria of ~10^{-3} (33), a bacterial population founded by a single cell will produce more than a million mutations at a typical stationary-phase density of 10^9. All subsequent phenotypic and genetic change therefore arises from natural selection among these newly occurring mutations. Tens or hundreds of generations might be required for beneficial mutants to reach high frequency in the population and appreciably affect the population mean phenotype, however, so the evolutionary response is slower than in populations seeded with initial genetic variation. After several hundreds or even thousands of generations of propagation in the laboratory, numerous properties of the evolutionary process may be studied in an open-ended (and not necessarily goal-directed) manner.

Because I will refer repeatedly to two long-term experiments throughout this chapter, I first provide a brief overview of these in particular. The first involves the long-term experimental evolution of 12 populations of *Escherichia coli* B, originally founded by Richard Lenski in 1988. The ancestral strain is prototrophic, but it is unable to use arabinose owing to mutation in the *ara* operon (60, 67). It also lacks any transmissible plasmids and viruses; as a result, all evolution is strictly asexual. A spontaneous mutant of the ancestor capable of using arabinose (Ara+) was used to found six of the populations, whereas the other six were founded with the Ara− ancestor. Arabinose utilization can be used to distinguish between populations on indicator plates, but it is neutral in the selective environment. The populations are maintained by the daily transfer of 0.1 ml of culture into 9.9 ml of fresh Davis minimal medium supplemented with 25 μg of glucose/ml. These conditions allow ~6.6 generations per day and ~5 × 10⁷ cells/ml at stationary phase. Growth occurs in a constant 37°C shaking incubator, but samples of each population were stored in a glycerol suspension at −80°C at 100-generation intervals through 2,000 generations and at 500-generation intervals thereafter. These lines, hereafter referred to as the Lenski long-term (LT) lines, have undergone more than 20,000 generations of evolution and have been studied comprehensively (24).

The second experiment of this review was derived from this first one as follows. After 2,000 generations of evolution, a clone from one LT population was used to found five separate experimental groups each consisting of six independent populations. Each group was subsequently maintained for an additional 2,000 generations at different temperatures: 20, 32, 37, and 42°C and temperatures of 32 and 42°C that alternated daily. This experiment was designed by Bennett and Lenski to investigate the dynamics and consequences of thermal adaptation, and the populations are hereafter referred to as the BL lines (6, 7).

DYNAMICS OF ADAPTATION
Evolution by natural selection requires two processes: (i) the production of heritable variation, and (ii) nonrandom differential survival or reproduction. If microbial populations are of the large sizes typical of laboratory culture, the *production* of variation is rarely limiting (but see references 31 and 47 for a more detailed discussion). The *efficiency* of the second step, on the other hand, can vary widely and ultimately depends upon the mean and variance in fitness of the population in its current environment. Populations whose phenotype(s) is far from some optimum may adapt more rapidly, whereas those close to their optimum may adapt more slowly. Also, genetically diverse

populations should respond more rapidly to natural selection. Theory predicts that genetic mixis (sexual recombination) and increased mutation rate may also accelerate adaptation, at least under certain conditions; tests of these predictions are discussed below.

Microbial populations introduced to novel laboratory environments typically undergo a period of rapid adaptation, but then the rate of adaptation slows. For example, the relative fitness (quantified in head-to-head competition with the ancestor as described above) of the LT lines improved ~25% over the first 1,000 generations, but only improved an additional 12% during the second 1,000 generations (71). The rate of adaptation continued to slow in these populations, such that an equivalent improvement required an additional 18,000 generations (24) (Fig. 1). While this degree of improvement is substantial by any measure, other populations introduced to drastically novel environments have undergone even more rapid improvement. For example, populations of a soil isolate of *Ralstonia eutropha* selected in laboratory environments containing 2,4-dichlorphenoxyacetic acid as the sole carbon source adapted roughly twice as quickly in the early going as during later stages (63). Higher rates of adaptation have also been observed in populations

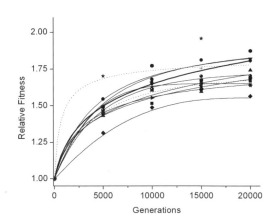

FIGURE 1 Trajectory for mean fitness of 12 *E. coli* populations during 20,000 generations in minimal glucose medium. Each point is the population mean measured relative to the ancestor with fivefold replication. Curves are the best fit of a hyperbolic model.

founded by strains with initially low fitness, such as those carrying deleterious mutations or harboring conditionally beneficial traits such as resistance to antibiotics or phage (4, 10, 66, 88). Finally, viral populations (and especially RNA viruses) may exhibit extreme rates of adaptation that, perhaps simply because of their short generation times and complex intracellular dynamics, are more rapid than any bacterial system (42, 92, 93).

On the other hand, the BL lines achieved relatively modest fitness increases during 2,000 generations of selection in novel temperatures, owing to the previous adaptation by the progenitor to all other environmental conditions besides the novel temperature. The greatest adaptation among the BL lines occurred in the extreme temperature groups because the ancestor was least fit in these environments. Thus, the rate of adaptation appears to be directly related to the distance from the optimum phenotype, given an adequate supply of beneficial genetic variation. While this distance is difficult to predict a priori, it is nonetheless reasonable to assume that freshly isolated "wild" microbes will usually adapt more rapidly to laboratory conditions than will more "domesticated" strains.

The efficiency of natural selection on a population may also be buffered by events in its previous history or by chance effects. Travisano et al. (118) asked whether "replaying life's tape" (49) repeatedly would result in distinct evolutionary outcomes in microbial populations, thus disentangling the contributions of chance and history. Single clones from each of the 12 LT lines were used to found three new populations in an environment that differed from the prior selective environment only in the use of maltose instead of glucose as the sole carbon source. Because the fitness of each LT line varied in the novel environment, the effect of this evolutionary *history* (or starting genetic condition) on subsequent adaptation could be quantified. Furthermore, any variation in fitness that arose among the replicates of each clone could be attributed to *chance*, or the stochastic fixation of different favorable, neutral, and even unfa-

vorable mutations among the replicates. Travisano et al. (118) quantified the fitness of each line after 1,000 generations in the maltose environment, and found that each population converged on a nearly equivalent level of adaptation regardless of its prior history or random mutations that accumulated during selection (Fig. 2). Thus, natural selection mostly obscured the effects of previous selection and chance events on further adaptation.

However, when the authors measured change in cell size, a morphological trait only loosely correlated with fitness, they found substantial effects of adaptation, chance, and history. For example, populations founded with small cells tended to remain relatively small, though replicates from the same ancestor diverged significantly. The authors emphasized two key conclusions. First, natural selection has the potential to erase the effects of prior evolutionary history and stochastic events when the element under selection (here, fitness itself) is tightly related to reproductive success. Second, in contrast, traits that arose for reasons other than natural selection (e.g., by genetic drift, mutation rates, or recombination) may remain etched in the organism and may contribute significantly to the path of future evolution. This basic framework might be instructive when evaluating the potential for various microbial populations to respond to ecological opportunities or pressures.

EVOLUTION OF GENETIC AND ECOLOGICAL DIVERSITY

One of the key objectives of establishing the LT lines was to determine the shape of the "fitness landscape," which is a theoretical or graphical relationship between genotypes and their reproductive success (Fig. 3). Fitness landscapes include peaks, combinations of genotypes that result in high fitness, and valleys, combinations that produce low fitness. An unresolved controversy is whether the landscape is dominated by a single adaptive peak that is evolutionarily accessible to all genotypes (as envisioned by Fisher [44a]), or whether it is composed of multiple peaks separated by maladaptive valleys that

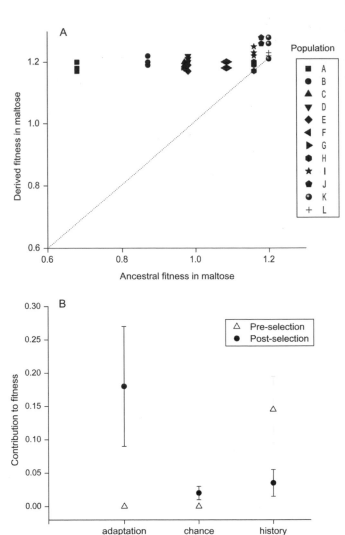

FIGURE 2 Evolution of fitness during 1,000 generations in maltose, after 2,000 generations of prior evolution in glucose. (A) Derived versus ancestral values for mean fitness in the 36 experimental populations. Symbols A through L reflect 12 different progenitor genotypes. (B) Relative contributions of adaptation, chance, and history to mean fitness (triangles) and fitness after (circles) 1,000 generations in maltose. Error bars represent 95% confidence intervals. Reprinted from reference 118 with permission.

restrict further evolution (as envisioned by Wright [132a]). If only one peak exists, then different populations adapting to a common environment should eventually converge in their genotypes and relative fitness. The more "rugged" the landscape, however, the greater the number of different adaptive solutions in a particular environment and the less likely that replicate populations will ever converge in genotype or relative fitness.

Evidence from the LT experiment as well as from several other long-term evolution experiments suggests that the genetic variance that accumulates among isolated replicate populations is sustained over time, which supports a Wrightian interpretation (7, 24, 73, 124). Each population acquires different sets of adaptive mutations early in its history due to chance, and some of these may be functionally equivalent. Also, much of the subsequent adaptation is contingent upon the first beneficial substitution in the population, which reinforces subsequent divergence. One factor that promotes and reinforces diversification among and even within replicate populations is physical structure (63, 101, 127). Environmental structure acts to

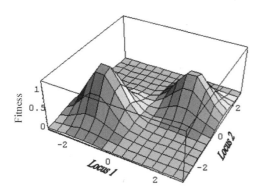

FIGURE 3 A Wrightian landscape, illustrating that maladaptive "valleys" may separate two adaptive "peaks" of unequal relative value. A Fisherian landscape, on the other hand, would be dominated by a single adaptive peak. See reference 99 for a more detailed discussion of these alternative population genetic models.

subdivide populations and increases the probability that unique mutations arise and produce heterogeneity. For instance, Korona et al. (63) investigated whether liquid or solid agar environments would favor greater diversity among experimental populations of *Ralstonia*. While significant variance evolved in both environments, the spatial structure afforded by the agar surface generated considerably more diversity in both mean fitness and colony morphology.

One contention is that bacterial evolution in particular is biased toward a Wrightian interpretation because recombination is extremely rare and prevents the eventual assembly of favorable mutations arising in separate populations. Experimental methods that promote recombination and competition between lineages might conceivably promote convergence toward a common peak and a Fisherian interpretation. A distinct but certainly relevant question is whether bacteria actually typically evolve as isolated clonal lineages, which remains a matter of debate (52).

Bacteriophages and other genetic parasites are potent capacitors of evolutionary diversification because of the strong selection they can generate and because resistance to infection is typically costly (9, 76). Lenski (67, 68) compared fitness of mutants resistant to infection by bacteriophage T4 relative to their susceptible ancestor in an environment lacking bacteriophages and found that all resistant mutants grew more slowly than their susceptible progenitor. The effects of the mutations that conferred resistance varied widely, however, because they altered other phenotypes (pleiotropy) and varied in their interaction with other genes (epistasis) (67, 68). Based on the observed trade-off between fitness and phage resistance, one may predict that susceptible bacteria will be maintained in nature even if phages are abundant because of their relative growth advantage. This in turn could lead to fluctuating cycles between populations of susceptible genotypes, resistant genotypes, and bacteriophages (69, 75). Thus, phages are expected neither to eliminate susceptible hosts nor to select completely for resistant mutants, and thus heterogeneous populations are maintained.

Bohannan and Lenski (8) tested these predictions in chemostat microcosms of phages and bacteria, and also studied the effects of altering the resource concentration (in this case, glucose) on the dynamics of these subpopulations. Increasing resource concentration led to (i) an increased equilibrium size of the bacteriophage population, (ii) only a slight increase in the number of susceptible bacteria, (iii) more rapid evolution of resistant bacteria, and (iv) a more erratic and severe cycling between the populations of bacteriophages and susceptible bacteria. These empirical findings matched the predictions of an elegant mathematical model that describes the behavior of a simple, prey-dependent (or host dependent) food chain. In this model, predator density is tied directly to prey density, as opposed to a more complex ratio of predators to prey. Studies such as this are especially useful because they explain the coexistence of phages and bacteria in microbial populations, and for their potential as models of ecosystem composition.

Remarkably, the evolution of different phenotypes from a single ancestor is sometimes predictable. Rainey and Travisano (101) studied the adaptive response of a strain of *P. fluorescens* to novel opportunities created by static (as opposed to continuously shaken) culture tubes.

Three different genotypes, described by their morphology as smooth, wrinkly spreader, and fuzzy spreader, predictably and repeatedly emerged in replicate populations. Because each morph bred true, these were clearly the product of stable genetic changes. These genotypes form a stable polymorphic population by exploiting distinct niches—the broth itself, the air-broth interface, and the tube walls. Furthermore, each genotype was able to invade these complex communities when rare. The genetic changes that produce these morphologies appear to be highly repeatable among replicate experiments, but remain incompletely resolved. In the case of the wrinkly spreader morph, at least, the expression of an operon involved in biofilm formation consistently becomes up-regulated, and the cells also undergo altered cell cycle control (114).

In other cases, the bacteria themselves generate environmental complexity despite an apparently uniform environment. One of the best examples involves the evolution of a population founded by a single clone of *E. coli* K-12 in a glucose-limiting chemostat over 773 generations, described in detail by Adams and colleagues (56, 64, 107, 121). This population rapidly became polymorphic as genetic variability arose in the genes important for the secretion and uptake of the secondary metabolites glycerol and acetate. "Wasteful" clones capable of rapid glucose uptake because they exported secondary substrates were the first to evolve, and were then followed by "specialist" clones that used these secretions. These specialists frequently acquired mutations in the regulatory region of the acetyl coenzyme A synthetase gene (*acs*), which enhances acetate uptake. Thus, a simple environment with a single resource became more complex through the action of the first genotype, which allowed additional genotypes to evolve and exploit the new niches. Rozenzweig et al. (107) and Kurlandzka et al. (64) further dissected the ecological and physiological roles of these genotypes and found that specializing in these new niches was accompanied by trade-offs in the use of other resources.

Rozen and Lenski (108) described the evolution of a polymorphism in the LT lines sustained over a longer evolutionary period. Two clones were isolated on the basis of their differing colony morphology (small, S; and large, L) after 6,000 generations of evolution, and their continual evolution was studied over a subsequent 14,000 generations. S clones were competitively inferior to L clones in fresh medium. However, in media "conditioned" by the growth of L clones, which were removed and replaced by the usual starting concentration of glucose, S clones were the superior competitors. This suggested that L clones excreted a substrate that promoted S growth. In addition, S clones were also shown to increase L clones' death rate. At any given evolutionary time point, coexistence of S and L clones was maintained by each clone's ability to invade a population of the other when rare (frequency-dependent selection), but equilibrial frequencies fluctuated over time.

The mechanisms responsible for this fluctuating equilibrium are unclear, but could represent alternative mechanisms of the coevolutionary process. One possible model suggests that S or L cells compete almost exclusively against *fellow* S or L cells for the limiting nutrients, but do not directly interact with one another. Given a shared pool of nutrients, fluctuations in the relative frequency of S and L cells result simply from a time lag between adaptations accumulating in each population. Another, more intriguing explanation of these fluctuations involves true coevolution and even antagonism. (This can be seen as a "Red Queen" interaction, in which each population must evolve as quickly as possible just to remain viable in competition with the other [123]. The Red Queen is a reference to Lewis Carroll's character in *Through the Looking Glass,* who explains to Alice, "Now, here, you see, it takes all the running you can do to keep in the same place" [14].) Under this scenario, consumer S cells evolve increasingly efficient strategies of using L secretions, perhaps even by promoting L-cell lysis. L cells counter this interaction by evolving defenses to S antagonism or by limiting the quantity of their secretions. Distinguishing between these alternatives would illustrate the poorly understood mechanisms of coevolution, which are clearly important to understand ecological complexity and interactions between hosts and pathogens. Furthermore, since it is becoming increasingly clear that many diseases are caused by polymicrobial interactions, further study of how such interactions evolve is certainly necessary and forthcoming.

PERIODIC SELECTION AND THE EFFECT OF RECOMBINATION

One key distinction between the population genetics of prokaryotes and many eukaryotes is the amount of sexual, or homologous, recombination that occurs. Most long-term experimental evolution has permitted little if any recombination between asexual clones, which confines adaptations to their source lineage and prevents mixing. This produces a pattern known as *periodic selection,* which is actually nothing more than the sequential replacement of clonal lineages by superior clones (much like "leapfrog"). However, interesting patterns of evolution can emerge if markers are linked to the competing lineages and followed over time. Atwood et al. (3) first described fluctuations in the frequency of histidine auxotrophs during long-term laboratory growth of *E. coli* populations. When beneficial mutations arose by chance on one mutant background (say, *his*+), these cells increased in frequency at the expense of the alternative mutant type (in this case, *his*−). If one lineage were able to completely exclude the other, one might expect complete elimination of the alternative *his* genotype, but in fact constant back-mutation to the alternative *his* genotype, combined with ongoing selection for beneficial mutations on *both* genetic backgrounds, prevents exclusion of either type. As a result, secondary loci, which are functionally unrelated but physically linked to beneficial mutations, can mark the rise of each beneficial mutation in the population and hence reflect adaptation.

This pattern of periodic selection proved especially obvious in one LT population (41). Prior experiments (73) suggested that adaptation in this population seemed to proceed not continuously, but rather in "fits and starts." These same experiments also demonstrated a correlation between cell size and relative fitness; fitter cells also tended to be larger. Closer examination, by measuring both cell size and relative fitness after every 100 generations, demonstrated a clear pattern of punctuated evolution in both cell size and fitness, these two phenotypes being almost perfectly correlated with one another (Fig. 4). In hindsight, such a pattern is to be expected during adaptation in a large population if recombination among lineages is rare or absent. In such populations, even highly beneficial alleles require several hundred generations to rise to a detectable frequency, but the selective "sweep," or the event when less fit clones are displaced from the majority (swept aside) by the adaptive lineage, occurs relatively rapidly. Sampling both alleles (winner and loser) is therefore possible only during a short interval, so when populations are sampled infrequently, they appear to change instantaneously. Thus, each beneficial allele that rose to fixation in this asexual population therefore produced a punctuated increase in cell size and fitness.

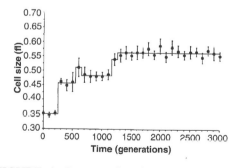

FIGURE 4 Punctuated evolution caused by periodic selection of beneficial mutations, which produced correlated increases in cell size. Data are from one population of *Escherichia coli* adapting to a minimal laboratory environment. Reprinted from reference 41 with permission.

This experiment demonstrated that a simple population genetic process such as periodic selection can account for relatively complex morphological evolution, and begs the more controversial question of whether seemingly complicated macroevolutionary patterns such as punctuated equilibria (50) may have simple explanations. Periodic selection may even explain punctuated evolution in sexually recombining populations if beneficial variation is relatively rare, because adaptive mutations would still arise separately in time and space and produce sudden phenotypic changes rather than being gradually recombined into a collective lineage.

The question of whether genetic recombination (as opposed to strict asexuality) accelerates adaptation in bacteria is equally contentious, though the apparent ubiquity of horizontal genetic exchange illustrated by genome sequencing projects is certainly compelling (19, 52, 53). Recombination has the power not only to generate novel variants but also to assemble existing beneficial alleles, formerly isolated in separate lineages, into a common genotype. A population undergoing evolution in a constant environment will over time typically experience a decelerating rate of adaptation, which is likely caused by the exhaustion of beneficial genetic variation. Allowing separate populations such as these to recombine could reaccelerate the process of adaptation. Souza et al. (113) tested this hypothesis by periodically introducing donor *E. coli* K-12 Hfr+ strains to *E. coli* B populations that were evolving in a simple environment. Contrary to their predictions, regular recombination opportunities did not accelerate adaptation, but instead only increased the genetic variance for fitness among the populations. One possibility why this experiment failed to speed up adaptation was that the donor K-12 strain had not adapted previously to the selective environment, thus reducing the possibility of introducing beneficial variation. Another possibility is that beneficial variation in these populations was never actually limiting, so

recombination would add no benefit; this hypothesis is discussed in greater detail below.

EVOLUTION OF MUTATION RATES

Is the mutation rate optimal or minimal? This long-standing question asks whether the amount of variation produced during reproduction is ideal for the long-term success of the lineage, or whether it is simply held at the limits of physiochemical boundaries (111). This question becomes all the more relevant considering that the mutation rate of related lineages within the same bacterial species may vary (65, 79), many of the "mutator" strains being pathogens. This association between high mutation rate and pathogenicity has been challenged as a product of biased sampling (79, 98), but pathogenic bacterial populations still seem to contain a greater frequency of mutator clones. For instance, both *E. coli* derived from urinary tract infections and *Pseudomonas aeruginosa* derived from cystic fibrosis patients seem to be composed of a high frequency of mutators (48, 95). Before we may properly evaluate the association between pathogenicity and high genomic mutation rates, we must first consider the selective forces acting on mutation rate.

Mutation rate evolves primarily through genetic hitchhiking, or physical linkage to other beneficial alleles (111). When beneficial genetic variation becomes limiting in a population, any genetic change that increases the mutation rate, and hence the supply of adaptive mutations, may become genetically linked to a different beneficial mutation. Natural selection should not directly increase mutation rates because, on average, the only outcome will be reduced offspring quality. Thus, mutators should only evolve when beneficial genetic variation is limiting, which may occur when population sizes are prohibitively small (so-called bottlenecking) or after a long period of sustained adaptation to a constant environment.

These hypotheses were subject of two elegant experiments by de Visser et al. (31) and by Giraud et al. (48), who collectively demonstrated that (i) mutators were only at an advantage in small or initially well-adapted populations, (ii) the selective advantage of mutator lineages disappeared over time as the nonmutator lineages achieved similar levels of fitness, and (iii) mutator lineages tended to accumulate defects when passaged in vivo that precluded survival in minimal environments. Furthermore, deVisser et al.(31) found that a speed limit on adaptation exists in asexual populations, no matter how abundant the beneficial genetic variation or how rapid the mutation rate. This speed limit arises from "clonal interference," which occurs when different beneficial lineages arise simultaneously in a population, compete with one another, and slow the eventual fixation of the best adapted lineage (47). To conclude, mutator lineages should only be favored when beneficial genetic variation becomes limiting, and perhaps then only transiently.

Nonetheless, the pathogenic lifestyle may include conditions favorable for the evolution of mutator lineages. A small number of pathogens are thought to initiate most infections, and establishing a successful infection probably requires an initial period of rapid adaptation. Thus, favorable variation may be limiting at the outset, and repair-deficient lineages should produce a greater frequency of better adapted offspring. The association between high mutation rates and pathogenicity may therefore predominate in certain situations, but lineages with lower mutation rates might eventually replace mutators over the longer term because they better avoid accumulating genetic defects. Nonpathogenic bacteria may also evolve high mutation rates when beneficial variation becomes limiting. For example, 4 of the 12 benign LT populations evolved 50- to 100-fold greater genomic mutation rates over the course of 20,000 generations, each having acquired defects in methyl-directed mismatch repair (112). Empirical and mathematical models have set boundaries on the conditions under which mutators should be advantageous, and have found that population size and the rate at which beneficial genetic variation is produced are the two key parameters. In large populations,

favorable mutations are typically not lacking, but in small populations, a decrease in the fidelity of replication could ultimately be advantageous by producing more beneficial variation (31, 115).

In the end, mutator populations appear not to achieve higher relative fitness; while certain mutator LT populations may have gained transient advantages, none of these persisted over time (V. Cooper and R. E. Lenski, unpublished data). These populations did in fact accumulate more mutations in the multiple loci sequenced from the LT clones (74), and extrapolation from these data (roughly 18 kb) suggests that roughly 250 substitutions have occurred in each mutator population, as compared with only (approximately) 3 substitutions per nonmutator population after 20,000 generations. While such low levels of mutation accumulation seem a discrepancy when compared with the overall genomic mutation rate of $\sim 10^{-3}$ per generation, the fixation of any of these mutations is an extremely rare event in a large population, occurring at a rate equivalent to the genomic mutation rate (60).

Several long-term evolution experiments, including those with the LT lines, and numerous other studies have demonstrated the importance of transposable elements in generating adaptive mutations (see, e.g., references 26, 64, 81, 96, and 109). Clearly, mobile elements, typically in the form of insertion sequences (ISs), represent an important class of mutations, and unusually active elements may significantly increase the raw material upon which natural selection may act. Bursts of IS activity may conceivably ease limits on beneficial genetic variation, but their relative contributions remain unclear. IS mobilizations are more readily detectable at the level of the genome than single substitutions, insertions, or deletions and may therefore be overrepresented. Furthermore, it is unclear whether ISs are most mobile when adaptation is most rapid, as an adaptive theory of IS mutations might suggest. In the case of the LT populations, most IS activity appeared once the rate of adaptation slowed, and the rapid adaptation may in fact have been caused mostly by single substitutions (109). In other evolving chemostat *E. coli* populations, adaptive mutations were only partly the product of IS movement (64, 81). Improvements in single nucleotide screening methods in bacteria should soon better describe the effects of single substitutions and clarify whether any particular class of mutations is more relevant to adaptation.

EVOLUTIONARY SPECIALIZATION AND GENETIC TRADE-OFFS

Changes correlated to adaptation, as opposed to those that are the direct consequence of the adaptive response, have been the focus of much experimental evolution (106, 120). Several groups have explored whether adaptation to the selective environment is accompanied by loss of adaptation to alternative environments, that is, whether specific adaptation produces ecological specialization (22, 24, 46, 117, 120). One might predict that the LT populations, evolving in a simple glucose-only medium, have undergone tremendous genetic streamlining to eliminate needless functions. Such a prediction is based on the premise that unused functions, and especially constitutively expressed ones, are energetically and physiologically quite costly to the cell. Bear in mind, however, that the cost of producing unused peptides is typically much too small to explain the large benefits measured when traits are eliminated in novel environments (35), so most loss of function needs to be explained on other grounds.

Genetic trade-offs caused by antagonistic pleiotropy provide a more realistic explanation of evolutionary specialization. Under antagonistic pleiotropy, the same mutation that produces adaptation in the selective environment also reduces performance in alternative environments. For example, mutations that increase the efficiency of transporting a particular resource into the cytoplasm might decrease the transport efficiency for less important or absent resources. Specialization by antagonistic pleiotropy is therefore driven by natural selection, and loss of function and adaptation are

expected to be quantitatively and temporally correlated.

An alternative cause of specialization is mutation accumulation, in which unused genes that are hidden from selection accumulate substitutions by genetic drift. Because genetic drift is a stochastic process, losses of function are expected to accumulate randomly (and slowly) for any given locus, and log-linearly over time across all unused loci. When specialization is caused by mutation accumulation, the mutations responsible for functional decay and those causing adaptation are distinct groups.

Travisano and others began the study of specialization in the LT populations by measuring fitness in a variety of growth media after 2,000 generations of evolution in minimal glucose medium (117, 120). They concluded that the populations had adapted to growth on glucose in particular, because they grew better when the carbon source was transported using the glucose pathway, but worse and more variably when the carbon source was transported by different mechanisms. We expanded upon this study by measuring the performance of each population on 95 different carbon sources over 20,000 generations (24). The longer evolutionary history not only provided greater resolution, but also allowed us to evaluate the relative importance of antagonistic pleiotropy and mutation accumulation in causing specialization. Average performance for the collection of all foreign substrates decayed over time in all populations, but importantly, not significantly more in mutator populations. Because an accelerated mutation rate increases the rate of substitutions by genetic drift, but mutator populations were not more specialized, mutation accumulation could not explain much of the observed specialization in this system. On the other hand, when the same loss occurs repeatedly in replicate populations adapting to a common environment, we can infer that this convergent evolution is tied to adaptation. In fact, 16 functions were lost or significantly impaired in all 12 replicate populations in the first 10,000 generations, and 9 of these accumulated during the first 2,000 generations of rapid adaptation. The tight association between adaptation and functional decay suggests that antagonistic pleiotropy produced much of the resource specialization in these populations, and a growing number of mechanistic studies (see below) support this inference (21, 26).

We (23) also quantified the evolution of thermal niche in the LT populations, which are maintained at a constant 37°C. Maximum growth rate increased for all moderate temperatures surrounding the selected temperature, but tended on average to decrease at extreme temperatures (20°C, >40°C). Because these two trends evolved coincidentally during the first few thousand generations (impaired growth at extreme temperatures mirrored adaptation to moderate temperatures almost exactly), antagonistic pleiotropy also likely shaped the thermal niche. The loss of any particular trait by genetic drift in populations containing 10^7 or more individuals typically requires tens of thousands of generations, so mutation accumulation was unlikely to constrain the thermal niche by generation 2,000.

The loss of a particular function, the ability to catabolize D ribose, in all 12 LT populations allowed (26) a more precise dissection of the population and molecular genetic mechanisms responsible (Fig. 5). A genetic screen for ISs in a single LT population revealed that one element, IS150, had been lost from the region containing the genes that allow ribose catabolism, the *rbs* operon, along with a 2.7-kb fragment. Further analysis proved that some or all of the operon was eliminated in all populations by IS duplication, transposition, and recombination. This highly mobile element explained the extreme mutation rate of this locus in ancestral populations, which became *rbs⁻* at rates 10^3 to 10^5 times faster than for other traits. Thus, the most obvious explanation was loss by mutation accumulation. However, complete loss of ribose function in these populations occurred roughly 10 times too rapidly if only mutation accumulation was involved.

Next, the fitness effect of the *rbs* deletions was quantified; seven independent mutations improved competitive ability relative to the

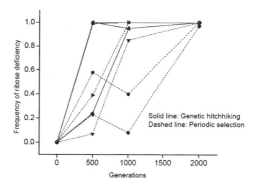

FIGURE 5 Frequency of Rbs⁻ cells over time in the 12 evolving LT populations. Seven of 12 populations became 100% Rbs⁻ by generation 500, which is best explained by genetic linkage to other "big-benefit" mutations (genetic hitchhiking). In the remaining five populations, ribose function acts as a marker for other selective sweeps (periodic selection), including positive selection on the Rbs⁻ mutation itself. Adapted from reference 26.

ancestor by 1 to 2%. Natural selection for these deletion mutants combined with their high rate of appearance would certainly lead to their eventual fixation, but this process would require an estimated 3,000 generations. To explain the complete loss of ribose function by generation 500 in seven populations, we must presume that *rbs* mutations became linked genetically with other mutations of greater benefit. Thus, the first selective sweeps in these experimental populations likely involved double mutants, in which small-benefit mutations hitchhiked to fixation with distinct large-benefit mutations. In summary, antagonistic pleiotropy, mutation accumulation, and genetic hitchhiking were all responsible for functional loss in this instance; this argues that the study of specialization (e.g., by a pathogen to a particular host) may frequently defy assumptions and require empirical evaluation.

The flip side to specialization is the retention of function and phenotypic flexibility in the face of directional, apparently streamlining selection. The LT lines actually maintained most of the diet breadth of the ancestor, and even improved in head-to-head competition versus the ancestor in some foreign environments (22).

Because these populations were forced to manufacture all cellular components using only glucose as a carbon source, auxotrophs could not evolve. If *E. coli* B were allowed instead to evolve in a resource-rich, ecologically complex environment, more extensive specialization may have evolved. Lacking a direct test at the moment, this hypothesis remains supported by plenty of microbiological folk wisdom (auxotrophs are commonly isolated during serial passage in rich broth) and by a compelling study of *E. coli* evolution in a mouse (48), in which 25% of mutator populations evolved auxotrophy after 300 days of in vivo passage. A more direct test of the relationship between ecological complexity and specialization is certainly worthy of further study. To summarize, the weight of evidence suggests that natural selection, and not an absence of selection, causes ecological specialization in large, evolving bacterial populations.

In small or bottlenecked populations, such as the founders of new infections, the case may be somewhat different. Genetic drift may operate more strongly and fix deficient mutants in the population, perhaps with long-term consequences for the pathogen. For example, mutants that grow less efficiently outside the host or in alternative hosts may randomly become numerically dominant, which could erode survival outside the host. Such specialization could also be favored by natural selection (antagonistic pleiotropy), but the smaller the population size, the less deterministic the evolutionary process and the more rapid the effects of drift. In small, asexual populations, the process of Müller's ratchet can increase the mutation load and decrease relative fitness. Müller's ratchet is the random but irreversible accumulation of mildly deleterious mutations in predominantly asexual populations; the ratchet "clicks" with each new mutation, leading to a progressive decline in functionality. This process has been confirmed during repeated population bottlenecks of laboratory *E. coli* populations, which have become functional specialists and inferior competitors (45, 59). Such experiments may reflect the processes that have generated the extreme specialization observed in obligate intracellular symbionts and pathogens (84–86). For example, the *Buchnera* symbionts of aphids are derived from Enterobacteriacae but retain less than one-half the genome of their free-living relatives (5, 84). Another extreme example of specialization is *Mycobacterium leprae,* whose closest relative is *M. tuberculosis.* Both are obligate pathogens, but *M. leprae* has barely half the functional genome of *M. tuberculosis* (20). At the moment, it is unclear whether the tissue specificity of *M. leprae* or its simplified genome evolved first, but a combination of antagonistic pleiotropy, mutation accumulation, permissive environments, and small effective population sizes probably provides the explanation.

MECHANISMS OF ADAPTATION

The more we understand how adaptation proceeds in vitro, the better we will understand how pathogens evolve. This section discusses selected examples in which the mechanisms and consequences of genetic adaptation were discovered. In many cases, the comparative method provided the key inference, where convergent evolution among replicate populations highlights specific targets of adaptation to a defined environment.

Following prolonged laboratory growth, adapted genotypes exhibit the following general trends. First, maximum growth rate increases; this is often the most significant component of fitness in both batch culture and chemostats (38, 124). Second, the duration of lag phase typically shortens in batch culture to permit an earlier start of exponential growth (124). Third, the resource affinity, which can be measured using Michaelis-Menton kinetics as the resource saturation constant K_s (this essentially describes the ability of the strain to uptake a limiting nutrient from the medium), has been shown to improve in chemostats but actually decrease slightly in batch culture (38, 124). This seeming contradiction is a product of more intense selection for maximal growth in batch culture, perhaps at the expense of efficiency, but strong selection for resource affinity at submaximal growth in chemostats. Lastly, and less predictably, a number of correlated responses to selection may evolve, including the secretion of metabolic by-products (56, 107, 108), increased cell size (73, 82), decreased phage susceptibility (9), variable death rate in stationary phase (124), and widely divergent fitness in alternative environments (22, 117, 120). While the *direct* physiological response to experimental evolution is often quite repeatable among replicates within a particular environment, the *correlated* responses are far less predictable.

Heterogeneous correlated responses to selection arise either from variation in the adaptive mechanisms or from separate, neutral substitutions that accumulate independently of direct selection. Even if the direct and correlated responses are temporally correlated, secondary mutations producing the correlated response could have hitchhiked along with selected mutations. These alternative scenarios complicate finding the genes that enhance fitness: is the phenotype in question the direct or the correlated response? The best solutions employ screens of multiple characters, use evolutionary convergence to select candidate loci, and take advantage of whole-genome technologies.

Using some of these methods, Notley-McRobb et al. identified different adaptive mutations in *E. coli* chemostat populations (78, 89–91). Adaptation consistently arose from mutations in the *mgl* operon, which increased the binding protein-dependent transport of glucose. However, the nature of these mutations differed across replicates: some were caused by base substitutions, and others by short duplications, small deletions, or IS*1* insertions in the ~1-kb *mgl* repressor *mglD*. The majority were actually found in the short *mgl* operator (*mglO*), involving single substitutions that greatly increased glucose affinity at low concentrations (91). Because each population harbored several beneficial lineages with distinct adaptive mutations, Notley-McRobb and Ferenci argued that this complexity was in conflict with the more conventional model of periodic selection (see above) that purges genetic variation (91). It remains to be seen whether

this diversity could be sustained over a longer period of time (by means of fine-scale environmental partitioning, for example) or whether the genetic variance amounts simply to unresolved competition between different adapted lineages (e.g., clonal interference [31, 47]).

More recently, the genetic bases of adaptation in the LT populations have been illuminated by means of expression microarrays (21). Parallel changes in two replicate populations after 20,000 generations of evolution were sought as an indicator of adaptation and to highlight genes for further study. When compared to the ancestor, the expression of 59 genes had changed significantly in the same direction in both populations, and most of these were members of the cyclic AMP-cyclic AMP receptor protein and guanosine tetraphosphate regulons (21). The authors then sequenced several candidate genes and identified a nonsynonymous mutation in *spoT*, which is involved in the phosphorylation of guanosine tetraphosphate, in one population but not the other. When this mutation was introduced into the ancestral background, it increased fitness and changed expression in some other genes of the 59-member group. However, the same mutation had no effect on fitness when introduced into the other evolved population, indicating that a mutation of similar effect was present already and confirming the hypothesis that multiple genetic solutions produced adaptation in these populations (21). A survey of all 12 populations revealed eight separately evolved *spoT* alleles, and illustrates the general importance of *spoT* in adaptation of the LT populations (Fig. 6).

Riehle et al. (103) described the role of insertions and deletions in evolutionary adaptation to high temperature by six *E. coli* BL populations. Here, the insertion sequence IS*186* produced a hot spot that led to duplications in three of six lines and implicated four genes previously shown to enhance survival under stressful and starvation conditions. In addition, the timing of the duplications coincided with the timing of increased fitness at high temperature. It remains to be seen whether these duplications alone

Line	Residue	A	R	Y	N	A	R	K	K
Ancestor		A	R	Y	N	A	R	K	K
Ara-1	662	-	-	-	-	-	-	-	I
Ara-2	455	-	-	-	-	D	-	-	-
Ara-4	389	-	-	C	-	-	-	-	-
Ara-6	607	-	-	-	-	-	-	T	-
Ara+2	575	-	-	-	-	-	L	-	-
Ara+3	189	V	-	-	-	-	-	-	-
Ara+4	209	-	H	-	-	-	-	-	-
Ara+6	454	-	-	-	I	-	-	-	-

FIGURE 6 Nonsynonymous mutations in *spoT* in eight independently evolved *E. coli* populations. Only the variable amino acid residues are shown, with the ancestor listed first and the eight mutant alleles shown below. Four other populations retained the ancestral sequence. Reprinted from reference 21 with permission.

improve high-temperature fitness in the naive ancestor, and whether they might also reduce fitness at moderate temperatures as a model of genetic trade-offs might predict.

Both the costs of specific adaptation and its unpredictability were elegantly demonstrated when the single-stranded DNA bacteriophage φX174 was grown on alternate bacterial hosts (27). Phage populations were cultured first on *Salmonella* and then on *Escherichia,* alternating every 11 days. The costs of adaptation to each host were not reciprocal: adaptation to *Salmonella* reduced growth on the traditional *Escherichia* host, but the reverse was not the case. Moreover, continued host switching did not alter this pattern because just two or three substitutions in a viral capsid gene caused all of the adaptation in *Salmonella,* but then reverted in *E. coli* (27). This repeated reversion might be more likely in viruses than in bacteria because their much smaller genomes have fewer targets, and because evidence suggests that fluctuating environments promote second-site, compensatory changes in bacteria, rather than reversion at the original mutational site (83).

With the exception of the examples presented in this chapter, genetic trade-offs have proved surprisingly difficult to find (46). Trade-off models provide the foundation of much of

behavioral ecology despite relatively little mechanistic analysis. The primitive social interactions (or at least cell-to-cell interaction) among the bacterium *Myxococcus xanthus* proved to be an ideal starting point. Velicer et al. (126–128) selected *M. xanthus* in conditions favoring asocial behavior—liquid batch culture—for 1,000 generations. All populations lost at least part of their social motility, losses that were partly explained by mutations in the *pil* gene cluster that forms a type IV pilus (128). When the ancestral *pil* genes were restored by complementation, social traits were regained and fitness in the asocial environment was reduced. Likewise, when defined *pil* mutants were constructed in the ancestor, asocial fitness improved (128). Because social interaction in *M. xanthus* is both evolutionarily labile and phenotypically costly when conditions favor asocial behavior, sociality is evidently under strong stabilizing selection in its natural environment. Otherwise, one might expect to find a high frequency of asocial *M. xanthus.*

Studying the mechanisms of evolutionary adaptation may never be more important than as a strategy to curb the epidemic of antibiotic resistance. It is widely assumed but poorly proven that antibiotic resistance is phenotypically costly and reduces competitive fitness when antibiotics are absent. This presumption has been perhaps the sole source of comfort in the face of the increasing problem of antimicrobial resistance. Unfortunately, two contradictory examples are clear: one involving a tetracycline-resistant plasmid (10, 72, 88), and the other involving chromosomal streptomycin resistance in *E. coli* (110). In both cases, resistance in a naive host background was costly, but after only a few hundred generations, the cost of resistance was eliminated. Even worse, the mechanisms of compensatory adaptation actually precluded reversion to antibiotic sensitivity, because genetically engineered sensitivity was toxic to the evolved host (10, 72, 88, 110). These models suggest that prolonged antibiotic usage could irrevocably purge antibiotic sensitivity from pathogenic and commensal bacterial populations.

In summarizing this section, it is clear that relatively few mutations accumulating early during microbial adaptation can have large phenotypic effects, and that these first mutations often involve genetic trade-offs. If this generality holds, then specialization by antagonistic pleiotropy may be inevitable. Thus, the actual paradox may be the existence of phenotypic generalists such as *Pseudomonas* and *Burkholderia,* for example. Furthermore, chance effects may also play a large role in the early adaptation of isolated microbial populations, with all subsequent substitutions being contingent upon the first, randomly arising beneficial mutation. These stochastic effects should be unique in every population and therefore may suggest that "rewinding life's tape" will always yield a different genetic outcome.

EMPIRICAL MODELS OF THE EVOLUTION OF VIRULENCE

Some of the best studies of the evolution of pathogens are the fruits of vaccine research. Attenuated vaccine development is predicated on the assumption that serial passage of a pathogen in a novel host or culturing system will lead to loss of adaptation in the affected host—in other words, that the vaccine population will undergo specialization that leads to "genetic paralysis." (Readers interested in an overview of serial passage experiments using parasites, including many vaccine trials, should consult Ebert's fine review [39].) The success of several attenuated vaccines for humans, including Theiler's yellow fever vaccine and Sabin's polio vaccine, suggests that this underlying assumption may sometimes be valid (39).

However, focused searches for weakened vaccine candidates may have obscured some of the subtle evolutionary conflicts that pathogens face. Despite many challenges to various trade-off models of pathogen evolution, it is probable that many directly transmitted pathogens face one fundamental life history trade-off (25): within-host competition versus between-host transmission. For example, competition among parasites for resources within a host can lead to escalating exploitation and hence increased virulence, whereas selection for transmission between hosts may (but not always) counter this escalation (28). More specifically, overly aggressive competition among pathogens may kill the host and prevent transmission between hosts, especially if they are rare or ecologically dispersed.

Thus, one reason why serial passage experiments have actually typically led to *increased* virulence in the selected host is that artificial transmission alleviates all requirements for transmission between hosts and permits extensive host exploitation. Other possible reasons include the genetic homogeneity and stasis of the host model, high initial pathogen diversity, and large pathogen populations. Increased fitness in the model host sometimes restricts host range, as it did in the study of bacteriophage φX174 noted above (27). In addition, prolonged serial transfer of vesicular stomatitis virus greatly enhanced fitness in a tissue culture analogue of a human host while compromising survival in tissue culture analogues of mouse or canine hosts (92). Furthermore, serial transfer of a nuclear polyhedrosis virus in a single moth species significantly reduced the infectious capacity of the virus in other insect species (39).

Somewhat surprisingly, few serial passaging experiments involving bacterial pathogens have been reported in detail in the English microbiology literature, but many have appeared in Russian and in specialist veterinary journals and have thus gone unrecognized. Two products of Russian bioweapons research deserve special mention because of their potential for future study. The first reported the enhancement and stabilization of *Yersinia pestis* virulence after serial transfer in guinea pig macrophages (32), generating a scary pathogen indeed. The second described stable avirulence of a natural isolate of *Francisella tularensis* despite 10 passages in laboratory mice (61), discovering perhaps an excellent candidate for vaccine research. Among the more conventional systems, the in vitro culture of *Bacillus anthracis* to produce attenuated vaccines for humans and livestock has selected strains lacking particular plasmid-borne virulence determinants (15). In another case, Mekalanos demonstrated that *Vibrio cholerae* strains with duplicated cholera toxin genes rapidly achieve numerical superiority during a few transfers in a rabbit model, with concomitant increased toxin production (79a). In this case, the duplication mechanism has since been shown to be mediated by transposition of a selfish element, which forms a functional filamentous phage in El Tor strains but not in the classical genotypes used in these experiments (129). Remarkably, the ancestral strain used in this study was itself the product of serial transfer in rabbits, the original progenitor being hypovirulent (34). To conclude, despite the brevity of this overview of a large applied field, it is apparent that the experimental evolution of pathogens can illuminate both adaptive potential and genotypic constraints. More hypothesis-driven studies should therefore become essential components of the development of predictive models of the evolution of pathogens.

I will conclude this section by highlighting three projects that used experimental evolution to empirically test models of the evolution of virulence. The first involved the filamentous bacteriophage f1, which infects only cells bearing an F pilus, and *E. coli* host cells that were either F^+ or F^-. Bull et al. (13) designed selection regimens to enforce either high host fidelity by providing no opportunities for f1 transmission between hosts, or low host fidelity by providing ample opportunities for f1 to infect new susceptible hosts. High fidelity should favor vertical viral transmission and hence low virulence, whereas low fidelity should favor horizontal transmission and greater virulence. Virulence or benevolence in this system was measured as the effect of the phage on the growth rate of the host bacterium. The basic predictions were confirmed: when evolved viruses competed in the absence of susceptible hosts, selection favored vertically transmitted viruses because they harmed the infected host significantly less. However, once susceptible hosts were introduced to the culture, the horizontally transmitted viruses gained a selective advantage. Thus, the mode of transmission (e.g., lysis versus lysogeny) is critical to the virulence evolution of pathogens, and the greater the density of susceptible hosts, the more infectious and potentially severe the pathogen may evolve.

In actuality, virulence may increase in evolving pathogens for several reasons, contrary to the long-standing assumption that microbial virulence is maladaptive. Even if the frequency of available hosts remains constant, the timing of transmission may affect the evolution of virulence (25, 40). For example, transmission between hosts during the early stages of an infection may favor more rapidly reproducing pathogens and hence increased virulence, while transmission during later stages may favor slower replicators and reduced virulence. An experiment in Paul Ewald's lab (25) tested this hypothesis by serially transferring a gypsy moth nuclear polyhedrosis virus in live larvae. One set of viral lineages was transmitted early, while another set was transmitted late during larval infections. Early-transmitted viruses evolved increased virulence, but they tended to kill their larval hosts sooner, when larvae were small, so total virus production declined. Late-transmitted viruses tended to be more benign and allowed additional larval growth and much greater viral production. Here, virulence evolution obeyed a trade-off that is governed by local ecology: sparsely distributed hosts will select for reduced virulence, but high densities of susceptible hosts will favor rapid replicators and greater severity.

Evolutionary scenarios for pathogens may become far more complex if multiple infections per host (superinfection) are common. Under these conditions, competition among pathogens within a host may become maladaptive (see, e.g., references 28, 29, 43, and 94), and not only because overly aggressive host exploitation may prevent transmission. In a fascinating study of intrahost pathogen competition, the RNA phage φ6 was propagated at either high or low multiplicity of infection in the host bacterium *Pseudomonas phaseolicola* (122). Phage grown at high multiplicity of infection first evolved increased fitness but then surprisingly became less fit. This pattern was clearly explained by a game theory model of the "prisoner's dilemma," in which selfish viral strategies evolve despite the greater fitness rewards of cooperation. The reduced viral fitness, or defection, likely resulted from selfish use of gene products that are normally shared (30). This strategy evolved only among genetically unrelated competitors, and not among clonal, highly related sister clones. Even the simplest parasites may therefore follow evolutionary strategies typically observed in animals competing in complex social environments.

PROSPECTUS: FUTURE DIRECTIONS

From the evidence presented here, the use of long-term laboratory culture to understand the evolution of microbial pathogens holds considerable promise. Nevertheless, this approach introduces its own challenges, such as choosing appropriate ancestral genotypes, defining amenable and relevant experimental conditions, and allowing sufficient evolutionary time for variation to arise and become detectable. Thankfully, technologies for strain detection, identifying selected mechanisms, and constructing relevant selective environments continue to improve apace. High-density hybridization and expression arrays are becoming increasingly available to assess the genomics of adaptation, microsatellites (57, 102) and other novel marker systems enhance detection and quantification (58), and innovative host models are on the upswing. Here I highlight four areas for future research that should be of interest to readers of this book.

One assumption that largely remains untested is that genes important for virulence are selectively *optimal* in particular hosts, genetic backgrounds, or environments. This is especially relevant when virulence traits are borne on plasmids or phages, because suboptimality may favor an unstable relationship between the host and the mobile element, and thus only occasionally produce pathogenicity. Suboptimal interactions between a complex of virulence genes and the remainder of the genome may also reflect inadequate coevolutionary history, as in the case of emerging or opportunistic pathogens, and thus should be followed closely. Optimality may be tested in defined laboratory culture by directly competing genotypes that differ only for these virulence genes. Furthermore, culture conditions can and should be varied to reflect the changing environment of the pathogen. We can also examine whether the cost of carrying a pathogenic element is ameliorated over longer term laboratory selection, which has already been demonstrated for elements encoding antibiotic resistance. Despite conventional thought that most human pathogens are well adapted to human hosts, predicting the evolutionary epidemiology of microbial pathogens hinges upon empirical estimates of the benefits of virulence mechanisms.

Of course, the success of this approach requires realistic models of the microbial environment, which is a tall order. Given the complexity that evolves even in the simplest systems, developing natural in vivo or "environmental" models has seemed intractable. Nevertheless, the future of experimental evolution must move beyond the simplest systems if the goal is to evaluate the role of a particular pathogen in nature. Indeed, "mice are not furry chemostats" (12), as some authors referenced in this chapter have demonstrated. Recently, a number of novel animal and plant models of pathogenesis have been used to assay different candidate genes, and these have often arrived at the somewhat surprising conclusion that mechanisms for virulence in *Arabidopsis* (for example) are frequently identical in animal models (mice or *Caenorhabditis elegans* [1, 77, 100, 116]). My group is currently using these findings as the basis for in vivo experimental evolution of species of the *Burkholderia cepacia* complex, and similar applications are ongoing in other laboratories.

Such use of novel laboratory culture systems may permit the study of many poorly understood microbes and better address classical questions. For example, it is frequently presumed that the evolutionary transition to pathogenicity is accompanied by niche specialization that compromises growth in other environments (131, 132). Experiments presented here have shown that prolonged growth in laboratory culture produces specialization, but it is unclear whether the evolution of virulence also must lead to specialization. The fact that parasites exhibit some of the most extraordinarily specialized life histories certainly supports this idea, and thus the extreme natural selection that occurs during host invasion and is in need of further study.

Finally, the evidence that important steps in microbial evolution have been driven significantly, and perhaps mostly, by interspecies recombination continues to grow. Comparative genomics shows that only 40% of the genome of *E. coli* is shared by three different sequenced strains (130), and abundant evidence for recombination in pathogenic lineages exists. The most frequent objection to previous experimental evolution, an absence of recombination, may prove to one of the most exciting avenues in the future. Natural competence and plasmid exchange rates vary widely in bacteria and are obvious targets for natural selection, but some species that feature large "integron islands" (55) may experience extreme levels of recombination. Do these species harbor extraordinary evolutionary flexibility and the potential for rapid adaptation? What are the evolutionary processes that maintain generalization? How do bacteria preserve the capacity for horizontal transfer, which on average should produce maladaptive offspring? These challenging questions may prove in the near future to be excellent candidates for study using more sophisticated long-term experimental evolution.

CHAPTER SUMMARY

- The most conspicuous product of evolution, adaptation, is surprisingly difficult to study in most systems. Experimental evolution using bacteria has shed light on this process by taking advantage of the large population sizes, rapid generation times, and relatively accessible genetics of microbial systems.

- Adaptation by bacterial populations to a novel environment is often initially rapid, and the sequential replacement of clones within the population can lead to punctuated dynamics known as periodic selection.

- Competitive exclusion is not inevitable, however, because stable polymorphisms may be maintained by cross feeding, environmental partitioning, interactions with bacteriophages, or toxin production.

- Adaptation is frequently accompanied by genetic trade-offs that compromise fitness in alternative environments. Selection may favor the silencing or deletion of certain genes, which has been associated with the transition to pathogenicity.

- Insertion sequences and other transposable elements are responsible for a large proportion of the genetic mechanisms of adaptation published to date.

- Some trade-offs may be overcome by compensatory evolution. In the case of antibiotic resistance, evolutionary trade-offs may preclude reversion to sensitivity.

- While increasing the mutation rate may lead to short-term advantages, it may also be detrimental in the long run, either because of enhanced mutation accumulation in small populations or the eventual loss of functionality in alternative environments.

- Experimental evolution remains a powerful but underutilized technique in the study of microbial pathogens and the evolution of virulence.

ACKNOWLEDGMENTS

I thank Richard Lenski for his help in organizing the material in this chapter and with editing a draft of this chapter.

Richard Lenski's funding from the National Science Foundation (currently DEB-9981397) supported much of the work that I have reviewed here. I thank the Michigan Society of Fellows for financial support.

REFERENCES

1. **Aballay, A., and F. M. Ausubel.** 2002. Caenorhabditis elegans as a host for the study of host-pathogen interactions. *Curr. Opin. Microbiol.* **5:**97–101.
2. **Adams, J., C. Paquin, P. W. Oeller, and L. W. Lee.** 1986. Physiological characterization of adaptive clones in evolving populations of the yeast *Saccharomyces cerevisiae. Genetics* **110:**173–185.
3. **Atwood, K. C., L. K. Schneider, and F. J. Ryan.** 1951. Periodic selection in *Escherichia coli. Proc. Natl. Acad. Sci. USA* **37:**146–155.
4. **Baquero, F., and J. Blazquez.** 1997. Evolution of antibiotic resistance. *Trends Ecol. Evol.* **12:**482–487.
5. **Baumann, P., N. A. Moran, and L. Baumann.** 1997. The evolution and genetics of aphid endosymbionts. *Bioscience* **47:**12–20.
6. **Bennett, A. F., and R. E. Lenski.** 1993. Evolutionary adaptation to temperature. II. Thermal niches of experimental lines of *Escherichia coli. Evolution* **47:**1–12.
7. **Bennett, A. F., R. E. Lenski, and J. E. Mittler.** 1992. Evolutionary adaptation to temperature. I. Fitness responses of *Escherichia coli* to changes in its thermal environment. *Evolution* **46:**16–30.
8. **Bohannan, B. J. M., and R. E. Lenski.** 1997. Effect of resource enrichment on a chemostat community of bacteria and bacteriophage. *Ecology* **78:**2303–2315.
9. **Bohannan, B. J. M., M. Travisano, and R. E. Lenski.** 1999. Epistatic interactions can lower the cost of resistance to multiple consumers. *Evolution* **53:**292–295.
10. **Bouma, J. E., and R. E. Lenski.** 1988. Evolution of a bacteria/plasmid association. *Nature* **335:**351–352.
11. **Bull, J. J., M. R. Badgett, H. A. Wichman, J. P.**

Huelsenbeck, D. M. Hillis, A. Gulati, C. Ho, and I. J. Molineux. 1997. Exceptional convergent evolution in a virus. *Genetics* **147:**1497–1507.
12. **Bull, J. J., and B. R. Levin.** 2000. Mice are not furry petri dishes. *Science* **287:**1409–1410.
13. **Bull, J. J., I. J. Molineux, and W. R. Rice.** 1991. Selection of benevolence in a host-parasite system. *Evolution* **45:**875–882.
14. **Carroll, L.** 2000. *Through the Looking Glass.* Project Gutenberg. [Online.] http://www.gutenberg.org/dins/etext91/lglass19.txt
15. **Cataldi, A., M. Mock, and L. Bentancor.** 2000. Characterization of *Bacillus anthracis* strains used for vaccination. *J. Appl. Microbiol.* **88:**648–654.
16. **Chao, L.** 1990. Fitness of RNA virus decreased by Muller's ratchet. *Nature* **348:**454–455.
17. **Chao, L., and B. R. Levin.** 1981. Structured habitats and the evolution of anticompetitor toxins in bacteria. *Proc. Natl. Acad. Sci. USA* **78:**6324–6328.
18. **Clarke, D. K., E. A. Duarte, S. F. Elena, A. Moya, E. Domingo, and J. Holland.** 1994. The red queen reigns in the kingdom of RNA viruses. *Proc. Natl. Acad. Sci. USA* **91:**4821–4824.
19. **Cohan, F. M.** 1995. Does recombination constrain neutral divergence among bacterial taxa? *Evolution* **49:**164–175.
20. **Cole, S. T., P. Supply, and N. Honore.** 2001. Repetitive sequences in Mycobacterium leprae and their impact on genome plasticity. *Lepr. Rev.* **72:**449–461.
21. **Cooper, T. F., D. E. Rozen, and R. E. Lenski.** 2003. Parallel changes in gene expression after 20,000 generations of evolution in *Escherichia coli. Proc. Natl. Acad. Sci. USA* **100:**1072–1077.
22. **Cooper, V. S.** 2002. Long-term experimental evolution in *Escherichia coli.* X. Quantifying the fundamental and realized niche. *BMC Evol. Biol.* **2:**12. [Online.] http://www.biomecentral.com/1471–2146/2/12
23. **Cooper, V. S., A. F. Bennett, and R. E. Lenski.** 2001. Evolution of thermal dependence of growth rate of *Escherichia coli* populations during 20,000 generations in a constant environment. *Evolution* **55:**889–896.
24. **Cooper, V. S., and R. E. Lenski.** 2000. The population genetics of ecological specialization in evolving *Escherichia coli* populations. *Nature* **407:**736–739.
25. **Cooper, V. S., M. H. Reiskind, J. A. Miller, K. A. Shelton, B. A. Walther, J. S. Elkinton, and P. W. Ewald.** 2002. Timing of transmission and the evolution of virulence of an insect virus. *Proc. R. Soc. Lond. B* **269:**1161–1165.
26. **Cooper, V. S., D. Schneider, M. Blot, and R. E. Lenski.** 2001. Mechanisms causing rapid and parallel losses of ribose catabolism in evolving

populations of *Escherichia coli* B. *J. Bacteriol.* **183:** 2834–2841.

27. **Crill, W. D., H. A. Wichman, and J. J. Bull.** 2000. Evolutionary reversals during viral adaptation to alternating hosts. *Genetics* **154:**27–37.

28. **Day, T.** 2001. Parasite transmission modes and the evolution of virulence. *Evolution* **55:**2389–2400.

29. **Day, T.** 2003. Virulence evolution and the timing of disease life-history events. *Trends Ecol. Evol.* **18:**113–118.

30. **Dennehy, J. J., and P. E. Turner.** 2004. Reduced fecundity is the cost of cheating in RNA virus varphi6. *Proc. R. Soc. Lond. B* **271:**2275–2282.

31. **de Visser, J., C. W. Zeyl, P. J. Gerrish, J. L. Blanchard, and R. E. Lenski.** 1999. Diminishing returns from mutation supply rate in asexual populations. *Science* **283:**404–406.

32. **Doroshenko, E. P., G. I. Vasileva, and A. K. Kiseleva.** 1996. The virulence of *Yersinia pestis* strains in serial-passage in guinea pig peritoneal macrophages. *Zh. Mikrobiol. Epidemiol. Immunobiol.* **1:**14–16.

33. **Drake, J. W.** 1991. A constant rate of spontaneous mutation in DNA-based microbes. *Proc. Natl. Acad. Sci. USA* **88:**7160–7164.

34. **Dutta, N. K., and M. K. Habbu.** 1955. Experimental cholera in infant rabbits: a method for chemotherapeutic investigation. *Br. J. Pharmacol. Chemother.* **10:**153–159.

35. **Dykhuizen, D.** 1978. Selection for tryptophan auxotrophs of *Escherichia coli* in glucose-limited chemostats as a test of the energy conservation hypothesis of evolution. *Evolution* **32:**125–150.

36. **Dykhuizen, D., and D. L. Hartl.** 1981. Evolution of competitive ability in *Escherichia coli*. *Evolution* **35:**581–594.

37. **Dykhuizen, D. E.** 1990. Experimental studies of natural selection in bacteria. *Annu. Rev. Ecol. Syst.* **21:**378–398.

38. **Dykhuizen, D. E., and D. L. Hartl.** 1983. Selection in chemostats. *Microbiol. Rev.* **47:**150–168.

39. **Ebert, D.** 1998. Evolution—experimental evolution of parasites. *Science* **282:**1432–1435.

40. **Ebert, D., and W. W. Weisser.** 1997. Optimal killing for obligate killers: the evolution of life histories and virulence of semelparous parasites. *Proc. R. Soc. Lond. B* **264:**985–991.

41. **Elena, S. F., V. S. Cooper, and R. E. Lenski.** 1996. Punctuated evolution caused by selection of rare beneficial mutations. *Science* **272:**1802–1804.

42. **Elena, S. F., F. Gonzalez-Candelas, I. S. Novella, E. A. Duarte, D. K. Clarke, E. Domingo, J. J. Holland, and A. Moya.** 1996. Evolution of fitness in experimental population of vesicular stomatitis virus. *Genetics* **142:**673–679.

43. **Ewald, P. W.** 1994. *Evolution of Infectious Disease.* Oxford University Press, New York, N.Y.

44. **Finkel, S. E., and R. Kolter.** 1999. Evolution of

microbial diversity during prolonged starvation. *Proc. Natl. Acad. Sci. USA* **96:**4023–4027.

44a. **Fisher, R. A.** 1930. *The Genetical Theory of Natural Selection.* Clarendon Press, Oxford, U.K.

45. **Funchain, P., A. Yeung, J. L. Stewart, R. Lin, M. M. Slupska, and J. H. Miller.** 2000. The consequences of growth of a mutator strain of *Escherichia coli* as measured by loss of function among multiple gene targets and loss of fitness. *Genetics* **154:**959–970.

46. **Futuyma, D. J., and G. Moreno.** 1988. The evolution of ecological specialization. *Annu. Rev. Ecol. Syst.* **19:**207–233.

47. **Gerrish, P. J., and R. E. Lenski.** 1998. The fate of competing beneficial mutations in an asexual population. *Genetica* **103:**127–144.

48. **Giraud, A., I. Matic, O. Tenaillon, A. Clara, M. Radman, M. Fons, and F. Taddei.** 2001. Costs and benefits of high mutation rates: adaptive evolution of bacteria in the mouse gut. *Science* **291:**2606–2608.

49. **Gould, S. J.** 1989. *Wonderful Life: The Burgess Shale and the Nature of History.* W. W. Norton & Co., New York, N.Y.

50. **Gould, S. J., and N. Eldredge.** 1993. Punctuated equilibrium comes of age. *Nature* **366:**223–227.

51. **Greig, D., E. J. Louis, R. H. Borts, and M. Travisano.** 2002. Hybrid speciation in experimental populations of yeast. *Science* **298:** 1773–1775.

52. **Guttman, D. S.** 1996. Recombination and clonality in natural populations of *Escherichia coli*. *Trends Ecol. Evol.* **12:**16–22.

53. **Guttman, D. S., and D. E. Dykhuizen.** 1994. Clonal divergence in *Escherichia coli* as a result of recombination, not mutation. *Science* **266:**1380–1383.

54. **Hartl, D. L., D. Dykhuizen, and A. M. Dean.** 1985. Limits of adaptation: the evolution of selective neutrality. *Genetics* **111:**655–674.

55. **Heidelberg, J. F., J. A. Eisen, W. C. Nelson, R. A. Clayton, M. L. Gwinn, R. J. Dodson, D. H. Haft, E. K. Hickey, J. D. Peterson, L. Umayam, S. R. Gill, K. E. Nelson, T. D. Read, H. Tettelin, D. Richardson, M. D. Ermolaeva, J. Vamathevan, S. Bass, H. Y. Qin, I. Dragoi, P. Sellers, L. McDonald, T. Utterback, R. D. Fleishmann, W. C. Nierman, O. White, S. L. Salzberg, H. O. Smith, R. R. Colwell, J. J. Mekalanos, J. C. Venter, and C. M. Fraser.** 2000. DNA sequence of both chromosomes of the cholera pathogen *Vibrio cholerae*. *Nature* **406:**477–483.

56. **Helling, R. B., C. Vargas, and J. Adams.** 1987. Evolution of *Escherichia coli* during growth in a constant environment. *Genetics* **116:**349–358.

57. **Imhof, M., and C. Schlotterer.** 2001. Fitness effects of advantageous mutations in evolving

Escherichia coli populations. *Proc. Natl. Acad. Sci. USA* **98:**1113–1117.

58. **Keim, P., L. B. Price, A. M. Klevytska, K. L. Smith, J. M. Schupp, R. Okinaka, P. J. Jackson, and M. E. Hugh-Jones.** 2000. Multiple-locus variable-number tandem repeat analysis reveals genetic relationships within *Bacillus anthracis. J. Bacteriol.* **182:**2928–2936. (Erratum, **182:**6862.)

59. **Kibota, T. T., and M. Lynch.** 1996. Estimate of the genomic mutation rate deleterious to overall fitness in E. coli. *Nature* **381:**694–696.

60. **Kimura, M.** 1983. *The Neutral Theory of Molecular Evolution.* Cambridge University Press, Cambridge, United Kingdom.

61. **Kormilitsnya, M. I., and I. S. Meshcheriakova.** 1996. The characteristics of a natural attenuated isolate of *Francisella tularensis. Zh. Mikrobiol. Epidemiol. Immunobiol.* **2:**3–6.

62. **Korona, R.** 1996. Genetic divergence and fitness convergence under uniform selection in experimental populations of bacteria. *Genetics* **143:**637–644.

63. **Korona, R., C. H. Nakatsu, L. J. Forney, and R. E. Lenski.** 1994. Evidence for multiple adaptive peaks from populations of bacteria evolving in a structured habitat. *Proc. Natl. Acad. Sci. USA* **91:**9037–9041.

64. **Kurlandzka, A., R. F. Rosenzweig, and J. Adams.** 1991. Identification of adaptive changes in an evolving population of *Escherichia coli:* The role of changes with regulatory and highly pleiotrophic effects. *Mol. Biol. Evol.* **8:**261–281.

65. **LeClerc, J. E., B. Li, W. L. Payne, and T. A. Cebula.** 1996. High mutation frequencies among *Escherichia coli* and *Salmonella* pathogens. *Science* **274:**1208–1211.

66. **Lenski, R. E.** 1997. The cost of antibiotic resistance—from the perspective of a bacterium. *Antibiot. Resist. Orig. Evol. Selection Spread* **207:**131–140.

67. **Lenski, R. E.** 1988. Experimental studies of pleiotropy and epistasis in *Escherichia coli.* I. Variation in competitive fitness among mutants resistant to virus T4. *Evolution* **42:**425–432.

68. **Lenski, R. E.** 1988. Experimental studies of pleiotropy and epistasis in *Escherichia coli.* II. Compensation for maladaptic pleiotropic effects associated with resistance to virus T4. *Evolution* **42:**433–440.

69. **Lenski, R. E., and B. R. Levin.** 1985. Constraints on the coevolution of bacteria and virulent phage: a model, some experiments, and the predictions for natural communities. *Am. Nat.* **125:**585–602.

70. **Lenski, R. E., J. A. Mongold, P. D. Sniegowski, M. Travisano, F. Vasi, P. J. Gerrish, and T. M. Schmidt.** 1998. Evolution of competitive fitness in experimental populations of E. coli: what makes one genotype a better competitor than another? *Antonie Leeuwenhoek* **73:**35–47.

71. **Lenski, R. E., M. R. Rose, S. C. Simpson, and S. C. Tadler.** 1991. Long-term experimental evolution in *Escherichia coli.* I. Adaptation and divergence during 2,000 generations. *Am. Nat.* **138:**1315–1341.

72. **Lenski, R. E., S. C. Simpson, and T. T. Nguyen.** 1994. Genetic analysis of plasmid-encoded, host genotype-specific enhancement of bacterial fitness. *J. Bacteriol.* **176:**3140–3147.

73. **Lenski, R. E., and M. Travisano.** 1994. Dynamics of adaptation and diversification: a 10,000-generation experiment with bacterial populations. *Proc. Natl. Acad. Sci. USA* **91:**6808–6814.

74. **Lenski, R. E., C. L. Winkworth, and M. A. Riley.** 2003. Rates of DNA sequence evolution in experimental populations of *Escherichia coli* during 20,000 generations. *J. Mol. Evol.* **56:**498–508.

75. **Levin, B. R., and R. E. Lenski.** 1985. Bacteria and phage: a model system for the study of the ecology and coevolution of hosts and parasites, p. 227–242. *In* D. Rollinson and R. M. Anderson (ed.), *Ecology and Genetics of Host-Parasite Interactions.* Academic Press, London, United Kingdom.

76. **Luria, S. E., and M. Delbruck.** 1943. Mutations of bacteria from virus sensitivity to virus resistance. *Genetics* **28:**491–511.

77. **Mahajan-Miklos, S., M. W. Tan, L. G. Rahme, and F. M. Ausubel.** 1999. Molecular mechanisms of bacterial virulence elucidated using a *Pseudomonas aeruginosa-Caenorhabditis elegans* pathogenesis model. *Cell* **96:**47–56.

78. **Manche, K., L. Notley-McRobb, and T. Ferenci.** 1999. Mutational adaptation of *Escherichia coli* to glucose limitation involves distinct evolutionary pathways in aerobic and oxygen-limited environments. *Genetics* **153:**5–12.

79. **Matic, I., M. Radman, F. Taddei, B. Picard, C. Doit, E. Bingen, E. Denamur, and J. Elion.** 1997. Highly variable mutation rates in commensal and pathogenic Escherichia coli. *Science* **277:**1833–1834.

79a. **Mekalanos, J. J.** 1983. Duplication and amplification of toxin genes in *Vibrio cholerae. Cell* **35:**253–263.

80. **Messenger, S. L., I. J. Molineux, and J. J. Bull.** 1999. Virulence evolution in a virus obeys a trade-off. *Proc. R. Soc. Lond. B* **266:**397–404.

81. **Modi, R. I., L. H. Castilla, S. Puskasrozsa, R. B. Helling, and J. Adams.** 1992. Genetic changes accompanying increased fitness in evolving populations of *Escherichia coli. Genetics* **130:**241–249.

82. **Mongold, J. A., and R. E. Lenski.** 1996. Experimental rejection of a nonadaptive expla-

nation for increased cell size in *Escherichia coli*. *J. Bacteriol.* **178:**5333–5334.

83. **Moore, F. B., D. E. Rozen, and R. E. Lenski.** 2000. Pervasive compensatory adaptation in Escherichia coli. *Proc. R. Soc. Lond. B* **267:** 515–522.

84. **Moran, N. A.** 2002. Genome evolution in symbiotic bacteria: genomic analysis opens path to analyzing obligate symbionts, among the most intriguing and varied of noncultivable bacteria. *ASM News* **68:**499–505.

85. **Moran, N. A.** 2002. Microbial minimalism: genome reduction in bacterial pathogens. *Cell* **108:**583–586.

86. **Moran, N. A.** 2002. The ubiquitous and varied role of infection in the lives of animals and plants. *Am. Nat.* **160:**S1–S8.

87. **Nakatsu, C. H., R. Korona, R. E. Lenski, F. J. De Bruijn, T. L. Marsh, and L. J. Forney.** 1998. Parallel and divergent genotypic evolution in experimental populations of Ralstonia sp. *J. Bacteriol.* **180:**4325–4331.

88. **Nguyen, T. N., Q. G. Phan, L. P. Duong, K. P. Bertrand, and R. E. Lenski.** 1989. Effects of carriage and expression of the Tn*10* tetracycline-resistance operon on the fitness of Escherichia coli K12. *Mol. Biol. Evol.* **6:**213–225.

89. **Notley-McRobb, L., and T. Ferenci.** 1999. Adaptive mgl-regulatory mutations and genetic diversity evolving in glucose-limited *Escherichia coli* populations. *Environ. Microbiol.* **1:**33–43.

90. **Notley-McRobb, L., and T. Ferenci.** 2000. Experimental analysis of molecular events during mutational periodic selections in bacterial evolution. *Genetics* **156:**1493–1501.

91. **Notley-McRobb, L., and T. Ferenci.** 1999. The generation of multiple co-existing mal-regulatory mutations through polygenic evolution in glucose limited populations of *Escherichia coli*. *Environ. Microbiol.* **1:**45–52.

92. **Novella, I. S., D. K. Clarke, J. Quer, E. A. Duarte, C. H. Lee, S. C. Weaver, S. F. Elena, A. Moya, E. Domingo, and J. J. Holland.** 1995. Extreme fitness differences in mammalian and insect hosts after continuous replication of vesicular stomatitis virus in sandfly cells. *J. Virol.* **69:**6805–6809.

93. **Novella, I. S., E. A. Duarte, S. F. Elena, A. Moya, E. Domingo, and J. J. Holland.** 1995. Exponential increases of RNA virus fitness during large population transmissions. *Proc. Natl. Acad. Sci. USA* **92:**5841–5844.

94. **Nowak, M. A., and R. M. May.** 1992. Superinfection and the evolution of parasite virulence. *Proc. R. Soc. Lond. B* **255:**81–89.

95. **Oliver, A., R. Canton, P. Campo, F. Baquero, and J. Blazquez.** 2000. High frequency of hypermutable *Pseudomonas aeruginosa* in cystic

fibrosis lung infection. *Science* **288:**1251–1253.

96. **Papadopoulos, D., D. Schneider, J. Meier-Eiss, W. Arber, R. E. Lenski, and M. Blot.** 1999. Genomic evolution during a 10,000-generation experiment with bacteria. *Proc. Natl. Acad. Sci. USA* **96:**3807–3812.

97. **Paquin, C., and J. Adams.** 1983. Frequency of fixation of adaptive mutations is higher in evolving diploid than haploid yeast populations. *Nature* **302:**495–500.

98. **Picard, B., P. Duriez, S. Gouriou, I. Matic, E. Denamur, and F. Taddei.** 2001. Mutator natural *Escherichia coli* isolates have an unusual virulence phenotype. *Infect. Immun.* **69:**9–14.

99. **Provine, W. B.** 2001. *The Origins of Theoretical Population Genetics*, 2nd ed. University of Chicago Press, Chicago, Ill.

100. **Rahme, L. G., F. M. Ausubel, H. Cao, E. Drenkard, B. C. Goumnerov, G. W. Lau, S. Mahajan-Miklos, J. Plotnikova, M. W. Tan, J. Tsongalis, C. L. Walendziewicz, and R. G. Tompkins.** 2000. Plants and animals share functionally common bacterial virulence factors. *Proc. Natl. Acad. Sci. USA* **97:**8815–8821.

101. **Rainey, P. B., and M. Travisano.** 1998. Adaptive radiation in a heterogeneous environment. *Nature* **394:**69–72.

102. **Read, T. D., S. L. Salzberg, M. Pop, M. Shumway, L. Umayam, L. X. Jiang, E. Holtzapple, J. D. Busch, K. L. Smith, J. M. Schupp, D. Solomon, P. Keim, and C. M. Fraser.** 2002. Comparative genome sequencing for discovery of novel polymorphisms in *Bacillus anthracis*. *Science* **296:**2028–2033.

103. **Riehle, M. M., A. F. Bennett, and A. D. Long.** 2000. Genetic analysis of the adaptation to temperature stress: a role for gene duplications. *Am. Zool.* **40:**1188–1189.

104. **Riley, M. A.** 1998. Molecular mechanisms of bacteriocin evolution. *Annu. Rev. Genet.* **32:**255–278.

105. **Riley, M. A., and J. E. Wertz.** 2002. Bacteriocins: evolution, ecology, and application. *Annu. Rev. Microbiol.* **56:**117–137.

106. **Riley, M. S., V. S. Cooper, R. E. Lenski, L. J. Forney, and T. L. Marsh.** 2001. Rapid phenotypic change and diversification of a soil bacterium during 1000 generations of experimental evolution. *Microbiology* **147:**995–1006.

107. **Rosenzweig, R. F., R. R. Sharp, D. S. Treves, and J. Adams.** 1994. Microbial evolution in a simple unstructured environment: genetic differentiation in *Escherichia coli*. *Genetics* **137:** 903–917.

108. **Rozen, D. E., and R. E. Lenski.** 2000. Long-term experimental evolution in *Escherichia coli*. VIII. Dynamics of a balanced polymorphism. *Am. Nat.* **155:**24–35.

109. **Schneider, D., E. Duperchy, E. Coursange,**

R. E. Lenski, and M. Blot. 2000. Long-term experimental evolution in *Escherichia coli*. IX. Characterization of insertion sequence-mediated mutations and rearrangements. *Genetics* **156**:477–488.

110. Schrag, S., V. Perrot, and B. Levin. 1997. Adaptation to the fitness costs of antibiotic resistance in *Escherichia coli*. *Proc. R. Soc. Lond. B* **264**:1287–1291.

111. Sniegowski, P. D., P. J. Gerrish, T. Johnson, and A. Shaver. 2000. The evolution of mutation rates: separating causes from consequences. *Bioessays* **22**:1057–1066.

112. Sniegowski, P. D., P. J. Gerrish, and R. E. Lenski. 1997. Evolution of high mutation rates in experimental populations of E. coli. *Nature* **387**:703–705.

113. Souza, V., P. E. Turner, and R. E. Lenski. 1997. Long-term experimental evolution in Escherichia coli. V. Effects of recombination with immigrant genotypes on the rate of bacterial evolution. *J. Evol. Biol.* **10**:743–769.

114. Spiers, A. J., S. G. Kahn, J. Bohannon, M. Travisano, and P. B. Rainey. 2002. Adaptive divergence in experimental populations of *Pseudomonas fluorescens*. I. Genetic and phenotypic bases of wrinkly spreader fitness. *Genetics* **161**:33–46.

115. Taddei, F., M. Radman, J. Maynard-Smith, B. Toupance, P. H. Gouyon, and B. Godelle. 1997. Role of mutator alleles in adaptive evolution. *Nature* **387**:700–702.

116. Tan, M. W., L. G. Rahme, J. A. Sternberg, R. G. Tompkins, and F. M. Ausubel. 1999. Pseudomonas aeruginosa killing of Caenorhabditis elegans used to identify P. aeruginosa virulence factors. *Proc. Natl. Acad. Sci. USA* **96**: 2408–2413.

117. Travisano, M., and R. E. Lenski. 1996. Long-term experimental evolution in *Escherichia coli*. IV. Targets of selection and the specificity of adaptation. *Genetics* **143**:15–26.

118. Travisano, M., J. A. Mongold, A. F. Bennett, and R. E. Lenski. 1995. Experimental tests of the roles of adaptation, chance, and history in evolution. *Science* **267**:87–90.

119. Travisano, M., and P. B. Rainey. 2000. Studies of adaptive radiation using model microbial systems. *Am. Nat.* **156**:S35–S44.

120. Travisano, M., F. Vasi, and R. E. Lenski. 1995. Long-term experimental evolution in *Escherichia coli*. III. Variation among replicate populations in correlated responses to novel environments. *Evolution* **49**:189–200.

121. Treves, D. S., S. Manning, and J. Adams. 1998. Repeated evolution of an acetate-crossfeeding polymorphism in long-term populations of *Escherichia coli*. *Mol. Biol. Evol.* **15**: 789–797.

122. Turner, P. E., and L. Chao. 1999. Prisoner's dilemma in an RNA virus. *Nature* **398**:441–443.

123. Van Valen, L. 1973. A new evolutionary law. *Evol. Theory* **1**:1–30.

124. Vasi, F., M. Travisano, and R. E. Lenski. 1994. Long-term experimental evolution in *Escherichia coli*. II. Changes in life-history traits during adaptation to a seasonal environment. *Am. Nat.* **144**:432–456.

125. Vasi, F. K., and R. E. Lenski. 1999. Ecological strategies and fitness tradeoffs in *Escherichia coli* mutants adapted to prolonged starvation. *J. Genet.* **78**:43–49.

126. Velicer, G. J., L. Kroos, and R. E. Lenski. 2000. Developmental cheating in the social bacterium *Myxococcus xanthus*. *Nature* **404**: 598–601.

127. Velicer, G. J., L. Kroos, and R. E. Lenski. 1998. Loss of social behaviors by *Myxococcus xanthus* during evolution in an unstructured habitat. *Proc. Natl. Acad. Sci. USA* **95**:12376–12380.

128. Velicer, G. J., R. E. Lenski, and L. Kroos. 2002. Rescue of social motility lost during evolution of *Myxococcus xanthus* in an asocial environment. *J. Bacteriol.* **184**:2719–2727.

129. Waldor, M. K., and J. J. Mekalanos. 1996. Lysogenic conversion by a filamentous phage encoding cholera toxin. *Science* **272**:1910–1914.

130. Welch, R. A., V. Burland, G. I. Plunkett, P. Redford, P. Roesch, D. A. Rasko, E. L. Buckles, S.-R. Liou, A. Boutin, J. Hackett, D. Stroud, G. F. Mayhew, D. J. Rose, S. Zhou, D. C. Schwartz, N. T. Perna, H. L. T. Mobley, M. S. Donnenberg, and F. R. Blattner. 2002. Extensive mosaic structure revealed by the complete genome sequence of uropathogenic *Escherichia coli*. *Proc. Natl. Acad. Sci. USA* **99**:17020–17024.

131. Woolhouse, M. E. J. 2002. Population biology of emerging and re-emerging pathogens. *Trends Microbiol.* **10**:S3–S7.

132. Woolhouse, M. E. J., L. H. Taylor, and D. T. Haydon. 2001. Population biology of multi-host pathogens. *Science* **292**:1109–1112.

132a. Wright, S. 1932. The roles of mutation in breeding, crossbreeding and selection in evolution. *Proc. 6th Int. Congr. Genet.* **1**:356–366.

133. Zamenhof, S., and H. H. Eichhorn. 1967. Study of microbial evolution through loss of biosynthetic functions: establishment of "defective" mutants. *Nature* **216**:456–458.

134. Zeyl, C., and G. Bell. 1997. The advantage of sex in evolving yeast populations. *Nature* **388**:465–468.

135. Zeyl, C., M. Mizesko, and J. de Visser. 2001. Mutational meltdown in laboratory yeast populations. *Evolution* **55**:909–917.

THE CONTRIBUTION OF PATHOGENICITY ISLANDS TO THE EVOLUTION OF BACTERIAL PATHOGENS

Bianca Hochhut, Ulrich Dobrindt, and Jörg Hacker

5

Within the last few years, the increasing knowledge of the organization of bacterial genomes and the availability of complete genome sequences has led to a new era of pathogen research. Generally, the typical bacterial genome consists of a core gene pool containing those genes that encode essential functions, such as DNA replication and cell division, and a flexible gene pool encompassing genes that are only required under certain environmental conditions. Core genes have characteristically a relatively homogeneous G+C content and are located in stable regions of the chromosome. The genomic organization of these regions in closely related species is very similar. In contrast, genes of the flexible gene pool are often located on mobile genetic elements or in variable regions of the chromosome. This is exemplified by various virulence-associated genes that have been found to be encoded on transposons, integrons, plasmids, or phages (27, 38, 50). They can be horizontally transferred by means of transformation, transduction, or conjugation, underscoring the importance of lateral gene transfer as one of the driving forces of evolution for the transformation of avirulent into virulent bacteria (Fig. 1) (99). In addition to the gain of new information due to horizontal gene transfer, gene loss has been shown to contribute to the formation of new pathogens (Fig. 1). "Evolution by reduction" especially occurs in intracellular and obligate pathogens that have adapted to the physiologically stable environments of their host by deleting genes no longer essential for the life within the host, but has also been detected in facultative pathogens (87; also see chapter 6). Furthermore, point mutations and DNA rearrangements contribute to constant evolution of bacterial pathogens.

The determination of the genome sequence of pathogenic *Escherichia coli* isolates revealed that virulence determinants were clustered in these strains in large regions of the chromosome that were not present in the chromosome of nonpathogenic isolates and that varied among different isolates. These regions were designated "pathogenicity islands" (PAIs) (47). PAIs have been defined as (i) large genomic regions that (ii) carry one or more virulence-associated gene, (iii) have a G+C content different from that of the rest of the chromosome, (iv) are frequently associated with tRNA genes, (v) are often flanked by repeat structures, (vi) contain mobility genes such as integrase genes and transposases, and (vii) are often unstable (48) (Fig. 2).

Bianca Hochhut, Ulrich Dobrindt, and Jörg Hacker, Institut für Molekulare Infektionsbiologie, Universität Würzburg, D-97070 Würzburg, Germany.

Evolution of Microbial Pathogens, Edited by H. S. Seifert and V. J. DiRita, © 2006 ASM Press, Washington, D.C.

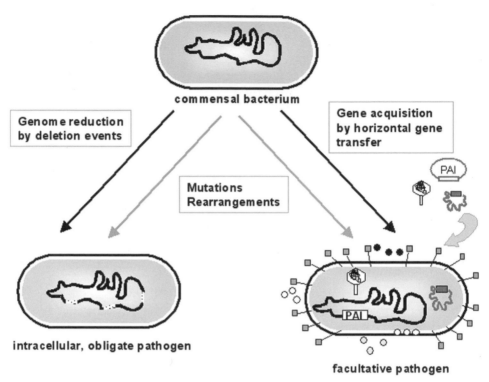

FIGURE 1 General mechanisms in evolution of bacterial pathogens. Genome evolution is based on loss (indicated by shaded areas) and acquisition of genetic information. Mobile genetic elements such as plasmids, bacteriophages, and PAIs encoding virulence traits (fimbriae, secreted toxins, etc.) that are horizontally transferred by transformation, transduction, and conjugation play an important role in gene acquistion. For more details, see text.

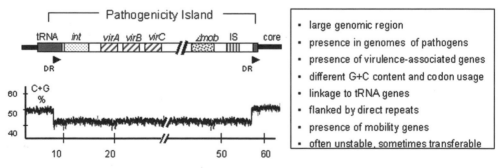

FIGURE 2 Features of pathogenicity islands (PAIs). The model illustrates the main features of PAIs that are listed in the box. Island-associated genes are shown as shaded boxes and the bacterial chromosome as a line (top). G+C content of the PAI and the core genome often differ from each other (bottom). Abbreviations: *int,* integrase gene; *vir,* virulence-associated gene; $\Delta mob,$ truncated mobility gene; IS, insertion sequence. Modified from reference 49.

Based on these characteristics, it has been assumed that PAIs have been acquired by horizontal gene transfer. Since the discovery of PAIs in extraintestinal as well as intestinal *E. coli* strains (13, 90), similar elements have been identified in the genomes of many other bacteria that are pathogens of humans, animals, and plants and that belong to different species and genera. In this chapter, the role of PAIs in the evolution of bacterial virulence will be discussed.

FEATURES OF PAIs

Virulence Traits

Pathogenicity islands that have been identified so far carry a variety of virulence factors that represent the entire spectrum of bacterial virulence-associated genes (for more detailed overviews, see references 51 and 119). As most PAIs often encode more than one virulence factor, their acquisition results in a severe change of the recipient's virulence potential. In the following paragraphs, the major bacterial virulence determinants that have been found on PAIs will be briefly introduced.

Adhesins play a critical role in colonization of the host by enabling the microbe to attach to specific eukaryotic receptor molecules. Examples are the PAIs of extraintestinal *E. coli* that carry the genes for P or P-related fimbriae (also called P pili) and S-fimbrial gene clusters (reviewed in reference 51). Another type of adhesin, an intimin, is encoded by the *eae* gene located on the locus of enterocyte effacement (LEE) PAI of enteropathogenic and enterohemorrhagic *E. coli* (EPEC and EHEC, respectively) (reviewed in reference 70). The LEE island also encodes the intimin receptor protein Tir, which is translocated from the bacterium into the host cell by type III secretion (also see below). A third example is the pathogenicity island VPI of *Vibrio cholerae* that encodes a type IV pilus, the toxin-coregulated pilus (TCP) (72). TCP also acts as the receptor for the cholera toxin encoding filamentous phage CTXφ (138).

Secretion systems are essential for the transport of virulence factors to the surface or directly into the host cell. Type III secretion systems have been identified on the *Salmonella enterica*-specific islands SPI-1 and SPI-2 (56, 93), on the LEE island of EHEC and EPEC isolates (with intimin-receptor Tir as one of the translocated substrates) (40, 104, 128), and on the Hrp PAIs of several plant pathogens (3, 30, 75). The translocated proteins have different modes of action (such as mediating invasion of epithelial cells; modulating activity of signal molecules such as Rac, Cdc42, and other GTPases; and rearranging the host cell cytoskeleton), with each mechanism reflecting the lifestyle of the respective pathogen. The type III effector genes are frequently located on the same island as their secretion apparatus, but there are also examples of type III effector proteins that are encoded by coresiding PAIs or plasmids (94, 144).

Type IV secretion systems are thought to be built from components of conjugation machines that are involved in the transfer of DNA from a donor to a recipient cell (28). They have been found to be essential for full virulence of several pathogens, such as *Helicobacter pylori, Bordetella pertussis, Legionella pneumophila, Agrobacterium tumefaciens,* and *Brucella suis* (see reference 21 for an overview). A recently described island in *Neisseria gonorrhoeae* encodes a putative type IV secretion system that is thought to release DNA as a source for transformation events (34). Furthermore, some variants of the island that are preferentially associated with disseminated infection isolates of *N. gonorrhoeae* confer production of a cytotoxin as well as serum resistance.

Toxin genes are frequently located on mobile genetic elements such as bacteriophages or plasmids, and consequently, they can also be associated with PAIs (reviewed in reference 38). PAIs or PAI-like structures may encode cytolysins, proteases, lipases, or enterotoxins (51, 126).

Acquisition of iron is required to multiply in the ecological niche of the eukaryotic host, and pathogenic microbes have to scavenge this essential nutrient in competition with their host. Examples of PAI-associated siderophore systems are aerobactin and yersiniabactin (Ybt) (24, 96, 137, 139). The *ybt* genes are located on the so-called high-pathogenicity island (HPI) that was initially discovered in *Yersinia* spp. This HPI consists of a Ybt-encoding core and additional loci that are characteristic for particular species (20).

Regulation of PAI-associated genes is in most cases well integrated into the global regulation mechanisms of the bacterial cell, and virulence genes on PAIs are coordinately expressed with genes of the core chromosome. Several PAIs encode regulator proteins that control their respective virulence genes but also act on loci outside the island. For example, ToxT is a transcriptional activator of the AraC family that is encoded on the *V. cholerae* VPI and that is involved in expression of the *tcp* gene cluster. ToxT also regulates cholera toxin production by activating expression of *ctxAB* that are part of the genome of CTXφ (76). In the case of fimbrial gene cluster expression in uropathogenic *E. coli* (UPEC) strains, PAI-encoded regulators influence genes encoded on another PAI, which was described as "cross-talk activation" (95). In UPEC strain 536, the two regulatory proteins encoded in the *prf* (P-related fimbria) gene cluster are able to activate not only the *prf* genes but also the S-fimbrial gene cluster that is found on PAI III$_{536}$ (36). Finally, the regulation of the LEE island of *E. coli* and SPI-1 of *S. enterica* have been investigated in great detail (for overviews, see references 71, 83, and 84).

Mobility Genes

Besides the presence of virulence-associated genes, PAIs are characterized by the fact that they often carry mobility genes such as genes that encode phage-related integrases and/or transposases, indicating that horizontal gene transfer processes have been involved in the evolution of PAIs. However, presence and functionality of these genes differ greatly among the various PAIs, and even though there are several examples of PAIs with intact and functional mobility genes, there are also cases of mutated genes encoding nonfunctional products or PAIs that do not seem to contain any mobility genes. The role of these genes and their products in stability and mobility of PAIs will also be discussed later in this chapter.

PAIs have been defined as distinct pieces of DNA integrated into the backbone of a core chromosome with boundaries that are often flanked by direct repeats (DR) of varying length (from 9 up to 135 bp), whereas in related strains or species that do not carry the respective island, only one copy of the DR sequence is present. It has been assumed that the duplication is caused by site-specific recombination between the chromosome and the element corresponding to the well-studied integration mechanism of lysogenic phages. The presence of phage-related integrases in many islands supports this model.

Insertion sequence (IS) elements and transposon sequences have been identified in various PAIs and are thought to have been involved in the original mobilization as well as in subsequent rearrangements within several elements. In case of the *cag* island of *H. pylori*, IS*605*-mediated rearrangements can be observed playing a major role in the ongoing adaptation between *H. pylori* and its human host (see overview in reference 100). Analysis of the DNA sequence of various PAIs in *Enterobacteriaceae* revealed the presence of open reading frames (ORFs) typical for IS elements or transposons of origins that were not restricted to the respective host genome of a PAI, but also included DNA sequences specific for IS elements of other species. This suggests that foreign DNA has been inserted into PAIs by recombination events involving mobile genetic elements.

Impact of tRNA Genes

In gram-negative bacteria, most of the known PAIs are inserted next to a tRNA gene or similar genes that encode small regulatory RNAs such as *ssrA*. It has long been known that the 3' ends of tRNA genes represent hot spots for site-specific recombination systems, and the finding that PAIs are also associated with these genes implies that PAIs or parts of PAIs may have evolved from lysogenic phages. A systematic screening of tRNA genes for the presence of foreign DNA can lead to the identification of novel PAIs. When it was applied to *Shigella flexneri* or *S. enterica,* SHI-2 and SPI-3, respectively, were discovered.

There has been speculation as to why tRNA genes are preferred integration sites of foreign DNA (113, 142). First, the nucleotide sequences of tRNA genes are generally highly conserved even among distantly related species, and their use as integration sites may increase the putative host range of a mobile genetic element. Second, tRNA genes are transcriptional active sites and may therefore serve as hot spots of recombination events. Third, tRNA genes exhibit symmetrical nucleotide sequences, facilitating the binding of integrases as well as other proteins that mediate the recombination process. Finally, it has been suggested that association with particular tRNAs, called minor tRNAs, that are less frequently used than others may have modulatory effects on the translational efficiency of transferred genes with a high number of minor tRNA-specific codons (minor codon hypothesis).

In most cases, integration of PAIs restores the ORF of the respective tRNA gene. Furthermore, PAIs normally insert into the 3' end of their target gene, leaving the promoter regions uninterrupted and expression of tRNA genes unaltered. Nevertheless, integration seems to occur preferentially into nonessential tRNA genes (such as *selC*) or tRNA genes that are present in more than one copy on the chromosome (such as *pheV* and *pheU*). Other PAIs (e.g., PAI II of UPEC strain 536), are located to minor tRNA genes such as *leuX*, which is truncated at its 3' end when PAI II$_{536}$ excises from the chromosome. It has been shown that the expression of the island-encoded α–hemolysin determinant as well as the expression of virulence genes outside the island are affected by the presence of an intact *leuX* allele and that a *leuX* mutant is less virulent than a *leuX*-positive derivative (37, 105, 114). Similarly, expression of fimbrial genes of *S. enterica* is influenced by

the minor tRNA *argU* (134). In summary, these results suggest that tRNA loci may play a key role in the evolution of bacterial pathogens.

Instability and Transferability

After acquisition of PAIs, most of these elements seem to have undergone modifications such as mutations and/or deletions of mobility genes as well as changes within the flanking DR repeats that resulted in a relatively stable association with the host chromosome, a process that has also been termed "homing" (51). However, certain PAIs still show a tendency for deletion of partial sequences or even of the complete island (92, 108, 133). In case of PAIs of *E. coli* 536, island-associated integrase genes play a role in these deletion events (our unpublished results). Middendorf et al. (92) analyzed the influence of various growth conditions on the stability of PAIs. They found an increase in the incidence of excision of PAI II$_{536}$ when cells were grown to stationary phase at low temperatures, indicating that environmental parameters may modulate the deletion process. Deletion of PAIs in UPEC strains may also play a role during transition of the pathogen from an acute state of infection to a chronic state wherein expression of highly antigenic factors may be disadvantageous. More generally, pathogens with a relatively high genetic flexibility may be more competent in the colonization of new ecological niches and may have a selective advantage over organisms with less flexible genomes.

In *Yersinia* spp., the deletion behavior of the HPI varies greatly within the different species (6, 18, 19). Whereas the HPI in *Y. pseudotuberculosis* excises from the chromosome by site-specific recombination between the flanking DRs, the HPI of *Y. enterocolitica* is relatively stable because it carries a mutation within the integrase gene and has no conserved 17-bp repeat on one end, therefore lacking the potential of precise deletion. In *Y. pestis,* HPI excision has been described as part of a bigger deletion of 102 kb including the adjacent pigmentation (*pgm*) locus at high frequencies that is probably mediated by recombination between two flanking IS*100* copies (54).

As HPI-like elements are widely distributed among enterobacteria, lateral transfer by a yet unknown mechanism has been postulated (109). Generally, little is known about the mechanisms that have been involved in the acquisition of PAIs, and there is nearly no evidence of mobilization in natural or laboratory settings. However, there are at least two examples of intercellular transfer of PAIs. The *V. cholerae* VPI is generally only present in disease-related strains of *V. cholerae*. Therefore, detection of nearly identical elements in *Vibrio mimicus* isolates that also carried a CTXφ-like prophage suggests recent gene transfer between *V. cholerae* and *V. mimicus* (15). Furthermore, VPI can be transferred among *V. cholerae* strains by generalized transduction involving vibriophage CP-T1 (102). Generalized transducing phages also mediate transfer of the SaPI1 family of elements in *Staphylococcus aureus*. These elements are not capable of self-transfer, but they can be propagated by staphylococcal phages φ80α and φ13 (82). When SaPI1 excises from the chromosome in the presence of φ80α, the circular intermediate is replicated and efficiently encapsulated into special small phage heads (116). This is reminiscent of the intimate relationship between the defective coliphage P4 and its helper phage P2 (81). As many of the enterobacterial PAIs encode P4- or CP4-like integrases, it has been speculated that P2 or related phages may have contributed to the mobilization of these elements. However, under laboratory conditions there has been no evidence for transfer of PAI-specific DNA by P2 bacteriophage.

PATHOGENICITY ISLANDS AND OTHER MOBILE GENETIC ELEMENTS

PAIs, Phages, Plasmids, and Conjugative Transposons

Mobilizable plasmids and bacteriophages represent key elements enabling prokaryotes to exchange genetic information by means of conjugation and transduction. Recent genomic research has revealed that, besides these two types of mobile genetic elements, PAIs have played a major role in the transformation of avirulent into virulent bacteria. Little to nothing is known about the origin of PAIs, but it has been speculated that they may have been derived from integrating plasmids or phages that had lost the genes required for replication and self-transfer in exchange for a more stable association and inheritance with the host chromosome (48) (Table 1). Evidence to support this model includes the finding that PAIs often encode phage-like integration systems. Most frequently, tyrosine recombinases of the P4 family are associated with PAIs. For example, related P4-like integrases have been identified in several PAIs in *Enterobacteriaceae* that are associated with either of the tRNA genes *pheV* or *pheU* (Table 2). Similarly, nearly identical CP4-like integrases are encoded by PAIs that are linked to *selC* (Table 2). This suggests a modular

TABLE 1 Properties of mobile genetic elements

Type of element	Example	Autonomous replication	Autonomous transfer	Mobilization	Integration	Excision
Large plasmid	RP4	+	+	+	+/−	+/−
Small plasmid	RSF1010	+	−	+/−	(−)	(−)
Prophage	λ	−[a]	(+)	+	+	+
Conjugative transposon[b]	SXT	−	+	+	+	+
Integron, superintegron	In1	−	−	−	+	+
PAIs/GEIs	PAI ll$_{536}$	−	−	(+)	(+)	+
Core genes	Various genes	−	−	−	−	−

[a]Most prophages are integrated into the chromosome with the exception of few phages (e.g., P1) that are maintained as extrachromosomal replicons.

[b]Including elements designated as integrative and conjugative elements or conjugative genomic islands.

TABLE 2 Pathogenicity islands (PAIs) or PAI-like structures of pathogenic enterobacteria[a]

Organism	Serotype	Designation	Encoded traits	Size (kb)	Junction	Integrase	Insertion site	Reference(s)
Escherichia coli 536 (UPEC)	O6:K15:H31	PAI I$_{536}$	α-Hemolysin, put. adhesins	75.8	DR 16 bp	CP4-like (cryptic?)	*selC*	36
E. coli 536 (UPEC)	O6:K15:H31	PAI II$_{536}$	α-Hemolysin, P fimbriae (P-f), put. adhesin	102	DR 18 bp	P4-like	*leuX*	36
E. coli 536 (UPEC)	O6:K15:H31	PAI III$_{536}$	S fimbriae (Sfal), *iro* siderophore system, hemoglobin protease	76.8	DR 46 bp	Sfx-like	*thrW*	36
E. coli 536 (UPEC)	O6:K15:H31	PAI V$_{536}$	K15 capsule	>75	DR ~40 bp	P4-like	*pheV*	121
E. coli J96 (UPEC)	O4:K−:H5	PAI I$_{J96}$	α-Hemolysin, P fimbriae (Pap)	>170	?	?	*pheV*	132
E. coli J96 (UPEC)	O4:K−:H5	PAI II$_{J96}$	α-Hemolysin, P fimbriae (Prs), cytotoxic necrotizing factor 1 (CNF1)	110	DR 135 bp	P4-like	*pheU*	132
E. coli CFT073 (UPEC)	O6:K2:H1	PAI I$_{CFT073}$	α-Hemolysin, P fimbriae (Pap)	58	DR 9 bp	P4-like	*pheV*	69, 139
E. coli CFT073 (UPEC)	O6:K2:H1	PAI II$_{CFT073}$	P fimbriae (Pap), iron acquisition	71	No DR	P4-like	*pheU*	110, 139
E. coli AL862		PAI I$_{AL862}$	*afa8* adhesin	61	DR 14 bp	P4-like	*pheU*	79
E. coli AL862		PAI II$_{AL862}$	*afa8* adhesin	61	DR 136 bp (imperfect)	P4-like	*pheV*	79
E. coli EV36	K1	*kps* PAI	K1 capsule	ND	?	?	*pheV*	29
E. coli C5	O18:K1:H7	PAI I$_{C5}$	α-Hemolysin, P fimbriae (Prs), cytotoxic necrotizing factor 1 (CNF1), heat-resistant hemagglutinin	~100	DR 18 bp	?	*leuX*	60
E. coli E2348/69 (EPEC)	O127:H6	LEE	Type III secretion, invasion	35	No DR	No	*selC*	40
E. coli RW1374 (STEC)	O·03:H2	LEE	Type III secretion, invasion, parts of the *she* PAI (*S. flexneri* 2a)	>80	?	No	*pheV*	68
E. coli (EPEC and EHEC)	O111:H8 O111:H− O26:H11 O26:H−	LEE	Type III secretion, invasion	?	?	?	*pheU*	128
E. coli EDL933 (EHEC)	O157:H7	LEE (01#148)	Type III secretion, invasion	43	No DR	CP4-like	*selC*	104
E. coli RDEC-1 (REPEC)	O15:H−	LEE	Type III secretion, invasion, put. adhesin	?	No DR	P4-like	*pheU*	147
E. coli 83/39 (REPEC)	O15:H−	LEE	Type III secretion, invasion, put. adhesin, enterotoxin	59.5	No DR	P4-like	*pheU*	133

Table 2 continues

TABLE 2 Pathogenicity islands (PAIs) or PAI-like structures of pathogenic enterobacteria[a] *(Continued)*

Organism	Serotype	Designation	Encoded traits	Size (kb)	Junction	Integrase	Insertion site	Reference(s)
E. coli 84/110-1 (REPEC)	O103:H2	LEE	Type III secretion, invasion	~85	DR 23 bp (imperfect)	P4-like	*pheV*	133
E. coli E2348/69 (EPEC)	O127:H7	EspC-PAI	Autotransporter/enterotoxin	15.2	No DR	No	*sstA*	91
E. coli 135/12 (EPEC)	O55:H⁻	EPEC Afa-PAI	Diffuse adherence adhesin	>11	?	P4-like	*pheV*	74
E. coli (EHEC)	O91:H⁻	Locus of proteolysis activity (LPA)	Serine protease (Espl), vitamin B_{12} receptor (BtuB), adhesin	33	No DR	CP4-like	*selC*	120
E. coli 10407 (ETEC)	O78:H11	TPAI-I	Invasion	46	DR 25 bp	Yes	*selC*	43
Pathogenic *E. coli*, non-pathogenic *Salmonella*		HPI (PAI IV$_{536}$)	Yersiniabactin synthesis, transport	31–43	No DR ?	P4-like	*asnT*	7,73,101,123
Yersinia enterocolitica Ye8081		HPI	Yersiniabactin synthesis, transport	45	DR 17 bp	P4-like	*asnT*	25
Y. pseudotuberculosis		HPI	Yersiniabactin synthesis, transport	36	DR 17 bp	P4-like	*asnT, asnU, asnW*	18
Y. pestis		HPI (*pgm* locus)	Yersiniabactin synthesis, transport, hemin uptake	102	IS *100* DR 17 bp	P4-like	*asnT*	19
Shigella flexneri		SHI-1 (*she*)	Enterotoxin (Set), protease (Pic)	46.6	DR 22 bp (imperfect)	P4-like	*pheV*	108
S. flexneri		SHI-2	Aerobactin synthesis, colicin V immunity	23–30	No DR	CP4-like	*selC*	96,137
S. flexneri		*Shigella* resistance locus (SRL)	Ferric dicitrate transport, antibiotic resistances	66	DR 14 bp	Yes	*serX*	85
S. flexneri		Shi-O	Genes involved in serotype conversion	11	No DR	Yes	*thrW*	2
Salmonella enterica sv. Typhimurium		SPI-1	Type III secretion, invasion into epithelial cells, apoptosis	40	No DR	No	Between *fhlA* and *mutS*	93
S. enterica		SPI-2	Type III secretion, invasion into monocytes	40	No DR	No	*valV*	56
S. enterica		SPI-3	Invasion, survival in macrophages	17	No DR	No	*selC*	11
S. enterica		SPI-4	Invasion, survival in monocytes	25	No DR	No	Put.tRNA gene	143
S. enterica		SPI-5	SPI-1 effector protein (SopB)	7	No DR	No	*serT*	59,144

[a]DR, direct repeat; ND, not determined; Put., putative; UPEC, uropathogenic *E. coli*; EPEC, enteropathogenic *E. coli*; EHEC, enterohemorrhagic *E. coli*; STEC, Shiga toxin-producing *E. coli*; REPEC, rabbit-specific enteropathogenic *E. coli*; ETEC, enterotoxigenic *E. coli*.

evolution of the different islands from precursors carrying the conserved integration module. Additional analysis of PAI-specific DNA sequences revealed the presence of regions with similarity to phage- and/or plasmid-related genes or sequences (27, 36, 64), which is another hint that PAIs may have evolved from other mobile genetic elements. A relation of PAIs and plasmids is corroborated by the fact that island-encoded properties have been located on plasmids in related species or a different isolate of the same species. Examples are aerobactin-encoding genes that are often part of plasmids that additionally encode colicin ColV. As the *aer* genes of *Shigella* island SHI-2 are associated with regions of sequence homology to ColV-specific genes, parts of SHI-2 may have evolved from an integrating plasmid (96, 137). Similarly, the *vap* region has been found to be plasmid encoded in a clinical isolate of *Dichelobacter nodosus*. Based on these findings, a model for the evolution of the *vap* genomic island has been proposed that involves integration of a plasmid and subsequent rearrangements (10).

However, in contrast to plasmids or phages that are able to mediate their own replication and can be actively transferred among populations, thereby playing an important role in the fast adaptation to changing environmental conditions, the acquisition mechanisms of PAIs are not well understood. As already discussed, SaPI1 and VPI are two examples of PAIs that are still mobilizable by means of transduction. Alternatively, some PAIs may have been acquired by mechanisms related to conjugation. In the last few years, an increasing number of elements (termed "conjugative transposons," "integrative conjugative elements," or "conjugative genomic islands") have been discovered in gram-negative and -positive bacteria that are normally integrated in the chromosome, but can excise in a precise manner to be subsequently transferred to recipient cells by conjugation (reviewed in references 22, 118, and 124). In gram-negative bacteria, some of these elements exhibit several features reminiscent of PAIs, including a site-specific recombi-

nase and the lack of autonomous replication (Table 1). In contrast to PAIs, they carry genes required for mating-pair formation and conjugative DNA metabolism that are related to plasmid-encoded conjugation systems (7a, 13a). An integrative conjugative elements as a putative progenitor of the HPI has been recently identified by Schubert and coworkers (122). This HPI derivative from an *E. coli* isolate carries an additional 35-kb region with similarity to conjugation genes.

PAIs, Transposons, IS Elements, and Integrons

IS elements contribute to genome variability by several means. First, they mediate DNA rearrangements by transpositional events as well as by homologous recombination between multiple copies of the same IS element within one genome. Second, IS elements can modulate fast changes in gene activity by reversible excision and integration events into target sequences within coding regions. Finally, they are involved in the mobilization of genetic information due to association and dissociation of chromosomal DNA segments to and from natural vectors such as plasmids (31).

Whereas some PAIs have a very compact structure, others possess a high percentage of regions that are related to sequences common to IS elements or transposons. For example, SHI-2 of *S. flexneri* contains numerous partial or complete IS elements that are clustered within the island and that are thought to have been involved in the assembly of the island as a unit, or, more likely, in a stepwise fashion. Additionally, variations within a PAI are often based on diverging types and numbers of IS elements present within the island (96, 137).

The finding that identical or closely related virulence genes can be associated with different types of genetic elements has raised the possibility that they are part of transposons enabling intermolecular transfer. However, location on a transposon has only been published for the *E. coli*-specific ST enterotoxin genes (127). Nevertheless, other virulence genes (e.g., those encoding α-hemolysin and cytotoxic necrotizing factor 1) are located next to IS elements, suggesting that they have been acquired by transposition events (reviewed in reference 38).

Integrons represent gene expression elements that are able to capture promoterless gene cassettes by site-specific recombination (Table 1). They have been shown to be important means for the propagation of antibiotic resistance genes (53) and are frequently associated with transposons and conjugative plasmids that mediate their spread. In addition to these resistance-mediating integrons, superintegrons occupy large regions in the chromosomes of several bacteria (88, 115). These may represent reservoirs of gene cassettes that can become part of integrons associated with mobile genetic elements. For example, a hemaglutinin determinant has been found to be associated with the superintegron that is part of the smaller of the two chromosomes of *V. cholerae* (88). Even though many PAIs are associated with site-specific recombinases, integron-like structures have not been located yet on PAIs. Further investigations will show whether integrons may have been a means of gene acquisition by PAIs.

Islands and Islets

Some bacterial pathogens carry insertions of smaller pieces of DNA that encode virulence-associated genes and that have been termed "pathogenicity islets" in contrast to the larger PAIs (129). Similar to PAIs, pathogenicity islets exhibit a G+C content that differs from the base composition of the core genome, and they are often flanked by DRs. These features suggest that the corresponding virulence genes have been introduced into the genome of their host by lateral gene transfer. In contrast to the islands, virulence genes on islets are generally not connected with a larger number of additional genes including mobility functions. Islets are typically found in the genomes of bacteria that have the capacity to take up DNA from the environment via natural transformation (e.g., *H. pylori, Streptococcus* spp., *Neisseria* spp.) and that may introduce preferentially small pieces of

DNA into the genome. Furthermore, discussion has focused on whether some islets may have derived from larger islands that have undergone severe deletion events.

Only a few examples of islets will be discussed here. In *Streptococcus pyogenes*, a 6-kb region encoding a C5a peptidase and M and M-like proteins has been identified that exhibits features of an islet (106). Several islets have been identified in the genome of *S. enterica* that seem to be required for full virulence (reviewed in reference 45): the 1.6-kb *sifA* region is flanked by 14-bp DRs and is inserted between the *potB* and *potC* genes at 27 min of the chromosome. At 41%, the G+C content of the *sifA* locus is significantly lower than that of the core genome, and the region is absent from the chromosome of nonpathogenic enteric bacteria. A region at 25 min comprises two putative virulence genes, *msgA* and *pagC*.

PATHOGENICITY ISLANDS AND THE EVOLUTION OF MICROBES

PAIs in Gram-Negative Human Pathogens

PAIs represent characteristic features of many gram-negative pathogens and seem to play a profound role in the evolution of different variants or pathotypes. These genetic entities were initially described in gram-negative organisms, and the current definition of PAIs results from these findings (52). In gram-negative microbes, a considerable fraction of the entire genome represents PAIs with significant structural and functional diversity. There are hardly any pathogenic enterobacterial species with only one PAI per strain, and the number of multiple PAIs detected in individual isolates is constantly increasing (46, 69, 79, 132). This situation is also corroborated by complete genome sequences confirming that even higher numbers of PAIs or PAI-like structures can be found in different gram-negative bacteria: in pathogenic *E. coli* strains, up to 13 PAI-like genetic entities have been identified in one strain (104, 139). In *S. enterica* serovar Typhimurium LT2, 15 PAI-like regions are associated with tRNA-encoding genes and 7 of them also carry a bacteriophage integrase gene (89), whereas in *S. enterica* serovar Typhi CT18, at least 5 more PAI-like regions have been detected in addition to the already described 5 SPIs (103). Nine chromosomal regions of *Y. pestis,* including the HPI, and eight regions in *S. flexneri* 2a exhibit some features of PAIs (33, 65). Lists of known PAIs of enterobacteria and other gram-negative pathogens (such as *V. cholerae, H. pylori,* or *N. gonorrhoeae*) are presented in Tables 2 and 3; some have already been discussed earlier in this chapter.

The growing sequence information on PAIs of different gram-negative species demonstrates that horizontal gene transfer and homologous recombination play pivotal roles in evolution of PAIs and enterobacteria. Based on the diseases that are caused by pathogenic *E. coli,* they have been classified into different pathotypes such as EPEC, EHEC, and UPEC, as well as enterotoxigenic and enteroinvasive *E. coli* (for a recent review, see reference 71). They are characterized by the presence of specific virulence factors that enable them to exploit new niches in their host and to change the normal host physiology. Many of these key virulence factors are located on PAIs of pathogenic *E. coli* or *Shigella* species, which underscores that the acquisition of PAIs has been an important step in the evolution of virulent variants from a benign ancestor. Whereas some types of PAIs are closely linked to certain pathotypes, the comparison of PAIs in enterobacteria reveals that identical or almost identical PAIs can also be detected in different enterobacterial species, pathotypes, or strains. Typical examples are the HPIs of pathogenic yersiniae and the LEE in EHEC and EPEC. HPI-related elements seem to be widely spread among *Enterobacteriaceae* because they have been identified in various pathotypes of *E. coli,* in *Citrobacter* and *Klebsiella* spp., in some *Salmonella* spp., and even in commensal *E. coli* isolates, where they contribute to the fitness of these organisms as well as to their adaptability to particular environments (7, 73, 101, 123). However, although many PAIs superficially

resemble each other with respect to the presence and/or genetic linkage of certain virulence determinants, a great variability exists with regard to PAI composition, structural organization, and chromosomal localization even among strains of the same patho- or serotype. Typical virulence factors of UPEC strains include the pore-forming toxin α-hemolysin, fimbrial adhesins, iron uptake systems, and capsule determinants, and these traits are encoded by PAIs that are similar to each other but not identical in different strains (36, 46, 67, 112). Interestingly, fimbrial gene clusters of UPEC strains are often linked to toxin genes, suggesting a coevolution of these two factors (13).

Another interesting aspect of PAI evolution may also be duplication of entire islands. The genome of the EHEC O157:H7 strain EDL933 contains two PAI-like structures (the so-called O-islands 43 and 48) inserted next to the *serW* and *serX* tRNA-encoding genes, which comprise 106 genes and include those for tellurite resistance and urease production (104). The sepsis strain AL862 carries two 61-kb PAIs that are located at *pheV* and *pheU* and contain the afimbrial adhesin variant 8 (*afa8*) gene cluster. Whether they are truly the result of a duplication event will have to be confirmed by sequence determination of both islands (79).

Similar to *E. coli,* the acquisition of PAIs has also been an important prerequisite for the pathogenic lifestyle of *Salmonella* species (45). Whereas SPI-1 of *Salmonella* is very ancient and has become a stable part of the chromosome, other islands such as SPI-3 still undergo evolutionary changes due to insertion of IS elements or retron phages (4).

Another example how PAIs have contributed to the formation of bacterial pathogens is the *cag* island of *H. pylori* (26). This island is prevalently found in type I strains that are associated with severe forms of gastroduodenal disease. The encoded type IV secretion apparatus delivers the CagA protein into host cells, where it induces growth changes typically observed in infections with type I strains (125).

TABLE 3 PAIs of other gram-negative bacteria

Organism	Designation	Encoded traits	Size (kb)	Junction[a]	Integrase	Insertion site	Reference
Vibrio cholerae	VPI-1	Type IV pilus (TCP), regulator	39.5	DR 30 bp	CP4-57 like	*ssrA*	72
V. cholerae	VPI-2	Neuraminidase	57	DR 7 bp	Yes	tRNA (Ser)	64
Helicobacter pylori	*cag* PAI	Type IV secretion, Cag antigen	37	DR 31 bp	No	*glr*	26
Neisseria gonorrhoeae	*atlA* locus	Serum resistance, cytotoxin	60–70	?	?	?	34
Bordetella pertussis	*ptx-ptl* locus	Pertussis toxin		No DR	No	tRNA (Asp)	5
Dichelobacter nodosus	*intA* region (*vap* regions 1 and 3)	Vap proteins	15	DR 19 bp	CP4-like	tRNA (Ser)	12
D. nodosus	*vrl* region	Vrl proteins	27	No DR	No	*ssrA*	9
Pseudomonas aeruginosa X24509	PAGI-1	Detoxification of reative oxygen species?	49	?	No	PA02217	80
Erwinia amylovora Ea321	*hrp* PAI	Type III secretion, effectors	~60	?	Yes	*pheV*	75
Pseudomonas syringae	*hrp* PAI	Type III secretion, effectors	~50	?	No	tRNA (Leu)	3, 30
Xanthomonas campestris pv. vesicatoria	*hrp* PAI	Type III secretion, effectors	~35	?	No	tRNA (Arg)	97

[a]DR, direct repeat.

PAIs in Gram-Positive Human Pathogens

PAIs that fulfill all the criteria defined for gram-negative bacteria are not as prevalent in gram-positive pathogens (reviewed in reference 52). Several hallmarks of gram-negative PAIs, such as flanking DRs, mobility genes (integrases, transposases, IS elements), and association with tRNA-encoding genes, are frequently absent from many PAI-like chromosomal regions of gram-positive pathogens. Bacteriophages, conjugative plasmids, and transposons seem to contribute more to evolution and genetic diversity than the PAI type of mobile genetic element. However, several examples of PAIs have been described, especially in *S. aureus* (98). In the complete genome sequences of *S. aureus* strains N315 and Mu50, three and four PAI-like regions (respectively) coding for toxins are detectable. Hiramatsu and coworkers argued that different families of PAIs exist in human and animal isolates that can be distinguished by the toxin type(s) encoded on these islands (e.g., toxic shock syndrome toxin 1 islands, exotoxin islands, and enterotoxin islands) (78). Other predominantly toxin-encoding PAI-like structures can be detected in pathogenic *Listeria* species, *Clostridium difficile,* and *Enterococcus faecalis*. In *Streptococcus pneumoniae*, a PAI-like genomic region contains genes coding for an ABC transporter involved in iron uptake (17). PAIs and PAI-like structures of gram-positive pathogens are listed in Table 4. Whereas the experimentally investigated staphylococcal PAIs seem to represent defective prophages that can be mobilized by different helper phages (82), the PAI described in *E. faecalis* meets most of the criteria of PAIs in gram-negative organisms.

PAIs in Veterinary and Plant Pathogens

PAIs should exist not only in human pathogens, but also in veterinary and plant pathogenic microbes. However, detailed knowledge on PAIs is so far mainly restricted to human isolates of pathogenic bacteria, some of which can also cause disease in animals. The best studied example of this is *E. coli*. Numerous *E. coli* vari-

ants belong to the commensal intestinal flora, whereas other subtypes are responsible for intestinal and extraintestinal infection in humans and many animals. Extraintestinal pathogenic *E. coli* (ExPEC) include UPEC, which cause urinary tract infections in humans, dogs, and cats, as well as *E. coli* strains associated with newborn meningitis or with septicemia in humans and other animals. Avian pathogenic *E. coli* resemble human ExPEC in their virulence factor repertoire. Although complete PAI structures of animal ExPEC variants have not been described so far, typical ExPEC virulence factors such as toxins (e.g., α-hemolysin, cytotoxic necrotizing factor 1, and cytolethal distending toxin), adhesins (e.g., type 1, S, and P fimbriae; afimbrial adhesins), proteases, siderophore systems, and capsules commonly encoded on PAIs of human ExPEC isolates are also expressed in animal pathogenic *E. coli* isolates (1, 44). That (i) several of these determinants are frequently combined on PAIs or plasmids, (ii) extraintestinal infection in humans and animals requires similar or even identical virulence mechanisms, and (iii) extraintestinal diseases such as urinary tract infection in humans, dogs, and cats may be caused by identical ExPEC clones (66, 140) imply that genomic regions with features typical of human ExPEC PAIs also exist in animal pathogenic strains. It is conceivable that these islands, although superficially similar to PAIs already isolated from human ExPEC, will also exhibit considerable diversity with regard to gene content and structural organization. One exciting question is whether animal ExPEC-specific genetic information determining host specificity can be identified or this is the result of more minor sequence variations leading to different receptor specificities, differences in regulation of gene expression, or specific virulence factor combinations. With regard to intestinal *E. coli* pathotypes, several adhesin determinants have been described that are absent from ExPEC (see also Table 2). Their chromosomal sequence context is often unknown. The LEE PAI has also been detected in several EHEC and EPEC isolates that can cause diarrhea in rabbits and shows some

TABLE 4 PAIs of gram-positive bacteria

Organism	Designation	Encoded traits	Size (kb)	Junction[a]	Integrase	Insertion site	Reference
Staphylococcus aureus RN4282	SapI1	Toxic shock syndrome toxin 1 (TSST-1)	15	DR 17 bp	Yes	Near *tyrB*	82
S. aureus RN3984	SapI2	TSST-1	?	?	?	Near *trp* gene cluster	82
S. aureus COL	SapI3	Enterotoxin serotypes B, K, Q	16	DR 17 bp	Yes	?	146
S. aureus RF122	SaPIbov	TSST-1, enterotoxin C	16	DR 74 bp	?	Intergenic	42
S. aureus TY114	*etd* PAI	Exfoliative toxin D, glutamyl endopeptidase	15	DR 5 bp	No	Intergenic	145
Enterococcus faecalis	*E. faecalis* PAI	Cytolysin, surface protein (Esp), aggregation substance	~150	DR 10 bp	Yes	Intergenic	126
Clostridium difficile	Pathogenicity locus (PaLoc)	Enterotoxin (TcdA), cytotoxin (TcdB)	19	No DR	No	Intergenic	16
Streptococcus pneumoniae, pathogenic *Listeria*	PPI1	Iron uptake system	27	No DR	Recombinase	*yefA*	17
	LIPI-1	PrfA-dependent virulence gene cluster (phospholipases, listeriolysin, ActA)	9	No DR	No	Intergenic	77
Listeria ivanovii	LIPI-2	Internalins, sphingomyelinase C	22	No DR	No	Intergenic	77

[a]DR, direct repeat.

96

variation with regard to size, gene content, and chromosomal insertion site in these isolates (128, 133, 147; see also Table 2). This suggests that LEE-like islands have been acquired independently more than one time. Similarly, members of the same PAI family can be detected in human and bovine isolates of *S. aureus* (78).

Knowledge of PAI-like structures in true animal pathogenic bacteria is scarce. The best known example is *D. nodosus,* the causative agent of foot rot in sheep and other ruminants. Two different genomic loci that are only present in virulent isolates of *D. nodosus* have been described. The 27.1-kb *vrl* region (9) differs with regard to G+C content from that of the host chromosome and is inserted into the end of the *ssrA* gene (55). Several of the *vrl*-encoded proteins have similarity to phage- or plasmid-encoded proteins; however, none of the genes located within this region is homologous to known virulence genes and none of their gene products has been recognized in experimental infection or vaccination studies (9). The *vap* regions represent PAI-like structures as well. Model strain A198 contains three copies. Two of them are juxtaposed on the chromosome and form the so-called *intA* element (141). They are chromosomally inserted into tRNA-encoding genes and encode an integrase, but they are not exclusively present in pathogenic *D. nodosus* strains and do not carry any known virulence-associated gene or contribute to virulence. Without further proof of their importance for virulence of *D. nodosus,* they may be rather considered as genomic islands, which will be discussed further below.

Several gram-negative plant pathogens use type III secretion systems to affect properties of the plant cells. The corresponding determinant belongs to a group of so-called *hrp* (hypersensitive response) or *hrc* (hypersensitive response and conserved) genes, which induce a plant tissue defense line including programmed cell death. The *hrp/hrc* gene clusters of plant pathogenic enterobacteria are closely related and form PAI-like genomic regions (reviewed in reference 75) that can be located on the chromosome but also on plasmids. They encode the type III apparatus as well as effector proteins secreted by the type III system and are frequently flanked by other regions coding for virulence-associated genes (3, 8, 23, 30, 32, 63, 97). Several homologues of virulence genes of human pathogens have been detected in complete genome sequencing projects of plant pathogens (117, 136). In the case of *Ralstonia solanacearum,* 93 alternative codon usage regions have been described whose G+C content differs more or less from that of the rest of the chromosome. Five of them have typical features of PAIs, including the presence of mobility- and virulence-associated genes as well as the association with tRNA-encoding genes or prophage sequences. These alternative codon usage regions contain not only the *hrp/hrc* gene cluster but also other putative ORFs coding for virulence factors described in human pathogens, such as hemagglutinin-like proteins (117).

PAIs and Genomic Islands

The number of PAIs and PAI-like structures described as distinct genetic entities in pathogenic bacteria is constantly increasing. Additionally, the growing knowledge of genetic diversity and whole-genome organization in bacteria shows that PAIs represent a subtype of a more general genetic element, termed a "genomic island" (GEI), that is widespread among pathogenic and nonpathogenic microbes (52). These findings mirror the importance of horizontal gene transfer as well as of gene acquisition and genome reduction events as fundamental mechanisms involved in evolution of bacterial variants. GEIs are part of the flexible gene pool and carry selfish genes (e.g., genes involved in recombination and transfer or modification/restriction of DNA), but also determinants that may be beneficial under certain conditions, thus increasing bacterial fitness and consequently their survival or transmission (Table 5). These islands can be divided into different subtypes depending on their contribution to the lifestyle of the microbe. If GEIs encode virulence-associated factors, they can be called "pathogenicity islands." "Symbiosis islands," "ecological islands," or "resistance islands" provide traits required for interaction with hosts or adaptation to specific growth conditions (39, 49). In some cases, GEIs can belong to different functional subtypes depending on the genetic background of the organism they are residing in, the ecological habitat of the host, and the genetic information carried on the island itself. The HPI of yersiniae is a "broad-host-range GEI" present in many pathogenic and nonpathogenic enterobacteria. Whereas it can be considered as a PAI in bacterial pathogens, it may be an "ecological" or "saprophytic" island in fecal *E. coli, Klebsiella* spp., or nonpathogenic *S. enterica* spp. (7, 101, 123). Type III secretion systems can be encoded on PAIs in pathogens that affect processes of eukaryotic cells (pathogenic salmonellae, shigellae, yersiniae, EHEC, EPEC, plant pathogens) but also can be encoded on a symbiosis island in, for example, *Sinorhizobium fredii*. Other GEIs carry genes required for resistance to antibiotics (the *mecA* locus in staphylococci and the NR1-like plasmid in *S. flexneri*), nitrogen fixation (*Mesorhizobium meliloti*), degradation of phenolic compounds (pseudomonads),

or sucrose uptake (*Salmonella senftenberg*) (58, 62, 111, 130).

Selection Criteria for PAIs and GEIs

According to Charles Darwin, an increase of fitness is the result of progressing evolution. If bacterial fitness is defined as properties that enhance survival and transmission of an organism within a specific niche (107), the evolutionary advantage of GEIs is that large numbers of genes (e.g., entire operons that confer new traits) may be horizontally transferred into the recipient's genome, resulting in dramatic changes of this strain's characteristics. This process has been termed "evolution in quantum leaps" (41). Accordingly, genomic or fitness islands may provide a selective advantage for the microbe under specific growth conditions as they may enhance transmission, colonization, or survival within a niche (107). Therefore, GEIs whose encoded traits increase directly or indirectly the adaptational capacity of their bacterial host underlie positive selection. Selected islands may be kept within the genome by inactivation or loss of mobility genes, resulting in immobilized variants of former mobile genetic

TABLE 5 Genomic islands (GEIs) and their encoded functions[a]

Organism	GEI subtype	Encoded traits	Reference(s)	Homologous PAIs
Fecal *Escherichia coli*	SAI	Iron uptake (yersiniabactin)	7, 123	HPI in pathogenic *Yersinia* spp., and pathogenic *E. coli*
Klebsiella spp.	ECI	Iron uptake (yersiniabactin)	7	
Salmonella enterica subgroups III and VI	ECI	Iron uptake (yersiniabactin)	101	
Fecal *E. coli*	SAI	Adhesins (F1C)	35	PAIs of uropathogenic *E. coli*
Salmonella enterica	ECI	Multidrug resistance	14	
Shigella flexneri	ECI	Multidrug resistance	108	
Staphylococcus aureus	ECI	Antibiotic resistance (MecA)	57, 61, 62	
Mesorhizobium meliloti	SYI	Nitrogen fixation	130, 131	
Pseudomonas putida	ECI	Degradation of phenolic compounds	135	
Salmonella senftenberg	ECI	Sucrose uptake and degradation	58	
Sinorhizobium fredii	SYI	Type III secretion system	86	PAIs of pathogenic enterobacteria and plant pathogenic bacteria

[a]PAI, pathogenicity island; SAI, saprophytic island; ECI, ecological island; SYI, symbiosis island; HPI, high-pathogenicity island.

elements (bacteriophages, plasmids, conjugative transposons) that may undergo further recombination processes.

PAIs in Nonpathogenic Organisms

As GEIs are grouped according to their effects within a specific organism living in a specific niche and not because of their encoded traits, they can be regarded as ecological islands when the bacterium lives in the environment, but also as PAIs if this organism enters a host and causes infection. Good examples for GEIs with a dual function are those carrying siderophore determinants (e.g., the HPI [see above]) or gene clusters coding for adhesins. Iron uptake systems can serve as fitness factors and promote cellular metabolism under iron-limiting conditions, either in the environment or in a host. In the latter case, the siderophore system serves as an additional virulence factor. In *E. coli*, GEIs coding for fimbrial adhesins (e.g., members of the P- and S-adhesin families) can be detected in commensal strains of the normal intestinal microflora, where they increase the ability to colonize the intestine. If these intestinal strains enter the urinary tract, the adhesins can also be involved in colonization of the new niche, thus promoting an infection. In this case, the corresponding GEI would be regarded as a PAI, although it has not originally been selected for increased colonization ability of this new niche.

GEIs have been described for more than 30 microbial species, and the ongoing discussion of their properties and definition as well as their significance for microbial evolution is reflected in this chapter. From our point of view, GEIs represent formerly transferred or still mobile genetic entities that have evolved from horizontal gene transfer and DNA recombination events. They are important factors for bacterial evolution and will contribute to an ongoing evolution of bacterial variants, including bacterial pathogens.

CONCLUSION

There is a wealth of evidence that evolution of pathogenic variants in several bacterial species results from the acquisition of defined genetic elements, some of which are self-transmissible. In addition, loss of genetic information is also involved in genetic diversification. Mobile or mobilizable genetic elements and cointegrates thereof may contribute to horizontal gene transfer and consequently to evolution of pathogens. The occurrence and genetic organization of PAIs mirror the importance of gene acquisition and genome reduction events for bacterial evolution as they exhibit several features of horizontally transferred as well as of accessory genetic elements. PAIs represent a subtype of distinct genetic entities designated genomic islands (GEIs) that may contribute to rapid evolution of new bacterial variants. GEI mobilization and horizontal gene transfer as well as continous reorganization of GEIs by recombination (e.g., mediated by multiple fragments of accessory DNA elements present on one or multiple GEIs) contribute to ongoing evolution of bacterial variants.

CHAPTER SUMMARY

- PAIs are large genomic regions that carry one or more virulence-associated genes, are flanked by direct repeats, and are frequently linked to tRNA genes. They are thought to have been acquired by horizontal gene transfer because their G+C content generally differs from that of the core genome, they may carry mobility genes such as integrases and transposases, and they are often unstable.

- PAIs that fulfill most of these criteria have been identified in the genomes of various gram-negative as well as gram-positive bacterial pathogens and may encode some of the key virulence factors of their respective hosts.

- Besides PAIs, an increasing number of related elements is found in the genome of pathogenic and nonpathogenic bacteria that have been termed "genomic islands" (GEIs). Depending on their encoded traits and their contribution to the adaptation of their host to its respective environment, GEIs can be divided into different subtypes, including PAIs.

- PAIs and GEIs in general have played an important role in evolution and formation of bacterial species. A continuous modulation of these elements due to recombination and deletion events seems to contribute to an ongoing adaptation and modification of bacterial pathogens.

REFERENCES

1. **Achtman, M., A. Mercer, B. Kusecek, A. Pohl, M. Heuzenroeder, W. Aaronson, A. Sutton, and R. P. Silver.** 1983. Six widespread bacterial clones among *Escherichia coli* K1 isolates. *Infect. Immun.* **39:**315–335.
2. **Adhikari, P., G. Allison, B. Whittle, and N. K. Verma.** 1999. Serotype 1a O-antigen modification: molecular characterization of the genes involved and their novel organization in the *Shigella flexneri* chromosome. *J. Bacteriol.* **181:** 4711–4718.
3. **Alfano, J. R., A. O. Charkowski, W. L. Deng, J. L. Badel, T. Petnicki-Ocwieja, K. van Dijk, and A. Collmer.** 2000. The *Pseudomonas syringae* Hrp pathogenicity island has a tripartite mosaic structure composed of a cluster of type III secretion genes bounded by exchangeable effector and conserved effector loci that contribute to parasitic fitness and pathogenicity in plants. *Proc. Natl. Acad. Sci. USA* **97:**4856–4861.
4. **Amavisit, P., D. Lightfoot, G. F. Browning, and P. F. Markham.** 2003. Variation between pathogenic serovars within *Salmonella* pathogenicity islands. *J. Bacteriol.* **185:**3624–3635.
5. **Antoine, R., D. Raze, and C. Locht.** 1998. The pertussis toxin locus has some features of a pathogenicity island. *Zentbl. Bakteriol.* **29**(Suppl.): 393–394.
6. **Bach, S., C. Buchrieser, M. Prentice, A. Guiyoule, T. Msadek, and E. Carniel.** 1999. The high-pathogenicity island of *Yersinia enterolytica* Ye8081 undergoes low-frequency deletion but not precise excision, suggesting recent stabilization in the genome. *Mol. Microbiol.* **67:** 5091–5099.
7. **Bach, S., A. de Almeida, and E. Carniel.** 2000. The *Yersinia* high-pathogenicity island is present in different members of the family *Enterobacteriaceae*. *FEMS Microbiol. Lett.* **183:**289–294.
7a. **Beaber, J. W., V. Burrus, B. Hochhut, and M. K. Waldor.** 2002. Comparison of SXT and R391, two conjugative integrating elements: definition of a genetic backbone for the mobilization of resistance determinants. *Cell. Mol. Life Sci.* **59:**2065–2070.
8. **Bell, K. S., A. O. Avrova, M. C. Holeva, L. Cardle, W. Morris, W. De Jong, I. K. Toth, R. Waugh, G. J. Bryan, and P. R. Birch.** 2002. Sample sequencing of a selected region of the genome of *Erwinia carotovora* subsp. atroseptica reveals candidate phytopathogenicity genes and allows comparison with *Escherichia coli*. *Microbiology* **148:**1367–1378.
9. **Billington, S. J., A. S. Huggins, P. A. Johanesen, P. K. Crellin, J. K. Cheung, M. E. Katz, C. L. Wright, V. Haring, and J. I. Rood.** 1999. Complete nucleotide sequence of the 27-kilobase virulence related locus (*vrl*) of *Dichelobacter nodosus*: evidence for extrachromosomal origin. *Infect. Immun.* **67:**1277–1286.
10. **Billington, S. J., M. Sinistaj, B. F. Cheetham, A. Ayres, E. K. Moses, M. E. Katz, and J. I. Rood.** 1996. Identification of a native *Dichelobacter nodosus* plasmid and implications for the evolution of the *vap* region. *Gene* **172:**111–116.
11. **Blanc-Potard, A. B., and E. A. Groisman.** 1997. The *Salmonella selC* locus contains a pathogenicity island mediating intramacrophage survival. *EMBO J.* **16:**5376–5385.
12. **Bloomfield, G. A., G. Whittle, M. B. McDonagh, M. E. Katz, and B. F. Cheetham.** 1997. Analysis of sequences flanking the *vap* region of *Dichelobacter nodosus*: evidence for multiple integration events, a killer system, and a new genetic element. *Microbiology* **143:**553–562.
13. **Blum, G., M. Ott, A. Lischewski, A. Ritter, H. Imrich, H. Tschäpe, and J. Hacker.** 1994. Excision of large DNA regions termed pathogenicity islands from tRNA-specific loci in the chromosome of an *Escherichia coli* wild-type pathogen. *Infect. Immun.* **62:**606–614.
13a. **Böltner, D., C. MacMahon, J. T. Pembroke, P. Strike, and A. M. Osborne.** 2002. R391: a conjugative integrating mosaic comprised of phage, plasmid, and transposon elements. *J. Bacteriol.* **184:**5158–5169.
14. **Boyd, D., G. A. Peters, A. Cloeckaert, K. S. Boumedine, E. Chaslus-Danca, H. Imberechts, and M. R. Mulvey.** 2001. Complete nucleotide sequence of a 43-kilobase genomic island associated with the multidrug resistance region of *Salmonella enterica* serovar Typhimurium DT104 and its identification in phage type DT120 and serovar Agona. *J. Bacteriol.* **183:**5725–5732.
15. **Boyd, E. F., K. E. Moyer, L. Shi, and M. K. Waldor.** 2000. Infectious CTXφ and the vibrio pathogenicity island prophage in *Vibrio mimicus*: evidence for recent horizontal transfer between *V. mimicus* and *V. cholerae*. *Infect. Immun.* **68:**1507–1513.
16. **Braun, V., T. Hundsberger, P. Leukel, M. Sauerborn, and C. von Eichel-Streiber.** 1996. Definition of the single integration site of the pathogenicity locus in *Clostridium difficile*. *Gene* **181:**29–38.
17. **Brown, J. S., S. M. Gilliland, and D. W.**

Holden. 2001. A *Streptococcus pneumoniae* pathogenicity island encoding an ABC transporter involved in iron uptake and virulence. *Mol. Microbiol.* **40:**572–585.

18. **Buchrieser, C., R. Brosch, S. Bach, A. Guiyoule, and E. Carniel.** 1998. The high-pathogenicity island of *Yersinia pseudotuberculosis* can be inserted into any of the three chromosomal *asn* tRNA genes. *Mol. Microbiol.* **30:**965–978.

19. **Buchrieser, C., M. Prentice, and E. Carniel.** 1998. The 102-kilobase unstable region of *Yersinia pestis* comprises a high-pathogenicity island linked to a pigmentation segment which undergoes internal rearrangement. *J. Bacteriol.* **180:**2321–2329.

20. **Buchrieser, C., C. Rusniok, L. Frangeul, E. Couve, A. Billault, F. Kunst, E. Carniel, and P. Glaser.** 1999. The 102-kilobase pgm locus of *Yersinia pestis:* sequence analysis and comparison of selected regions among different *Yersinia pestis* and *Yersinia pseudotuberculosis* strains. *Infect. Immun.* **67:**4851–4861.

21. **Burns, D. L.** 1999. Biochemistry of type IV secretion. *Curr. Opin. Microbiol.* **2:**25–29.

22. **Burrus, V., G. Pavlovic, B. Decaris, and G. Guédon.** 2002. Conjugative transposons: the tip of the iceberg. *Mol. Microbiol.* **46:**601–610.

23. **Buttner, D., and U. Bonas.** 2002. Getting across—bacterial type III effector proteins on their way to the plant cell. *EMBO J.* **21:**5313–5322.

24. **Carniel, E.** 2001. The *Yersinia* high-pathogenicity island: an iron-uptake island. *Microbes Infect.* **3:**561–569.

25. **Carniel, E., I. Guilvout, and M. Prentice.** 1996. Characterization of a large chromosomal "high-pathogenicity island" in biotype 1B *Yersinia enterocolitica. J. Bacteriol.* **178:**6743–6751.

26. **Censini, S., C. Lange, Z. Xiang, J. E. Crabtree, P. Ghiara, M. Borodovsky, R. Rappuoli, and A. Covacci.** 1996. cag, a pathogenicity island of *Helicobacter pylori*, encodes type-I specific and disease-associated virulence factors. *Proc. Natl. Acad. Sci. USA* **93:**14648–14653.

27. **Cheetham, B. F., and M. E. Katz.** 1995. A role for bacteriophages in the evolution and transfer of bacterial virulence determinants. *Mol. Microbiol.* **18:**201–208.

28. **Christie, P. J.** 2001. Type IV secretion: intercellular transfer of macromolecules by systems ancestrally related to conjugation machines. *Mol. Microbiol.* **40:**294–305.

29. **Cieslewicz, M., and E. Vimr.** 1997. Reduced polysialic acid capsule expression in *Escherichia coli* K1 mutants with chromosomal defects in *kpsF. Mol. Microbiol.* **26:**237–249.

30. **Collmer, A., J. L. Badel, A. O. Charkowski, W. L. Deng, D. E. Fouts, A. R. Ramos, A. H. Rehm, D. M. Anderson, O. Schneewind, K.**

van Dijk, and J. R. Alfano. 2000. *Pseudomonas syringae* Hrp type III secretion system and effector proteins. *Proc. Natl. Acad. Sci. USA* **97:**8770–8777.

31. **Craig, N. L.** 1996. Transposition, p. 2339–2362. *In* F. C. Neidhardt, R. Curtiss III, J. L. Ingraham, E. C. C. Lin, K. B. Low, B. Magasanik, W. S. Reznikoff, M. Riley, M. Schaechter, and H. E. Umbarger (ed.), Escherichia coli *and* Salmonella: *Cellular and Molecular Biology,* vol. 2. ASM Press, Washington D.C.

32. **da Silva, A. C., J. A. Ferro, F. C. Reinach, C. S. Farah, L. R. Furlan, R. B. Quaggio, C. B. Monteiro-Vitorello, M. A. Van Sluys, N. F. Almeida, L. M. Alves, A. M. do Amaral, M. C. Bertolini, L. E. Camargo, G. Camarotte, F. Cannavan, J. Cardozo, F. Chambergo, L. P. Ciapina, R. M. Cicarelli, L. L. Coutinho, J. R. Cursino-Santos, H. El-Dorry, J. B. Faria, A. J. Ferreira, R. C. Ferreira, M. I. Ferro, E. F. Formighieri, M. C. Franco, C. C. Greggio, A. Gruber, A. M. Katsuyama, L. T. Kishi, R. P. Leite, E. G. Lemos, M. V. Lemos, E. C. Locali, M. A. Machado, A. M. Madeira, N. M. Martinez-Rossi, E. C. Martins, J. Meidanis, C. F. Menck, C. Y. Miyaki, D. H. Moon, L. M. Moreira, M. T. Novo, V. K. Okura, M. C. Oliveira, V. R. Oliveira, H. A. Pereira, A. Rossi, J. A. Sena, C. Silva, R. F. de Souza, L. A. Spinola, M. A. Takita, R. E. Tamura, E. C. Teixeira, R. I. Tezza, M. Trindade dos Santos, D. Truffi, S. M. Tsai, F. F. White, J. C. Setubal, and J. P. Kitajima.** 2002. Comparison of the genomes of two *Xanthomonas* pathogens with differing host specificities. *Nature* **417:**459–463.

33. **Deng, W., V. Burland, G. Plunkett III, A. Boutin, G. F. Mayhew, P. Liss, N. T. Perna, D. J. Rose, B. Mau, S. Zhou, D. C. Schwartz, J. D. Fetherston, L. E. Lindler, R. R. Brubaker, G. V. Plano, S. C. Straley, K. A. McDonough, M. L. Nilles, J. S. Matson, F. R. Blattner, and R. D. Perry.** 2002. Genome sequence of *Yersinia pestis* KIM. *J. Bacteriol.* **184:**4601–4611.

34. **Dillard, J. P., and H. S. Seifert.** 2001. A variable genetic island specific for *Neisseria gonorrhoeae* is involved in providing DNA for natural transformation and is found more often in disseminated infection isolates. *Mol. Microbiol.* **41:**263–277.

35. **Dobrindt, U., G. Blum-Oehler, T. Hartsch, G. Gottschalk, E. Z. Ron, R. Fünfstück, and J. Hacker.** 2001. S-fimbria-encoding determinant sfa_1 is located on pathogenicity island III_{536} of uropathogenic *Escherichia coli* strain 536. *Infect. Immun.* **69:**4248–4256.

36. **Dobrindt, U., G. Blum-Oehler, G. Nagy, G. Schneider, A. Johann, G. Gottschalk, and J. Hacker.** 2002. Genetic structure and distribution

of four pathogenicity islands (PAI I$_{536}$-PAI IV$_{536}$) of uropathogenic *Escherichia coli* strain 536. *Infect. Immun.* **70:**6365–6372.

37. **Dobrindt, U., L. Emödy, I. Gentschev, W. Goebel, and J. Hacker.** 2002. Efficient expression of the α-haemolysin determinant in the uropathogenic *Escherichia coli* strain 536 requires the *leuX*-encoded tRNA$_5$^{Leu}. *Mol. Genet. Genomics* **267:**370–379.

38. **Dobrindt, U., and J. Hacker.** 1999. Plasmids, phages and pathogenicity islands: lessons on the evolution of bacterial toxins, p. 3–23. *In* J. Alouf and J. Freer (ed.), *The Comprehensive Sourcebook of Bacterial Protein Toxins.* Academic Press, New York, N.Y.

39. **Dobrindt, U., B. Hochhut, U. Hentschel, and J. Hacker.** 2004. Genomic islands in pathogenic and environmental microorganisms. *Nat. Rev. Microbiol.* **2:**414–424.

40. **Elliott, S. J., L. A. Wainwright, T. K. McDaniel, K. G. Jarvis, Y. K. Deng, L. C. Lai, B. P. McNamara, M. S. Donnenberg, and J. B. Kaper.** 1998. The complete sequence of the locus of enterocyte effacement (LEE) from enteropathogenic *Escherichia coli* E2348/69. *Mol. Microbiol.* **28:**1–4.

41. **Falkow, S.** 1996. The evolution of pathogenicity in *Escherichia, Shigella,* and *Salmonella,* p. 2723–2729. *In* F. C. Neidhardt, R. Curtiss III, J. L. Ingraham, E. C. C. Lin, K. B. Low, B. Magasanik, W. S. Reznikoff, M. Riley, M. Schaechter, and H. E. Umbarger (ed.), Escherichia coli *and* Salmonella: *Cellular and Molecular Biology,* vol. 2. ASM Press, Washington D.C.

42. **Fitzgerald, J. R., S. R. Monday, T. J. Foster, G. A. Bohach, P. J. Hartigan, W. J. Meaney, and C. J. Smyth.** 2001. Characterization of a putative pathogenicity island from bovine *Staphylococcus aureus* encoding multiple superantigens. *J. Bacteriol.* **183:**63–70.

43. **Fleckenstein, J. M., D. J. Kopecko, R. L. Warren, and E. A. Elsinghorst.** 1996. Molecular characterization of the tia invasion locus from enterotoxigenic *Escherichia coli. Infect. Immun.* **64:**2256–2265.

44. **Girardeau, J. P., L. Lalioui, A. M. Said, C. De Champs, and C. Le Bouguenec.** 2003. Extended virulence genotype of pathogenic *Escherichia coli* isolates carrying the *afa-8* operon: evidence of similarities between isolates from humans and animals with extraintestinal infections. *J. Clin. Microbiol.* **41:**218–226.

45. **Groisman, E. A., and H. Ochman.** 1997. How *Salmonella* became a pathogen. *Trends Microbiol.* **5:**343–349.

46. **Guyer, D. M., J. S. Kao, and H. L. Mobley.** 1998. Genomic analysis of a pathogenicity island in uropathogenic *Escherichia coli* CFT073: distribu-

tion of homologous sequences among isolates from patients with pyelonephritis, cystitis, and catheter-associated bacteriuria and from fecal samples. *Infect. Immun.* **66:**4411–4417.

47. **Hacker, J., L. Bender, M. Ott, J. Wingender, B. Lund, R. Marre, and W. Goebel.** 1990. Deletions of chromosomal regions coding for fimbriae and hemolysins occur *in vitro* and *in vivo* in various extraintestinal *Escherichia coli* isolates. *Microb. Pathog.* **8:**213–225.

48. **Hacker, J., G. Blum-Oehler, I. Mühldorfer, and H. Tschäpe.** 1997. Pathogenicity islands of virulent bacteria: structure, function and impact on microbial evolution. *Mol. Microbiol.* **23:**1089–1097.

49. **Hacker, J., and E. Carniel.** 2001. Ecological fitness, genomic islands and bacterial pathogenicity. *EMBO Rep.* **2:**376–381.

50. **Hacker, J., U. Hentschel, and U. Dobrindt.** 2003. Prokaryotic chromosomes and disease. *Science* **301:**790–793.

51. **Hacker, J., and J. B. Kaper.** 2000. Pathogenicity islands and the evolution of microbes. *Annu. Rev. Microbiol.* **54:**641–679.

52. **Hacker, J., and J. B. Kaper (ed.).** 2002. *Pathogenicity Islands and the Evolution of Pathogenic Microbes.* Springer, Berlin, Germany.

53. **Hall, R. M., and C. M. Collis.** 1995. Mobile gene cassettes and integrons: capture and spread of genes by site-specific recombination. *Mol. Microbiol.* **15:**593–600.

54. **Hare, J. M., and K. A. McDonough.** 1999. High-frequency RecA-dependent and -independent mechanisms of Congo red binding mutations in Yersinia pestis. *J. Bacteriol.* **181:**4896–4904.

55. **Haring, V., S. J. Billington, C. L. Wright, A. S. Huggins, M. E. Katz, and J. I. Rood.** 1995. Delineation of the virulence-related locus (*vrl*) of *Dichelobacter nodosus. Microbiology* **141:**2081–2089.

56. **Hensel, M., T. Nikolaus, and C. Egelseer.** 1999. Molecular and functional analysis indicates a mosaic structure of *Salmonella* pathogenicity island 2. *Mol. Microbiol.* **31:**489–498.

57. **Hiramatsu, K., Y. Katayama, H. Yuzawa, and T. Ito.** 2002. Molecular genetics of methicillin-resistant *Staphylococcus aureus. Int. J. Med. Microbiol.* **292:**67–74.

58. **Hochhut, B., K. Jahreis, J. W. Lengeler, and K. Schmid.** 1997. CTnscr94, a conjugative transposon found in enterobacteria. *J. Bacteriol.* **179:**2097–2102.

59. **Hong, K. H., and V. L. Miller.** 1998. Identification of a novel *Salmonella* invasion locus homologous to Shigella *ipgDE. J. Bacteriol.* **180:**1793–1802.

60. **Houdouin, V., S. Bonacorsi, N. Brahimi, O. Clermont, X. Nassif, and E. Bingen.** 2002. A uropathogenicity island contributes to the patho-

genicity of *Escherichia coli* strains that cause neonatal meningitis. *Infect. Immun.* **70**:5865–5869.

61. **Ito, T., Y. Katayama, K. Asada, N. Mori, K. Tsutsumimoto, C. Tiensasitorn, and K. Hiramatsu.** 2001. Structural comparison of three types of staphylococcal cassette chromosome *mec* integrated in the chromosome in methicillin-resistant *Staphylococcus aureus. Antimicrob. Agents Chemother.* **45**:1323–1336.

62. **Ito, T., Y. Katayama, and K. Hiramatsu.** 1999. Cloning and nucleotide sequence determination of the entire mec DNA of pre-methicillin-resistant *Staphylococcus aureus* N315. *Antimicrob. Agents Chemother.* **43**:1449–1458.

63. **Jackson, R. W., E. Athanassopoulos, G. Tsiamis, J. W. Mansfield, A. Sesma, D. L. Arnold, M. J. Gibbon, J. Murillo, J. D. Taylor, and A. Vivian.** 1999. Identification of a pathogenicity island, which contains genes for virulence and avirulence, on a large native plasmid in the bean pathogen *Pseudomonas syringae* pathovar phaseolicola. *Proc. Natl. Acad. Sci. USA* **96**:10875–10880.

64. **Jermyn, W. S., and E. F. Boyd.** 2002. Characterization of a novel *Vibrio cholerae* pathogenicity island (VPI-2) encoding neuraminidase (*nanH*) among toxigenic *Vibrio cholerae* isolates. *Microbiology* **148**:3681–3693.

65. **Jin, Q., Z. Yuan, J. Xu, Y. Wang, Y. Shen, W. Lu, J. Wang, H. Liu, J. Yang, F. Yang, X. Zhang, J. Zhang, G. Yang, H. Wu, D. Qu, J. Dong, L. Sun, Y. Xue, A. Zhao, Y. Gao, J. Zhu, B. Kan, K. Ding, S. Chen, H. Cheng, Z. Yao, B. He, R. Chen, D. Ma, B. Qiang, Y. Wen, Y. Hou, and J. Yu.** 2002. Genome sequence of *Shigella flexneri* 2a: insights into pathogenicity through comparison with genomes of *Escherichia coli* K12 and O157. *Nucleic Acids Res.* **30**:4432–4441.

66. **Johnson, J. R., N. Kaster, M. A. Kuskowski, and G. V. Ling.** 2003. Identification of urovirulence traits in *Escherichia coli* by comparison of urinary and rectal *E. coli* isolates from dogs with urinary tract infection. *J. Clin. Microbiol.* **41**:337–345.

67. **Johnson, J. R., T. T. O'Bryan, M. Kuskowski, and J. N. Maslow.** 2001. Ongoing horizontal and vertical transmission of virulence genes and *papA* alleles among *Escherichia coli* blood isolates from patients with diverse-source bacteremia. *Infect. Immun.* **69**:5363–5374.

68. **Jores, J., L. Rumer, S. Kießling, J. B. Kaper, and L. H. Wieler.** 2001. A novel locus of enterocyte effacement (LEE) pathogenicity island inserted at *pheV* in bovine shiga toxin-producing *Escherichia coli* strain O103:H2. *FEMS Microbiol. Lett.* **204**:75–79.

69. **Kao, J. S., D. M. Stucker, J. W. Warren, and H. L. Mobley.** 1997. Pathogenicity island sequences

of pyelonephritogenic *Escherichia coli* CFT073 are associated with virulent uropathogenic strains. *Infect. Immun.* **65**:2812–2820.

70. **Kaper, J. B., L. J. Gansheroff, W. R. Wachtel, and A. D. O'Brien.** 1998. Intimin-mediated adherence of shiga toxin producing *Escherichia coli* and attaching-and-effacing pathogens, p. 148–156. *In* J. B. Kaper and A. D. O'Brien (ed.), Escherichia coli *O157:H7 and Other Shiga Toxin-Producing* E. coli *Strains.* ASM Press, Washington, D.C.

71. **Kaper, J. B., J. P. Nataro, and H. L. Mobley.** 2004. Pathogenic Escherichia coli. *Nat. Rev. Microbiol.* **2**:123–140.

72. **Karaolis, D. K. R., J. A. Johnson, C. C. Bailey, E. C. Boedeker, J. B. Kaper, and P. R. Reeves.** 1998. A *Vibrio cholerae* pathogenicity island associated with epidemic and pandemic strains. *Proc. Natl. Acad. Sci. USA* **95**:3134–3139.

73. **Karch, H., S. Schubert, D. Zhang, W. Zhang, H. Schmidt, T. Olschlager, and J. Hacker.** 1999. A genomic island, termed high-pathogenicity island, is present in certain non-O157 Shiga toxin-producing *Escherichia coli* clonal lineages. *Infect. Immun.* **67**:5994–6001.

74. **Keller, R., J. G. Ordonez, R. R. de Oliveira, L. R. Trabulsi, T. J. Baldwin, and S. Knutton.** 2002. Afa, a diffuse adherence fibrillar adhesin associated with enteropathogenic *Escherichia coli*. *Infect. Immun.* **70**:2681–2689.

75. **Kim, J. F., and J. R. Alfano.** 2002. Pathogenicity islands and virulence plasmids of bacterial plant pathogens. *Curr. Top. Microbiol. Immunol.* **264**(II): 127–147.

76. **Klose, K. E.** 2001. Regulation of virulence in *Vibrio cholerae. Int. J. Med. Microbiol.* **291**:81–88.

77. **Kreft, J., J. A. Vazquez-Boland, S. Altrock, G. Dominguez-Bernal, and W. Goebel.** 2002. Pathogenicity islands and other virulence elements in *Listeria. Curr. Top. Microbiol. Immunol.* **264**(II): 109–125.

78. **Kuroda, M., T. Ohta, I. Uchiyama, T. Baba, H. Yuzawa, I. Kobayashi, L. Cui, A. Oguchi, K. Aoki, Y. Nagai, J. Lian, T. Ito, M. Kanamori, H. Matsumaru, A. Maruyama, H. Murakami, A. Hosoyama, Y. Mizutani-Ui, N. K. Takahashi, T. Sawano, R. Inoue, C. Kaito, K. Sekimizu, H. Hirakawa, S. Kuhara, S. Goto, J. Yabuzaki, M. Kanehisa, A. Yamashita, K. Oshima, K. Furuya, C. Yoshino, T. Shiba, M. Hattori, N. Ogasawara, H. Hayashi, and K. Hiramatsu.** 2001. Whole genome sequencing of methicillin-resistant *Staphylococcus aureus. Lancet* **357**:1225–1240.

79. **Lalioui, L., and C. Le Bouguenec.** 2001. *afa-8* gene cluster is carried by a pathogenicity island inserted into the tRNA(Phe) of human and bovine pathogenic *Escherichia coli* isolates. *Infect. Immun.* **69**:937–948.

80. Liang, X., X. Q. Pham, M. V. Olson, and S. Lory. 2001. Identification of a genomic island present in the majority of pathogenic isolates of *Pseudomonas aeruginosa. J. Bacteriol.* **183**: 843–853.

81. Lindqvist, B. H., G. Deho, and R. Calendar. 1993. Mechanisms of genome propagation and helper exploitation by satellite phage P4. *Microbiol. Rev.* **57**:683–702.

82. Lindsay, J. A., A. Ruzin, H. F. Ross, N. Kurepina, and R. P. Novick. 1998. The gene for toxic shock toxin is carried by a family of mobile pathogenicity islands in *Staphylococus aureus. Mol. Microbiol.* **29**:527–543.

83. Lostroh, C. P., and C. A. Lee. 2001. The *Salmonella* pathogenicity island-1 type III secretion system. *Microbes Infect.* **3**:1281–1291.

84. Lucas, R. L., and C. A. Lee. 2000. Unravelling the mysteries of virulence gene regulation in *Salmonella typhimurium. Mol. Microbiol.* **36**: 1024–1033.

85. Luck, S. N., S. A. Turner, K. Rajakumar, H. Sakellaris, and B. Adler. 2001. Ferric dicitrate transport system (Fec) of *Shigella flexneri* 2a YSH6000 is encoded on a novel pathogenicity island carrying multiple antibiotic resistance genes. *Infect. Immun.* **69**:6012–6021.

86. Marie, C., W. J. Broughton, and W. J. Deakin. 2001. *Rhizobium* type III secretion systems: legume charmers or alarmers? *Curr. Opin. Plant Biol.* **4**: 336–342.

87. Maurelli, A. T., R. E. Fernandez, C. A. Bloch, C. K. Rode, and A. Fasano. 1998. 'Black holes' and bacterial pathogenicity: a large genomic deletion that enhances virulence of *Shigella* spp. and enteroinvasive *Escherichia coli. Proc. Natl. Acad. Sci. USA* **95**:3943–3948.

88. Mazel, D., B. Dychinco, V. A. Webb, and J. Davies. 1998. A distinctive class of integron in the *Vibrio cholerae* genome. *Science* **280**:605–608.

89. McClelland, M., K. E. Sanderson, J. Spieth, S. W. Clifton, P. Latreille, L. Courtney, S. Porwollik, J. Ali, M. Dante, F. Du, S. Hou, D. Layman, S. Leonard, C. Nguyen, K. Scott, A. Holmes, N. Grewal, E. Mulvaney, E. Ryan, H. Sun, L. Florea, W. Miller, T. Stoneking, M. Nhan, R. Waterston, and R. K. Wilson. 2001. Complete genome sequence of *Salmonella enterica* serovar Typhimurium LT2. *Nature* **413**:852–856.

90. McDaniel, T. K., K. G. Jarvis, M. S. Donnersberg, and J. B. Kaper. 1995. A genetic locus of enterocyte effacement conserved among diverse enterobacterial pathogens. *Proc. Natl. Acad. USA* **92**:1664–1668.

91. Mellies, J. L., F. Navarro-Garcia, I. Okeke, J. Frederickson, J. P. Nataro, and J. B. Kaper. 2001. espC pathogenicity island of enteropathogenic *Escherichia coli* encodes an enterotoxin. *Infect. Immun.* **69**:315–324.

92. Middendorf, B., B. Hochhut, K. Leipold, U. Dobrindt, G. Blum-Oehler, and J. Hacker. 2004. Instability of pathogenicity islands in uropathogenic Escherichia coli 536. *J. Bacteriol.* **186**:3086–3096.

93. Mills, D. M., V. Bajaj, and C. A. Lee. 1995. A 40 kb chromosomal fragment encoding *Salmonella typhimurium* invasion genes is absent from the corresponding region of the *Escherichia coli* K-12 chromosome. *Mol. Microbiol.* **15**:749–759.

94. Mirold, S., W. Rabsch, M. Rohde, S. Stender, H. Tschäpe, H. Russmann, E. Igwe, and W. D. Hardt. 1999. Isolation of a temperate bacteriophage encoding the type III effector protein SopE from an epidemic *Salmonella typhimurium* strain. *Proc. Natl. Acad. Sci. USA* **96**:9845–9850.

95. Morschhäuser, J., V. Vetter, L. Emödy, and J. Hacker. 1994. Adhesin regulatory genes within large, unstable DNA regions of pathogenic *Escherichia coli*: cross-talk between different adhesin gene clusters. *Mol. Microbiol.* **11**:555–566.

96. Moss, J. E., T. J. Cardozo, A. Zychlinsky, and E. A. Groisman. 1999. The selC-associated SHI-2 pathogenicity island of *Shigella flexneri. Mol. Microbiol.* **33**:74–83.

97. Noel, L., F. Thieme, D. Nennstiel, and U. Bonas. 2002. Two novel type III-secreted proteins of *Xanthomonas campestris* pv. vesicatoria are encoded within the *hrp* pathogenicity island. *J. Bacteriol.* **184**:1340–1348.

98. Novick, R. P., P. Schlievert, and A. Ruzin. 2001. Pathogenicity and resistance islands of staphylococci. *Microbes Infect.* **3**:585–594.

99. Ochman, H., J. G. Lawrence, and E. A. Groisman. 2000. Lateral gene transfer and the nature of bacterial innovation. *Nature* **405**: 299–304.

100. Odenbreit, S., and R. Haas. 2002. *Helicobacter pylori*: impact of gene transfer and the role of the *cag* pathogenicity island for host adaptation and virulence. *Curr. Top. Microbiol. Immunol.* **264**(II): 1–22.

101. Ölschläger, T. A., D. Zhang, S. Schubert, E. Carniel, W. Rabsch, H. Karch, and J. Hacker. 2003. The high pathogenicity island is absent in human pathogens of *Salmonella enterica* subspecies I but present in isolates of subspecies III and VI. *J. Bacteriol.* **185**:1107–1111.

102. O'Shea, Y. A., and E. F. Boyd. 2002. Mobilization of the *Vibrio* pathogenicity island between *Vibrio cholerae* isolates mediated by CP-T1 generalized transduction. *FEMS Microbiol. Lett.* **214**:153–157.

103. Parkhill, J., G. Dougan, K. D. James, N. R. Thomson, D. Pickard, J. Wain, C. Churcher, K. L. Mungall, S. D. Bentley, M. T. Holden, M. Sebaihia, S. Baker, D. Basham, K. Brooks, T. Chillingworth, P. Connerton, A.

Cronin, P. Davis, R. M. Davies, L. Dowd, N. White, J. Farrar, T. Feltwell, N. Hamlin, A. Haque, T. T. Hien, S. Holroyd, K. Jagels, A. Krogh, T. S. Larsen, S. Leather, S. Moule, P. O'Gaora, C. Parry, M. Quail, K. Rutherford, M. Simmonds, J. Skelton, K. Stevens, S. Whitehead, and B. G. Barrell. 2001. Complete genome sequence of a multiple drug resistant *Salmonella enterica* serovar Typhi CT18. *Nature* **413**:848–852.

104. Perna, N. T., G. Plunkett III, V. Burland, B. Mau, J. D. Glasner, D. J. Rose, G. F. Mayhew, P. S. Evans, J. Gregor, H. A. Kirkpatrick, G. Posfai, J. Hackett, S. Klink, A. Boutin, Y. Shao, L. Miller, E. J. Grotbeck, N. W. Davis, A. Lim, E. T. Dimalanta, K. D. Potamousis, J. Apodaca, T. S. Anantharaman, J. Lin, G. Yen, D. C. Schwartz, R. A. Welch, and F. R. Blattner. 2001. Genome sequence of enterohaemorrhagic *Escherichia coli* O157:H7. *Nature* **409**:529–533.

105. Piechaczek, K., U. Dobrindt, A. Schierhorn, G. S. Fischer, M. Hecker, and J. Hacker. 2000. Influence of pathogenicity islands and the minor *leuX*-encoded tRNA$_5^{Leu}$ on the proteome pattern of the uropathogenic *Escherichia coli* strain 536. *Int. J. Med. Microbiol.* **290**:75–84.

106. Podbielski, A., M. Woischnik, B. Pohl, and K. H. Schmidt. 1996. What is the size of the group A streptococcal *vir* regulon? The Mga regulator affects expression of secreted and surface virulence factors. *Med. Microbiol. Immunol.* **185**:171–181.

107. Preston, G. M., B. Haubold, and P. B. Rainey. 1998. Bacterial genomics and adaptation to life on plants: implications for the evolution of pathogenicity and symbiosis. *Curr. Opin. Microbiol.* **1**:589–597.

108. Rajakumar, K., C. Sasakawa, and B. Adler. 1997. Use of a novel approach, termed island probing, identifies the *Shigella flexneri she* pathogenicity island which encodes a homolog of the immunoglobulin A protease-like family of proteins. *Infect. Immun.* **65**:4606–4614.

109. Rakin, A., C. Noelting, P. Schropp, and J. Heesemann. 2001. Integrative module of the high-pathogenicity island of *Yersinia*. *Mol. Microbiol.* **39**:407–415.

110. Rasko, D. A., J. A. Phillips, X. Li, and H. L. Mobley. 2001. Identification of DNA sequences from a second pathogenicity island of uropathogenic *Escherichia coli* CFT073: probes specific for uropathogenic populations. *J. Infect. Dis.* **184**:1041–1049.

111. Ravatn, R., S. Studer, A. J. Zehnder, and J. R. van der Meer. 1998. Int-B13, an unusual site-specific recombinase of the bacteriophage P4 integrase family, is responsible for chromosomal insertion of the 105-kilobase clc element of *Pseudomonas* sp. strain B13. *J. Bacteriol.* **180**:5505–5514.

112. Redford, P., and R. A. Welch. 2002. Extraintestinal *Escherichia coli* as a model system for the study of pathogenicity islands. *Curr. Top. Microbiol. Immunol.* **264**:15–30.

113. Reiter, W.-D., P. Palm, and S. Yeats. 1989. Transfer RNA genes frequently serve as integration sites for prokaryotic genetic elements. *Nucleic Acids Res.* **17**:1907–1914.

114. Ritter, A., D. L. Gally, P. B. Olsen, U. Dobrindt, A. Friedrich, P. Klemm, and J. Hacker. 1997. The PAI-associated *leuX* specific tRNA$_5^{Leu}$ affects type 1 fimbriation in pathogenic *E. coli* by control of FimB recombinase expression. *Mol. Microbiol.* **25**:871–882.

115. Rowe-Magnus, D. A., A.-M. Guerout, P. Ploncard, B. Dychinco, J. Davies, and D. Mazel. 2001. The evolutionary history of chromosomal super-integrons provides an ancestry for multiresistant integrons. *Proc. Natl. Acad. Sci. USA* **98**:652–657.

116. Ruzin, A., J. Lindsay, and R. P. Novick. 2001. Molecular genetics of SaPI1—a mobile pathogenicity island in *Staphylococcus aureus*. *Mol. Microbiol.* **41**:365–377.

117. Salanoubat, M., S. Genin, F. Artiguenave, J. Gouzy, S. Mangenot, M. Arlat, A. Billault, P. Brottier, J. C. Camus, L. Cattolico, M. Chandler, N. Choisne, C. Claudel-Renard, S. Cunnac, N. Demange, C. Gaspin, M. Lavie, A. Moisan, C. Robert, W. Saurin, T. Schiex, P. Siguier, P. Thebault, M. Whalen, P. Wincker, M. Levy, J. Weissenbach, and C. A. Boucher. 2002. Genome sequence of the plant pathogen *Ralstonia solanacearum*. *Nature* **415**:497–502.

118. Salyers, A. A., N. B. Shoemaker, A. M. Stevens, and L.-Y. Li. 1995. Conjugative transposons: an unusual and diverse set of integrated gene transfer elements. *Microbiol. Rev.* **59**:579–590.

119. Schmidt, H., and M. Hensel. 2004. Pathogenicity islands in bacterial pathogenesis. *Clin. Microbiol. Rev.* **17**:14–56.

120. Schmidt, H., W. L. Zhang, U. Hemmrich, S. Jelacic, W. Brunder, P. I. Tarr, U. Dobrindt, J. Hacker, and H. Karch. 2001. Identification and characterization of a novel genomic island integrated at *selC* in locus of enterocyte effacement-negative, Shiga toxin-producing *Escherichia coli*. *Infect. Immun.* **69**:6863–6873.

121. Schneider, G., U. Dobrindt, H. Brüggemann, G. Nagy, B. Janke, G. Blum-Oehler, C. Buchrieser, G. Gottschalk, L. Emödy, and J. Hacker. 2004. The pathogenicity island-associated K15 capsule deter-

minant exhibits a novel genetic structure and correlates with virulence in uropathogenic *Escherichia coli* strain 536. *Infect. Immun.* **72:** 5993–6001.

122. **Schubert, S., S. Dufke, J. Sorsa, and J. Heesemann.** 2004.A novel integrative and conjugative element (ICE) of Escherichia coli: the putative progenitor of the Yersinia high-pathogenicity island. *Mol. Microbiol.* **51:**837–848.

123. **Schubert, S., A. Rakin, H. Karch, E. Carniel, and J. Heesemann.** 1998. Prevalence of the 'high-pathogenicity island' of *Yersinia* species among *Escherichia coli* strains that are pathogenic to humans. *Infect. Immun.* **66:**480–485.

124. **Scott, J. R., and G. G. Churchward.** 1995. Conjugative transposition. *Annu. Rev. Microbiol.* **49:**367–397.

125. **Selbach, M., S. Moese, R. Hurwitz, C. R. Hauck, T. F. Meyer, and S. Backert.** 2003. The Helicobacter pylori CagA protein induces cortactin dephosphorylation and actin rearrangement by c-Src inactivation. *EMBO J.* **22:**515–528.

126. **Shankar, N., A. S. Baghdayan, and M. S. Gilmore.** 2002. Modulation of virulence within a pathogenicity island in vancomycin-resistant *Enterococcus faecalis. Nature* **417:**746–750.

127. **So, M., and B. J. McCarthy.** 1980. Nucleotide sequence of the bacterial transposon Tn*1681* encoding a heat-stable (ST) toxin and its identification in enterotoxigenic *Escherichia coli* strains. *Proc. Natl. Acad. Sci. USA* **77:**4011–4015.

128. **Sperandio, V., J. B. Kaper, M. R. Bortolini, B. C. Neves, R. Keller, and L. R. Trabulsi.** 1998. Characterization of the locus of enterocyte effacement (LEE) in different enteropathogenic *Escherichia coli* (EPEC) and Shiga-toxin producing *Escherichia coli* (STEC) serotypes. *FEMS Microbiol. Lett.* **164:**133–139.

129. **Stein, M. A., K. Y. Leung, M. Zwick, F. Garcia-del Portillo, and B. B. Finlay.** 1996. Identification of a *Salmonella* virulence gene required for formation of filamentous structures containing lysosomal membrane glycoproteins within epithelial cells. *Mol. Microbiol.* **20:** 151–164.

130. **Sullivan, J. T., and C. W. Ronson.** 1998. Evolution of rhizobia by acquisition of a 500 kb symbiosis island that integrates into a phe-tRNA gene. *Proc. Natl. Acad. Sci. USA* **95:**5145–5149.

131. **Sullivan, J. T., J. R. Trzebiatowski, R. W. Cruickshank, J. Gouzy, S. D. Brown, R. M. Elliot, D. J. Fleetwood, N. G. McCallum, U. Rossbach, G. S. Stuart, J. E. Weaver, R. J. Webby, F. J. De Bruijn, and C. W. Ronson.** 2002. Comparative sequence analysis of the symbiosis island of *Mesorhizobium loti* strain R7A. *J. Bacteriol.* **184:**3086–3095.

132. **Swenson, D. L., N. O. Bukanov, D. E. Berg, and R. A. Welch.** 1996. Two pathogenicity islands in uropathogenic *Escherichia coli* J96: cosmid cloning and sample sequencing. *Infect. Immun.* **64:**3736–3743.

133. **Tauschek, M., R. A. Strugnell, and R. M. Robins-Browne.** 2002. Characterization and evidence of mobilization of the LEE pathogenicity island of rabbit-specific strains of enteropathogenic *Escherichia coli. Mol. Microbiol.* **44:** 1533–1550.

134. **Tinker, J. K., and S. Clegg.** 2001. Control of FimY translation and type 1 fimbrial production by the arginine tRNA encoded by *fimU* in *Salmonella enterica* serovar Typhimurium. *Mol. Microbiol.* **40:**757–768.

135. **van der Meer, J. R., R. Ravatn, and V. Sentchilo.** 2001. The clc element of *Pseudomonas* sp. strain B13 and other mobile degradative elements employing phage-like integrases. *Arch. Microbiol.* **175:**79–85.

136. **Van Sluys, M. A., C. B. Monteiro-Vitorello, L. E. Camargo, C. F. Menck, A. C. Da Silva, J. A. Ferro, M. C. Oliveira, J. C. Setubal, J. P. Kitajima, and A. J. Simpson.** 2002. Comparative genomic analysis of plant-associated bacteria. *Annu. Rev. Phytopathol.* **40:**169–189.

137. **Vokes, S. A., S. A. Reeves, A. G. Torres, and S. M. Payne.** 1999. The aerobactin iron transport system genes in *Shigella flexneri* are present within a pathogenictiy island. *Mol. Microbiol.* **33:**63–73.

138. **Waldor, M. K., and J. J. Mekalanos.** 1996. Lysogenic conversion by a filamentous phage encoding cholera toxin. *Science* **272:**1910–1914.

139. **Welch, R. A., V. Burland, G. Plunkett III, P. Redford, P. Roesch, D. Rasko, E. L. Buckles, S. R. Liou, A. Boutin, J. Hackett, D. Stroud, G. F. Mayhew, D. J. Rose, S. Zhou, D. C. Schwartz, N. T. Perna, H. L. Mobley, M. S. Donnenberg, and F. R. Blattner.** 2002. Extensive mosaic structure revealed by the complete genome sequence of uropathogenic *Escherichia coli. Proc. Natl. Acad. Sci. USA* **99:** 17020–17024.

140. **Whittam, T. S., M. L. Wolfe, and R. A. Wilson.** 1989. Genetic relationships among *Escherichia coli* isolates causing urinary tract infections in humans and animals. *Epidemiol. Infect.* **102:**37–46.

141. **Whittle, G., G. A. Bloomfield, M. E. Katz, and B. F. Cheetham.** 1999. The site-specific integration of genetic elements may modulate thermostable protease production, a virulence factor in *Dichelobacter nodosus,* the causative agent of ovine footrot. *Microbiology* **145:**2845–2855.

142. **Williams, K. P.** 2002. Integration sites for genetic elements in prokaryotic tRNA

and tmRNA genes: sublocation preference of integrase subfamilies. *Nucleic Acids Res.* **30:** 866–875.

143. **Wong, K. K., M. McClelland, L. C. Stillwell, E. C. Sisk, S. J. Thurston, and J. D. Saffer.** 1998. Identification and sequence analysis of a 27-kilobase chromosomal fragment containing a *Salmonella* pathogenicity island located at 92 minutes on the chromosome map of *Salmonella enterica* serovar Typhimurium LT2. *Infect. Immun.* **66:**3365–3371.

144. **Wood, M. W., M. A. Jones, P. R. Watson, S. Hedges, T. S. Wallis, and E. E. Galyov.** 1998. Identification of a pathogenicity island required for *Salmonella* enteropathogenicity. *Mol. Microbiol.* **29:**883–891.

145. **Yamaguchi, T., K. Nishifuji, M. Sasaki, Y. Fudaba, M. Aepfelbacher, T. Takata, M.** Ohara, H. Komatsuzawa, M. Amagai, and M. Sugai. 2002. Identification of the *Staphylococcus aureus etd* pathogenicity island which encodes a novel exfoliative toxin, ETD, and EDIN-B. *Infect. Immun.* **70:**5835–5845.

146. **Yarwood, J. M., J. K. McCormick, M. L. Paustian, P. M. Orwin, V. Kapur, and P. M. Schlievert.** 2002. Characterization and expression analysis of *Staphylococcus aureus* pathogenicity island 3. Implications for the evolution of staphylococcal pathogenicity islands. *J. Biol. Chem.* **277:**13138–13147.

147. **Zhu, C., T. S. Agin, S. J. Elliott, L. A. Johnson, T. E. Thate, J. B. Kaper, and E. C. Boedeker.** 2001. Complete nucleotide sequence and analysis of the locus of enterocyte effacement from rabbit diarrheagenic *Escherichia coli* RDEC-1. *Infect. Immun.* **69:**2107–2115.

BLACK HOLES AND ANTIVIRULENCE GENES: SELECTION FOR GENE LOSS AS PART OF THE EVOLUTION OF BACTERIAL PATHOGENS

William A. Day and Anthony T. Maurelli

6

Microbial pathogens are generally believed to have evolved from ancestral strains that were once commensal inhabitants of the hosts in which they now cause disease. Underlying this belief is the assumption that microbes, as the earliest life forms whose appearance on earth preceded plants and animals, evolved to exploit these latter life forms as novel environments to populate. At some point, variants of these commensals acquired traits that proved beneficial to the microbes but harmful for the host. In our host-centered view, these variants are no longer the peaceful, coexisting residents of higher animals and plants but pathogens to be avoided lest they cause damage or death of the host. While this viewpoint may not be universally applicable, it provides a useful starting point for studies on pathogen evolution.

Within the last 2 decades, our understanding of the mechanisms of bacterial pathogen evolution has undergone nothing short of a revolution. Several technological advances, including molecular cloning of genes encoding virulence traits and the advent of whole-genome sequencing, have fueled this revolution. These advances have permitted discovery of unexpected evolutionary mechanisms that transform benign bacteria into organisms capable of invading and surviving in host tissues, often resulting in disease. These new insights have greatly enhanced our understanding of bacterial pathogen evolution as well as mechanisms that generate new bacterial species.

In this chapter, we will discuss the concept of gene loss in the evolution of bacterial pathogens from commensals as a mechanism of fine-tuning pathogen genomes for maximal fitness in new host environments. Specifically, we will describe the nature of antivirulence genes and the pressures that drive selection for gene inactivation and examine how this process complements the mechanisms of pathogen evolution through gene acquisition discussed in other chapters of this book.

EVOLUTION OF BACTERIAL PATHOGENS FROM COMMENSALS

Shortly after the discovery of the microbial world, it was recognized that bacteria associated with disease shared numerous morphological and biochemical characteristics with nonpathogenic organisms. These characteristics included metabolic pathways shared by a number of organisms occupying a common niche (such as

William A. Day, Bacteriology Division, U.S. Army Medical Research Institute of Infectious Diseases, Fort Detrick, MD 21702. *Anthony T. Maurelli,* Department of Microbiology and Immunology, F. Edward Hébert School of Medicine, Uniformed Services University of the Health Sciences, Bethesda, MD 20814-4799.

the mammalian intestine) as well as other characteristics that were expressed by a narrower population. Clustering of organisms based on these natural characteristics provided an early framework that illustrated the apparent close relationship of bacteria with very different virulence potentials. These relationships were further supported by studies that used methods including sequence analysis of 16S ribosomal RNA genes, gene linkage analysis, and electrophoretic analysis of enzymes involved in widely shared biochemical reactions. For example, these characteristics in four *Shigella* species, all of which are pathogens that cause bacillary dysentery, are nearly identical to those of nonpathogenic *Escherichia coli* (7). The broad matching of these genotypic and phenotypic characteristics indicates that the pathogenic shigellae are, in fact, a subset of nonpathogenic *E. coli* (29). Studies of other bacterial pathogens and their nonpathogenic relatives have revealed similar genealogies. For instance, *Bacillus anthracis,* the causative agent of anthrax, is in fact a single clone of the ubiquitous nonpathogenic soil bacterium *Bacillus cereus* (12). These observations are striking when one considers the very different virulence potentials of the two pathogens relative to their respective ancestors. *Shigella* and *B. anthracis* invade and thrive in host tissues. On the other hand, commensal bacteria cannot invade, let alone survive in, new host niches where bacteria may encounter new selective pressures such as nutrient deprivation and immune molecules and cells unique to hostile host environments. Pathogens that evolved from commensal strains must therefore have acquired new biochemical pathways and whole systems of novel traits (encoded by multiple genes) that enable access to and survival in these unique environments. Moreover, the close relationship between the pathogen and commensal bacteria suggests that virulence traits evolve rapidly, outpacing genetic drift associated with genotypic differences that define different species. This prediction was incompatible with classical views of bacterial evolution.

Bacterial evolution proceeds via mutation and selection. Only those mutations that confer a growth advantage to the organism are selected and survive within a population. For decades classical models held that, as in eucaryotes, evolution of new bacterial traits was accomplished by the slow process of random nucleotide changes in established genes. When one considers the nature of mutations, it is clear that single mutational events within a genome, whether base pair changes, deletions, or rearrangements, have a limited potential for generating completely novel phenotypic changes. These mutations may result in incremental improvements in fitness within a particular niche, but even accumulation of multiple, independent events may not be sufficient to allow an organism to colonize a new niche (24). Quite simply, this slow pathway cannot account for the rapid evolution of novel biochemical functions or complex traits observed in pathogenic bacteria derived from commensal organisms.

Horizontal transfer of blocks of genes via conjugation or transduction is a more powerful engine of evolution with the potential to radically alter the phenotypic profile of an organism in a single step. Such alterations include expressions of complex new metabolic capabilities and colonization factors that can extend the host range of an organism and improve its ability to exploit a new niche. The evolution of bacterial pathogens from their commensal ancestors is believed to occur by this type of gene acquisition that allows the organism to colonize a new ecological niche. A "quantum leap" in the evolution of a bacterium occurs when new genes are acquired en bloc via horizontal transfer of genes in the form of plasmids or bacteriophages (11). The presence of virulence genes in "pathogenicity islands" in a pathogen reflects this form of gene acquisition (16; also see chapter 5 in this volume]. Thus, horizontal gene transfer can drastically transform an organism from a benign resident of a eucaryotic host into a pathogen capable of colonizing a new niche within the host and, incidentally, causing harm to the host.

Commensal organisms that acquire new biochemical pathways and traits (e.g., virulence factors) have the potential to breach host defenses and access new niches within the host, often resulting in disease. This opportunity may present a significant advantage for the new pathogen. Microbial competition is often minimal or absent in these uncolonized tissues. Since these tissues are not normally exposed to a microbial challenge, the host may not have evolved mechanisms to restrict access to essential nutrients in these environments. Thus, if the new pathogen can survive the new selective pressures presented by host immune molecules and cells, as well as unique nutrient limitations such as iron sequestration, then the organism may multiply to sufficient numbers to guarantee transmission to another suitable niche (often a second host) and achieve evolutionary success. A new pathogen is born. However, the newly evolved pathogen, which expresses the full complement of ancestral traits as well as virulence factors, may not yet be optimally suited for this new pathogenic lifestyle.

It is simplistic to assume that gene acquisition alone is sufficient to create a successful pathogen. New pathogens often live in niches very different from those occupied by their nonpathogenic ancestors. For example, E. coli (the commensal) resides in the lumen of the colon, while Shigella (the closely related pathogen) is a facultative intracellular parasite that lives within colonic epithelial cells. B. cereus (the nonpathogenic soil organism) resides in soil, while B. anthracis (the closely related pathogen) replicates exclusively within mammalian blood and tissues. Selective pressures that shaped the ancestor for fitness in its original niche may be very different than those present in the new environment. Thus, it is very unlikely that the genome of the newly evolved pathogen is maximally fit for the new selective pressures presented by the new niche. Indeed, the evolutionary model of antagonistic pleiotrophy predicts that genes required for fitness in one niche may actually inhibit fitness in another environment that presents new selective pressures (33). Therefore, some ancestral traits may interfere with expression or function of factors required for survival within host tissues. The response to this new selective pressure is pro-

gressive adaptation by the organism to the new niche by mutation and selection for improved fitness. These modifications to the genome of the new pathogen are termed "pathoadaptive mutations." The process of pathoadaptive evolution serves as a complement to bacterial pathogen evolution by gene acquisition (39).

An important element of pathoadaptive evolution is the selection of "black holes" in pathogen genomes, that is, the inactivation or loss of genes that are incompatible with, and even antagonistic to, the new pathogenic lifestyle. These incompatible genes, which we define as antivirulence genes, are present in the genome of a nonpathogenic ancestor but absent or inactive in the pathogen (4). Deletion or mutational inactivation of antivirulence genes is strongly selected because expression of antivirulence genes in the pathogen is detrimental to expression of some virulence phenotype. Mutation of an antivirulence gene results in enhanced pathogenicity. Thus, modification of antivirulence genes allows the newly evolved pathogen to adapt to its new lifestyle and attain optimal fitness in the new host environment.

SHIGELLA AS A MODEL FOR PATHOADAPTIVE MUTATION BY GENE LOSS AND GENE INACTIVATION

Bacteria of the genus Shigella are gram-negative rods that are the causative agents of bacillary dysentery or shigellosis. The bacteria are highly host adapted and cause disease only in humans and primates. Shigella invade cells of the colonic epithelium, replicate intracellularly, spread from cell to cell, and cause abscesses and ulcerations of the intestinal lining leading to the bloody mucoid stools characteristic of dysentery. Bacterial invasion and replication also lead to an intense inflammatory response that serves both the host and the pathogen (see reference 35 for model). Studies of the virulence factors that contribute to the pathogenic makeup of Shigella have benefited from the availability of genetic tools for manipulation of the pathogen and model systems to assay different facets of virulence. For example, the capacity of *Shigella* to invade mammalian cells is measured in tissue culture monolayers, and these assays can be modified to measure intracellular replication and cell-to-cell spread as well. These features, plus its close genetic relatedness with *E. coli*, make *Shigella* an excellent model system for testing theories of pathogen evolution and pathoadaptive mutation.

As mentioned above, the four species of *Shigella* are so closely related to *E. coli* that they should be included in a single species. The chromosomes of these organisms are largely colinear, and the genomes are more than 90% homologous (2, 14). Many studies using a variety of methods have demonstrated that *Shigella* strains do not form a single subgroup of *E. coli*, as would be expected of a distinct genus, but are instead derived from separate *E. coli* strains (25, 28, 29, 32). The majority of *Shigella* strains fall into three main clusters within *E. coli* (Fig. 1), though seven different *Shigella* lineages have been identified through sequence analysis of a number of chromosomal loci (15). Therefore, the shigellae are a group of pathogenic *E. coli*.

What distinguishes *Shigella* from the non-pathogenic commensal *E. coli* is a plasmid. The hallmarks of *Shigella* virulence—invasion, intracellular replication, intercellular spread, and induction of an inflammatory response—are mediated by pathogenic determinants encoded on a large plasmid that is found in all species of *Shigella*. The clustering of these virulence genes and their low G+C content also suggest that they constitute a pathogenicity island within the plasmid. Thus, horizontal transfer of the virulence plasmid to commensal *E. coli* has occurred multiple times, on each occasion giving rise to new *Shigella* clones (29). Further evidence of independent horizontal gene transfer in the evolution of *Shigella* comes from the finding of distinct pathogenicity islands in the genomes of *S. flexneri* and *S. boydii*. Among the genes encoded on these islands are genes for an enterotoxin and an iron transport system (22, 30, 31, 40).

These findings suggest that traits unique to and shared by *Shigella* species are the result of convergent evolution driven by unique selective forces present within the new host niche (inside colonocytes) that were encountered by each newly evolved *Shigella* clone. These unique *Shigella* traits arose either through gain-of-function mutations (horizontal transfer of the virulence plasmid) or loss-of-function mutations (deletion of traits expressed by ancestral *E. coli* strains). Thus, the convergent evolution of the seven *Shigella* lineages presents a unique opportunity for the identification and study of antivirulence genes and pathoadaptive mutations as well as the study of pathogen evolution.

Antagonistic pleiotrophy predicts that ancestral traits that interfere with virulence are lost from the newly evolved pathogen genome early on as increased fitness of adapted clones fixes these beneficial mutations in the newly or recently evolved pathogen population. Therefore, traits absent in all pathogenic clones of a species, but commonly expressed in the closely related commensal ancestor species, are strong candidates for pathoadaptive mutations that have arisen by convergent evolution. Evidence in support of this new model of pathogen evolution was first provided by comparison of *Shigella* with its commensal ancestor *E. coli*. As mentioned earlier, while *Shigella* and *E. coli* share many biochemical traits, there are some characteristic markers that have proved useful over the years to differentiate *Shigella* from *E. coli*. One of these is lysine decarboxylase (LDC) activity, which is encoded by the *cadA* gene in *E. coli*. LDC is expressed in >90% of *E. coli* isolates. In contrast, none of the *Shigella* clones expresses LDC activity (7). Moreover, pathogenic enteroinvasive strains of *E. coli* that cause a disease clinically indistinguishable from dysentery caused by *Shigella* also lack LDC activity (38). Lack of LDC activity in the shigellae is consistent with the expected pattern of a pathoadaptive mutation and suggests that *cadA* may be an antivirulence gene for *Shigella*.

Experimental evidence for the antivirulence nature of the *cadA* gene was demonstrated by examination of the virulence phenotypes of a strain of *S. flexneri* 2a transformed with the *cadA*

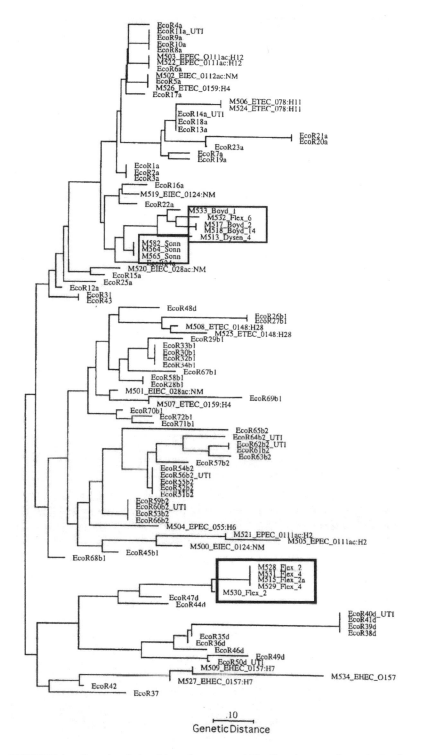

FIGURE 1 Genetic relationships of commensal *E. coli* strains to pathogenic *E. coli* strains and *Shigella*. The three major clusters of *Shigella* are shown boxed. *S. dysenteriae* serotypes 1, 8, and 10 fall outside the three main clusters (but within the population structure of *E. coli*) and are not shown on this tree. ECOR, *E. coli* reference strain. Adapted from reference 28.

gene from *E. coli* K-12. The LDC-producing *Shigella* is still invasive, but it fails to produce the wild-type level of enterotoxic activity in the rabbit ileal loop and the Ussing chamber assays (18). Further analysis showed that cadaverine, the product of the decarboxylation of lysine, is an inhibitor of the virulence plasmid-encoded *Shigella* enterotoxins. Cadaverine is also responsible for the block in the ability of an LDC-expressing *S. flexneri* to elicit transepithelial migration of polymorphonuclear neutrophils in a polarized tissue culture model system for the inflammatory response (19). This phenotype appears to be due to a failure of the bacteria to escape the phagolysosome after invasion of the polarized cells (8). Attenuation of these virulence-associated phenotypes is linked to expression of LDC and production of cadaverine in the *S. flexneri* 2a strain transformed with the *cadA* gene from *E. coli* K-12. Therefore, *cadA* behaves as an antivirulence gene for *Shigella*.

Genomic analysis suggested that the chromosomal region to which *cadA* maps in *E. coli* K-12 has undergone a large deletion in *S. flexneri* 2a (18). Sequence analysis of the *cadA* region of four *Shigella* lineages revealed novel genetic arrangements that were distinct in each strain examined (4). Insertion sequences, a phage genome, and/or loci from different positions on the ancestral *E. coli* chromosome displaced the *cadA* locus to form distinct genetic linkages unique to each *Shigella* lineage (Fig. 2). None of these novel gene arrangements was observed in representatives of all *E. coli* phylogenies. In the case of *S. boydii,* the *cadA* region is deleted and replaced with a pathogenicity island that encodes an iron uptake system (30). However, it is not possible to determine whether acquisition of the pathogenicity island occurred prior to, coincident with, or after deletion of the *cadA* antivirulence gene. Collectively, these observations indicate that inactivation of the *cadA* antivirulence gene occurred independently in each *Shigella* lineage and suggest that, following evolution from commensal *E. coli,* strong pressures in host tissues selected *Shigella* clones with increased fitness and virulence through the loss of an ancestral trait (LDC). These observations strongly support the role of pathoadaptive mutation as an important pathway in the evolution of pathogenic organisms and validate the use of *Shigella* as a model for the study of this evolutionary mechanism.

Another example of pathoadaptive mutation in *Shigella* spp. is the absence of curli expression. Curli are thin aggregative surface fibers encoded by *csg* genes that are expressed by strains of *E. coli* and *Salmonella enterica* serovar Typhimurium. Curli mediate binding to a variety of extracellular matrix proteins and the formation of biofilms on inert surfaces (27). They also mediate internalization by eucaryotic cells (9). Curli are reported to be capable of inducing an inflammatory response in sepsis. Invasive strains of bacteria tend to not produce curli. A survey of *csg* genes in all four species of *Shigella* found that the *csg* loci were disrupted by insertions or deletions in a wide variety of isolates of diverse serotypes and geographical origin (34). Even isolates of enteroinvasive *E. coli* were found to contain *csg* loci that were mutated by insertion or deletion. By contrast, curli are expressed by 60% of environmental isolates of *E. coli* (26). These observations suggest the effects of strong pathoadaptive selective pressure against expression of this surface appendage in *Shigella* and thus present the possibility that curli genes are antivirulence genes.

The *ompT* gene of *E. coli* K-12, which encodes an outer membrane protease (10), provides another example of a gene expressed by a nonpathogen that is incompatible with virulence when expressed in a pathogen. OmpT protease activity destroys the surface-expressed IcsA protein of *Shigella* when *icsA* is cloned and expressed in *E. coli* K-12 (23). IcsA is required for actin-based intracellular motility and cell-to-cell spread postinvasion (1). Introduction and expression of *ompT* from *E. coli* K-12 into *S. flexneri* abolishes cell-to-cell spread in tissue culture and the ability to produce conjunctivitis in the Sereny test (23, 36), an in vivo assay for damage caused by cell-to-cell spread of *Shigella*. These two phenotypes are dependent on IcsA expression in the outer membrane. Thus,

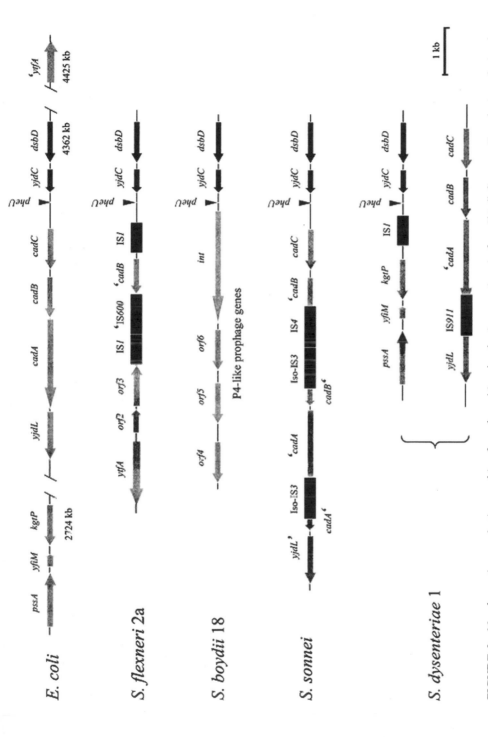

FIGURE 2 Novel genetic organization resulting from the *cadA* pathoadaptive mutations in four *Shigella* lineages. Gene loci are depicted as arrows, insertion sequences as black rectangles, and the *pheU* tRNA locus as an inverted triangle; truncated open reading frames (ORFs) and insertion sequences are indicated by an apostrophe. The chromosomal maps are aligned at the *yjdC* locus to facilitate comparison. The locations (in kilobase pairs) of *kgtP*, *dsbD*, and *'ytfA* on the *E. coli* K-12 chromosome are indicated below each ORF. The *S. dysenteriae* 1 *cad* operon, which is displaced and not linked to *yjdC*, is depicted below the region CCW to *yjdC*. Reprinted from reference 4.

115

expression of *ompT* is incompatible with *Shigella* virulence as it destroys a critical outer membrane protein essential for postinvasion virulence phenotypes. The *ompT* locus is contained within a 21-kb cryptic prophage in *E. coli* K-12 (17) that is absent in all four species of *Shigella* as well as in enteroinvasive *E. coli* (23). *E. coli* strains that represent lineages from which the different groups of *Shigella* evolved do not contain this cryptic prophage either. This observation suggests that the absence of the antivirulence gene *ompT* from *Shigella* is not the result of a pathoadaptive mutation but rather may have resulted because OmpT expression imposed a limitation on the likely ancestral strains capable of giving rise to the successful *Shigella* we see today.

EXTENDING THE PARADIGM

Antagonistic pleiotropy predicts that fitness in any single niche, where selective pressures are static, is compromised by the action of elements required for survival in other environments. Thus, fitness in any given niche is balanced against the cost of maintaining fitness in a dynamic environment. Bacteria often live in dynamic environments that present ever-changing selective pressures, and they have numerous genomic loci encoding a wide range of biochemical pathways that enable response and survival in these fluid niches. Pathogenic bacteria must balance fitness in the host against maintaining fitness in the wider ancestral niche. One may predict that an equilibrium exists in which increases in virulence (through loss of antivirulence genes) are weighed against the costs of niche adaptation and the corresponding negative effects on fitness in the ancestral environment. That said, more efficient interaction with host cells and tissues may minimize exposure to the ancestral niche. Thus, a pathogen highly adapted to life in a particular host (reflected by narrow host range and/or tissue specificity) may have traded fitness in the ancestral niche for fitness in host tissues. This critical phase of pathogen evolution can be traced in other organisms that occupy a narrow host range (or niche), demonstrating the important role of pathoadaptive mutation in bacterial pathogen evolution.

As previously discussed, *Bacillus anthracis* evolved from a nonpathogenic soil organism, *B. cereus*, following acquisition of two plasmids encoding several virulence traits. These quantum leaps in evolution enabled this soil organism to access and survive in mammalian blood and tissues, resulting in the disease anthrax. Clearly, the anthrax pathogen lives in an environment that presents very different selective pressures from those that shaped the ancestral organism. Several observations suggest that *B. anthracis* has become highly adapted for maximum fitness in this narrow niche. First, *B. anthracis* is not known to grow in soil (6). Instead, when the pathogen exits animal tissues, it forms an environmentally resistant spore that is metabolically inactive. This characteristic is in sharp contrast to the closely related nonpathogenic ancestor *B. cereus*, which grows in soil. This key observation suggests that *B. anthracis* has traded fitness in the new host niche (blood) for fitness in the ancestral niche (soil). Indeed, several traits expressed by the nonpathogenic ancestor *B. cereus* are not expressed by the pathogen. Given the enormous difference in the two environments, loss of one or more of these traits may reflect deletion of antivirulence genes through pathoadaptive mutation. Experimental evidence supporting antagonistic pleiotrophy as a mechanism in *B. anthracis* niche adaptation has been provided. Several traits, including hemolysin, lipase, and lecithinase activity, expressed by *B. cereus* are not expressed by *B. anthracis*. Genes encoding each of these traits, as well as many others, are members of a pleiotropic global regulon that is positively regulated by the transcription factor PlcR. Examination of genes encoding hemolysin, lipase, and lecithinase in *B. anthracis* revealed full-length open reading frames encoding proteins nearly identical to those encoded in several *B. cereus* isolates, suggesting that lack of each trait in *B. anthracis* is not due to mutation of each locus (20). However, examination of the *B. anthracis plcR* gene revealed a nonsense mutation one-third of the way from the end of the allele. Expression of this allele in a *B. cereus plcR* mutant does not result in hemolysin, lipase, or lecithinase expression. Furthermore, expression of the wild-type *plcR* allele from *B. cereus* in *B. anthracis* restores each of these enzymatic activities, indicating that lack of expression of each of these traits is due to the observed mutation in the *plcR* gene of *B. anthracis*. The antivirulence properties of PlcR were observed as expression of a wild-type *plcR* allele in *B. anthracis* inhibited sporulation (20); wild-type *B. cereus* strains harbor functional *plcR* alleles and are able to sporulate. Since *B. anthracis* evolved from *B. cereus,* this observation suggests that traits unique to *B. anthracis* are incompatible with ancestral sporulation pathways. Experimental evidence supporting this hypothesis identified AtxA as the source of the incompatability. AtxA is a regulator of *B. anthracis* gene expression required for toxin production and encoded within the pathogenicity island on one of the plasmids. A null mutation in the gene encoding AtxA enables an anthrax strain carrying a wild-type *plcR* allele to efficiently sporulate.

These studies suggest the following model for pathoadaptation of *B. anthracis.* After acquisition of the anthrax virulence plasmids by horizontal gene transfer, *B. anthracis* gained access to a new niche and a new pathogenic lifestyle. This lifestyle allowed amplification to high numbers in animal tissues and blood and a return to the environment in the form of spores following death of the host, to await interaction with a new host through cutaneous infection, inhalation, or ingestion. The new pathogen was not optimally fit for this pathogenic lifestyle as ancestral traits—expression of PlcR-regulated genes—were incompatible with the virulence systems. This led to mutation of an ancestral antivirulence gene *(plcR)* to ensure survival outside the host. Inactivation of this locus thus represents a pathoadaptive mutation in the evolution of *B. anthracis.* Moreover, the nature of the effect of this antivirulence gene on *B. anthracis* fitness (i.e., blocking sporulation) expands the model of antivirulence genes, and the pressures that drive pathoadaptive mutation, to include those that affect all aspects of pathogen fitness, including traits required for fitness outside host tissues.

Additional *B. anthracis* pathoadaptive mutations may affect the responsiveness of the organism's spore to germinant signals. As previously noted, *B. anthracis* does not grow in soil. In contrast, the ubiquitous, nonpathogenic ancestor *B. cereus* grows and thrives in soil worldwide. Nearly all strains of *B. cereus* express traits associated with the PlcR regulon; thus, it is likely that the many traits encoded by the regulon may enhance fitness in the soil. Likewise, if these traits were required for soil fitness, then loss of expression of these traits (as in *B. anthracis*) would decrease the ability to compete in this niche. Accordingly, loss of genes encoding factors that direct germination of these organisms in response to signals in soil would be beneficial as they would ensure that the endospore does not germinate in an environment in which the organism is not fit. Consistent with this prediction, germination signals that signal spore outgrowth differ between *B. anthracis* and *B. cereus* (13).

Significant environmental changes that often accompany a pathogenic lifestyle (and corresponding changes in selective pressures) potentially generate antivirulence genes in each newly evolved pathogen. These loci may be eliminated by pathoadaptive mutations to maximize fitness in the virulence niche, possibly at the expense of fitness in the ancestral niche. Likewise, pathogens that exhibit a narrow or altogether new host or tissue range relative to their nonpathogenic ancestors exhibit characteristics consistent with those predicted to result from elimination of antivirulence genes. Not coincidentally, pathogens that exhibit these characteristics are often more virulent than even pathogenic relatives. For example, *Burkholderia mallei,* an equine and human pathogen acquired through mucosal membranes that causes a fatal systemic disease, evolved from *Burkholderia pseudomallei,* a soil organism that is capable of causing an opportunistic localized infection in a number of animal hosts (41, 42). Importantly, *B. mallei* is not found in soil, and many traits associated with *B.*

pseudomallei, including motility and multidrug efflux pumps, are not expressed by *B. mallei.* Moreover, comparison of the recently deciphered genomes of the two organisms has not revealed operons or biochemical systems unique to *B. mallei* (indicative of gain-of-function mutations acquired through horizontal gene transfer that may increase fitness in the host and virulence). Rather, the 6.0-Mbp *B. mallei* genome appears to be a subset of the 7.2-Mbp *B. pseudomallei* genome, suggesting that the significant increase in virulence and narrowing of host range observed in *B. mallei* are associated with loss of multiple ancestral loci (antivirulence genes).

Of note, the antivirulence activity of an operon encoding arabinose catabolic enzymes has been demonstrated for *B. pseudomallei* (21). This operon, encoded within the nonpathogenic *B. pseudomallei* ancestor *B. thailandensis,* has been deleted from the pathogen's genome. Reintroduction of this operon into *B. pseudomallei* permits growth on arabinose but significantly reduces virulence in the Golden Syrian hamster model (21). The precise nature of the antivirulence effect has not been determined, but preliminary data suggest that the presence of the operon reduces expression of several *B. pseudomallei* virulence factors, including a type III secretion system required for virulence in animals. Thus, the arabinose utilization locus harbors antivirulence genes for pathogenic *Burkholderia.*

GENOMIC STRATEGIES TO REVEAL PUTATIVE ANTIVIRULENCE GENES

The recognition that each pathogen clone of *Shigella* lacks trait(s) expressed in the nonpathogenic ancestor led to identification of the antivirulence genes described earlier (18). Additional traits expressed by nonpathogenic ancestors, but absent in closely related pathogens, may be identified in the future by using phenotypic arrays that examine hundreds of phenotypes (and the functionality of thousands of genes encoding these traits) in a single experiment. Cooper et al. demonstrated the utility of this approach as phenotypic arrays revealed defects in metabolism of ribose sugars in several distinct *E. coli* cultures adapted to growth in a static environment (minimal glucose) (3). Increased fitness of the adapted clones, relative to the nonadapted ancestor, indicated negative selection of genes encoding ribose catabolic pathways through an antagonistic pleiotrophic mechanism. Thus, identification of unrecognized variations in phenotypes expressed by pathogens and their cognate commensals may permit discovery of additional pathoadaptive mutations in *Shigella* spp. as well as other bacterial pathogens.

Thousands of genes in each sequenced bacterial genome encode completely unknown functions even in well-characterized organisms such as *E. coli.* Thus, phenotypes observed in the laboratory represent only a subset of all the potential phenotypes expressed by an organism. Methods that do not focus on laboratory phenotypes will prove useful for the identification of additional pathoadaptive mutations. Undoubtedly, these methods will include functional genomic strategies that exploit data provided by genome sequencing studies. For example, comparison of the sequence of a pathogen genome to that of its nonpathogenic ancestor provides a direct means of identifying loci acquired through horizontal gene transfer as well as ancestral genes that have been inactivated or deleted from the pathogen genome. Inactivated ancestral genes may represent pathoadaptive mutations. The challenge is determining which of the inactivated genes encode factors that inhibit fitness in the virulence niche.

Gene distribution analyses may employ microarrays containing each of the nonpathogenic ancestor's genes. The arrays may be screened in hybridization studies to identify genes that are absent in the closely related pathogen. This type of analysis, termed "comparative genomic hybridization" (CGH), identifies genes deleted from the pathogen genome. The independent and convergent evolution of each *Shigella* lineage provides powerful reagents for CGH studies of these pathogens since deletion of an ancestral gene from each distinct

Shigella lineage strongly suggests negative selection through an antagonistic pleiotrophic mechanism. CGH analysis of the shigellae using a microarray containing all genes comprising the genome of a laboratory *E. coli* strain identified several ancestral genes deleted from each of the *Shigella* genomes (W. A. Day and A. T. Maurelli, unpublished observations). These putative pathoadaptive mutations target genes encoding several *E. coli* surface structures, suggesting that, as the pathogen acquired new mechanisms of interacting with host cells (such as the ability to invade colonocytes), ancestral surface factors required for adherence in the gut lumen were eliminated as they may interfere with the function of virulence traits. More recently, Dobrindt et al. performed an analysis of genome plasticity in *E. coli* isolates by use of DNA arrays (5). They found that up to 10% of the *E. coli* K-12–specific genes were absent in different pathogenic and commensal strains of *E. coli*. For example, the *fec* operon, encoding a ferric citrate uptake system in K-12, is absent in a strain of uropathogenic *E. coli* and in all four strains of enterohemorrhagic *E. coli* tested. Several genes involved in cold shock adaptation are also not present in some of the pathogenic *E. coli* tested. It should be noted that, while the microarray method provides a powerful genome-wide screen, missense or nonsense mutations that may inactivate rather than delete an antivirulence gene cannot be identified using CGH. Thus, identification of the full range of pathoadaptive mutations in an organism will require the application of several different screening techniques.

Antivirulence genes are eliminated from the ancestral genome following acquisition of traits that permit access to a new environment. Thus, an additional method of identifying pathoadaptive mutations may include reconstruction of the newly evolved pathogen by introduction of virulence genes into the nonpathogenic ancestor and subsequent passage through the virulence niche. Pathoadaptive mutations that benefit the new pathogen would enhance fitness of clones that have eliminated antivirulence genes. Thus, those clones harboring

beneficial mutations would become over-represented in the virulence niche. A recently described functional genomics technique termed "transposon site hybridization" (TraSH) may permit a means of readily identifying clones harboring transposon insertion mutations in antivirulence genes that enhance fitness of the reconstructed pathogen (37).

FUTURE PERSPECTIVES

Pathogens evolve through the acquisition of genetic information by horizontal gene transfer in the form of plasmids, bacteriophages, or pathogenicity islands. Subsequent to this quantum leap, pathoadaptive mutation results in the loss or inactivation of genes incompatible with the pathogenic lifestyle of the newly evolved pathogen. Thus, the consequence of selective pressures in the new niche is elimination or inactivation of genes to achieve optimal fitness in this niche. *Shigella* spp. represent the index model in which this paradigm of pathogen evolution has been established (Fig. 3). Pathoadaptive mutations also played a critical role in *B. anthracis* evolution and provide further evidence of the important contribution of this evolutionary pathway in niche adaptation and the generation of maximally fit pathogen clones.

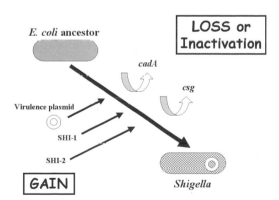

FIGURE 3 Model of the evolution of *Shigella* from an ancestral *E. coli*. Horizontal gene transfer and pathoadaptive mutation events are shown. SHI-1 and SHI-2 are the *Shigella* pathogenicity islands located on the chromosome. *cadA* and *csg* represent the genes for lysine decarboxylase and synthesis of curli, respectively.

The recognition that pathoadaptive mutations play a central role in the evolution of new pathogens strongly supports the value of identifying and studying nonpathogenic relatives and ancestors of pathogenic organisms. Furthermore, the observations on antivirulence genes in *Shigella* suggest criteria for the identification of antivirulence genes:

1. The antivirulence gene must be present and expressed in closely related or ancestral species occupying the nonvirulent ancestral niche but absent (or mutated) from pathogenic clones living in host tissues.

2. Expression of the antivirulence gene by the pathogen in host tissues must attenuate virulence and inhibit fitness.

These criteria form a type of converse Koch's postulates. Application of the converse Koch's postulates holds great promise for identification of antivirulence genes lost by pathoadaptive mutation. These genes should provide us with new insights into the ecology and evolution of bacterial pathogens as well as identify new products that can block the activity of virulence factors required for pathogen survival in host tissues. Thus, the study of antivirulence genes holds the potential for discovery of new pathogen-specific therapies and the development of safer, attenuated vaccine strains.

CHAPTER SUMMARY
- Pathoadaptive mutation via gene loss complements bacterial pathogen evolution by gene acquisition.
- The evolutionary model of antagonistic pleiotrophy predicts that genes required for fitness in one niche may actually inhibit fitness in another environment that presents new selective pressures.
- "Black holes" in pathogen genomes are formed by inactivation or loss of ancestral genes that are incompatible with, and even antagonistic to, the pathogenic lifestyle. These incompatible genes are defined as antivirulence genes.

- *Shigella* serves as a model for pathoadaptive mutation by gene loss and gene inactivation.
- Converse Koch's postulates are proposed as criteria for identification of antivirulence genes.
- New techniques such as phenotypic arrays, comparative genomic hybridization, and transposon site hybridization will improve our ability to identify pathoadaptive mutations in an organism.

ACKNOWLEDGMENT
The opinions or assertions contained herein are the private ones of A.T.M. and are not to be construed as official or reflecting the views of the Department of Defense or the Uniformed Services University of the Health Sciences.

REFERENCES
1. **Bernardini, M. L., J. Mounier, H. d'Hauteville, M. Coquis-Rondon, and P. J. Sansonetti.** 1989. Identification of *icsA,* a plasmid locus of *Shigella flexneri* that governs bacterial intra- and intercellular spread through interaction with F-actin. *Proc. Natl. Acad. Sci. USA* **86:** 3867–3871.
2. **Brenner, D. J., G. R. Fanning, K. E. Johnson, R. V. Citarella, and S. Falkow.** 1969. Polynucleotide sequence relationships among members of Enterobacteriaceae. *J. Bacteriol.* **98:** 637–650.
3. **Cooper, V. S., D. Schneider, M. Blot, and R. E. Lenski.** 2001. Mechanisms causing rapid and parallel losses of ribose catabolism in evolving populations of *Escherichia coli* B. *J. Bacteriol.* **183:** 2834–2841.
4. **Day, W. A., Jr., R. E. Fernandez, and A. T. Maurelli.** 2001. Pathoadaptive mutations that enhance virulence: genetic organization of the *cadA* regions of *Shigella* spp. *Infect. Immun.* **69:**7471–7480.
5. **Dobrindt, U., F. Agerer, K. Michaelis, A. Janka, C. Buchrieser, M. Samuelson, C. Svanborg, G. Gottschalk, H. Karch, and J. Hacker.** 2003. Analysis of genome plasticity in pathogenic and commensal *Escherichia coli* isolates by use of DNA arrays. *J. Bacteriol.* **185:**1831–1840.
6. **Dragon, D. C., and R. P. Rennie.** 1995. The ecology of anthrax spores: tough but not invincible. *Can. Vet. J.* **36:**295–301.
7. **Ewing, E. H.** 1986. *Edwards and Ewing's Identification of Enterobacteriacae,* 4th ed. Elsevier Science Publishing Co. Inc., New York, N.Y.
8. **Fernandez, I. M., M. Silva, R. Schuch, W. A. Walker, A. M. Siber, A. T. Maurelli, and B. A.**

McCormick. 2001. Cadaverine prevents the escape of *Shigella flexneri* from the phagolysosome: a connection between bacterial dissemination and neutrophil transepithelial signaling. *J. Infect. Dis.* **184:**743–753.

9. **Gophna, U., M. Barlev, R. Seijffers, T. A. Oelschlager, J. Hacker, and E. Z. Ron.** 2001. Curli fibers mediate internalization of *Escherichia coli* by eukaryotic cells. *Infect. Immun.* **69:** 2659–2665.

10. **Grodberg, J. and J. J. Dunn.** 1988. *ompT* encodes the *Escherichia coli* outer membrane protease that cleaves T7 RNA polymerase during purification. *J. Bacteriol.* **170:**1245–1253.

11. **Groisman, E. A., and H. Ochman.** 1996. Pathogenicity islands: bacterial evolution in quantum leaps. *Cell* **87:**791–794.

12. **Helgason, E., O. A. Økstad, D. A. Caugant, H. A. Johansen, A. Fouet, M. Mock, I. Hegna, and A.-B. Kolstø.** 2000. *Bacillus anthracis, Bacillus cereus,* and *Bacillus thuringiensis*—one species on the basis of genetic evidence. *Appl. Environ. Microbiol.* **66:** 2627–2630.

13. **Ireland, J. A., and P. C. Hanna.** 2002. Amino acid- and purine ribonucleoside-induced germination of *Bacillus anthracis* △Sterne endospores: *gerS* mediates responses to aromatic ring structures. *J. Bacteriol.* **184:**1296–1303.

14. **Jin, Q., Z. Yuan, J. Xu, Y. Wang, Y. Shen, W. Lu, J. Wang, H. Liu, J. Yang, F. Yang, X. Zhang, J. Zhang, G. Yang, H. Wu, D. Qu, J. Dong, L. Sun, Y. Xue, A. Zhao, Y. Gao, J. Zhu, B. Kan, K. Ding, S. Chen, H. Cheng, Z. Yao, B. He, R. Chen, D. Ma, B. Qiang, Y. Wen, Y. Hou, and J. Yu.** 2002. Genome sequence of *Shigella flexneri* 2a: insights into pathogenicity through comparison with genomes of *Escherichia coli* K12 and O157. *Nucleic Acids Res.* **30:**4432–4441.

15. **Lan, R., and P. R. Reeves.** 2002. *Escherichia coli* in disguise: molecular origins of *Shigella. Microbes Infect.* **4:**1125–1132.

16. **Lee, C. A.** 1996. Pathogenicity islands and the evolution of bacterial pathogens. *Infect. Agents Dis.* **5:**1–7.

17. **Lindsey, D. F., D. A. Mullin, and J. R. Walker.** 1989. Characterization of the cryptic lambdoid prophage DLP12 of *Escherichia coli* and overlap of the DLP12 integrase gene with the tRNA gene *argU. J. Bacteriol.* **171:**6197–6205.

18. **Maurelli, A. T., R. E. Fernandez, C. A. Bloch, C. K. Rode, and A. Fasano.** 1998. "Black holes" and bacterial pathogenicity: a large genomic deletion that enhances the virulence of *Shigella* spp. and enteroinvasive *Escherichia coli. Proc. Natl. Acad. Sci. USA* **95:**3943–3948.

19. **McCormick, B. A., M. I. Fernandez, A. M. Siber, and A. T. Maurelli.** 1999. Inhibition of *Shigella flexneri*-induced transepithelial migration of polymorphonuclear leucocytes by cadaverine. *Cell Microbiol.* **1:**143–155.

20. **Mignot, T., M. Mock, D. Robichon, A. Landier, D. Lereclus, and A. Fouet.** 2001. The incompatibility between the PlcR- and AtxA-controlled regulons may have selected a nonsense mutation in *Bacillus anthracis. Mol. Microbiol.* **42:** 1189–1198.

21. **Moore, R. A., S. Reckseidler-Zenteno, H. Kim, W. Nierman, Y. Yu, A. Tuanyok, J. Warawa, D. DeShazer, and D. E. Woods.** 2004. Contribution of gene loss to the pathogenic evolution of *Burkholderia pseudomallei* and *Burkholderia mallei. Infect. Immun.* **72:**4172–4187.

22. **Moss, J. E., T. J. Cardozo, A. Zychlinsky, and E. A. Groisman.** 1999. The *selC*-associated SHI-2 pathogenicity island of *Shigella flexneri. Mol. Microbiol.* **33:**74–83.

23. **Nakata, N., T. Tobe, I. Fukuda, T. Suzuki, K. Komatsu, M. Yoshikawa, and C. Sasakawa.** 1993. The absence of a surface protease, OmpT, determines the intercellular spreading ability of *Shigella:* the relationship between the *ompT* and *kcpA* loci. *Mol. Microbiol.* **9:**459–468.

24. **Ochman, H., J. G. Lawrence, and E. A. Groisman.** 2000. Lateral gene transfer and the nature of bacterial innovation. *Nature* **405:** 299–304.

25. **Ochman, H., T. S. Whittam, D. A. Caugant, and R. K. Selander.** 1983. Enzyme polymorphism and genetic population structure in *Escherichia coli* and *Shigella. J. Gen. Microbiol.* **129** (Pt. 9):2715–2726.

26. **Olsen, A., A. Arnqvist, M. Hammar, S. Sukupolvi, and S. Normark.** 1993. The RpoS sigma factor relieves H-NS-mediated transcriptional repression of *csgA,* the subunit gene of fibronectin-binding curli in *Escherichia coli. Mol. Microbiol.* **7:**523–536.

27. **Olsen, A., A. Jonsson, and S. Normark.** 1989. Fibronectin binding mediated by a novel class of surface organelles on *Escherichia coli. Nature* **338:**652–655.

28. **Pupo, G. M., D. K. Karaolis, R. Lan, and P. R. Reeves.** 1997. Evolutionary relationships among pathogenic and nonpathogenic *Escherichia coli* strains inferred from multilocus enzyme electrophoresis and *mdh* sequence studies. *Infect. Immun.* **65:**2685–2692.

29. **Pupo, G. M., R. Lan, and P. R. Reeves.** 2000. Multiple independent origins of *Shigella* clones of *Escherichia coli* and convergent evolution of many of their characteristics. *Proc. Natl. Acad. Sci. USA* **97:**10567–10572.

30. **Purdy, G. E., and S. M. Payne.** 2001. The SI II-3 iron transport island of *Shigella boydii* 0-1392

carries the genes for aerobactin synthesis and transport. *J. Bacteriol.* **183**:4176–4182.

31. **Rajakumar, K., C. Sasakawa, and B. Adler.** 1997. Use of a novel approach, termed island probing, identifies the *Shigella flexneri she* pathogenicity island which encodes a homolog of the immunoglobulin A protease-like family of proteins. *Infect. Immun.* **65**:4606–4614.

32. **Rolland, K., N. Lambert-Zechovsky, B. Picard, and E. Denamur.** 1998. *Shigella* and enteroinvasive *Escherichia coli* strains are derived from distinct ancestral strains of *E. coli. Microbiology* **144**(Pt. 9):2667–2672.

33. **Rose, M., and B. Charlesworth.** 1980. A test of evolutionary theories of senescence. *Nature* **287**:141–142.

34. **Sakellaris, H., N. K. Hannink, K. Rajakumar, D. Bulach, M. Hunt, C. Sasakawa, and B. Adler.** 2000. Curli loci of *Shigella* spp. *Infect. Immun.* **68**:3780–3783.

35. **Sansonetti, P. J., J. Arondel, M. Huerre, A. Harada, and K. Matsushima.** 1999. Interleukin-8 controls bacterial transepithelial translocation at the cost of epithelial destruction in experimental shigellosis. *Infect. Immun.* **67**:1471–1480.

36. **Sansonetti, P. J., T. L. Hale, G. J. Dammin, C. Kapfer, H. H. Collins, Jr., and S. B. Formal.** 1983. Alterations in the pathogenicity of *Escherichia coli* K-12 after transfer of plasmid and chromosomal genes from *Shigella flexneri. Infect. Immun.* **39**:1392–1402.

37. **Sassetti, C. M., D. H. Boyd, and E. J. Rubin.** 2001. Comprehensive identification of conditionally essential genes in mycobacteria. *Proc. Natl. Acad. Sci. USA* **98**:12712–12717.

38. **Silva, R. M., M. R. Toledo, and L. R. Trabulsi.** 1980. Biochemical and cultural characteristics of invasive *Escherichia coli. J. Clin. Microbiol.* **11**:441–444.

39. **Sokurenko, E. V., D. L. Hasty, and D. E. Dykhuizen.** 1999. Pathoadaptive mutations: gene loss and variation in bacterial pathogens. *Trends Microbiol.* **7**:191–195.

40. **Vokes, S. A., S. A. Reeves, A. G. Torres, and S. M. Payne.** 1999. The aerobactin iron transport system genes in *Shigella flexneri* are present within a pathogenicity island. *Mol. Microbiol.* **33**:63–73.

41. **Woods, D. E.** 2002. The use of animal infection models to study the pathogenesis of melioidosis and glanders. *Trends Microbiol.* **10**:483–484.

42. **Woods, D. E., D. DeShazer, R. A. Moore, P. J. Brett, M. N. Burtnick, S. L. Reckseidler, and M. D. Senkiw.** 1999. Current studies on the pathogenesis of melioidosis. *Microbes Infect.* **1**:157–162.

ENVIRONMENT AND THE EVOLUTION OF MICROBIAL PATHOGENS

PART II OVERVIEW

Roberto Kolter and Deborah A. Hogan

7

The second section of this book presents five chapters that discuss the general principles of pathogen evolution (chapters 8 and 9) and the mechanisms by which specific bacterial virulence determinants may have evolved (chapters 10, 11, and 12). The discussion on environmental settings that provided selection pressures for the evolution of certain virulence determinants focuses on soil (chapter 8, by Muir and Tan) and the human gut (chapter 9, by McFall-Ngai and Gordon). The actual evolutionary pathways and mechanisms are explored more specifically for toxins (chapter 10, by Stine and Nataro), transporters (chapter 11, by Planet et al.), and antibiotic resistance (chapter 12, by Rowe-Magnus and Mazel). What can be summed up from the foregoing presentations? In the following paragraphs, we attempt to bring forth some of the key "take home" messages that arise from these chapters. We emphasize one idea in particular: many of the determinants that contribute to a microbe's ability to become a clinically relevant pathogen likely evolve and persist in environmental settings, in microbial communities, or in mutualistic associations.

In chapter 8, Muir and Tan discuss how the selective pressures in soil likely drove the evolution of factors associated with bacterial virulence in mammals. The authors focus on two aspects of life in the soil: low nutrient availability and predation. For example, the high-affinity metal acquisition systems that bacteria likely use in soil environments are also essential for survival in the host, where the concentrations of free iron and manganese are very low. The authors go on to describe how factors that likely help bacteria avoid predation or killing by other soil organisms, such as protozoa, nematodes, and fungi, also participate in bacterial pathogenesis in humans. These findings support the idea that pathogenesis toward humans is not the only, or even the predominant, selective pressure for the evolution of many factors that are studied in the context of disease. As discussed in subsequent chapters, there are also important symbiotic interactions between bacteria and eukaryotes in the soil that involve factors that, in other settings, can also play a role in virulence. Examples include bacterial nodulation of plant roots, bacterial-fungal interactions in degradative communities, or bacterial symbiosis with insect hosts (mediated by cell surface components and type III secreted effectors) (2, 3).

Roberto Kolter, Department of Microbiology and Molecular Genetics, Harvard Medical School, Boston, MA 02115. *Deborah A. Hogan,* Department of Microbiology and Immunology, Dartmouth Medical School, Hanover, NH 03755.

Evolution of Microbial Pathogens, Edited by H. S. Seifert and V. J. DiRita, © 2006 ASM Press, Washington, D.C.

The concept of pathogenesis arising within the context of ongoing and coevolving *beneficial* associations between microbes and their eukaryotic hosts is emphasized in chapter 9. In presenting pathogen evolution this way, McFall-Ngai and Gordon likely challenge readers to rethink many widely held views on microbial pathogenesis. As a legacy of the enormously important "germ theory of disease," developed late in the 19th century, much of 20th-century thinking vis-à-vis host-microbe interactions was dominated by the concept that "microbes cause disease." Add to that our inevitably self-preserving anthropocentric perspective, which greatly biases which microbes have been the subject of investigation, and it is easy to understand why many of us might have developed skewed views on microbial virulence—views that might lead us to the perception that pathogens have evolved specifically to cause disease. McFall-Ngai and Gordon present a different view. Symbiont evolution is driven by selection of organisms that achieve reproductive success by exploiting the available niches afforded by another organism. But, by and large, the "winners" of such interactions are those that can thrive through beneficial interactions. This makes sense, as in the long run it is counterproductive for the symbiont to destroy its source of nutrition or to promote the evolution of host responses designed to eradicate the bacterial colonizer. Thus, pathogenesis might be considered a transient evolutionary "mistake" in the process of correction.

What we, through our limited perspective, see as a "virulence factor" need not always be such. A clear example of this is the fact that tracheal cytotoxin (a fragment of peptidoglycan), long known for its tissue-damaging effects in mammals, is released by the beneficial squid symbiont *Vibrio fischeri* to trigger tissue development that aids in the establishment of the mutualistic symbiosis (8). Certain instances of pathogenesis are due to an otherwise beneficial organism being "in the wrong place at the wrong time." For example, normal flora gut microbes, which are greatly beneficial in the gastrointestinal tract, can cause serious infec-

tions when physical damage introduces these organisms into other regions of the body. Clearly, a complete view of the evolution and action of "virulence" determinants can only be achieved by examining their role in both health and disease settings.

The study of microbial activities during a "beneficial interaction" is remarkably complex. Witness the previously unsuspected complexity of our own microbial symbionts. Work by Eckburg et al. makes evident the gargantuan diversity of the human gut microflora, which contains mostly unknown microbes and displays much interindividual variability (4). To begin to analyze these complicated and dynamic microbial communities and how they contribute to health and disease will certainly necessitate the development of approaches quite different from those developed to specifically focus on bacterial pathogenesis. Such approaches are in their infancy, and thus we are only beginning to understand the breadth of nonpathogenic molecular interactions between microbes and humans.

While the first two chapters focus on the selective pressures that drive the evolution of factors that can contribute to disease, the third chapter, by Stine and Nataro, focuses on the mechanistic question of how one class of bacterial virulence determinants (exotoxins) evolved and moved between different microbial species. They start by approaching the question of how the toxin-coding genes might end up residing in particular genomes. The answer to this is rather clear for a multitude of toxins. Horizontal gene transfer, be it conjugation, transduction, or transformation, appears largely responsible for the dissemination of many toxins. Whether the toxin-coding genes are present in phage genomes, in plasmids, and/or within transposable DNA elements, these can generally be recognized as recent acquisitions based on G+C content and codon usage.

More tantalizing and much more difficult to answer with certainty are questions relating to the adaptive functions of toxins and the original selective conditions that gave rise to these proteins. The advantages for damaging the host utilizing a toxin are largely enigmatic. Take the example of the clostridial neurotoxins. Despite their exquisite specificity for interfering with mammalian neurotransmitter release, it is highly unlikely that their initial evolution occurred in the context of mammalian infections. The unmet challenge, however, is to find probable settings where production of these toxins clearly could have provided a selective advantage to the producer microorganisms. One attractive hypothesis is that some of the mammalian mechanisms that are hampered by toxins have close homologs in microscopic eukaryotes. Thus, toxins might have evolved in the setting of competition for resources in natural settings, such as soil, where encounters between bacteria and microscopic eukaryotes (or even small animals such as nematodes) are far more numerous and have been occurring for much longer. In the context of that hypothesis, it is possible to consider the drastic effects that many toxins have on humans as rather accidental, evolutionary "mistakes" that are on their way to attenuation or extinction. This, however, does not make the fact that such toxins can have devastating effects on humans any easier to tolerate.

Some toxins may have initially evolved as factors participating in microbe-microbe interactions or microbe-surface interactions. After all, microbes had over 2 billion years of ongoing evolution in the absence of any potential multicellular hosts. For example, the *Staphylococcus aureus* alpha-toxin, a secreted, multimeric, hemolytic toxin encoded by the *hla* gene, plays an integral role in biofilm formation (1). The *hla* mutant was unable to fully colonize plastic surfaces under both static and flow conditions. Based on microscopy studies, it was proposed that alpha-hemolysin is required for cell-to-cell interactions during biofilm formation. This finding suggests that some toxins may have initially evolved to enhance microbe-microbe interactions.

Extracellular factors, including toxins, degradative enzymes, and signaling molecules, involved in a microbe's interaction with its local environment, must be translocated across one or more membranes to reach their external target. Both free-living and host-associated microbes, including all pathogens, achieve this with a number of diverse strategies for the export of macromolecules. Because such translocation mechanisms are not exclusively found in microbes with pathogenic potential, it is interesting to investigate their evolutionary histories. In many cases, phylogenetic analyses can yield important insights into the natural histories of these export systems. Planet et al. have done this, focusing on gram-negative microbes, and discuss their findings in the fourth chapter of this section.

There are several systems that microbes utilize to solve the problem of translocating macromolecules across their two membranes. There is some disagreement and confusion regarding the classification and nomenclature of these systems in the literature. The numbering system used is, of course, completely arbitrary and reflects the historical context of when these systems were classified rather than representing a functional hierarchy.

None of the six transport systems known in bacteria are likely exclusively used for the transport of virulence factors. Type I secretion, involving a three-component apparatus with an ATP-binding cassette domain, transports proteins across both bacterial membranes in a single step. These are thought to have evolved from very ancient import/export systems essential for the translocation of small molecules such as sugars and metal ions. Type II secretion enables extracellular proteins to cross the cytoplasmic membrane via the signal sequence-dependent *sec* or *tat* systems. Here again, the systems able to translocate virulence factors probably arose from more ancient systems that translocate enzymes involved in nutrient acquisition and systems involved in the assembly of surface-attachment organelles such as the type IV pili. While in many cases these pili are recognized as virulence determinants, many of them serve to attach to abiotic surfaces and likely were extant prior to the appearance of eukaryotes. Contact-dependent type III secretion systems translocate diverse effector molecules in a single step across both bacterial membranes and often directly into a eukaryotic cell's cytoplasm. The most striking feature of these systems is that their 20 or so component protein subunits display remarkable sequence similarity to the basal body structures of the highly conserved bacterial flagellar apparatus. This similarity has prompted the hypothesis that type III secretion systems, which appear to have been largely disseminated through horizontal gene transfer, evolved from the more ancient flagellar system that does not appear to move horizontally. While phylogenetic analyses cannot conclusively support this evolutionary history, it does at least suggest that the divergence of the type III secretion system and the flagellar basal body occurred very early. Type III secretion systems are well studied for their role in pathogenesis; their participation in symbiotic interactions between bacteria and higher eukaryotes have been documented but are much less well described (2, 5). The type IV conjugation-dependent systems bear striking sequence similarity to the proteins involved in plasmid transfer between bacteria. The evolutionary relationship between conjugation and type IV protein secretion remains an unresolved matter, but the current phylogenetic relationships presented in chapter 11 favor a "conjugation-first" hypothesis. It is certainly true that the potential to transfer DNA between bacteria predated the existence of eukaryotes. Type V secretion involves autotransporters, or single polypeptides with all the information necessary to translocate across the outer membrane. While most of the autotransporters described to date indeed encode virulence factors, analyses of fully sequenced genomes does reveal the existence of many predicted autotransporters with no specific function known (7). Lastly, type VI secretion is characterized by chaperone/usher systems that are used in the assembly of some adhesion pili. The protein subunits that are eventually assembled as pili first reach the periplasm via the *sec* system. There they are received by a dedicated chaperone that delivers them to the usher proteins, which form an outer membrane pore and facilitate pilus assembly. Again, the chaperone/usher-secreted

pili have been shown to play roles in bacterial interactions with both biotic and abiotic surfaces (6, 10, 12).

There are two important points to take home regarding the evolution of these macromolecular export systems. First, in no case is it evident that the initial selective conditions in which they arose were necessarily a pathogenic interaction with a host. Second, none of these export systems appear to play functions that are solely seen in the setting of pathogenesis.

The last topic treated in this section, in chapter 12 (by Rowe-Magnus and Mazel), is the evolution of antibiotic resistance. While not directly an attribute of pathogens, antibiotic resistance is one of the most important problems in dealing with the effects of pathogens in the clinical setting. As the authors state, resistance to antibiotics can arise through the acquisition of resistance genes by horizontal gene transfer or by mutation of resident bacterial genes.

Consistent with the theme that evolution of factors that participate in clinically relevant pathogens first occurred within microbial communities, many of the genes involved in antibiotic resistance likely evolved within soil communities. For example, the authors describe how the *arr-2* gene, which confers resistance to rifampin, a derivative of rifamycin, was identified in *Pseudomonas aeruginosa*, where it likely enabled this strain to persist in communities with rifamycin-producers such as *Amycolatopsis mediterranei* (11). The majority of antibiotics in use today were first identified in bacterial and fungal cultures, thus it stands to reason that transferable mechanisms of antibiotic resistance also evolved in these settings. A significant reservoir of antibiotic resistance genes, with greater genetic diversity than that observed in clinical strains, was identified by using culture-independent methods to survey antibiotic resistance mechanisms in soil communities (9). These findings underscore the likelihood that most mechanisms for antibiotic resistance probably evolve in environmental settings.

Apart from acquisition of antibiotic resistance mechanisms by horizontal gene transfer, the authors describe the rise of antibiotic-resistant strains by mutation. Mutation can cause changes in the drug target, up-regulation of efflux pumps or target-encoding genes, inactivation of enzymes required to activate pro-drugs, or modification of resistance mechanisms to broaden resistance specificity. The authors also discuss the frequency with which strains with increased rates of mutation are isolated upon challenge with antibiotics. While it has been proposed that increased mutation rates might aid in the development of antibiotic resistance, this hypothesis has not been critically tested.

In closing this section's summary, we wish to remind the readers of three important points:

1. Pathogens constitute a remarkably minute fraction of the microbes with which humans interact.

2. In the context of the much greater number of beneficial associations between microbes and their hosts, much of virulence could be considered a transient evolutionary "mistake."

3. Pathogen evolution is taking place among a myriad of beneficial interactions between hosts and the microbes and between microbes and their environment.

Thus we as a community of scientists interested in human health will do well by placing great emphasis on understanding the molecular interactions between host and microbe in the context of the nonpathogenic and beneficial microbial interactions that occur both in the environment and within the human body. This perspective on virulence may give us insight into novel ways by which pathogenic interactions can be manipulated or prevented.

REFERENCES

1. **Caiazza, N. C., and G. A. O'Toole.** 2003. Alpha-toxin is required for biofilm formation by *Staphylococcus aureus. J. Bacteriol.* **185:**3214–3217.

2. **Dale, C., S. A. Young, D. T. Haydon, and S. C. Welburn.** 2001. The insect endosymbiont *Sodalis glossinidius* utilizes a type III secretion system for cell invasion. *Proc. Natl. Acad. Sci. USA* **98:** 1883–1888.

3. **Dorr, J., T. Hurek, and B. Reinhold-Hurek.** 1998. Type IV pili are involved in plant-microbe and fungus-microbe interactions. *Mol. Microbiol.* **30:**7–17.

4. **Eckburg, P. B., E. M. Bik, C. N. Bernstein, E. Purdom, L. Dethlefsen, M. Sargent, S. R. Gill, K. E. Nelson, and D. A. Relman.** 2005. Diversity of the human intestinal microbial flora. *Science* **308:**1635–1638.

5. **Freiberg, C., R. Fellay, A. Bairoch, W. J. Broughton, A. Rosenthal, and X. Perret.** 1997. Molecular basis of symbiosis between *Rhizobium* and legumes. *Nature* **387:**394–401.

6. **Friedman, L., and R. Kolter.** 2004. Genes involved in matrix formation in *Pseudomonas aeruginosa* PA14 biofilms. *Mol. Microbiol.* **51:**675–690.

7. **Henderson, I. R., F. Navarro-Garcia, M. Desvaux, R. C. Fernandez, and D. Ala' Aldeen.** 2004. Type V protein secretion pathway: the autotransporter story. *Microbiol. Mol. Biol. Rev.* **68:**692–744.

8. **Koropatnick, T. A., J. T. Engle, M. A. Apicella, E. V. Stabb, W. E. Goldman, and M. J. McFall-Ngai.** 2004. Microbial factor-mediated development in a host-bacterial mutualism. *Science* **306:** 1186–1188.

9. **Riesenfeld, C. S., R. M. Goodman, and J. Handelsman.** 2004. Uncultured soil bacteria are a reservoir of new antibiotic resistance genes. *Environ. Microbiol.* **6:**981–989.

10. **Sauer, F. G., M. Barnhart, D. Choudhury, S. D. Knight, G. Waksman, and S. J. Hultgren.** 2000. Chaperone-assisted pilus assembly and bacterial attachment. *Curr. Opin. Struct. Biol.* **10:** 548–556.

11. **Tribuddharat, C., and M. Fennewald.** 1999. Integron-mediated rifampin resistance in Pseudomonas aeruginosa. *Antimicrob. Agents Chemother.* **43:**960–962.

12. **Vallet, I., J. W. Olson, S. Lory, A. Lazdunski, and A. Filloux.** 2001. The chaperone/usher pathways of Pseudomonas aeruginosa: identification of fimbrial gene clusters (cup) and their involvement in biofilm formation. *Proc. Natl. Acad. Sci. USA* **98:**6911–6916.

EVOLUTION OF PATHOGENS IN SOIL

Rachel Muir and Man-Wah Tan

8

The soil is a particularly complex environment and is one of the most dynamic sites of biological interactions in nature. It is not merely a static physicochemical matrix, but a biological system in a continuous dynamic equilibrium. In just 1 g of soil, there can be as many as 4,000 species of both prokaryotic and eukaryotic organisms. Among the various groups of soil-dwelling organisms, such as bacteria, fungi, protozoa, actinomycetes, algae, and nematodes, bacteria are by far the most abundant. The number of organisms found in the zone of soil located in the closest proximity to plant roots, the rhizosphere, can reach numbers exceeding 10^9/g. The tremendously dense numbers of organisms found in some soils act as a continuous selective pressure for the emergence of a number of competitive and symbiotic interactions between bacteria and the other soil inhabitants.

Interestingly, some of the abiotic and biotic challenges faced by bacteria in the soil are similar to those encountered when these bacteria attempt to colonize a plant or an animal host. In the following, we will briefly discuss the genetic diversity within the soil environment and some of the mechanisms that generate

genetic diversity within soil-dwelling bacteria. Next, we will highlight, with some examples, how the physical and chemical (abiotic) properties of the soil and the living organisms (biotic) within the soil might act as selective forces on existing genetic variations, and how they contribute to the evolution of bacterial pathogens in the soil. Lastly, we discuss broadly conserved community behaviors intrinsic to the survival of soil bacteria and their relevance to pathogenesis.

GENETIC DIVERSITY IN SOIL-DWELLING BACTERIA

The availability of complete genome sequences from a large number of bacteria has provided significant insights into the genetic diversity of bacteria. There is considerable variation in the size and organization of bacterial genomes, which range from 580 kb for *Mycoplasma genitalium,* with 480 predicted genes (16), to 8667 kb for *Streptomyces coelicolor,* with 7,825 predicted genes (2). Comparative genomic analyses, achieved either by comparing complete genome sequences or by whole-genome comparisons using DNA microarrays, indicate that there is great genome heterogeneity and genetic diversity among closely related strains and underline the fact that both the acquisition and deletion of DNA elements are important

Rachel Muir and Man-Wah Tan, Departments of Genetics and of Microbiology and Immunology, Stanford University School of Medicine, Stanford, CA 94305.

Evolution of Microbial Pathogens, Edited by H. S. Seifert and V. J. DiRita, © 2006 ASM Press, Washington, D.C.

processes involved in the evolution of bacteria. These studies also demonstrate that bacterial genomes are organized from two gene pools, "the core and the flexible gene pools" (23). The core gene pool consists of the bacterial chromosome and the flexible gene pool consists of genomic islands, integrons, plasmids, transposons, and phages. In general, genes encoding proteins necessary for basic cellular functions form the core gene pool, exhibiting rather homogeneous G+C contents and codon usage. In contrast, DNA constituents of the flexible gene pool, which have features characteristic of transferred elements (different G+C content and codon usage, presence of mobility genes), encode additional functions that are not essential for bacterial growth. Differences in genome size and organization among bacterial species reflect size variations of the flexible gene pool. The genetic components within the flexible gene pool are subject to selection. Those elements that provide selective advantages under particular conditions, such as changes in the environment and entry into a new host, will be retained.

MECHANISMS THAT GENERATE GENETIC DIVERSITY

What are the genetic mechanisms leading to the acquisition or loss of genomic DNA? By far the most potent mechanism that brings about substantial genetic change is horizontal transfer, which is the transfer of flexible gene pool elements between genetically distinct organisms. Horizontal (or lateral) gene transfer represents a cornerstone of bacterial evolution; it is the creative force that is largely responsible for the patterns of similarities and differences we see between prokaryotic microbes. Horizontal gene transfer has led to dramatic changes in the composition of microbial genomes over relatively short time periods (48). Because the amount of horizontally acquired genetic elements (plasmids, phages, and genomic islands) is disproportionately high among bacterial pathogens, it is likely that horizontal gene transfer plays an important role in the adaptive evolution of different pathogenic bacteria. There is

also evidence of horizontal gene transfer between pathogens and symbionts. For example, the symplasmid of *Rhizobium*, which carries essential genes for symbiotic competence, might have been derived from the plant pathogen *Agrobacterium tumefaciens* (18). The genetic material from the flexible gene pool can be horizontally transferred through three processes: transduction, conjugation, and natural transformation.

Transduction

Transduction is mediated by bacterial viruses, in which bacterial DNA along with viral sequences are transferred from donor to recipient cells. It is not rare for bacteria to contain multiple prophages in their chromosomes, which account for a sizable part of the total bacterial DNA. When mRNA expression patterns were studied with microarrays in lysogenic bacteria that underwent physiologically relevant changes in growth conditions, prophage genes figured prominently in the mRNA species that changed their expression pattern. This indicates that prophages are not a passive genetic cargo of the bacterial chromosome, but are likely to be active players in cell physiology. Indeed, the acquisition of prophages can lead to increased competitive fitness of the host strain, either by growing lytically and destroying bacteria from rival strains or by haboring virulence factors that allow the bacterial hosts to be pathogenic on their eukaryotic hosts. As an example of the former, a recent study showed that a *Salmonella enterica* serovar Typhimurium strain that harbors prophages in its genome spontaneously releases a small titer of phage. When cocultured with a competing nonlysogenic strain, the released phage kill off the competing strain. Thus, at the population level, the lysogenic strain is more competitively fit than the nonlysogenic strain (3).

There is good evidence that some of these prophages may affect the pathogenicity of the bacteria within which they reside and that phage-mediated transduction is the most prominent mechanism of pathogenicity gene transfer. For example, biological experiments conducted over 30 years ago established that lysogenization of *Clostridium botulinum* by some bacteriophages with contractile tails converted nontoxigenic strains into toxigenic isolates. Curing of the prophage leads to concomitant loss of the toxigenicity (1). Similarly, the only difference between pathogenic and harmless strains of the ubiquitous soil bacteria *Corynebacterium diphtheriae* is the presence of a bacteriophage (17). Both the corynephage β and the corynephage ω secrete a toxin that ribosylates the host cell EF2 protein, resulting in the destruction of host cells. Recent work suggests that the emergence of epidemic salmonellosis in cattle and human is a consequence of horizontal transfer of the *sopE1* gene by the lysogenic bacteriophage sopE1phi (43, 74). The Gifsy-2 prophage within the *S. enterica* serovar Typhimurium encodes several proteins that are required for systemic infection in mice (13). It was postulated that this role of prophages as vectors for lateral transfer between bacteria is not limited to pathogenic bacteria, but that some adaptations of nonpathogenic bacterial strains to their ecological niches may also have been mediated by prophage genomes (6).

Conjugation

Conjugation is the transfer of DNA, usually in the form of a broad host range plasmid, and requires direct contact between donor and recipient cells. Conjugal transfer of plasmids has been shown to occur in a variety of environmental conditions, including those within an animal, in the rhizosphere, on leaves, and in soil. Many plasmids contain antibiotic resistance genes and virulence determinants. In many instances, acquisition of such plasmids allows the recipient strain to possess novel traits that promote adaptation to new environments. For example, although the soil bacteria *Bacillus cereus* and *B. thuringiensis* are derivatives of a single species and molecular analysis shows that they share the same genetic background, they manifest distinct pathogenic properties (28, 52). *B. cereus* is an opportunistic pathogen associated with food poisoning and periodontal disease, whereas *B. thuringiensis* is a virulent insect

pathogen that produces a plasmid-encoded crystalline pore-forming toxin. The variation in pathogenetic properties between the two *Bacillus* strains is due in part to the presence of the virulence plasmid in *B. thuringiensis*. This distinction in pathogenicity is lost when the virulence plasmid is introduced into *B. cereus;* intrahemocelic administration of either plasmid-containing species into susceptible insect larvae produced a similar lethal septicemia. Moreover, plasmid-cured *B. thuringiensis* is known to cause a *B. cereus*-like infection in mice (56). *B. anthracis* is another closely related soil bacillus that is a human pathogen primarily because of two large plasmids it carries, the toxin-encoding pXO1 and the capsule-encoding pXO2 (49). These virulence plasmids are not self-transmissible; however, in a laboratory setting plasmids from other *Bacillus* species, which are capable of transferring themselves by conjugation, have been shown to provide the mating functions, *in trans,* for moving the *B. anthracis* virulence plasmids. It is possible that such transfer also occurs in the natural soil setting.

Natural Genetic Transformation

There is an increasing body of evidence indicating that natural genetic transformation is an important mechanism for increasing genetic diversity and is widespread among Bacteria and Archaea domains (11, 39). Transformation appears to take place in a variety of ecosystems where bacteria live, such as the marine, freshwater, soil, and plant milieus. Despite the sensitivity of DNA to nucleases, DNA is relatively common in these environments, where it is excreted by both living and actively dying organisms. An exposed DNA molecule can be stabilized through its adsorption to sand and clay particles, rendering it more resistant to DNase while retaining its transforming ability. Natural transformation within the soil has been demonstrated for *Pseudomonas stutzeri, Pseudomonas fluorescens,* and the plant pathogen *A. tumefaciens* (10, 58).

The factors that contribute to genetic variability are countered by mechanisms that ensure genome stability, such as DNA repair, transfer barriers, and modifications by restriction endonucleases. Together, these opposing mechanisms generate the driving force for bacterial evolution. The subsequent genotypes created by the pressures that affect genomic stability and diversity are rapidly sorted and shaped by selection to give rise to new phenotypes. While acknowledging the role of drift in maintaining molecular variation, the focus of the rest of this chapter is on the ecological—both biotic and abiotic—factors in the soil that affect the patterns of genetic diversity found among bacteria. In particular, aspects of the soil milieus that contribute to the generation of new variants that are more suitably adapted to survive either among their competitors or within their selective environments will be discussed. Thus, diversity arises and is maintained through interplay between ecological and genetic factors.

ADAPTATIONS FOR SURVIVAL IN THE SOIL AND IN A LIVING HOST

Many bacterial pathogens of vertebrates are either members or evolutionarily close relatives of the natural soil microflora. Some of these pathogens are able to survive outside their vertebrate hosts, either as soil saprophytes or within invertebrate hosts. For example, although the primary habitats of S. enterica and Escherichia coli are vertebrate hosts, they are known to exists as normal flora of soil and certain tropical ecosystems, respectively (71). Pseudomonas aeruginosa is principally a soil microbe that is able to survive and infect vertebrate hosts (27). In order to survive within the soil, these bacteria have had both to adapt to the physicochemical properties of the soil and to escape predation by bacteria-feeding protozoans and nematodes in the soil. Others, such as Legionella pneumophila, live within amoebae (5). Thus, the evolution of these bacterial pathogens is shaped by the cyclic lifestyle consisting of passage through the vertebrate host into the environment (or alternative host, in the case of L. pneumophila) and back to the host. In

the following sections, we discuss how their interactions with the soil and with alternative hosts could provide selective pressures that lead to the evolution of strains that are pathogenic to mammalian hosts.

Selective Pressures from the Abiotic Components in the Soil

Within an animal host, a bacterial pathogen encounters a warm, constant temperature, as well as high concentrations of free amino acids and sugars, which are conducive to growth. However, there exist challenges or limitations (collectively referred to as abiotic stresses) that have to be overcome in order to survive within the animal host. Interestingly, some of the abiotic stresses encountered by bacteria within their hosts, such as limited availability of micronutrients and high osmolarity, are also encountered in the soil.

IRON

Bacteria require soluble iron for their metabolism. Iron is an essential cofactor for many proteins, including components of the respiratory chain (cytochromes, cytochrome oxidase), tricarboxylic acid cycle (aconitase, succinate dehydrogenase), and oxidative defense systems (catalase, peroxidase, superoxide dismutase). Although iron is abundant in the soil, it is found predominantly in the ferric (Fe^{3+}) form, and the extremely low solubility of Fe^{3+} at pH 7 means that precious little is available. Similarly, within eukaryotic cells, the readily soluble ferrous (Fe^{2+}) iron is sequestered tightly by iron-binding proteins and cofactors, thereby restricting its availability to invading organisms. Thus, the ability of bacteria to wrest iron from the host is fundamental to the pathogenesis of many infectious diseases (4, 53). The primary storage compounds of most animals and plants are ferritins and phytoferritins, respectively. The limited supply of soluble iron necessitates that bacteria evolve both intricate iron transport and iron regulatory systems to guarantee a sufficient pool of iron for growth and development. However, unbound ferrous iron is especially noxious within cells, as Fe^{2+} ions catalyze Fenton-type reactions that lead to the production of damaging hydroxyl radicals. Since prokaryotic cells lack internal compartmentalization, which functions in eukaryotic cells to provide safe intracellular storage for iron, tight regulation of iron flux across the cytoplasmic membrane has to be maintained.

Bacteria have evolved three principal iron acquisition systems to solve the iron supply problem. In the first system, the pathogen makes direct contact with the host's iron-bound component, and acquires iron either by directly abstracting it at the cell surface or, as with heme, importing entire iron-containing molecules into the cytoplasm. Acquisition of iron by *Porphyromonas gingivalis,* a gram-negative bacterium associated with periodontal disease, represents a unique mechanism of iron/heme utilization employed by bacterial pathogens (50). *P. gingivalis* first adheres to its iron source, red blood cells, using hemagglutinins. Proteases are then used by the pathogen to lyse the red blood cells, releasing hemoglobin. The freed hemoglobin is seized by bacterial cell surface receptors and degraded by gingipain proteases to generate heme. The heme is then transported into the bacteria via the iron import system. *P. gingivalis* also has the advantage of being able to stock a surplus of heme and subsequently iron on its cell surface, allowing the pathogen access to a safely stored iron supply. The second system involves the synthesis of ultrahigh-affinity iron chelators, known as siderophores, which physically capture iron from host proteins by virtue of their superior binding strength. Finally, anaerobes, such as *Clostridium perfringens,* acquire iron by creating their own microanaerobic environment in a host tissue that permits ferric iron in molecules such as transferrin or lactoferrin to be reduced to soluble Fe^{2+}. Soluble Fe^{2+} is then taken up without the aid of iron chelators, most likely imported via an active transport system common to other divalent metal ions. Whether the microbe is a benign soil inhabitant or a mammalian pathogen, the ability to acquire iron and

to effectively maintain its homeostasis are possibly the key determinants as to whether the microorganism can successfully sustain itself in the soil or within its host.

MANGANESE

Although not limiting in the soil environment, manganese is essential for normal physiology of prokaryotic and eukaryotic organisms. In bacteria, Mn^{2+} is an essential cofactor for many enzymes, some of which—manganese superoxide dismutase (encoded by *sodA*), for example—are essential for bacterial growth and survival under oxidative stress. The functions provided by such Mn^{2+}-containing enzymes are particularly important during infection of eukaryotic hosts. For example, inactivation of the *sodA* gene in *Streptococcus pneumoniae* reduces virulence in intranasal infection of mice (72). Reactive oxygen species (ROS) are known to play a vital role in host defense against bacterial infection. Thus, it is logical to hypothesize that an essential function of Mn^{2+} sequestration by infecting bacteria is to activate pathogen defense systems against external, host-derived ROS in addition to internally generated ROS.

Manganese homeostasis in bacteria depends largely upon the regulation of Mn^{2+} transport. There are at least two types of Mn^{2+} import systems: (i) the ABC-type transporter of the LraI family of ABC transporters and (ii) the MntH (proton-dependent manganese transporter)/ Nramp (natural resistance-associated macrophage protein) family (30, 32). These Mn^{2+} import systems are also capable of transporting other divalent metals. The expression of the LraI family of ABC transporters is upregulated under low Mn^{2+} concentrations, such as that found in serum. Unsurprisingly, these transporters have been shown to play essential roles in the virulence of several pathogens, including *Enterococcus faecalis* (60) and *S. enterica* serovar Typhimurium (31). The roles for the bacterial MntH family type of transporters in pathogenicity are less well established. The *mntH* mutant in *Salmonella* is only marginally attenuated in virulence in mice and is more sensitive to H_2O_2 relative to the wild-type strain (33). However, when both transport systems are inactivated in *Salmonella,* the double mutant is significantly attenuated in virulence, suggesting that manganese acquisition is required for the full virulence of the organism (73).

Interestingly, in many eukaryotic hosts the Nramp family of divalent cation symporters plays an important role in innate immunity (15). Nramp1 is recruited to the membrane of microbe-containing phagosomes, where it functions as an efflux pump to deplete the phagosomal space of divalent cations, such as Mn^{2+}, in a pH-dependent manner. This suggests that the bacterial Nramp homolog MntH and the macrophage Nramp1 transporters may directly compete for Mn and possibly other divalent metals within the phagosome (8).

OSMOADAPTATION

Inhabitants of the soil are exposed to periods of low and high rainfall. Similarly, uropathogens are frequently met with fluctuations in urine concentration and dilution. In order to survive in the soil or within animal hosts, bacteria have to adjust to dramatic changes in extracellular osmolarity. Both soil and pathogenic bacteria have evolved structural and physiological responses to changes in the osmolarity of their surroundings. One means by which bacteria adapt to increased osmotic pressure is through the accumulation of specific solutes (known as compatible solutes) that are either imported or synthesized de novo (62). Such compatible solutes include K^+, amino acids (e.g., glutamate, proline), amino acid derivatives (peptides, *N*-acetylated amino acids), quaternary amines (e.g., glycine betaine, carnitine), sugars (e.g., sucrose, trehalose), and tetrahydropyrimidines (ectoines). Important features of compatible solutes are that they can accumulate to high levels without interfering with vital cellular processes and are effective at stabilizing enzymes. Thus, compatible solutes play a dual role in osmoregulating cells—helping to restore cell volume while also protecting protein struc-

ture and function under adverse environmental conditions (62). This mechanism has also been shown to provide protection against high temperature, freeze-thawing, and drying.

There is increasing evidence to suggest that, in addition to their role in osmotic tolerance, compatible solutes, together with their transport and synthesis systems, are essential for adaptation of pathogenic bacteria, such as *Listeria monocytogenes* and uropathogenic *E. coli,* to their host environments. *L. monocytogenes* is a ubiquitous food-borne pathogen found widely distributed in nature. This ubiquity can be partly explained by the ability of the organism to grow at high osmolarity. *L. monocytogenes* is able to resist high osmotic stress (NaCl concentrations of up to 10%) by accumulating the compatible solutes glycine betaine and carnitine, both of which are provided by the mammalian host. This adaptation to osmotic stress likely contributes to the ability of *Listeria* to infect human hosts, particularly given the elevated osmolarity of the bloodstream (equivalent to 0.15 M NaCl) and gastrointestinal tract (equivalent to 0.3 M NaCl). The importance of betaine and carnitine uptake to *Listeria* survival is illustrated by the existence of at least two unrelated systems for each of the osmolytes. Betaine uptake occurs through the Na^+-dependent BetL transporter and the ATP-dependent GbuABC transporter, whereas the primary uptake systems for carnitine are the OpuC and OpuB transporters (61). Significantly, *Listeria* mutants in which the osmolyte transport systems are inactivated by mutation exhibit a substantial decrease in growth rate when grown under high osmotic conditions, and are attenuated in their ability to cause systemic infection following peroral coinoculation with the wild-type strain (63). The presence of homologous uptake systems in *B. subtilis* suggests that the systems may have evolved to cope with osmotic stresses in the abiotic environment and were subsequently co-opted by pathogenic *L. monocytogenes,* providing a means for adaptation within its host. Similarly, in *E. coli,* the osmoregulatory transporters ProP and ProU mediate the use of betaines as osmoprotectants (62). Given that glycine betaine and proline betaine are present in mammalian urine, the ProP system may facilitate the growth of *E. coli* in the urinary tract. Indeed, the uropathogenic *E. coli* strain HU734, haboring a deletion in the *proP* locus, is defective both in its growth capacity in human urine and in its ability to colonize the murine urinary tract (9).

In response to low osmolarity, gram-negative bacteria increase the production of a family of periplasmic oligosaccharides, the osmoregulated periplasmic glucans (OPGs). In *E. coli*, these OPGs are synthesized by the *mdo* genes. Although the role of OPGs in adaptation to changes in osmolarity remains unclear, several genes that are homologous to the *E. coli mdo* genes have been identified in pathogenicity screens and shown to play vital roles in virulence. For example, a homolog of the *E. coli mdoH* gene is essential for full virulence of *P. aeruginosa* in mouse, *Arabidopsis*, and *Caenorhabditis elegans* (41). A *Salmonella* mutant carrying an insertion *mudJ*, a homolog of the *E. coli mdoB*, is also highly attenuated in virulence (68).

Not all adaptations for survival in the soil translate to more suitable adaptations for survival within a host. For example, *Salmonella* has a periplasmic D-Ala–D-Ala dipeptidase encoded by *pcgL*. PcgL is required for scavenging D-Ala–D-Ala, which is released from the cell wall of dead bacteria or during peptidoglycan remodeling. *pcgL* mutants are hypervirulent in mice, but defective for survival in nutrient-poor conditions. There appear to be conflicting needs for *pcgL*, and *Salmonella* may have retained this gene because it is required to maintain fitness in nonhost environments (45). Similarly, mutator strains of *E. coli* represent a small fraction of natural isolates, despite their advantage in colonizing the mammalian gut. This has been ascribed to the reduced fitness of mutator bacteria in secondary environments, such as soil and water. It seems likely that bacterial pathogens may retain genes that reduce virulence, if such genes contribute significantly to

the overall fitness of the organism in both the host and nonhost environments (71).

Selective Pressures from the Biotic Components in the Soil

Many soil eukaryotes, such as protozoa and nematodes, demonstrate a voracious appetite for bacteria. Coexistence between predator and prey necessitates that the bacteria develop ways to avoid death by digestion, while still sharing the same ecological niche with their predators. Some, such as *Legionella*, have evolved mechanisms to survive within protozoan cells. Others, such as *S. enterica*, *Serratia marcescens*, and *P. aeruginosa* have evolved genes that allow them to colonize and eventually kill their nematode hosts. Various studies that examined the molecular interactions between bacterial pathogens and their mammalian, protozoan, and nematode hosts revealed that common sets of virulence determinants are required to infect these evolutionarily divergent organisms (67).

How might a universal virulence factor be conserved through evolution? A possible explanation comes from the analysis of phenazines, an interesting group of effector molecules identified as diffusible toxins used by *P. aeruginosa* to kill *C. elegans* (41). Phenazines belong to a group of tricyclic secondary products produced by *P. aeruginosa* that are cytotoxic to a variety of eukaryotic and prokaryotic cells. The cytotoxic effect of these molecules is partially due to their ability to undergo redox cycling. The deployment of phenazines as chemical weapons by the present day pathogen may have evolved much earlier than our modern world. This common survival strategy may have originated from an ancestral system used by microbes before the presence of multicellular eukaryotes, perhaps as a means of protection against bacteria-feeding protozoa or as antimicrobials to eliminate competing microorganisms in their natural environment. Using *P. aeruginosa* strains that produce pyocyanin and other phenazines, several studies have shown that amoebae that engulf these bacteria either encyst or die. In some cases, the phenazine-producing bacteria are not eaten (22, 59). Interestingly, phenazines have also been shown to be important virulence determinants of *P. aeruginosa* in burn sepsis and lung infections in mice (38, 41). Together, these data raise the possibility that this virulence determinant was first used for survival against simple eukaryotes and was later co-opted over the course of evolution for use during mammalian infections. The selective advantage attained from producing phenazines is so great that it has been retained at the expense of growth in some species. For example, the phenazine-producing *Pseudomonas phenazinium* forms smaller colonies and lower maximum cell densities (but does not have a lower growth rate) compared to mutants deficient in phenazine synthesis. In addition, mutants that lack phenazine production have greater survival rates than the parent strain when grown in a nutrient-limiting milieu. Yet, when grown together, the phenazine-producing parents out-compete the nonproducing mutants (42) and, by extension, could potentially out grow other nonproducing competitors of other species. This example illustrates that a virulence determinant that is as effective in aiding a pathogen's survival against a diversity of hosts as it is in assisting the organism's growth among competitors will be strongly selected for and maintained.

A further problem facing soil bacteria is the diversity of eukaryotic hosts they encounter, with each host species potentially posing a different selective environment to the bacteria. In theory, the adaptations that maximize fitness of the bacteria in one host may be the exact qualities selected against in an alternative host. Thus, particular adaptations may not be appropriate for all host types. Interestingly, a body of work in the second half of the 1990s revealed that the innate immune system among eukaryotic organisms is conserved. Therefore, coevolution of soil bacteria with their protozoan, nematode, and insect hosts, all of which possess the highly conserved innate immune system, may have led to the selection for a similar set of adaptations that, in addition to allowing growth within the

relatively simple eukaryotes, permits successful infection of mammalian hosts.

PROTOZOA

Protozoa are single-celled eukaryotes, many of which demonstrate a voracious appetite for bacteria. Predatory protozoa that utilize bacteria as their main food source appear to take up and consume their energy source in a manner remarkably similar to the engulfment and destruction of bacteria by mammalian macrophages. Molecular mechanisms employed by a number of prokaryotes to evade intracellular degradation by protozoans have been found to provide the same organisms with resistance to phagolysosomal-induced destruction within macrophages (26, 44, 64, 65). Apparently, the primitive eukaryote is more similar to the mammalian innate immunity cell than one would have guessed based on phylogenetic lineage alone.

The intracellular pathogen *Listeria pneumophila* is just one of a number of emerging prokaryotes that has made the jump from being a protozoan parasite to a significant human pathogen. It flourishes naturally in freshwater as a parasite of amoebae, but it can also replicate within alveolar macrophages (12, 36). The billions of years *L. pneumophila* spent coevolving with their protozoan predators, enduring a selective pressure from under which intracellular growth emerged as the most favorable survival strategy, clearly appears to have primed them to become successful human pathogens. *L. pneumophila* is a gram-negative, opportunistic, intracellular human pathogen that, when inhaled, can cause an acute alveolitis and bronchiolitis. In the most extreme cases, infection of aveolar macrophages by *L. pneumophila* results in a severe pneumonia, especially among immunocompromised patients. Human exposure to *L. pneumophila* is largely attributed to the organism's ability to survive and multiply within environmentally ubiquitous protozoa (14). *L. pneumophila* is unable to replicate in the extracellular environment and appears to be dependent on intraprotozoan replication for its survival and dispersal throughout the natural world (12). Transmission of the pathogen occurs through inhalation of infectious *L. pneumophila*-containing particles produced by infected protozoa found living within aquatic sources such as air-conditioning units, shower-heads, and drinking water systems (46).

L. pneumophila demonstrates a broad protozoal host spectrum; it can invade more than 15 species of protozoa, in addition to mammalian phagocytes, fibroblasts, and epithelial cells. There are several similarities, at both the phenotypic and molecular levels, between the infection of mammalian and protozoan cells that argue strongly for protozoa to play a central role in the transition of *L. pneumophila* into a human pathogen. The uptake of *L. pneumophila* by both its protozoan and mammalian hosts occurs through engulfment of the bacteria by coiling phagosomes. Once internalized, the virulent microbes redirect trafficking of the phagosomal vacuole in which they reside away from its progression through the host's endocytic pathway to the autophagic pathway. In the endocytic pathway, endosomes acquire lysosomal proteinase and become phagolysosomes in which the engulfed pathogen is destroyed. However, *L. pneumophila*-containing endosomes, instead of maturing into phagolysosomes, are fused with early autophagosomes and deposit the bacteria into the autophogosome compartment. Thus, by avoiding the endocytic pathway, *L. pneumophila* escapes killing by lysosomes. By residing instead in the permissive environment of the autophagosome-like vacuoles, this intracellular pathogen is exposed to host cell proteins that are normally sequestered for degradation, and these proteins may provide the nutrients for growth.

The endosome and autophagosome pathways are conserved between protozoa and mammals. This argues that the molecular nature of the interactions between the bacterium and its protozoan and mammalian host should also be similar. Indeed, work from several laboratories has shown that persistence of the pathogen within both aveolar macrophages and protozoa is strictly dependent on the *dot/icm* (defective for organelle trafficking/intracellular multiplication) genes, which encode the type IV virulence secretion system (26, 44, 64, 65). Mutants defective in type IV secretion are unable to establish residence within a protective autophagosomal-like vacuole and are instead targeted to the host's endocytic pathway upon phagocytic entry.

In addition to the analogous modes used to infect mammalian and protozoan cells, *L. pneumophila* also uses similar mechanisms to kill and exit its two evolutionarily distant hosts (26, 44, 64, 65). As *L. pneumophila* exhausts its nutrient supply, it transitions from a replicative form into its infective transmissive form. *L. pneumophila* is one of a number of bacterial pathogens that have co-opted the broadly conserved stringent response pathway to coordinate events pertinent to their survival. For *L. pneumophila*, these events include the exit from a deteriorating environment and the entry into its next host. Accumulation of the second messenger (p)ppGpp (the stringent response alarm signal) in response to a depleting amino acid supply induces cytotoxicity, osmotic resistance, motility, and the capacity to evade the endocytic pathway. Coordinate with the expression of the transmissive traits is the generation of a pore-forming activity used to kill and egress from both mammalian and protozoan cells. *L. pneumophila* exiting a depleted host cell are short, thick, and highly motile, and are more resistant to antibiotics than the vacuole-bound replicative form.

In addition to *L. pneumophila*, protozoa have been shown to function as a persistent reservoir for numerous infectious microbes (5). Several facultative bacterial intracellular pathogens, notably *Mycobacterium avium*, *Chlamydia pneumoniae*, and *L. monocytogenes*, have been shown to survive as endosymbionts or to infect free-living amoebae such as *Acanthamoeba*, *Hartmannella*, and *Naegleria*. Amoebae in the environment have also been found to harbor several other pathogenic bacteria, including *Escherichia coli* O157, *P. aeruginosa*, *Vibrio*,

Burkholderia cepacia, and *Francisella.* These findings suggest a role for protozoa as a significant microbial reservoir and as an important host in the evolution of these bacteria. Resistance to digestion by predatory protozoa serves as an evolutionary precursor of pathogenicity of bacteria in their mammalian host.

NEMATODES AND INSECTS

Like protozoa, many insects and free-living soil nematodes use bacteria as food. Due to the antagonistic nature of this association, it is reasonable to hypothesize that both the nematodes and bacteria have evolved strategies to combat each other.

For many multicellular organisms, the antimicrobial functions of the innate immune response provide the only means of cellular-based protection against invading microbes. Only vertebrates harbor a second cellular-based defense system, the acquired immune system, which is attained through exposure to infectious agents over their lifetime (hence "acquired"). The acquired immune response is mediated by lymphocytes that, through somatic gene rearrangements and a sophisticated diversification process, are capable of recognizing the bewildering array of different antigen epitopes presented by insulting pathogens. The vertebrate innate immune system first works to prevent the growth and spread of microbial invaders. Lymphocytes known as B cells and T cells then carry out the highly specific adaptive immune responses typically required for the complete elimination of pathogens. The pathogen-specific mechanisms B cells and T cells utilize to rid the host of infectious microbes are more efficient on the second exposure to the same pathogen, giving immunological memory to the acquired immune response—an extremely advantageous attribute that the ancient innate immune system lacks.

The innate immune response, on the other hand, operates constantly, without evocation, by nonspecific mechanisms to prevent the establishment of virulent organisms and is just as effective at combating the unwanted intruders on its first encounter as it is on subsequent encounters with the same organism. The innate immune response is an immediate first, and for invertebrates the only, line of cellular-based defense against virulent pathogens. Work in the last few years has provided compelling evidence that many of the components and the signaling mechanisms that comprise the innate immune responses are conserved across different phyla. Related proteins in the defense-associated pathways are present in diverse species ranging from nematodes and insects to plants and mammals, suggesting that the workings of the innate immune system evolved before the divergence of plants and animals.

A striking example of phylogenetic conservation of the innate immune system is the signaling pathway mediated by Toll-like receptor (TLR) proteins (66). The TLR family encodes transmembrane proteins containing extracellular leucine-rich repeats and an intracellular domain that is now known as the Toll/interleukin receptor domain because of its significant homology to the intracellular domain of the interleukin-1 receptor (55). First elucidated in *Drosophila,* the Toll pathway functions in dorsoventral patterning during embryonic development and in activating defense responses in adult flies upon challenge by infectious agents (29). In mammals, the leucine-rich repeat domains of TLRs are involved in the recognition of conserved molecular patterns on pathogens, leading to the activation of the innate immune response (66). Molecules that bear similarity to the TLRs and some of the downstream components are also present in nematodes and plants. *C. elegans* has a Toll homolog, *tol-1,* that is essential both for development and for recognition of a bacterial pathogen (51).

The mitogen-activated protein kinase (MAPK) cassette is another innate immune pathway that is conserved in phylogenetically diverse organisms. The MAPK cassette has a core unit consisting of a three-member protein cascade. MAPKs are activated by MAPK kinases (MKKs), dual-specificity kinases that catalyze the phosphorylation of MAPKs on both tyrosine and threonine residues (37). The

MKKs are themselves phosphorylated and activated by serine/threonine kinases that function as MKK kinases. The evolutionarily conserved MAPKs can be divided into three subgroups: the p38 kinases, the c-Jun N-terminal kinase (JNK, also known as stress-activated protein kinase), and the extracellular signal-regulated kinase. Typically, the p38 and JNK pathways are activated in response to stress stimuli or pathogens, whereas the extracellular signal-regulated kinase pathway transduces the signals from growth factors or mitogens. A wealth of cell biological and biochemical data have implicated a critical role for mammalian p38 MAPK signaling in cellular immune response. Cell biological studies have also implicated p38 and JNK MAPKs in the modulation of the *Drosophila* immune response (25). Genetic analysis using *C. elegans* as a host has provided direct evidence that the p38 MAPK pathway is required during the immune response (34).

The functionality of the phylogenetically conserved innate immune response has provided many eukaryotes with the means to establish themselves in a world dominated by prokaryotic life forms, including countless bacterial pathogens. However, immune pathways also serve as a common selective force that possibly led to the maintenance of universal virulence determinants in a variety of pathogens. Virulence determinants that are used to overcome a conserved cellular function will provide selective advantage to the pathogen, even when it is encountering alternative hosts. The utilization of common signaling pathways for initiation of innate immunity by all multicellular eukaryotes, including humans, in their defense against bacterial pathogens suggests that the coevolution of soil bacteria with their neighboring invertebrates may continue to provide a means of selection for virulence on mammalian hosts.

COMMUNITY BEHAVIORS IN THE SOIL AND ON A LIVING HOST

The ability of bacteria to colonize new territories, be it through interactions with soil substrates or eukaryotic hosts, requires their ability to adhere. It has become increasingly more evident that both plant and animal pathogens utilize common mechanisms to adhere to and infect their host, and that these virulence mechanisms are adapted from structures utilized by soil bacteria to interact with the external milieu. Similarly, the advantages of growth in biofilms, now known to be the principal mode of existence of most soil bacteria in nature, facilitate the pathogenic behavior of a number of microbes. Communal lifestyles and interactions first utilized by ancient prokaryotes to colonize the Earth's soils and vegetation have been employed by modern-day pathogens. In this section, examples will be presented that illustrate how some highly conserved bacterial community behaviors have allowed some soil microbes to successfully make the transition to human pathogens.

Colonization

Bacterial colonization of eukaryotic tissue occurred early in evolution. Land plants appeared on Earth more than 400 million years prior to the appearance of humans, and yet very similar strategies used by soil microbes to attach and adhere to the two evolutionarily divergent multicellular eukaryotes have been recently uncovered. Interestingly, the functionally conserved mechanisms of attachment have been co-opted for their use in pathogenesis.

It has been generally accepted that colonization of the host is a necessary first step in microbial-induced pathogenesis as well as in many host-beneficial interactions, such as those provided to us and many plant species by the normal resident microflora. In fact, bacterial genes encoding external structures that are utilized during the well-studied plant-beneficial interactions established between the gram-negative, root-colonizing bacterium *P. aeruginosa* and its plant hosts have also been implicated to play a role in the colonization of various human tissues by pathogenic microbes (7, 40). Not surprisingly, these are the same means by which soil bacteria colonize new fertile terrestrial environments. Flagella and pili or fimbriae are some of the commonly encoded external protein assemblies known to contribute significantly to the successful colonization of both plant and animal hosts by bacterial pathogens. For many microbes, motility provided by polarly localized or peritrichous flagella increases the likelihood of establishing contact with a potential host. Initial contact between a bacterium and the surface of its target host is often instigated through long, somewhat flexible appendages called pili or fimbriae. Closer contact and tighter binding to the host's surface than either flagella or pili offer the microorganisms are mediated through surface proteins called afimbrial adhesins and also through nonprotein components such as lipopolysaccharide and teichoic acids that comprise the outer surfaces of gram-negative and gram-positive bacteria, respectively. Significant decreases in the ability to colonize their respective hosts have been reported for numerous clinically relevant microbes suffering defects in any one of the surface structures described above (7, 40).

One strategy to prevent bacterial infection is to prevent the pathogen's initial adherence and subsequent colonization of the host. A notable finding is the beneficial effects cranberry juice consumption has in preventing urinary tract infections. Cranberries were found to contain two compounds, fructose and proanthocyanidin, that have antiadherence properties that prevent fimbriated *E. coli* from adhering to uroepithelial cells. Subsequent findings show not only cranberry, but lemon, lime, and blueberry juices to have antiadherence as well as antiproliferative effects on the human pathogens *E. coli* O157:H7, *L. monocytogenes,* and *Salmonella* (47, 54, 57). The activities of these plant-derived antimicrobial compounds underlines the importance of inhibiting bacterial attachment in the prevention of disease.

Biofilms

Most prokaryotes found throughout the Earth's soils live not as single planktonic cells, but in populations of biofilms. Microbial biofilms are surface-attached communities of bacteria typically encased within an extracellular polymeric substance (EPS) matrix composed of secreted protein, carbohydrate, and DNA. Recent findings suggest the ability to form biofilms is an ancient and fundamental behavior of prokaryotes. In fact, the fossil record shows evidence of microbial biofilms occurring 3.3 billion to 3.4 billion years ago (70). Although it has been understood for some time that biofilms are the predominant form within which bacteria in the natural environment survive, the significance of biofilms in infectious disease is just recently being understood.

It is now believed that more than 60% of the bacterial infections treated by physicians involve biofilm formation (19). Apparently, the advantages afforded by a biofilm mode of growth within the soil have been selected and maintained for growth within and on a human host. What evolutionarily conserved advantages does growth in a biofilm offer soil-dwelling and infectious microbes over the free-living planktonic lifestyle? It is hypothesized that growth within biofilms may have provided homeostasis among the extreme conditions of primitive Earth (24). Biofilms may have protected their microbial inhabitants from varying temperatures, alterations in pH, dehydration, and exposure to ultraviolet light and possibly allowed the beneficial concentration of nutrients. Similarly, survival within biofilms residing in a human host protects bacterial pathogens from host defenses such as phagocytes, secreted antibodies, and hydrogen peroxide, all of which are unable to successfully penetrate the EPS. For example, *P. aeruginosa* biofilms produce an exceptionally thick mucoid EPS in the lungs of cystic fibrosis patients. Overproduction of the exopolysaccharide alignate contributes to the resistance of the infection to host defenses and numerous antibiotics (21, 35). Biofilms might have provided an environment amenable to the development of sophisticated interactions between closely associated individual bacteria, such as the quorum-sensing and chemotactic motility signaling pathways, two regulatory pathways known to control the expression of virulence traits in a number of modern-day pathogens. Additionally, the reduced metabolic rate of bacteria existing within a biofilm decreases their susceptibility to antibiotics both in the natural environment and within a human host. The fact that biofilm formation is so prevalent clearly reflects the selective advantage growth upon a surface must provide.

Until recently, *Staphylococcus epidermidis,* a member of our normal skin flora, was not considered an opportunistic pathogen. It was only the extensive use of medical implants on which *S. epidermidis* was found to form biofilms that resulted in its reclassification as a human pathogen. Biofilm formation of streptococci, staphylococci, and *Pseudomonas* on medical implants eventually led to the characterization of the infectious disease chronic polymer-associated infection (20, 69). For these microbes, which were previously believed to be benign, the ability to form biofilms essentially functioned as a virulence mechanism, enabling them to cause disease and be deemed relevant human pathogens.

CONCLUSIONS

Most bacteria species exist in the soil as biofilms, an environment that brings many different strains of bacteria into close contact. These microorganisms will have ample opportunity to transfer genetic material by transformation, conjugation, or transduction. Indeed, gene transfers between bacteria on surfaces of soil particles have been well documented. It is well known that the acquisition of plasmids encoding genes that allow the bacteria to degrade xenobiotics is a response to the selective pressure of xenobiotic pollutants in the soil. Many of the selective pressures, in the form of biotic and abiotic stress, that operate in the soil and within the human body are remarkably similar. Mechanisms utilized by soil bacteria to adapt to their ever-changing environments and those required to successfully compete for limited resources appear to be the same ones necessary to combat the harsh environment of a eukaryotic host. Therefore, acquisition and selection of genes to cope with survival in the soil or in and among soil organisms, such as plants, protozoa, and nematodes, could lead to selection for bacteria that are better adapted to the human host as well.

CHAPTER SUMMARY

- Many bacterial pathogens of vertebrates are either members or evolutionarily close relatives of the natural soil microflora.
- Some of the same abiotic stresses encountered by bacteria within their hosts are also encountered in the soil.
- Bacteria have evolved three principal iron acquisition systems: direct contact and import of host iron-bound components, synthesis of ultrahigh-affinity iron chelators (siderophores), and creation of microanaerobic environments that permit iron absorption.
- Bacteria adapt to increased osmotic pressure through the accumulation of compatible solutes.
- Findings suggest a role for protozoa as a significant microbial reservoir and as an important host in the evolution of pathogenic bacteria.
- For many multicellular organisms, the antimicrobial functions of the innate immune response provide the only means of cellular-based protection against invading microbes.
- Utilization of common innate immunity signaling pathways by multicellular eukaryotes suggests that coevolution of soil bacteria with invertebrates may provide a means of selection for virulence on mammalian hosts.
- Biofilms are the predominant mode of growth for most prokaryotes; 60% of treated bacterial infections involve biofilm formation.

REFERENCES
1. **Barksdale, L., and S. B. Arden.** 1974. Persisting bacteriophage infections, lysogeny, and phage conversions. *Annu. Rev. Microbiol.* **28:**265–299.

2. **Bentley, S. D., K. F. Chater, A. M. Cerdeno-Tarraga, G. L. Challis, N. R. Thomson, K. D. James, D. E. Harris, M. A. Quail, H. Kieser, D. Harper, A. Bateman, S. Brown, G. Chandra, C. W. Chen, M. Collins, A. Cronin, A. Fraser, A. Goble, J. Hidalgo, T. Hornsby, S. Howarth, C. H. Huang, T. Kieser, L. Larke, L. Murphy, K. Oliver, S. O'Neil, E. Rabbinowitsch, M. A. Rajandream, K. Rutherford, S. Rutter, K. Seeger, D. Saunders, S. Sharp, R. Squares, S. Squares, K. Taylor, T. Warren, A. Wietzorrek, J. Woodward, B. G. Barrell, J. Parkhill, and D. A. Hopwood.** 2002. Complete genome sequence of the model actinomycete *Streptomyces coelicolor* A3(2). *Nature* **417:**141–147.

3. **Bossi, L., J. A. Fuentes, G. Mora, and N. Figueroa-Bossi.** 2003. Prophage contribution to bacterial population dynamics. *J. Bacteriol.* **185:**6467–6471.

4. **Braun, V.** 2001. Iron uptake mechanisms and their regulation in pathogenic bacteria. *Int. J. Med. Microbiol.* **291:**67–79.

5. **Brown, M. R. W., and J. Barker.** 1999. Unexplored reservoirs of pathogenic bacteria: protozoa and biofilms. *Trends Microbiol.* **7:**46–50.

6. **Brussow, H., C. Canchaya, and W. D. Hardt.** 2004. Phages and the evolution of bacterial pathogens: from genomic rearrangements to lysogenic conversion. *Microbiol. Mol. Biol. Rev.* **68:**560–602, table of contents.

7. **Cao, H., R. L. Baldini, and L. G. Rahme.** 2001. Common mechanisms for pathogens of plants and animals. *Annu. Rev. Phytopathol.* **39:**259–284.

8. **Cellier, M. F., I. Bergevin, E. Boyer, and E. Richer.** 2001. Polyphyletic origins of bacterial Nramp transporters. *Trends Genet.* **17:**365–370.

9. **Culham, D. E., C. Dalgado, C. L. Gyles, D. Mamelak, S. MacLellan, and J. M. Wood.** 1998. Osmoregulatory transporter ProP influences colonization of the urinary tract by Escherichia coli. *Microbiology* **144:**91–102.

10. **Demaneche, S., E. Kay, F. Gourbiere, and P. Simonet.** 2001. Natural transformation of Pseudomonas fluorescens and Agrobacterium tumefaciens in soil. *Appl. Environ. Microbiol.* **67:**2617–2621.

11. **Dubnau, D.** 1999. DNA uptake in bacteria. *Annu. Rev. Microbiol.* **53:**217–244.

12. **Fields, B.** 1996. The molecular ecology of legionellae. *Trends Microbiol.* **4:**286–290.

13. **Figueroa-Bossi, N., and L. Bossi.** 1999. Inducible prophages contribute to *Salmonella* virulence in mice. *Mol. Microbiol.* **33:**167–176.

14. **Fliermans, C. B., W. B. Cherry, L. H. Orrison, S. J. Smith, D. L. Tison, and D. H. Pope.** 1981. Ecological distribution of *Legionella pneumophila*. *Appl. Environ. Microbiol.* **41:**9–16.

15. **Forbes, J. R., and P. Gros.** 2001. Divalent-metal transport by NRAMP proteins at the interface of host-pathogen interactions. *Trends Microbiol.* **9:**397–403.

16. **Fraser, C. M., J. D. Gocayne, O. White, M. D. Adams, R. A. Clayton, R. D. Fleischmann, C. J. Bult, A. R. Kerlavage, G. Sutton, J. M. Kelley, et al.** 1995. The minimal gene complement of *Mycoplasma genitalium*. *Science* **270:**397–403.

17. **Freeman, V. J.** 1951. Studies on the virulence of bacteriophage-infected strains of *Corynebacterium diphtheriae*. *J. Bacteriol.* **61:**675–688.

18. **Freiberg, C., R. Fellay, A. Bairoch, W. J. Broughton, A. Rosenthal, and X. Perret.** 1997. Molecular basis of symbiosis between *Rhizobium* and legumes. *Nature* **387:**394–401.

19. **Fux, C. A., J. W. Costerton, P. S. Stewart, and P. Stoodley.** 2005. Survival strategies of infectious biofilms. *Trends Microbiol.* **13:**34–40.

20. **Gotz, F.** 2002. *Staphylococcus* and biofilms. *Mol. Microbiol.* **43:**1367–1378.

21. **Govan, J. R., and V. Deretic.** 1996. Microbial pathogenesis in cystic fibrosis: mucoid *Pseudomonas aeruginosa* and *Burkholderia cepacia*. *Microbiol. Rev.* **60:**539–574.

22. **Groscop, J. A., and M. M. Brent.** 1964. The effects of selected strains of pigmented microorganisms on small free-living amoebae. *Can. J. Microbiol.* **10:**579–584.

23. **Hacker, J., and E. Carniel.** 2001. Ecological fitness, genomic islands and bacterial pathogenicity. A Darwinian view of the evolution of microbes. *EMBO Rep.* **2:**376–381.

24. **Hall-Stoodley, L., J. W. Costerton, and P. Stoodley.** 2004. Bacterial biofilms: from the natural environment to infectious diseases. *Nat. Rev. Microbiol.* **2:**95–108.

25. **Han, Z. S., H. Enslen, X. Hu, X. Meng, I. H. Wu, T. Barrett, R. J. Davis, and Y. T. Ip.** 1998. A conserved p38 mitogen-activated protein kinase pathway regulates *Drosophila* immunity gene expression. *Mol. Cell. Biol.* **18:**3527–3539.

26. **Harb, O. S., L. Y. Gao, and Y. A. Kwaik.** 2000. From protozoa to mammalian cells: a new paradigm in the life cycle of intracellular bacterial pathogens. *Environ. Microbiol.* **2:**251–265.

27. **Hardalo, C., and S. C. Edberg.** 1997. *Pseudomonas aeruginosa*: assessment of risk from drinking water. *Crit. Rev. Microbiol.* **23:**47–75.

28. **Helgason, E., O. A. Okstad, D. A. Caugant, H. A. Johansen, A. Fouet, M. Mock, I. Hegna, and A.-B. Kolsto.** 2000. *Bacillus anthracis, Bacillus cereus*, and *Bacillus thuringiensis*—one species on the basis of genetic evidence. *Appl. Environ. Microbiol.* **66:**2627–2630.

29. **Hoffmann, J. A.** 2003. The immune response of *Drosophila*. *Nature* **426:**33–38.

30. **Jakubovics, N. S., and H. F. Jenkinson.** 2001. Out of the iron age: new insights into the critical role of manganese homeostasis in bacteria. *Microbiology* **147:**1709–1718.

31. **Janakiraman, A., and J. M. Slauch.** 2000. The putative iron transport system SitABCD encoded on SPI1 is required for full virulence of *Salmonella typhimurium*. *Mol. Microbiol.* **35:**1146–1155.

32. **Kehres, D. G., and M. E. Maguire.** 2003. Emerging themes in manganese transport, biochemistry and pathogenesis in bacteria. *FEMS Microbiol. Rev.* **27:**263–290.

33. **Kehres, D. G., M. L. Zaharik, B. B. Finlay, and M. E. Maguire.** 2000. The NRAMP proteins of *Salmonella typhimurium* and *Escherichia coli* are selective manganese transporters involved in the response to reactive oxygen. *Mol. Microbiol.* **36:**1085–1100.

34. **Kim, D. H., R. Feinbaum, G. Alloing, F. E. Emerson, D. A. Garsin, H. Inoue, M. Tanaka-Hino, N. Hisamoto, K. Matsumoto, M. W. Tan, and F. M. Ausubel.** 2002. A conserved p38 MAP kinase pathway in *Caenorhabditis elegans* innate immunity. *Science* **297:**623–626.

35. **Koch, C., and N. Hoiby.** 1993. Pathogenesis of cystic fibrosis. *Lancet* **341:**1065–1069.

36. **Kwaik, Y. A., L. Y. Gao, B. J. Stone, and O. S. Harb.** 1998. Invasion of mammalian and protozoan cells by *Legionella pneumophila*. *Bull. Inst. Pasteur* **96:**237–247.

37. **Kyriakis, J. M., and J. Avruch.** 2001. Mammalian mitogen-activated protein kinase signal transduction pathways activated by stress and inflammation. *Physiol. Rev.* **81:**807–869.

38. **Lau, G. W., H. Ran, F. Kong, D. J. Hassett, and D. Mavrodi.** 2004. *Pseudomonas aeruginosa* pyocyanin is critical for lung infection in mice. *Infect. Immun.* **72:**4275–4278.

39. **Lorenz, M. G., and W. Wackernagel.** 1994. Bacterial gene transfer by natural genetic transformation in the environment. *Microbiol. Rev.* **58:**563–602.

40. **Lugtenberg, B. J., L. Dekkers, and G. V. Bloemberg.** 2001. Molecular determinants of rhizosphere colonization by *Pseudomonas*. *Annu. Rev. Phytopathol.* **39:**461–490.

41. **Mahajan-Miklos, S., M.-W. Tan, L. G. Rahme, and F. M. Ausubel.** 1999. Molecular mechanisms of bacterial virulence elucidated using a *Pseudomonas aeruginosa-Caenorhabditis elegans* pathogenesis model. *Cell* **96:**47–56.

42. **Messenger, A. J., and J. M. Turner.** 1981. Effect of secondary metabolite production on the growth rate and variability of a pseudomonad. *Soc. Gen. Microbiol. Quarterly* **8:**2263–2264.

43. **Mirold, S., W. Rabsch, M. Rohde, S. Stender, H. Tschape, H. Russmann, E. Igwe, and W. D. Hardt.** 1999. Isolation of a temperate bacteriophage encoding the type III effector protein SopE from an epidemic Salmonella typhimurium strain. *Proc. Natl. Acad. Sci. USA* **96:**9845–9850.

44. **Molofsky, A. B., and M. S. Swanson.** 2004. Differentiate to thrive: lessons from the *Legionella pneumophila* life cycle. *Mol. Microbiol.* **53:**29–40.

45. **Mouslim, C., F. Hilbert, H. Huang, and E. A. Groisman.** 2002. Conflicting needs for a *Salmonella* hypervirulence gene in host and non-host environments. *Mol. Microbiol.* **45:**1019–1027.

46. **Muder, R. R., V. L. Yu, and A. H. Woo.** 1986. Mode of transmission of *Legionella pneumophila*. *Arch. Intern. Med.* **146:**1607–1612.

47. **Nogueira, M. C., O. A. Oyarzabal, and D. E. Gombas.** 2003. Inactivation of *Escherichia coli* O157:H7, *Listeria monocytogenes,* and *Salmonella* in cranberry, lemon, and lime juice concentrates. *J. Food Prot.* **66:**1637–1641.

48. **Ochman, H., J. G. Lawrence, and E. A. Groisman.** 2000. Lateral gene transfer and the nature of bacterial innovation. *Nature* **405:**299–304.

49. **Okinaka, R., K. Cloud, O. Hampton, A. Hoffmaster, K. Hill, P. Keim, T. Koehler, G. Lamke, S. Kumano, D. Manter, Y. Martinez, D. Ricke, R. Svensson, and P. Jackson.** 1999. Sequence, assembly and analysis of pX01 and pX02. *J. Appl. Microbiol.* **87:**261–262.

50. **Olczak, T., W. Simpson, X. Liu, and C. A. Genco.** 2005. Iron and heme utilization in *Porphyromonas gingivalis*. *FEMS Microbiol. Rev.* **29:**119–144.

51. **Pujol, N., E. M. Link, L. X. Liu, C. L. Kurz, G. Alloing, M. W. Tan, K. P. Ray, R. Solari, C. D. Johnson, and J. J. Ewbank.** 2001. A reverse genetic analysis of components of the Toll signaling pathway in *Caenorhabditis elegans*. *Curr. Biol.* **11:**809–821.

52. **Radnedge, L., P. G. Agron, K. K. Hill, P. J. Jackson, L. O. Ticknor, P. Keim, and G. L. Andersen.** 2003. Genome differences that distinguish *Bacillus anthracis* from *Bacillus cereus* and *Bacillus thuringiensis*. *Appl. Environ. Microbiol.* **69:**2755–2764.

53. **Ratledge, C., and L. G. Dover.** 2000. Iron metabolism in pathogenic bacteria. *Annu. Rev. Microbiol.* **54:**881–941.

54. **Raz, R., B. Chazan, and M. Dan.** 2004. Cranberry juice and urinary tract infection. *Clin. Infect. Dis.* **38:**1413–1419.

55. **Rock, F. L., G. Hardiman, J. C. Timans, R. A. Kastelein, and J. F. Bazan.** 1998. A family of human receptors structurally related to *Drosophila* Toll. *Proc. Natl. Acad. Sci. USA* **95:**588–593.

56. **Salamitou, S., F. Ramisse, M. Brehelin, D. Bourguet, N. Gilois, M. Gominet, E.**

Hernandez, and D. Lereclus. 2000. The plcR regulon is involved in the opportunistic properties of *Bacillus thuringiensis* and *Bacillus cereus* in mice and insects. *Microbiology* **146**(Pt. 11)**:**2825–2832.

57. **Schmidt, B. M., A. B. Howell, B. McEniry, C. T. Knight, D. Seigler, J. W. Erdman, Jr., and M. A. Lila.** 2004. Effective separation of potent antiproliferation and antiadhesion components from wild blueberry (*Vaccinium angustifolium* Ait.) fruits. *J. Agric. Food Chem.* **52**:6433–6442.

58. **Sikorski, J., S. Graupner, M. G. Lorenz, and W. Wackernagel.** 1998. Natural genetic transformation of Pseudomonas stutzeri in a non-sterile soil. *Microbiology* **144**(Pt. 2)**:**569–576.

59. **Singh, B. N.** 1945. The selection of bacterial food by soil amoeba, and the toxic effects of bacterial pigments and other products on soil protozoa. *Br. J. Exp. Pathol.* **26:**316–325.

60. **Singh, K. V., T. M. Coque, G. M. Weinstock, and B. E. Murray.** 1998. *In vivo* testing of an *Enterococcus faecalis efaA* mutant and use of *efaA* homologs for species identification. *FEMS Immunol. Med. Microbiol.* **21:**323–331.

61. **Sleator, R. D., C. G. Gahan, and C. Hill.** 2003. A postgenomic appraisal of osmotolerance in *Listeria monocytogenes. Appl. Environ. Microbiol.* **69:**1–9.

62. **Sleator, R. D., and C. Hill.** 2001. Bacterial osmoadaptation: the role of osmolytes in bacterial stress and virulence. *FEMS Microbiol. Rev.* **26:** 49–71.

63. **Sleator, R. D., J. Wouters, C. G. Gahan, T. Abee, and C. Hill.** 2001. Analysis of the role of OpuC, an osmolyte transport system, in salt tolerance and virulence potential of *Listeria monocytogenes. Appl. Environ. Microbiol.* **67:**2692–2698.

64. **Steinert, M., U. Hentschel, and J. Hacker.** 2002. *Legionella pneumophila:* an aquatic microbe goes astray. *FEMS Microbiol. Rev.* **26:**149–162.

65. **Swanson, M. S., and B. K. Hammer.** 2000. *Legionella pneumophila* pathogenesis: a fateful journey from amobae to macrophages. *Annu. Rev. Microbiol.* **54:**567–613.

66. **Takeda, K., and S. Akira.** 2004. TLR signaling pathways. Semin. Immunol. **16:**3–9.

67. **Tan, M.-W.** 2002. Cross-species infections and their analysis. *Annu. Rev. Microbiol.* **56:**539–565.

68. **Valentine, P. J., B. P. Devore, and F. Heffron.** 1998. Identification of three highly attenuated *Salmonella typhimurium* mutants that are more immunogenic and protective in mice than a prototypical aroA mutant. *Infect. Immun.* **66:**3378–3383.

69. **von Eiff, C., C. Heilmann, M. Herrmann, and G. Peters.** 1999. Basic aspects of the pathogenesis of staphylococcal polymer-associated infections. *Infection* **27**(Suppl. 1)**:**S7–S10.

70. **Westall, F., M. J. de Wit, J. Dann, S. van der Gaast, C. E. J. de Ronde, and D. Gerneke.** 2001. Early Archean fossil bacteria and biofilms in hydrothermally-influenced sediments from the Barberton greenstone belt, South Africa. *Precambrian Res.* **106:**93–116.

71. **Winfield, M. D., and E. A. Groisman.** 2003. Role of nonhost environments in the lifestyles of *Salmonella* and *Escherichia coli. Appl. Environ. Microbiol.* **69:**3687–3694.

72. **Yesilkaya, H., A. Kadioglu, N. Gingles, J. E. Alexander, T. J. Mitchell, and P. W. Andrew.** 2000. Role of manganese-containing superoxide dismutase in oxidative stress and virulence of *Streptococcus pneumoniae. Infect. Immun.* **68:** 2819–2826.

73. **Zaharik, M. L., V. L. Cullen, A. M. Fung, S. J. Libby, S. L. Kujat Choy, B. Coburn, D. G. Kehres, M. E. Maguire, F. C. Fang, and B. B. Finlay.** 2004. The *Salmonella enterica* serovar Typhimurium divalent cation transport systems MntH and SitABCD are essential for virulence in an Nramp1G169 murine typhoid model. *Infect. Immun.* **72:**5522–5525.

74. **Zhang, S., R. L. Santos, R. M. Tsolis, S. Mirold, W. D. Hardt, L. G. Adams, and A. J. Baumler.** 2002. Phage mediated horizontal transfer of the sopE1 gene increases enteropathogenicity of *Salmonella enterica* serotype Typhimurium for calves. *FEMS Microbiol. Lett.* **217:**243–247.

EXPERIMENTAL MODELS OF SYMBIOTIC HOST-MICROBIAL RELATIONSHIPS: UNDERSTANDING THE UNDERPINNINGS OF BENEFICENCE AND THE ORIGINS OF PATHOGENESIS

Margaret J. McFall-Ngai and Jeffrey I. Gordon

9

All biological systems are the result of particular evolutionary histories. To understand them fully, it is necessary to examine the entire scope of their past, considering what forces may have shaped their present-day genotypes and phenotypes. In this chapter, we take the position that pathogenesis arises within the context of pre-existing, coevolved beneficial associations between animal and plant species and their microbial partners. We first consider the evolutionary framework within which beneficial associations arose and describe what is known about the function of such relationships in selected plant and invertebrate model systems. In each case, we reflect upon known similarities and differences between beneficial and pathogenic associations. We then consider the molecular foundations of host-microbial symbioses in a mammalian model.

The study of beneficial associations of plants and animals with microorganisms is in its infancy. Thus, our chapter describes the very beginnings of a characterization. The understandable historical focus on determining the basis of devastating pathogenic diseases, as well as technical impediments to studying the dynamic and complex interactions between microbial communities and their hosts, have hindered our ability to obtain an accurate understanding of the relationships of animals and plants with the microbial world. However, advances such as the advent of convenient and cost-effective molecular methods for enumerating a microbiota, rapid sequencing and accurate annotation of microbial genomes, plus use of functional genomic methods to comprehensively profile the transcriptional responses of defined cellular populations, are helping to open this field so that we can define the contributions of indigenous microbial communities to the development of plant and animal species, and to their adult physiology.

DEFINITION OF TERMS

> Words are, of course, the most powerful drug used by mankind.
> Rudyard Kipling

The most widely accepted definition of the word "symbiosis" was formulated by Anton de Bary in 1879 as "the living together of two differently named organisms." Under this broader term, three types of symbioses are recognized: mutualistic (beneficial), commensal,

Margaret J. McFall-Ngai, Department of Medical Microbiology and Immunology, University of Wisconsin, Madison, WI 53706. *Jeffrey I. Gordon,* Center for Genome Sciences, Washington University School of Medicine, St. Louis, MO 63108.

Evolution of Microbial Pathogens, Edited by H. S. Seifert and V. J. DiRita, © 2006 ASM Press, Washington, D.C.

TABLE 1 The types of symbioses based on the effect of the association on the fitness of the partners[a]

Organism	Mutualism	Commensalism	Pathogenic
Host	+	+ or 0	− or +
Microbe	+	0 or +	+ or −

[a] +, increased fitness; 0, no effect on fitness; −, decreased fitness.

and pathogenic (parasitic). The characterization of symbioses within this trichotomy refers to the effect that a given association has on the fitness (number of offspring) of the host and its microbial partner (Table 1). It is often difficult to determine such effects, in which case the more general classification "symbiosis" is often applied. The term "commensal" has been widely used in the past to describe microbes in associations with vertebrates (such as the gut microbiota of mammals), and suggests that the microbes have no influence on the fitness of the host. This prior usage was an indication of our tendency to be conservative in the absence of specific knowledge. However, its continued usage reflects a denial of major conclusions reported in an emerging body of literature. Numerous studies in recent years have demonstrated that these bacteria are essential to the health of the host—findings that should compel biologists to no longer to consider themselves agnostic with regard to these associations.

BEYOND THE ENDOSYMBIOSIS THEORY

The widespread nature of coevolved associations of animals and plants with microbes is supported by theoretical considerations of the history of the biosphere and analyses of the patterns of occurrence of such associations. Within this context, dynamic, coevolved animal-bacterial alliances have formed that persist from generation to generation as specific and complex symbioses, providing hosts animals with unique physiological and biochemical capabilities (54). For decades, biologists have embraced theories that espouse the endosymbiotic origin of the eukaryotic cell (51). Did the profound impact of environmental microbes on evolutionary radiations stop with the advent of eukaryotes? In the study of the evolution of multicellularity, thus far the greatest emphasis has been placed on abiotic selection pressures (e.g., levels of atmospheric oxygen). However, when one considers the theoretical landscape, the most parsimonious explanation is that microbes are likely to have been, and continue to be, a significant selective force on the evolution of the biosphere. Specifically, multicellular organisms appeared on the scene somewhere between 600 million and 1,000 million years ago, within aquatic environments that had been the evolutionary "playground" of microbes for the previous 2+ billion years. All evidence suggests that metabolically versatile microbes were abundant in the seawater of that era, at hundreds of thousands to millions of cells per milliliter, just as they are in the oceans of today. Theoretically, with this environmental backdrop, it appears highly likely that multicellular organisms have always formed specific relationships with environmental bacteria, such that the natural situation is to occur as an array of communities integrated into a complex coevolving ecosystem. What is unexplored are the possible reciprocal impacts of such biotic pressure on the major milestones of animal evolution, e.g., the advent of gastrulation and, later, that of the complete gut or the celom (an advance that functionally separated the body wall from the gut), and invasion of terrestrial habitats. How would alliances with microbes influence, and be influenced by, these and other evolutionary events affecting host organisms?

Strong correlations for the occurrence of coevolved associations can be found in the patterns of radiation of specific taxonomic groups. One of the more dramatic examples is the water-to-land transition of plants. This transition is strongly correlated with the evolution of the root-associated mycorrhizae: i.e., fungi that mobilize inorganic phosphate and make it available to the plant (68). The persistent association of mycorrhizae with terrestrial plants through the course of their evolution, and the occurrence of such symbioses in the vast majority of modern-day land plants, strongly suggest that the association was a key innovation that led to the radiation of plants in terrestrial environments. Similarly, the presence of root nodules with nitrogen-fixing bacteria (rhizobia) is a shared derived characteristic of leguminous plants (18). Molecular studies of these systems over the last several decades have provided strong evidence for their coevolution (26, 76).

Although evidence of animal-microbial interactions is not generally preserved in the fossil record, many conspicuous examples of symbiosis-correlated radiations have occurred during animal evolution (16, 52). As in the legume-rhizobium (LR) associations, these symbioses have provided animal hosts with the ability to use resources that are inaccessible without the metabolic capabilities of their microbial partners. For example, the association of modern reef-building corals with their intracellular algal partners has been a principal force in their domination of tropical and subtropical oceanic habitats. In termites and ruminants, complex gut consortia have permitted the efficient use of plant products, a capacity that has been critical to the evolutionary success of these lineages.

One of the challenges for biologists armed with genomic tools is to determine how prevalent such phenomena are in the subtler associations. In recent years, these studies have begun by focusing principally on human and mouse systems, such as complex consortia in various regions of the alimentary canal (e.g., oral cavity, stomach, and intestine).

These few examples represent a sampling of data available suggesting that microbes are principal forces in the evolution of multicellular organisms. To take the argument one step further, how would the persistent influence of microbes over long geological time periods be reflected in the evolution of molecular programs and metabolic pathways? In the late 1990s, the field of cellular microbiology emerged (8, 30). This discipline recognizes that biologists can learn about the function of eukaryotic cells through an analysis of the effects of microorganisms on cellular processes. For example, the contributions of cAMP, cGMP, and calcium to cellular biology, as well as the behavior of the cytoskeleton, have been deduced in part through a characterization of the ways certain microbes alter the "normal" condition. Thus far, the microbes most commonly associated with these alterations are pathogens, and often their products that perturb eukaryotic cells are toxins (e.g., those produced by *Pseudomonas aeruginosa, Shigella* spp., *Yersinia enterocolitica,* and *Vibrio cholerae*).

The interaction of microbial pathogens with multicellular organisms is most commonly depicted as an "arms race." However, if coevolved associations with microbes began early in the evolution of multicellularity, the interactions would have imposed selection pressure on these pathways. The cell biology of present-day multicellular organisms would be the result of a shared history with associating microorganisms. Thus, the toxins of pathogens, and the responses to these toxins, may be a small part of a much larger molecular dialogue that is simply the set of mechanisms by which animal and plant cells converse with microbes. In this conceptualization, the outcome of the dialogue, whether a persistent beneficial association or the acute onset of pathology, is the result of how the genes and gene products are used in a given circumstance, by a given set of partners, in a given susceptible site, at a particular time in the life history of the host. These ideas are largely speculative at present, but increasing our knowledge of the molecular foundations of beneficial associations promises to provide new perspectives on exactly what biochemical and physiological processes establish and sustain host-symbiont interactions.

TRENDS IN BENEFICIAL ASSOCIATIONS

Evolution has created a remarkable variety of symbiotic associations. These are variously classified and described according to their mode of transmission, the physical relationship of partner cells, the principal products exchanged, and the complexity of the community. With rare exceptions, such as the associations in which light emission is the bacterial product used by the host, the basis of the symbiosis is nutritional: i.e., the partners exchange specific nutrients, or provide an environment where nutrients can be concentrated, such as in the gut.

Beneficial associations between microbes and multicellular organisms display a number of features that are likely to be critical to their evolutionary patterns. The mode of transmission between generations, for example, has profound effects on the symbiosis. Broadly speaking, the microbial symbiont(s) exhibit either horizontal (environmental) or vertical (transovarian) transmission. In other words, they are either acquired at each generation from an environmental reservoir of the microorganisms, or they are passed directly (vertically) by provision of the microbes with the eggs of the female host, respectively. Notable examples include the vertically transmitted bacteriocyte symbioses that are characteristic of at least 10 to 15% of insect species (14), and the horizontally transmitted consortial associations of many, if not all, mammals (e.g., reference 20).

Horizontally transmitted symbioses must evolve mechanisms to ensure that the juveniles recognize the appropriate environmental symbiont cells. In contrast, while vertically transmitted symbioses do not require this capability, they must evolve mechanisms to ensure that the symbiont is incorporated into the proper organ system during host embryogenesis. The cellular and molecular mechanisms by which these processes occur remain largely unknown, with the exception of a few horizontally transmitted symbioses, such as the LR and squid-vibrio (SV) alliances (see below).

The two different modes of transmission also appear to have an impact on the evolution of the microbial partner's genome size. Recent studies of insect-bacteriocyte associations have shown that the genome of the bacterial partner undergoes significant reduction, becoming increasingly like an organelle of the host cells (15). Apparently, the more ancient the vertically transmitted association, the greater the genome size reduction. For example, in the aphid-Buchnera symbioses, which are thought to date back about 200 million years to the mid-Mesozoic, the genome size of some microbial strains is less than 600 kbp, thus exhibiting a reduction size similar to that of many intracellular microbial pathogens (57). Analyses of these genomes have disclosed that they contain no unique genes (all have homologs in Escherichia coli). By contrast, in horizontally transmitted symbioses, the bacterial symbiont often inhabits more than one ecological niche. This complexity in lifestyle correlates with a significantly larger genome size—generally at least 8 to 10 times greater than in strains of Buchnera. For example, Mesorhizobium loti, the rhizobial species that is symbiotic in nitrogen-fixing root nodules of the lotus plant, has a 6.7-Mbp genome with a "symbiotic element" of 500 kbp that is larger than the entire genome of some Buchnera strains (43).

The location of a symbiont in relation to the host cell can vary from being embedded in an overlying mucus layer to being intracellular, free in the host's cytoplasm. Location does not necessary reflect the degree of metabolic interchange (commerce) between host and symbiont. An intracellular symbiont, although physically intimate with the host cell, may be quiescent, while an extracellular symbiont may be exporting products that profoundly influence host cell behavior. There is no apparent correlation between the cellular relationship and mode of transmission of symbionts between host generations. For example, the coral-photosynthetic algal (zooxanthellae) symbioses, in which the microbial partner is intracellular, have evolved to be either horizontally or vertically transmitted, depending on the association (70). Similarly, among the obligate associations between intracellular sulfur-oxidizing bacteria and the invertebrates that are nutritionally dependent upon them, some are horizontally transmitted (e.g., the vent tube worm Riftia pachyptila and the bivalve Codakia *costata*) while others are subject to vertical transmission (e.g., the bivalves *Solemya* spp. and *Calptogena elongata*) (6, 47). In the symbioses between extracellular bacteria and animals, examples can be found of horizontal transmission (e.g., the squid-vibrio association) and vertical transmission (e.g., the bryozoan *Bugula neritina* and its bacterial symbiont *Endobugula sertula* [28, 75]).

Associations may be consortial or binary (i.e., one host and one microbial species). Consortia usually exist as dozens to hundreds of microbial species that are extracellular and horizontally transmitted between host generations. Exceptions to this dichotomy are unusual and include a few invertebrates that have vertically transmitted symbioses involving two to three species of bacteria within host cells (e.g., a hydrothermal vent mussel host that has both thioautotrophic and methanotrophic bacterial symbionts coexisting within one host cell [12]).

In the case of consortial symbioses in terrestrial animals, the adult populations often help facilitate transmission between generations. For example, colony mates feed juvenile termites the symbiont-containing feces of adult animals. Many consortial symbioses colonize tissues that remain exposed to the environment throughout the lifespan of the host. Thus, one of the challenges to studying these alliances is to distinguish between "resident" coevolved (autochthonous) partners, and "tourists" (allochthonous partners), and to determine the relative contribution of each subset of the community to the overall "economy" of a given association.

Before careful analyses were performed, it was generally assumed that vertically transmitted, intracellular symbioses were more ancient and more tightly controlled alliances: i.e., there had been an evolutionary progression from looser, extracellular symbioses that were environmentally transmitted to more highly evolved, intracellular, vertically transmitted associations. A pattern of congruence between the phylogenies of host species and their microbial partners within related symbioses (i.e., one in which the phylogenetic trees of host species

and those of their symbionts mirror one another) strongly suggests a tightly coevolved set of associations. However, studies have revealed congruence as well as lack of congruence in the host and symbiont phylogenies in both horizontally and vertically transmitted associations. For example, the solemyid clams (a family of hydrothermal vent mollusks) do not exhibit congruence in their host and symbiont phylogenies, despite the fact that the associations are intracellular and vertically transmitted (46). This finding suggests that at least some of the symbioses in this group are relatively recently, and independently, acquired, or that they have been lost and reacquired several times. Another example can be found in associations involving an intracellular pathogen of insects, *Wolbachia*. Biologists have witnessed this association sweep through populations of *Drosophila* species in California, although it is vertically transmitted once acquired (71). In contrast, the extracellular, horizontally transmitted squid-vibrio symbioses do exhibit strong congruence in the phylogenies of the host species and symbiont strains (58). Furthermore, experiments testing the ability of strains of the microbial symbiont to colonize host animals have supported the hypothesis that the squid-vibrio symbioses are highly specific associations resulting from a prolonged period of coevolution between the partners (58).

In addition to these trends in beneficial associations, a pattern may also be emerging in the types of animal-microbe symbioses that generally occur in invertebrates and vertebrates. Invertebrates more often have binary, intracellular symbioses that rarely, if ever, occur in vertebrates. In contrast, vertebrates appear more often to have complex extracellular consortia. An exception in the invertebrates occurs in the hindguts of termites and cockroaches, which harbor very complex coevolved consortia. Some other invertebrate species have microbe-rich guts transiently (during feeding) or may associate with large concentrations of environmental microbes, although perhaps not coevolved partners. However, these differences between vertebrates and invertebrates could simply be a reflection of our lack of extensive comparative data, and therefore may not hold when more information becomes available.

BINARY PLANT AND INVERTEBRATE MODEL SYSTEMS: THE LEGUME-RHIZOBIUM AND SQUID-VIBRIO EXPERIMENTAL SYMBIOSES

Just as biologists have relied on a variety of model organisms to characterize the basic mechanisms of development (e.g., sea urchin, fruit fly, nematode, and mouse), a comprehensive understanding of the diverse mechanisms by which microbes associate with multicellular organisms requires investigation of a number of experimental systems. The LR system has been studied for over 100 years by dozens of laboratories, yielding a rich database of thousands of publications. In contrast, the SV association has been under intense investigation for less than 15 years, in only a handful of laboratories, producing several dozen reports. Nonetheless, comparative analyses of both associations have begun to reveal some basic principles of eukaryotic-prokaryotic interactions, and to identify properties that are unique to either plant-microbe or animal-microbe alliances (33). Because the LR and SV systems have been the subject of a number of recent reviews, we will only consider those aspects of the associations relevant to comparisons with pathogenesis.

The critical feature in both the LR and SV associations that renders them amenable to experimental study is the ability to culture and manipulate both partners, independently, under laboratory conditions. This capability stems from the nature of each association. The LR symbioses can be considered "facultative" in that they are only obligate to the host under conditions of nitrogen limitation in the soil; i.e., although rhizobia occur as free-living members of the rhizosphere microbial community, when sufficient nitrogen is available to the plant, nodules do not form (49). This feature, along with the ability to culture and genetically manipulate both the rhizobium and, more recently, its host, has allowed biologists to begin to decipher the dialogue that takes place between plant and bacterial partners. In contrast, the SV symbiosis is likely to be obligate under field conditions. While the precise function of the light organ symbiosis remains to be determined, its morphology strongly suggests that the host uses bacterial light as a camouflaging, antipredatory strategy. The symbiosis is always present in field-caught animals, and selection pressure has occurred on the host embryonic period for development of a nascent light organ that is poised to be colonized immediately upon hatching (55). These features of the association suggest that it is essential to the host's biology in nature. However, luminescence, as the principal bacterial product used by the animal host, is not critical to the host under laboratory conditions, where potential predators are not present. The physiology of the squid does not seem to be compromised by the absence of its microbial partner, which is not a source of nutrition as is common in many obligate symbioses. Furthermore, the luminous symbiont *Vibrio fischeri* is easily cultured under laboratory conditions, and genetic manipulations of this bacterium have become routine.

Beneficial Associations as Highly Predictable Interactions: Evidence from the LR and SV Symbioses

Many aspects of the onset and persistence of pathogenic associations are predictable. However, while the host must be prepared for the possibility of infection, the plant or animal has not coevolved to anticipate that a particular pathogenic symbiont will be engaged at a given time in its life history. The pathogenic symbiont may have a narrow host range, but variation exists between individuals both in terms of their susceptibility to infection, and in the course of the disease. In contrast, studies of the LR and SV symbioses have revealed that they are genetically programmed, developing as the result of a reciprocal conversation between the partners that has a predictable progression (69, 74). For the association to ensue and to successfully function, all components of both partners must come into play in the correct temporal sequence, and in the appropriate location within a host tissue. In each case, the anatomy (morphology) and physiological chemistry of the host are altered dramatically. Not only is the progression of these beneficial symbioses predictable within an individual, the course of colonization by the symbiont and the development of host tissues vary little between individuals. This relative lack of variation in host response permits these associations to be studied under genetic and environmental conditions that are relatively natural. To reveal basic underlying principles, it is not critical to have genetically manipulated hosts, such as those often used in studies of pathogenesis, to generate uniform responses.

Initiation of a Specific Symbiosis

As in many pathogenic associations, colonization of host tissues by beneficial bacteria is restricted to a site where conditions are expressed for initiation of the symbiosis. Two principal challenges characterize the initial stages of horizontally transmitted beneficial symbioses: (i) bringing potential, often rare, symbionts to susceptible host niches, and (ii) recognizing the appropriate symbiont against a background that includes a large number of nonspecific, sometimes closely related microbial species. In the LR symbiosis (72), would-be symbionts occur at densities as low as 100 cells per gram of soil, and only form nodules by initiating a symbiosis with root hairs positioned within a restricted portion of the root. Interactions between the partners are essential for transforming the morphology and physiology of host tissues so that they are conducive to efficient functioning of the nodule. For example, roots secrete flavonoids that are chemoattractants of rhizobia, acting to maximize the possibility of interaction between the partners. These flavonoids induce expression of the *nod* genes in the microbial partner. The *nod* genes direct synthesis of nod factors (*N*-acetylglucosamine oligomers) that trigger much of the early developmental program of the nodule. The host flavonoids have some bacterial strain specificity. Rhizobial nod factors vary in the details of their structures, which

confers host specificity. In addition, bacterial cell adhesin-host glycan interactions also appear to lend specificity to the association. Nonetheless, although these various factors lend a certain degree of specificity in the LR symbioses, recent analyses suggest that they may be generally less tightly coevolved than previously thought (64).

In the SV symbiosis, much less is understood about the precise nature of the host-microbe dialogue, but the broad outlines of the colonization events have been described (Fig. 1; for a review, see reference 61). Unlike the LR symbiosis, nascent symbiotic tissues are formed embryonically. Thus, in addition to mechanisms that encourage colonization with *V. fischeri*, mechanisms must also exist to dissuade colonization of the nascent tissue by "nonspecific" environmental bacteria. In the SV association, only specific strains of *V. fischeri* are capable of fully colonizing host tissues; when they are absent from the bacterioplankton, the light organ remains sterile. Unlike soil, the relatively chaotic nature of the aquatic environment renders chemoattraction of symbiotic partners an unlikely strategy for enriching for the microbial partner in the early stages of the initial interaction. Specificity is established in a stepwise fashion during the first few hours after the host hatches, and within a volume of about 10 nl in the area adjacent to sites of colonization (59, 62). At hatching, the juvenile animal immediately begins to ventilate. This activity draws environmental water into the body cavity and across the organs. The ventilated water contains an array of bacterioplankton at about 1 million cells/ml, only few of which (<0.01%) are *V. fischeri*. In a nonspecific response to the peptidoglycan (PGN) of environmental bacteria, the squid secretes mucus from a complex ciliated field of cells located on the surface of the nascent light organ, which lies in the center of the body cavity (59). The activity of the cilia entrains the mucus into foci above the sites of colonization. Whereas PGN of both gram-positive and gram-negative bacteria induce host mucus secretion, only gram-negative cells become attached to the mucus. Furthermore,

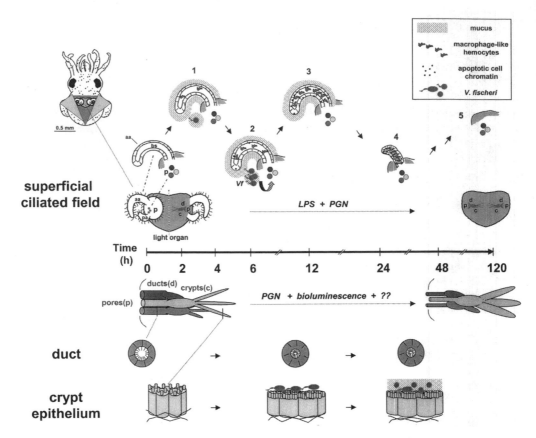

FIGURE 1 Symbiont-induced development of the host tissues in the squid–vibrio association. (Upper left) Diagram of a ventral dissection of a newly hatched *E. scolopes,* revealing the position of the light organ in the animal's body cavity (dashed line to an expanded view of the organ). (Upper half, light organ surface) Each complex ciliated field on the lateral surface of the organ is composed of an anterior appendage (aa) and a posterior appendage (pa), which are single layers of epithelial cells overlying a blood sinus (bs). At the base of these appendages is a ciliated field that surrounds the three pores (p) where the symbionts will enter host tissues. This ciliated epithelium serves two functions: the beat of the cilia entrains environmental bacteria into the vicinity of the pores, and the cells of the field secrete mucus in which symbionts will be harvested. Both nonspecific environmental bacteria and bacterial symbionts induce a series of dramatic alterations in this superficial ciliated epithelium in the hours to days following hatching of the host from the egg. First (1), interactions with nonspecific environmental bacteria and their associated peptidoglycan induce mucus shedding from the ciliated epithelium. Gram-negative bacteria begin to aggregate in this mucus and, concomitantly, macrophagelike hemocytes traffic into the blood sinuses underlying the superficial epithelium. In a second phase (2), symbiont cells (*Vf*) become numerically dominant in the mucus. They then enter pores on the organ surface (arrow) and travel down ducts (d) into crypts (c), where the symbiont population grows to fill to the crypt spaces. Hemocyte number continues to increase in the blood sinuses, and the first signs of apoptosis in the ciliated epithelium occur around the time that the aggregated symbionts are in the ducts of the organ. Once inside the crypt spaces (3), *V. fischeri* cells induce regression of the superficial ciliated epithelium of the light organ, which is remote from the population of colonizing symbionts. By 12 hours, a large proportion of the epithelial cells are undergoing apoptosis, and the blood sinus is filled with hemocytes. Upon continued colonization of the crypts with symbionts (4), further mucus production and harvesting of symbionts ceases, although this behavior can be restored by antibiotic-curing the light organ of its symbionts. By 4 to 5 days following colonization (5), the ciliated epithelium of the light organ has been completely lost. The lipopolysaccharide (LPS) and peptidoglycan (PGN) of the symbiont act synergistically to induce the complete regression of these ciliated fields. (Lower half, light organ interior) In response to interactions with the symbionts, the ducts constrict, a behavior that can be mimicked by exposure to PGN alone. The crypt cells exhibit a dramatic increase in the density of the microvilli. In addition, they show a fourfold increase in volume in response to interactions with the symbiont. *V. fischeri* mutants defective in light production do not induce cell swelling and are incapable of maintaining a persistent normal symbiosis.

although *V. fischeri* makes up only a small proportion of the bacteria in the environment, over the first 2 h of interaction with host mucus, it establishes its dominance in this matrix (60). Thus, the first site at which symbiont specificity becomes expressed is outside of the light organ. After approximately 3 h, in response to some as-yet-undescribed signal, the symbionts migrate to the pores of the light organ, and down long ciliated ducts into crypt spaces where they will reside throughout the lifetime of the host. In the crypts, the bacterial symbionts interact with two host cell types, the epithelium and a population of macrophage-like hemocytes.

When *V. fischeri* is absent, other gram-negative bacteria will aggregate and migrate to the pores, but are inhibited from traveling further than the pore-duct interface by physical and biochemical barriers. Cilia along the ducts leading to the crypt spaces beat in an outward direction. Studies of *V. fischeri* mutants have shown that flagella-driven motility is required to make the journey into the duct (24). The duct is also a region of considerable oxidative stress, with high levels of both nitric oxide and hydrogen peroxide (10, 65). As in the LR symbioses, and in common with many pathogenic associations, adhesin-glycan interactions between the partners are also critical to establishing the SV partnership (53).

The Developmental Programs of the LR and SV Symbioses

Development of the LR and SV associations involves dramatic changes in the structure and function of host tissues. One principal difference lies in the time course of the events. Although responses occur in the partners within minutes of first contact, formation of a functional symbiosis occurs over several days to weeks in the LR alliances (72), whereas the SV association is established within 6 to 12 h (74). In the LR association, interactions with the symbiont remodel preexisting host tissues, whereas embryogenesis in the host squid results in the development of a preformed set of tissues that foster immediate interaction with *V. fis-*

cheri. Nonetheless, in both instances, the symbionts induce alterations both in tissues with which they interact directly, and in more remote tissues.

The first responses in the LR symbiosis involve the deformation and curling of root hairs, and increased cortical cell division deep in the root tissue (72). Much of the early developmental program of this symbiosis is induced by the specific nod factor of the rhizobial partner. The symbionts enter at the site of root hair curling through an infection thread. Formation of the infection thread requires contact of the symbionts with the host cells and production of exopolysaccharides by the microbial partner. Studies of mutants in rhizobia indicate that components of the symbiont's lipopolysaccharide (LPS) are also important in inducing normal infection thread formation and the eventual release of the symbionts into host cortical cells (11, 23). Rhizobia that are deposited into nodule cells, which are surrounded by a host-derived peribacteroid membrane, eventually transform into nitrogen-fixing bacteroids.

Many of the host cellular events induced by *V. fischeri* in the initial stages of its relationship are similar to those that characterize pathogenic associations, including mucus secretion, blood cell trafficking to the area, and programmed cell death (Fig. 1) (45, 74). At 4 to 6 h following hatching and exposure to environmental *V. fischeri*, the harvested symbiont cells enter the ducts, which respond by narrowing, a behavior that can be mimicked by exposure of the host to purified PGN. This constriction correlates with a change in the synthesis of actin in the apical regions of ductal epithelial cells (44). Once symbionts enter the organ, they begin to grow until their population fills the crypt spaces. At about 12 h, the microbes send an irreversible signal (i.e., not reversed by antibiotic curing of the organ) that triggers a 4-day developmental program of regression of the superficial ciliated epithelial field (13). The induction of this regression does not involve direct interaction of symbiont cells with the superficial ciliated cells. The signal is somehow transmitted from the crypt to the surface through several layers of tissue. Exposure of the animal to bacterial LPS and PGN causes apoptosis and regression of these tissues in a manner similar to that induced by the specific symbiont (45). Although any bacterial PGN and LPS will induce the developmental events in the duct and superficial field, because these tissues are only exposed naturally to critical concentrations of these bioactive molecules when they interact with *V. fischeri,* the response is functionally specific.

The bacterial symbionts also affect the host cells with which they directly interface (74). They cause a swelling of the crypt epithelial cells and an increase in the density of apical microvilli. The overall effect is a gradual increase in the intimacy of the association between crypt epithelium and symbiont over the first several days following colonization. However, in contrast to the regression of the superficial field of cells, these events are reversible by antibiotic curing of the light organ. How bacteria induce a change in the microvilli is currently unknown. However, *V. fischeri* mutant in light production do not persist in the light organ, and also do not induce swelling of host cells (73).

Host "Defense" as "Offense"

Overall, a remarkable number of host mechanisms used to avoid infection by pathogenic microbes, such as production of reactive oxygen species (ROS) and "antimicrobial" proteins and peptides, appear to play significant roles in the LR and SV associations (33). These beneficial associations are limited to specific host locations, suggesting that mechanisms have evolved to restrict the interactions. In the LR symbiosis, the number of functional nodules that form is tightly controlled. Whereas successful nodules elicit a very limited defense response, aborted nodules elicit responses similar to those induced by plant pathogens, including accumulation of ROS and phytoalexins. Recent studies of hypernodulation (17) have revealed that legumes have homologs of *Arabidopsis* CLAVATA1, a serine/threonine kinase that restricts the activity of floral meristem. When

these genes are disrupted, the plant loses its ability to suppress hypernodulation, suggesting that hypernodulation is inhibited by suppression of the activity of the root cortical meristem where nodules form. The relationship between suppression of hypernodulation by CLAVATA1 homologs and the induction of host defense responses remains to be determined.

In the SV symbiosis, the nascent light organs of newly hatched, uninfected juveniles appear to have a heightened degree of defense (59). In the first minutes after hatching, the crypts are "open" to bacteria and bacteria-sized particles. During this early permissive phase, no bacteria, including *V. fischeri,* are capable of persisting and growing in the crypt spaces: all bacterial cells and particles that enter are immediately cleared. Only after *V. fischeri* cells aggregate in host-secreted mucus on the outside of the light organ do they become capable of migrating into and colonizing the host crypts. Colonization of the crypts shuts down mucus shedding from the light organ surface and attenuates the production of high levels of ROS that are characteristic of the hatchling light organ ducts.

Instructive analogies can be drawn from host responses to strains with defects in genes that are central to the functional symbiosis (i.e., *fix⁻* or *lux⁻* mutants in the LR and SV symbioses, respectively). These mutants, which occupy host tissues but do not perform their function, elicit responses similar to those induced by plant pathogens, such as a heightened plant defense response, and formation of vestigial nodules (69). In the SV symbiosis, colonization with *lux⁻* mutants results in the trafficking of large numbers of macrophage-like hemocytes into the crypt spaces and concomitant clearance of the microbe from the organ (M. J. McFall-Ngai, unpublished data).

Finally, to control symbiont number or invasion of other tissues, the plant host in the LR association sequesters rhizobia within a peribacteroid membrane. In the SV symbiosis, symbiont number is controlled in the persistent association by expulsion of 95% of the bacterial culture into the surrounding environment at dawn (25), when the host animal buries itself in the sand for its diurnal quiescent period.

Taken together, the available data on the LR and SV symbioses suggest that interactions between the partners involve molecules traditionally associated with host defense, although they appear to be modulated differently in these beneficial associations. Many of the responses appear to be ancient (shared by plants and animals) and may not have evolved as "antimicrobial" or "defense" mechanisms per se, but rather as a cellular and molecular language to be shared by all types of symbiotic interactions.

A Binary Mammalian Model System: the Human/Mouse-*Bacteroides thetaiotaomicron* Symbiosis

The number of microbial cells that colonize our adult bodies is believed to exceed the number of our somatic and germ cells by at least an order of magnitude. The gastrointestinal tract is home to our largest collection of symbionts. There are an estimated 500 to 1,000 species, although the true extent of diversity is presently unknown. The aggregate genome size of the gut microbiota (the "microbiome") may equal the size of our own genome, and the total number of microbial genes embedded in the microbiome may exceed the number of *Homo sapiens* genes by as much as 2 orders of magnitude. Regional differences in community structure and population density occur, with densities approaching 10^{11} organisms/ml of luminal contents in the proximal colon (2, 67). As noted above, some members of the gut microbiota are coevolved residential (autochthonous) partners, while others are transient tourists (allochthonous partners) (67). This imposes a further challenge in defining the structure of these microbial communities and the contributions of their members to overall function.

One of the driving forces in human evolution has been the ability to improve the efficiency with which we gather food and the flexibility of our diet. These adaptations have helped sustain expansion of the size of a brain that has large energy requirements (1, 48). Our gut microbiota has provided metabolic traits that allow us to access energy sources from our diet, such as plant polysaccharides, that would otherwise be unavailable because we have not evolved the required repertoire of enzymes needed to process these nutrients (e.g., glycoside hydrolases). Our Neolithic ancestors were innovators who oversaw a remarkable transition from the nomadic existence of Paleolithic humanoids to the development of agriculture and the raising of domesticated animals. Studies of the coevolution and coadaptation of humans and their microbial communities present an opportunity to gain new understanding about how our ancient migrations, dietary changes, and social innovations helped shaped our current biology, and how they influenced the origins of, our susceptibilities to, and the spread of various pathogenic symbioses (4, 19). The important concepts are that (i) a comprehensive view of ourselves as a life form should take into account genetic and metabolic traits provided by our microbial partners; (ii) in this early phase of the current revolution in applied genomics, the gut microbiota should be evaluated as an important environmental factor that influences host gene expression; and (iii) as in the LR and SV symbioses, features of postnatal mammalian gut development should be viewed as manifestations of beneficial symbioses.

A Gnotobiotic Mouse Model for Studying Beneficial Symbiotic Relationships in the Intestinal Ecosystem

Assembly of the gut microbiota produces a multilineage, spatially patterned "microbial organ." This organ operates through a cascade of inter- and intraspecies signal exchange and nutrient sharing. The overall complexity of the system defies imagination. It is also unmanageable when it comes to experimentally dissecting how this environmentally transmitted symbiosis is initiated and sustained, characterizing the molecular features of microbial-microbial and microbial-host communications, and identifying the contributions of members of the alliance to the overall functioning of the ecosystem. Using individuals with varying degrees of genetic relatedness represents one strategy for addressing a subset of these experimental challenges. For example, recent enumeration studies of the fecal flora of small numbers of humans have shown that community membership is more similar in monozygotic twins than in their marital partners (79). Another approach is to use inbred stains of mice, raised under germfree conditions (i.e., without any bacteria) and then colonized with one or more prominent members of the human and mouse gut microbiota (37). This gnotobiotic ("known life") system provides a simplified, environmentally and genetically defined experimental model for examining the principles underlying beneficial mammalian-bacterial symbioses.

A binary system has been established that involves colonization of adult germfree mice with *B. thetaiotaomicron*. This anaerobe was selected for several reasons. *B. thetaiotaomicron* can degrade host mucopolysaccharides and otherwise undigestable dietary plant polysaccharides (38). It is genetically manipulatable and easy to cultivate (66). It is a predominant member of the distal intestinal microbiota of humans (56) and mice. It gains prominence in the microbiota when the diet switches from mother's milk to one rich in polysaccharides (50), thereby providing an opportunity to examine the contributions of a component of the microbiota to a key transition in postnatal gut maturation.

Establishing Residency in the Intestine

Unlike the SV and LR symbioses, details of how *Bacteroides,* and other genera, gain a foothold in the gut microbiota remain obscure. Studies in gnotobiotic mice indicate that epithelial glycans may play an important role.

The inner core structures of many glycans have been highly conserved during evolution and mediate a number of important intracellular functions (e.g., those *N*-linked to proteins). In contrast, outer chains of mammalian glycans exhibit enormous structural complexity and diversity, as well as a high degree of cellular and developmental specificity. This reflects the nontemplate combinatorial nature of carbohydrate biosynthesis and modification, as well as the diverse repertoire and complex regulation of genes encoding members of the "glycobiome" [see the Carbohydrate Active Enzymes (CAZy) database (http://afmb.cnrs-mrs.fr/~cazy/CAZY/index.html)].

One source of selective pressure for maintaining outer chain diversity may be the need to evade pathogens (21, 34). For example, a pathogen can initiate interactions with its host through interactions of its adhesin(s) with glycan receptors expressed on the surface of target cells. The host could counter by eliminating expression of the functional receptor, either through inactivation of the glycosyltransferases necessary for its synthesis, or through activation of a glycosyltransferase that utilizes the glycan structure as an acceptor, thereby obscuring the receptor.

Another source of selective pressure for evolving the capacity to generate glycan diversity may be the need to create and sustain beneficial symbiotic relationships. This latter concept is illustrated by comparative studies of germfree mice from an inbred strain and their conventionally raised counterparts (i.e., mice that naturally acquire a microbiota beginning at birth). In conventionally raised mice belonging to the NMRI inbred strain, Fucα1,2Galβ-containing glycans are expressed in the distal small intestinal (ileal) epithelium beginning at postnatal day 21 (P21). Initially, glycan production is limited to scattered members of the enterocytic lineage overlying a few ileal villi (the fingerlike projections that decorate the luminal surface of the small intestine). During the 7-day interval from P21 to P28, weaning is completed, the composition of the microbiota evolves from a predominance of facultative anaerobes to a predominance of obligate anaerobes, and fucosylated glycan expression generalizes to all enterocytes overlying all ileal villi. Glycan production is then sustained throughout adulthood. Germfree mice are able to initiate synthesis of ileal Fucα1,2Galβ epitopes at the same time as their conventionally raised counterparts, but production is not sustained: synthesis is completely extinguished in the self-renewing epithelium by P28, and Fucα1,2Galβ-glycan-positive enterocytes are discarded. Introduction of an unfractionated distal intestinal microbiota, harvested from conventionally raised mice, into adult germfree recipients (a process termed "conventionalization"), or colonization with *B. thetaiotaomicron* alone (monoassociation), induces Fucα1, 2Galβ-glycan expression in a fashion that recapitulates the temporal evolution and cellular/regional specificity of what is observed during normal postnatal development (3). *B. thetaiotaomicron* is able to harvest monomeric fucose from these epithelial glycans using its secreted α-fucosidases (39, 76). Its ability to induce expression of host α1,2-fucosyltransferases (*FUT* genes), and synthesis of enterocytic fucosylated glycans is dependent upon achieving a critical microbial density in the intestinal lumen, is not associated with direct bacterial binding to the epithelium, and is not a general effect of colonization (at least two other components of the normal microbiota, *Peptostreptococcus micros* and *Bifidobacterium infantis*, are unable to elicit expression of Fucα1,2Galβ epitopes [3]). Moreover, microbial induction of host glycans with harvestable terminal α-linked fucose is coordinated with fucose availability: genetic disruption of the bacterium's fucose utilization operon results in constitutive signaling to the host to produce fucosylated epithelial glycans (39).

These observations prompt the following speculations about this environmentally transmitted symbiosis. Epithelial glycans, produced during the perinatal period, function as signposts, directing early colonizers to a particular location along the length of the intestine. Early colonizers are able to harvest sugar residues from these glycans for use as nutrient sources. The metabolic milieu of the developing gut subsequently evolves in a manner conducive to entry of other symbionts. A bioreactor is created as successive waves of colonization produce a consortium whose members are able to break down complex polysaccharides, generating products for themselves and their host.

B. thetaiotaomicron regulation of carbohydrate production may also have another important function. Colonization of germfree mice does not elicit an immunoinflammatory response (3, 35). One potential explanation for the absence of such a response is that *B. thetaiotaomicron* may be able to match carbohydrate availability in its developing intestinal niche with the types of capsular polysaccharides it expresses and the types of epithelial glycan structures it helps to synthesize (76). This hypothesis can be tested in gnotobiotic mice by assaying the effects of host and bacterial glycosyltransferase gene disruptions.

The simplified binary model of the intestinal ecosystem has also disclosed another mechanism that can help dictate establishment of an environmentally transmitted symbiosis. *B. thetaiotaomicron* colonization induces expression of an antimicrobial protein belonging to the RNase superfamily in one of the principal epithelial cell lineages of the small intestine—Paneth cells. This protein (Ang4) is secreted into the gut lumen and has species-selective bactericidal activity. For example, it has potent activity against *Listeria monocytogenes*, the gram-positive pathogen that causes food-borne gastroenteritis, but not against its benign relative, *L. innocua*. In contrast, gram-negative intestinal symbionts, such as *E. coli* and *B. thetaiotaomicron*, are relatively resistant to this protein antibiotic (38). The ability of *B. thetaiotaomicron* to induce synthesis and release of Ang4 into the gut lumen is a feature that distinguishes Ang4 from other Paneth cell-derived microbicidal proteins, such as the defensins, which are constitutively expressed when germfree mice are conventionalized or are monoassociated with *B. thetaiotaomicron*. In conventionally raised mice, *Ang4* undergoes a marked induction at the suckling-weaning transition, providing additional evidence for its microbial regulation (38).

By regulating secretion of a protein with species-selective bactericidal activity, resistant intestinal symbionts gain a measure of control over the composition of their evolving microbial community during postnatal development. The host, in turn, gains a measure of protection from exposure to pathogens, and is able to fortify its mucosal barrier.

A Microbial Genomics View of the Symbiosis

The 6.26-Mbp *B. thetaiotaomicron* genome has been sequenced (76). The composition of its 4,776 member proteome provides insights about molecular foundations of its beneficial symbiosis (76, 77). The most markedly expanded paralogous groups are involved in polysaccharide uptake and degradation, capsular polysaccharide biosynthesis (e.g., glycosyltransferases), and environmental sensing/signal transduction (e.g., hybrid two-component systems, extracytoplasmic function [ECF]-type sigma factors).

The *B. thetaiotaomicron* proteome contains 226 predicted glycoside hydrolases (more than any other sequenced bacteria in the public domain; http://afmb.cnrs-mrs.fr/~cazy/CAZY/index.html). Over half of these enzymes are predicted to be located in the periplasm, outer membrane, or extracellular space, suggesting that they may not only help satisfy the nutrient needs of *B. thetaiotaomicron,* but also shape the metabolic milieu of the habitat occupied by this anaerobe.

The largest paralogous group consists of 106 proteins with homology to an outer membrane protein (OMP) known as SusC, while a 57-member group has homology to another OMP known as SusD. SusC and SusD are part of an eight-component *B. thetaiotaomicron* starch utilization system (Sus). These OMPs mediate binding of starches to the bacterial cell surface so that they can then be processed by outer membrane and periplasmic α-amylases. Fifty-six of the 57 SusD homologs are paired together with a SusC homolog. Twenty of these clusters contain both SusC/SusD and an upstream open reading frame specifying an ECF-type sigma factor (also known as sigma-70 factor). Twelve of the 20 clusters also contain genes encoding glycoside hydrolases and other enzymes involved in sugar metabolism.

When adjusted for genome size, *B. thetaiotaomicron* has more sigma factors (fifty-four) than any other fully sequenced prokaryotic genome. This reflects a dramatic expansion in the number of ECF-type sigma factors (fifty). ECF-type sigma factors are often cotranscribed with a transmembrane anti-sigma factor that binds to and inhibits the sigma factor (29). Upon receipt of an environmental cue, the ECF-type sigma factor is released, binds to RNA polymerase, and regulates transcription of target genes (29). In *B. thetaiotaomicron,* 16 of 20 SusC/SusD-containing clusters with an ECF-type sigma factor also have a gene encoding a predicted transmembrane protein interposed between the ECF-type sigma factor and SusC.

Given the environmental sensing functions of these factors, it seems likely that different SusC/SusD homologs are regulated in response to changes in nutrient (polysaccharide) availability. This would allow *B. thetaiotaomicron* to function as a "grazer," harvesting a variety of sugars depending upon their availability in ingested dietary polysaccharides and in host mucopolysaccharides. This capacity has ecological implications: adaptive foraging promotes persistence of communities (78).

MOLECULAR CHARACTERISTICS IN BENEFICIAL AND PATHOGENIC ASSOCIATIONS

Genomic studies of the legume symbiont *Sinorhizobium meliloti* have revealed, among other things, a number of genes with homologs to virulence determinants of animal and plant pathogens (5). Annotation of the 4.2-Mbp *V. fischeri* genome is currently underway (http://ergo.integratedgenomics.com/Genomes/VFI/) and can be expected to provide a global picture of the proteome this symbiont has developed as an adaptation to its association.

Bacterial symbionts in beneficial and pathogenic associations employ homologous gene products, as well as similar genomic elements (e.g., plasmids, phages), to mediate their interactions with host cells (e.g., see references 31 and 32) (Fig. 2). For example, a number of beneficial symbionts, such as *V. fischeri,* use quorum sensing to control gene expression at high cell densities. Elements of a two-component regulatory system have been found in the symbiosis between *R. pachyptila* (the hydrothermal vent tube worm) and its sulfur-oxidizing bacterial partner (40). Recently, a type III secretion system has been described in the mutualistic symbiosis between the weevil and its bacterial endosymbiont, where it functions as a critical element in the transfer of the microbe to specific host cells during development (9). YopJ, a *Yersinia pestis* protein delivered to host cells through a type III secretion system, has

orthologs that act in a similar manner in plant symbionts and pathogens (7). As noted above, surface molecules and appendages, such as LPS and fimbriae, are involved in the LR and SV symbioses.

The Nods (not to be confused with nodulins, which are host proteins in the LR system induced by the symbiosis) are a family of proteins that regulate innate immune responses in animals. They may have functions similar to plant R proteins involved in resistance to pathogens (42). Mutations affecting human NOD2 (now named CARD15) have been

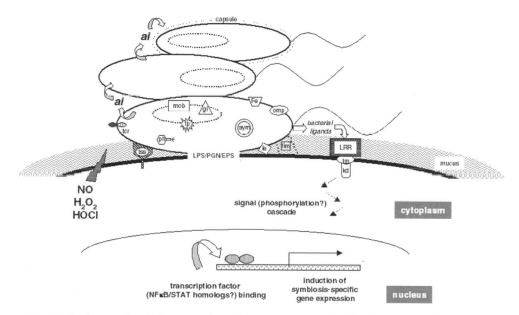

FIGURE 2 Composite of characters shared between mutualistic and pathogenic symbiotic associations. In both types of associations, the bacterial partners may have genomic elements that are involved in the dynamics of the symbiosis, including plasmids (sym), phages (ph), genomic (pathogenicity) islands (gi), transposons (tp), and mobilization loci (mob). In addition, the induction of similar, if not homologous, mechanisms for sensing and responding to the environment have been reported, including two-component regulatory systems (tcr), iron acquisition (Fe), and specific outer membrane proteins (omp), and autoinducers (ai) that enable the bacteria to sense and respond to being at high population density. The bacterial partner may interact directly with the host cells through conserved bacterial surface molecules such as lipopolysaccharide (LPS) and peptidoglycan (PGN), and/or through more specific exopolysaccharides (EPS), a type III secretion system (tss), lectins (le), or fimbriae (fim). Studies thus far on host cells demonstrate shared responses to mutualistic or pathogenic associations. In a number of cases, various bacterial ligands have been shown to interact with receptor proteins on host cell surfaces that include an extracellular leucine-rich repeat domain (LRR), a transmembrane domain (tm), and a kinase domain (kd). Circumstantial evidence exists that signal transduction pathways similar to the NF-κB and JAK/STAT pathways, which mediate responses to pathogens, are also present in beneficial associations. Reactive oxygen species, including nitric oxide (NO), hydrogen peroxide (H_2O_2), and hypohalous acid (HOCl), are host molecules also involved in the communication between host and symbiont in both beneficial and pathogenic associations.

associated with susceptibility to Crohn's disease, one form of inflammatory bowel disease (63, 41, 27). Inflammatory bowel disease is characterized by aberrant immunoimflammatory responses to components of the normal intestinal microbiota. NOD2/CARD15 is normally expressed in monocytes/macrophages. This intracellular protein senses bacterial cell wall peptidoglycans through its recognition of muramyl dipeptide: PGN sensing, in turn, activates the nuclear factor-$_k$B proinflammatory signaling pathway. The most common NOD2/CARD15 mutation, 3020insC, produces insensitivity to muramyl dipeptide, and thus disruption of the proper regulation of mucosal barrier activities (22).

Until more data are available about the molecular and biochemical similarities and differences between beneficial and pathogenic associations, we cannot make generalizations about the evolutionary origin or differential function of convergent features in the two types of symbioses. Because considerably more data are available on pathogenic associations, many authors have posited that beneficial symbioses co-opted these characters. However, if beneficial associations with microbes are the rule rather than the exception, it may be the pathogens that have co-opted or perverted aspects of the dialogue between hosts and their microbial partners. Thus, at this early stage in our knowledge, we should keep an open mind about these mechanisms of host-symbiont interaction, so that we can allow for the discovery of the true meaning of these convergences.

CHAPTER SUMMARY
- Three types of symbiosis are recognized: mutualistic, commensal, and pathogenic, wherein the fitness (genetic contribution to future generations) of the partners is positively affected, unaffected, or negatively affected, respectively.
- "Commensalism," a term signifying that one of the partners is unaffected by the association, should not be used in situations in which the effects on the fitness (genetic contribution to future generations) of the partners have not been determined, such as the association of mammals with their gut microbiota.
- Symbioses are characterized by their mode of transmission, the complexity of the stable community, and the types of exchange that occurs between the partners. Symbioses of all types emerged early in the evolution of multicellularity and have had an important influence on the adaptive radiation of animals and plants.
- Microbial pathogens not only threaten the health of the plant or animal host, but can compromise the integrity of the entire community, which is composed of the host and its coevolved microbiota. To understand the true nature of pathogenesis, biologists and physicians must first understand the dynamics of the normal interactions between the partners of a symbiosis.
- The development and exploitation of a variety of model systems of host-microbe interaction are critical to creating an in-depth understanding of what factors are shared by all such relationships (i.e., are primitive) and, conversely, what factors have directed the evolution of the vast diversity of associations (i.e., are derived or specific to a given relationship).

ACKNOWLEDGMENTS
Work cited from our labs was supported by grants from the National Science Foundation, the National Institutes of Health, and W. M. Keck Foundation.

We thank the people in our groups, including Catherine Brennan, Wendy Crookes, Seana Davidson, Judy Doino Lemus, Jamie Foster, Mike Goodson, Bernadette Janssens, Jennifer Kimbell, Tanya Koropatnick, Renate Kossmeyl, Laurence Lamarcq, Mary Montgomery, Spencer Nyholm, Andrea Small, Jennifer Stewart, Josh Troll, Virginia Weis, Cory Yap, Lynn Bry, Lora Hooper, Thad Stappenbeck, Jian Xu, Magnus Bjursell, Herb Chiang, Lynn Carmichael, Su Deng, Justin Himrod, Justin Sonnenburg, David O'Donnell, and Maria Karlsson for their contributions; and our collaborators, particularly Ned Ruby, Pete Greenberg, Mike Apicella, Eric Stabb, Brad Gibson,

Nancy Phillips, Bento Soares, Rex Gaskins, Per Falk, and Tore Midtvedt.

REFERENCES

1. **Aiello, L. C., and P. Wheeler.** 1995. The expensive-tissue hypothesis. *Curr. Anthropol.* **36:** 199–221.

2. **Berg, R.** 1996. The indigenous gastrointestinal microflora. *Trends Microbiol.* **4:**430–435.

3. **Bry, L., P. G. Falk, T. Midtvedt, and J. I. Gordon.** 1996. A model of host-microbial interactions in an open mammalian ecosystem. *Science* **273:**1380–1383.

4. **Cano, R. J., F. Tiefenbrunner, M. Ubaldi, C. del Cueto, S. Luciani, T. Cox, P. Orkand, K. H. Kunzel, and F. Rollo.** 2000. Sequence analysis of bacterial DNA in the colon and stomach of the Tyrolean iceman. *Am. J. Phys. Anthropol.* **112:** 297–309.

5. **Capela, D., F. Barloy-Hubler, J. Gouzy, G. Bothe, F. Ampe, J. Batut, P. Boistard, A. Becker, M. Boutry, E. Cadieu, S. Dreano, S. Gloux, T. Godrie, A. Goffeau, D. Kahn, E. Kiss, V. Lelaure, D. Masuy, T. Pohl, D. Portetelle, A. Puhler, B. Purnelle, U. Ramsperger, C. Renard, P. Thebault, M. Vandenbol, S. Weidner, and F. Galibert.** 2001. Analysis of the chromosome sequence of the legume symbiont Sinorhizobium meliloti strain 1021. *Proc. Natl. Acad. Sci. USA* **98:**9877–9882.

6. **Cary, S. C., and S. J. Giovannoni.** 1993. Transovarial inheritance of endosymbiotic bacteria in clams inhabiting deep-sea hydrothermal vents and cold seeps. *Proc. Natl. Acad. Sci. USA* **90:** 5695–5699.

7. **Ciesiolka, L. D., T. Hwin, J. D. Gearlds, G. V. Minsavage, R. Saenz, M. Bravo, V. Handley, S. M. Conover, H. Zhang, J. Caporgno, N. B. Phengrasamy, A. O. Toms, R. E. Stall, and M. C. Whalen.** 1999. Regulation of expression of avirulence gene avrRxv and identification of a family of host interaction factors by sequence analysis of avrBsT. *Mol. Plant Microbe Interact.* **12:**35–44.

8. **Cossart, P., S. Boquet, S. Normark, and R. Rappuoli (ed.).** 2000. *Cellular Microbiology.* ASM Press, Washington, D.C.

9. **Dale, C., G. R. Plague, B. Wang, H. Ochman, and N. Moran.** 2002. Type III secretion systems and the evolution of mutualistic endosymbioses. *Proc. Natl. Acad. Sci. USA* **99:**12397–12402.

10. **Davidson, S. K., T. A. Koropatnick, R. Kossmehl, L. Sycuro, and M. J. McFall-Ngai.** 2004. NO means 'yes' in the squid-vibrio symbiosis: nitric oxide (NO) during the initial stages of a beneficial association. *Cell Microbiol.* **6:**1139–1151.

11. **Dazzo, F. B., G. L. Truchet, R. I. Hollingsworth, E. M. Hrabak, H. S. Pankratz, S. Philip-Hollingsworth, J. L. Salzwedel, K. Chapman, L. Appenzeller, and A. Squartini.** 1991. Rhizobium lipopolysaccharide modulates infection thread development in white clover root hairs. *J. Bacteriol.* **173:**5371–5384.

12. **Distel, D. L., H. K.-W. Lee, and C. M. Cavanaugh.** 1995. Intracellular coexistence of methano- and thioautotrophic bacteria in a hydrothermal vent mussel. *Proc. Natl. Acad. Sci. USA* **92:**9598–9602.

13. **Doino J. A., and M. J. McFall-Ngai.** 1995. A transient exposure to symbiosis-competent bacteria induces light organ morphogenesis in the host squid. *Biol. Bull.* **189:**347–355.

14. **Douglas, A. E.** 1989. Mycetocyte symbiosis in insects. *Biol. Rev.* **69:**409–434.

15. **Douglas, A. E.** 1997. Parallels and contrasts between symbiotic bacteria and bacterial-derived organelles: evidence from Buchnera, the bacterial symbiont of aphids. *FEMS Microbiol. Ecol.* **24:**1–9.

16. **Douglas, A. E.** 1994. *Symbiotic Interactions.* Oxford University Press, Oxford, United Kingdom.

17. **Downie, J. A., and M. Parniske.** 2002. Fixation with regulation. *Nature* **420:**369–370.

18. **Doyle, J. J.** 1994. Phylogeny of the legume family: an approach to understanding the origin of nodulation. *Annu. Rev. Ecol. Syst.* **25:**325–349.

19. **Falush, D., T. Wirth, B. Linz, J. K. Pritchard, M. Stephens, M. Kidd, M. J. Blaser, D. Y. Graham, S. Vacher, G. I. Perez-Perez, Y. Yamaoka, F. Megraud, K. Otto, U. Reichard, E. Katzowitsch, X. Wang, M. Achtman, and S. Suerbaum.** 2003. Traces of human migrations in *Helicobacter pylori* populations. *Science* **299:** 1582–1585.

20. **Favier, C. F., E. E. Vaughan, W. M. De Vos, and A. D. L. Akkermans.** 2002. Molecular monitoring of succession of bacterial communities in human neonates. *Appl. Environ. Microbiol.* **68:** 219–236.

21. **Gagneux, P., and A. Varki.** 1999. Evolutionary considerations in relating oligosaccharide diversity to biological function. *Glycobiology* **9:**747–755.

22. **Girardin, S. E., I. G. Boneca, J. Viala, M. Chamaillard, A. Labigne, G. Thomas, D. J. Philpott, and P. J. Sansonetti.** 2003. Nod2 is a general sensor of peptidoglycan through muramyl dipeptide (MDP) detection. *J. Biol. Chem.* **278:** 8869–8872.

23. **Goosen-de Roo, L., R. A. de Maagd, and B. J. Lugtenberg.** 1991. Antigenic changes in lipopolysaccharide I of *Rhizobium leguminosarum* bv. viciae in root nodules of *Vicia sativa* subsp. *nigra* occur during release from infection threads. *J. Bacteriol.* **173:**3177–3183.

24. **Graf, J., P. V. Dunlap, and E. G. Ruby.** 1994. Effect of transposon-induced motility mutations on colonization of the host light organ by *Vibrio fischeri. J. Bacteriol.* **176:**6986–6991.

25. **Graf, J., and E. G. Ruby.** 1998. Characterization of the nutritional environment of a symbiotic light organ using bacterial mutants and chemical analyses. *Proc. Natl. Acad. Sci. USA* **95:**1818–1822.

26. **Gualtieri, G., and T. Bisseling.** 2000. The evolution of nodulation. *Plant Mol. Biol.* **42:**181–194.

27. **Hampe, J., A. Cuthbert, P. J. Croucher, M. M. Mirza, S. Mascheretti, S. Fisher, H. Frenzel, K. King, A. Hasselmeyer, A. J. MacPherson, S. Bridger, S. van Deventer, A. Forbes, S. Nikolaus, J. E. Lennard-Jones, U. R. Foelsch, M. Krawczak, C. Lewis, S. Schreiber, and C. G. Mathew.** 2001. Association between insertion mutation in NOD2 gene and Crohn's disease in German and British populations. *Lancet* **357:**1925–1928.

28. **Haygood, M. G., and S. K. Davidson.** 1997. Small-subunit rRNA genes and *in situ* hybridization with oligonucleotides specific for the bacterial symbionts in the larvae of the bryozoan *Bugula neritina* and proposal of "*Candidatus* endobugula sertula". *Appl. Environ. Microbiol.* **63:**4612–4616.

29. **Helmann, J. D.** 2002. The extracytoplasmic function (ECF) sigma factors. *Adv. Microb. Physiol.* **46:**47–110.

30. **Henderson, B., M. Wilson, R. McNab, and A. J. Lax.** 1999. *Cellular Microbiology. Bacteria-Host Interactions in Health and Disease.* Wiley and Sons, Chicester, United Kingdom.

31. **Hentschel, U., and J. Hacker.** 2001. Pathogenicity islands: the tip of the iceberg. *Microbes Infect.* **3:**545–548.

32. **Hentschel, U., M. Steinert, and J. Hacker.** 2000. Common molecular mechanisms of symbiosis and pathogenesis. *Trends Microbiol.* **8:**226–231.

33. **Hirsch, A., and M. J. McFall-Ngai.** 2000. Fundamental concepts in symbiotic interactions. *J. Plant Growth Regul.* **19:**113–130.

34. **Hooper, L., and J. I. Gordon.** 2001. Glycans as legislators of host-microbial interactions: spanning the spectrum from symbiosis to pathogenicity. *Glycobiology* **11:**1R–10R.

35. **Hooper, L., M. Wong, A. Thelin, L. Hansson, P. Falk, and J. I. Gordon.** 2001. Molecular analysis of commensal host-microbial relationships in the intestine. *Science* **291:**881–884.

36. **Hooper, L. V., T. Midtvedt, and J. I. Gordon.** 2002. How host-microbial interactions shape the nutrient environment of the mammalian intestine. *Annu. Rev. Nutr.* **22:**283–307.

37. **Hooper, L. V., J. C. Mills, K. A. Roth, T. S. Stappenbeck, M. H. Wong, and J. I. Gordon.** 2002. Combining gnotobiotic mouse models with functional genomics to define the impact of the microflora on host physiology. *Methods Microbiol.* **31:**559–589.

38. **Hooper, L. V., T. S. Stappenbeck, C. V. Hong, and J. I. Gordon.** 2003. Angiogenins: a new class of microbicidal proteins involved in innate immunity. *Nat. Immunol.* **4:**269–273.

39. **Hooper, L. V., J. Xu, P. G. Falk, T. Midtvedt, and J. I. Gordon.** 1999. A molecular sensor that allows a gut commensal to control its nutrient foundation in a competitive ecosystem. *Proc. Natl. Acad. Sci. USA* **96:**9833–9838.

40. **Hughes, D. S., H. Felbeck, and J. L. Stein.** 1997. A histidine protein kinase homolog from the endosymbiont of the hydrothermal vent tubeworm *Riftia pachyptila. Appl. Environ. Microbiol.* **63:** 3494–3498.

41. **Hugot, J. P., M. Chamaillard, H. Zouali, S. Lesage, J. P. Cezard, J. Belaiche, S. Almer, C. Tysk, C. A. O'Morain, M. Gassull, V. Binder, Y. Finkel, A. Cortot, R. Modigliani, P. Laurent-Puig, C. Gower-Rousseau, J. Macry, J. F. Colombel, M. Sahbatou, and G. Thomas.** 2001. Association of NOD2 leucine-rich repeat variants with susceptibility to Crohn's disease. *Nature* **411:**599–603.

42. **Inohara, N., Y. Ogura, and G. Nunez.** 2002. Nods: a family of cytosolic proteins that regulate the host response to pathogens. *Curr. Opin. Microbiol.* **5:**76–80.

43. **Kaneko, T., Y. Nakamura, S. Sato, E. Asamizu, T. Kato, S. Sasamoto, A. Watanabe, K. Idesawa, A. Ishikawa, K. Kawashima, T. Kimura, Y. Kishida, C. Kiyokawa, M. Kohara, M. Matsumoto, A. Matsuno, Y. Mochizuki, S. Nakayama, N. Nakazaki, S. Shimpo, M. Sugimoto, C. Takeuchi, M. Yamada, and S. Tabata.** 2000. Complete genome structure of the nitrogen-fixing symbiotic bacterium Mesorhizobium loti. *DNA Res.* **7:**331–338.

44. **Kimbell, J. R., and M. J. McFall-Ngai.** 2002. Symbiont-induced changes in host cytoskeletal actin. *Mol. Biol. Cell. Suppl.* **13:**450a.

45. **Koropatnick, T. A., J. T. Engle, M. A. Apicella, E. V. Stabb, W. E. Goldman, and M. J. McFall-Ngai.** 2004. Microbial factor-mediated development in a host-bacterial mutualism. *Science* **306:**1186–1188.

46. **Krueger, D. M., and C. M. Cavanaugh.** 1997. Phylogenetic diversity of bacterial symbionts of *Solemya* hosts based on comparative sequence analysis of 16S rRNA genes. *Appl. Environ. Microbiol.* **63:**91–98.

47. **Krueger, D. M., R. G. Gustafson, and C. M. Cavanaugh.** 1996. Vertical transmission of

chemoautotrophic symbionts in the bivalve *Solemya velum* (Bivalvia: Protobranchia). *Biol. Bull.* **190:**195–202.

48. **Leonard, W. R.** 2002. Food for thought: dietary change was a driving force in human evolution. *Sci. Am.* **287:**108–115.

49. **Lum, M. R. and A. M. Hirsch.** 2003. Roots and their symbiotic microbes: strategies to obtain nitrogen and phosphorus in a nutrient-limiting environment. *J. Plant Growth Regul.* **21:**368–382.

50. **Mackie, R. I., A. Sghir, and H. R. Gaskins.** 1999. Developmental microbial ecology of the neonatal gastrointestinal tract. *Am. J. Clin. Nutr.* **69:** 1035S–1045S.

51. **Margulis, L.** 1970. *Origin of Eukaryotic Cells.* Yale University Press, New Haven, Conn.

52. **Margulis, L., and R. Fester (ed.).** 1991. *Symbiosis as a Source of Evolutionary Innovation.* The MIT Press, Cambridge, Mass.

53. **McFall-Ngai, M., C. Brennan, V. Weis, and L. Lamarcq.** 1998. Mannose adhesin-glycan interactions in the *Euprymna scolopes-Vibrio fischeri* symbiosis, p. 273–277. In Y. LeGal and H. O. Halvorson (ed.), *New Developments in Marine Biology.* Plenum Publishing Co., New York, N.Y.

54. **McFall-Ngai, M. J.** 2001. Identifying prime suspects: symbioses and the evolution of multicellularity. *Comp. Biochem. Physiol.* **129:**711–723.

55. **Montgomery, M. K., and M. J. McFall-Ngai.** 1993. Embryonic development of the light organ of the sepiolid squid *Euprymna scolopes* Berry. *Biol. Bull.* **184:**296–308.

56. **Moore, W. E., and L. V. Holdeman.** 1974. Human fecal flora: the normal flora of 20 Japanese Hawaiians. *Appl. Microbiol.* **27:**961–979.

57. **Moran, N. A.** 2002. Microbial minimalism: genome reduction in bacterial pathogens. *Cell* **108:**583–586.

58. **Nishiguchi, M. K., E. G. Ruby, and M. J. McFall-Ngai.** 1998. Competitive dominance among strains of luminous bacteria provides an unusual form of evidence for parallel evolution in the sepiolid squid vibrio symbioses. *Appl. Environ. Microbiol.* **64:**3209–3213.

59. **Nyholm, S. V., B. Deplancke, H. R. Gaskins, M. A. Apicella, and M. J. McFall-Ngai.** 2002. Roles of *Vibrio fischeri* and nonsymbiotic bacteria in the dynamics of mucus secretion during symbiont colonization of the *Euprymna scolopes* light organ. *Appl. Environ. Microbiol.* **68:**5113–5122.

60. **Nyholm, S. V., and M. J. McFall-Ngai.** 2003. Dominance of *Vibrio fischeri* in secreted mucus outside the light organ of *Euprymna scolopes:* the first site of symbiont specificity. *Appl. Environ. Microbiol.* **69:**3932–3937.

61. **Nyholm, S. V., and M. J. McFall-Ngai.** 2004.

The winnowing: establishing the squid-vibrio symbiosis. *Nat. Rev. Microbiol.* **2:**632–642.

62. **Nyholm, S. V., E. V. Stabb, E. G. Ruby, and M. J. McFall-Ngai.** 2000. Harvesting symbiotic vibrios: imposing a magnet on the environmental haystack. *Proc. Natl. Acad. Sci. USA* **97:** 10231–10294.

63. **Ogura, Y., D. K. Bonen, N. Inohara, D. L. Nicolae, F. F. Chen, R. Ramos, H. Britton, T. Moran, R. Karaliuskas, R. H. Duerr, J. P. Achkar, S. R. Brant, T. M. Bayless, B. S. Kirschner, S. B. Hanauer, G. Nunez, and J. H. Cho.** 2001. A frameshift mutation in NOD2 associated with susceptibility to Crohn's disease. *Nature* **411:**603–606.

64. **Perret, X., C. Staehelin, and W. J. Broughton.** 2000. Molecular basis of symbiotic promiscuity. *Microbiol. Mol. Biol. Rev.* **64:**180–201.

65. **Ruby, E. G., and M. J. McFall-Ngai.** 1999. The many roles of oxygen in the symbiotic bacterial colonization of an animal epithelium. *Trends Microbiol.* **7:**414–419.

66. **Salyers, A. A., G. Bonheyo, and N. B. Shoemaker.** 2000. Starting a new genetic system: lessons from bacteroides. *Methods* **20:**35–46.

67. **Savage, D. C.** 1977. Microbial ecology of the gastrointestinal tract. *Annu. Rev. Microbiol.* **31:** 107–133.

68. **Smith, S. E., and F. A. Read.** 1997. *Mycorrhizal Symbiosis.* Academic Press, London, United Kingdom.

69. **Stougaard, J.** 2000. Regulators and regulation of legume root nodule development. *Plant Physiol.* **124:**532–539.

70. **Trench, R. K.** 1987. Dinoflagellates in non-parasitic symbioses, p. 530–570. In F. J. R. Taylor (ed.), *The Biology of Dinoflagellates.* Blackwell Scientific Publishers, Oxford, United Kingdom.

71. **Turelli, M., and A. A. Hoffmann.** 1991. Rapid spread of an inherited incompatibility factor in California *Drosophila. Nature* **353:**440–442.

72. **Van Rhijn, P., and J. Vanderleyden.** 1995. The *Rhizobium*-plant symbiosis. *Microbiol. Rev.* **59:**124–142.

74. **Visick, K. L., J. S. Foster, J. Doino Lemus, M. J. McFall-Ngai, and E. G. Ruby.** 2000. *Vibrio fischeri lux* genes play an important role in colonization and development of the host light organ. *J. Bacteriol.* **182:**4578–4586.

74. **Visick, K.L., and M. J. McFall-Ngai.** 2000. An exclusive contract: specificity in the *Vibrio fischeri-Euprymna scolopes* partnership. *J. Bacteriol.* **182:**1779–1787.

75. **Woollacott, R. M.** 1981. Association of bacteria with bryozoan larvae. *Mar. Biol.* **65:**155–158.

76. **Xu, J., M. K. Bjursell, J. Himrod, S. Deng, L.**

K. Carmichael, H. C. Chiang, L. V. Hooper, and J. I. Gordon. 2003. A genomic view of the human-*Bacteroides thetaiotaomicron* symbiosis. *Science* **299:**2074–2076.

77. Xu, J., and J. I. Gordon. 2003. Honor thy symbionts. *Proc. Natl. Acad. Sci. USA* **100:** 10452–10459.

78. Yachi, S., and M. Loreau. 1999. Biodiversity and ecosystem productivity in a fluctuating environment: the insurance hypothesis. *Proc. Natl. Acad. Sci. USA* **96:**1463–1468.

79. Zoetendal, E. G., A. D. L. Akkermans, W. M. Akkermans-van Vliet, J. A. G. M. deVisser, and W. M. deVos. 2001. The host genotype affects the bacterial community in the human gastrointestinal tract. *Microb. Ecol. Health Dis.* **13:**129–134.

THE EVOLUTION OF BACTERIAL TOXINS

O. Colin Stine and James P. Nataro

10

BACTERIAL TOXINS: AN EVOLUTIONARY PERSPECTIVE

Toxins are among the most important virulence factors of bacterial pathogens. As with all virulence factors, the basic phylogenetic roadmap of bacterial toxin development is thought to comprise the evolution of a functional progenitor molecule, followed by adaptive radiation of the gene to and within other strains or species. This latter process comprises evolutionary "finetuning," which takes the form of modified catalytic efficiency or substrate specificity, or altered interactions with target cells. As will be seen below, dissemination of toxin genes occurs by a large number of highly efficient mechanisms. The study of toxin evolution and phylogeny provides a highly instructive testing ground for theories on the evolution of bacterial pathogens.

Basic Concepts

The prevailing paradigm of bacterial evolution is clonal descent with periodic modification, punctuated with discrete occurrences of horizontal genetic transmission. Although bacterial reproduction by binary fission produces identical progeny, a bacterium is subject to spontaneous point mutations that can modify any gene in the genome. These mutations would presumably accumulate at a constant frequency, but whether they are retained in progeny is subject to pressure toward conservation of function, or to diversification that promotes immune evasion. The best genetic example of descent with modification may be the 16S ribosomal RNA gene. Phylogenetic trees developed using 16S rRNA gene sequences recapitulate the trees based on morphological evidence from classical microbiology (67, 170). While the 16S rRNA gene can be used to develop trees across large taxonomic distances (because it is perhaps the most highly conserved gene in bacteria), other genes are necessary to provide the finer branches within and between congeneric species.

This paradigm predicts that all genes in the genome of a bacterium will show similar phylogenetic relationship with its closest ancestor, i.e., the dendrogram has the same basic configuration regardless of which genes are studied. We have learned, however, that while this is true for most bacterial genes, it does not hold for all, and exceptions may be particularly evident for bacterial virulence factors. The unexpected

O. Colin Stine, Department of Epidemiology and Preventive Medicine and Department of Pediatrics, University of Maryland School of Medicine, Baltimore, MD 21201. James P. Nataro, Department of Pediatrics, Department of Medicine, Department of Microbiology and Immunology, and Center for Vaccine Development, University of Maryland School of Medicine, Baltimore, MD 21201.

Evolution of Microbial Pathogens, Edited by H. S. Seifert and V. J. DiRita, © 2006 ASM Press, Washington, D.C.

finding of highly similar genes across great phylogenetic distances is considered to represent evidence of horizontal genetic transfer. Unfortunately, there is no reliable "rule of thumb" for identifying a likely horizontal transfer event, but the more complete the phylogram, the easier it is to recognize this phenomenon. It should also be noted that horizontal transmission is not limited to single genes. Commonly blocks of genes (including pathogenicity islands and plasmids) travel together. In addition, segments of genes may be inserted or exchanged by recombination, suggesting a different phylogeny for different parts of a molecule. This latter phenomenon, termed "mosaicism," is reported with increasing frequency among bacterial toxins.

Horizontal transfer can occur within a species, as is the case for the hemolysin-encoding *lktA* gene of *Mannheimia (Pasteurella) haemolytica* and for many virulence genes of pathogenenic *Escherichia coli*, or it may occur between closely related species, as in the case of the movement of Shiga toxin genes between *E. coli* and *Shigella dysenteriae*. Sometimes introduction of a new gene involves the complete or partial replacement of an incumbent gene (the mechanism giving rise to mosaicism), but in most cases, it involves genes that were not previously in the recipient genome. In some cases, a new gene may be acquired by an organism that already carries a similar allele and both copies may be retained. This is the likely mechanism leading to the development of paralogs (related genes with different functions), as opposed to orthologs (related alleles serving the same function).

An extreme example of paralogous duplication is seen in *Vibrio cholerae*, where 12.8% of the genes are more closely related to other cholera genes than they are to genes from any other known species (40, 72). Remarkably, *V. cholerae* carries over 40 copies of methyl-accepting chemotaxic protein paralogs (72). Multiple copies of this gene have also been observed in other genomes, and in most cases these genes are similarly more closely related to other genes from the same organism than to those of other genomes. Thus, duplication within a genome probably occurs frequently. Examples of paralogous toxin genes include the case of toxins A and B from *Clostridium difficile* and the autotransporter toxins (see below).

Mechanisms of Horizontal Transmission

Each of the principal mechanisms of horizontal gene transmission in bacteria has been documented for bacterial toxins, including phage transduction, transposition, conjugation of plasmids, and simple recombination.

Shiga toxin-producing *E. coli* (STEC) O157:H7 serves as an example of a patchwork pathogen that has acquired virulence genes by multiple mechanisms. Based on molecular phylogenic analyses, including pulsed-field gel electrophoresis and multilocus sequence analysis, Donnenberg and Whittam have proposed a stepwise evolution of STEC, culminating in the hypervirulent clone *E. coli* O157:H7 (38). According to this scheme, first *stx2*- and then *stx1*-converting phages entered populations of attaching and effacing *E. coli* in two separate and distinct events in the evolution of O157:H7. Between these two events, the organism is thought to have acquired the ca. 60-MDa enterohemorrhagic *E. coli* plasmid. The STEC paradigm suggests the occurrence of multiple molecular "experiments," each the result of the random introduction of a fully functional genetic element. The resulting higher virulence of the recipient strain produced a selection favoring retention and pathogen propagation.

Remarkably, comparison of the O157:H7 genomic sequence with that of *E. coli* K–12 revealed that ca. 1,500 genes (out of about 5,000) are specific to the pathogenic strain. The occurrence of these multiple chance insertions in *E. coli* O157:H7 is likely to be the mechanism of increased virulence of this serotype, rather than any inherent advantage to the serotypic markers themselves. In a similar vein, it should be noted that the *V. cholerae* O1 antigen, so clearly linked to pandemicity, was replaced in recent years in one clone by the O139 antigen gene complex without significant diminution of virulence (119). Similarly, in *Vibrio parahaemolyticus* the pandemic clone O3:K6 has evolved to include serotypes O4:K68, O1:KUT, and O1:K25 (16).

Whereas the introduction of toxin-converting phage constituted an evolutionary milestone in the development of STEC, the natural history of toxin-converting phage in *Corynebacterium diphtheriae* depicts a different scenario (117, 131). Here, introduction of the phage is thought to be a dynamic event, as otherwise isogenic toxinogenic and nontoxinogenic strains can be detected in the same human population at the same time. This observation suggested that the epidemiology of *C. diphtheriae* represents a dynamic ecosystem, comprising the human host, its bacterial parasite, and the bacterium's own invader, the toxin-converting phage. It has been suggested that, in the nonimmune host, the presence of the toxin-converting phage is adaptive in its ability to facilitate spread among human hosts, by virtue of the dramatic respiratory pathology incited by toxinogenic strains (131). However, in toxin-immune hosts, the presence of the phage is maladaptive for the bacterium, and toxin-negative strains predominate. Presumably, the phage can be gained or lost, and therefore it is difficult to ascertain whether a particular host has been infected with toxin-negative strains or whether the host's bacteria have suffered spontaneous phage cure.

In *V. cholerae*, virulent clones have apparently evolved more stable cholera toxin genes, yet transduction of the cholera toxin phage can be recapitulated in vitro (48, 95, 163), and the toxin phage receptor, the toxin-coregulated pilus, is itself acquired by the bacterium in a pathogenicity island (VPI). The VPI has been reported to comprise its own phage element (33, 34, 110, 162), though this observation has been questioned (49). In *V. cholerae*, the VPI can be transferred to other non-O1/non-O139 strains, and the CTX phage may subsequently follow. This inference is based on the observation that many isolates have VPI only and some have both VPI and CTX, but none has CTX alone.

Toxins may also be acquired as transposable elements. So and colleagues demonstrated that the heat-stable toxin (ST) of enterotoxigenic *E. coli* (ETEC) is embedded within a functional transposon, and the presence of ST on widely variable plasmids supports this as the dominant mechanism for ongoing transfer (140–142). All members of the serine protease autotransporter proteins of enterobacteriaceae (the SPATEs; discussed in detail below) are flanked by remnants of related transposable elements, presumably accounting for their promiscuity among *E. coli* and *Shigella* strains (77). As described below, however, the data suggest that these SPATE elements are most likely nonfunctional, and transposition has not been documented in the laboratory.

Bacterial toxins are commonly located on plasmids, some of which are conjugative. The large conjugative virulence plasmid (pAA) of enteroaggregative *E. coli* (EAEC) commonly encodes an autotransporter toxin called Pet, as well as an adjacent ST-like toxin called EAST (128, 129). Both the ST and the heat-labile toxins of ETEC are usually plasmid-borne (123). The three-component toxin of anthrax is encoded on two plasmids that are typically coinherited (96).

Adaptive Functions of Toxins

Toxins are generally thought to execute one of two principal pathogenic functions: host avoidance and host damage. However, a prominent theme of bacterial toxin research in the last decade is the identification of multiple pathogenetic functions for bacterial toxins. Pertussis toxin, for example, has been suggested to function in host damage, immune avoidance, and colonization (4, 8, 125, 135, 153, 156). The adaptive advantage of host avoidance is clear: to facilitate initial colonization and, later, multiplication of the pathogen within the host. A myriad of bacterial toxins has been implicated in immune evasion (98), and even toxins previously considered to function as host-damaging molecules have now been shown to have strong immunomodulatory effects; examples of this phenomenon include cholera toxin (18) and

Shiga toxin (150). In terms of evolution, it may be most efficient to adopt virulence factors from another pathogenic organism, or to embue an existing one with additional functions.

The advantage of host damage to the pathogen is sometimes enigmatic. Factors that contribute to diarrheagenicity facilitate the spread of the pathogen to new hosts, which is the fundamental requirement of the pathogenic lifestyle. A vigorous cough, as induced by *Bordetella pertussis* (in part via its pertussis toxin), for example, would presumably serve a similar role for this bacterium. But the advantages conferred by other bacterial toxins are not as apparent. The ability of the clostridial neurotoxins to kill a host is unlikely to be the role for which these toxins were evolved. It may be that some bacterial toxins have evolved to confer advantages outside the human host, perhaps in other species. We must recognize as well that the advantages of toxin production to the bacterium may be very subtle, and not appreciable in animal models or within individual human infections.

EVOLUTION WITHIN TOXIN FAMILIES

The Heat-Stable Toxins of *E. coli*

The STs of ETEC and related organisms represent a diverse family of potent toxins (reviewed in references 123 and 139). STs were initially defined by their resistance to inactivation by boiling for 30 min. All STs are low-molecular-weight, poorly immunogenic proteins, which are presumed to act at the surface of the eukaryotic cell. STs are assigned to one of two families: STa and STb. STb toxin is not related to STa, and no STb variants have been described; therefore, it will not be considered further. STa, in contrast, comprises a family with both prokaryotic and eukaryotic members (Table 1), and presents an interesting evolutionary case study.

STa family members are single polypeptide chains of approximately 2 kDa. All members of the family are synthesized as larger precursor molecules (prepro-STa) that are cleaved in two steps, the first being processing of a signal sequence by the inner membrane Sec apparatus, and the second being the removal of a stabilizing peptide in the periplasm. The resultant mature toxin polypeptide passes through the TolC outer membrane channel to attain its extracellular location. The mechanism of action of mature STa toxins is still debated. The classical view is that the toxins act by binding to guanylate cyclase C (GC-C) in the apical plasma membrane of the intestinal epithelial cell (36). By this model, STa binding results in dimerization of the GC-C and initiation of a signaling cascade that includes protein kinase C, cGMP-dependent protein kinase II, and the

TABLE 1 The STa family of toxins

Toxin and host	No. of amino acids	Sequence	Reference
STaH ETEC	19	N-S-S-N-Y-C-C-E-L-C-C-N-P-A-C-T-G-C-Y	2
STaP ETEC	18	N-T-F-Y-C-C-E-L-C-C-N-P-A-C-A-G-C-Y	147
Citrobacter freundii	18	N-T-F-Y-C-C-E-L-C-C-N-P-A-C-A-G-C-Y	66
Yersinia enterocolitica	30	. . S-S-D-Y-D-C-C-D-Y-C-C-N-P-A-C-A-G-C	148
Vibrio cholerae non-O1	17	I-D-C-C-E-I-C-C-N-P-A-C-T-G-C-L-N	171
V. cholerae non-O1 Hataka	18	L-I-D-C-C-E-I-C-C-N-P-A-C-T-G-C-L-N	5
Vibrio mimicus	17	I-D-C-C-E-I-C-C-N-P-A-C-T-G-C-L-N	6
E. coli EAST-1	38	...A-S-S-Y-A-S-C-I-W-C-T---T-A-C-A-S-C-H-G	137
Conus geographus 13	13	E-C-C-N-P-A-C-G-R-H-Y-S-C	60
Guanylin (human)	15	P-G-T-C-E-I-C-A-Y-A-A-C-T-G-C	61

cystic fibrosis transmembrane conductance regulator, a principle Cl^- channel in the enterocyte (9, 26, 27, 116, 139). This cascade results in both enhanced Cl^- secretion and reduced Na^+-coupled Cl^- absorption.

A large family of STa-related toxins has been identified in various organisms. All share similar size (ranging from 15 to 30 amino acids) and a highly conserved 13-amino-acid C-terminal region, which is essential for toxicity. Four contiguous and conserved amino acids (N-P-A-C; indicated in boldface in Table 1) mediate binding to the membrane GC-C (61). Two prototype STs are recognized, STaH and STaP, designated according to their derivation from human and porcine ETEC strains, respectively. STaH (19 amino acids) and STaP (18 amino acids) are very similar, differing by only four amino acids. The STa family includes related toxins from several other enteric spp. (Table 1); these members are typically more diverse. The three-dimensional structure of STa reveals a spiral structure with three β turns, stabilized by three disulfide bonds (130). Most members of the family exhibit these same three disulfide bridges.

The complexity of STa downstream effects, all executed from an extracellular site, led investigators to search for an endogenous signaling ligand with parallels to the STa cascade. In 1992, Currie et al. reported the discovery of guanylin, a 15-amino-acid intestinal hormone that serves as the endogenous activator of intestinal guanylate cyclase (29, 169).

The phylogeny of the STa family is not readily apparent, but several models can be envisioned. STa is a small molecule with an existing receptor, thus it can be envisioned that the original progenitor of STa could have evolved de novo to exploit the gaunylin pathway, or could represent capture of the gaunylin gene from the mammalian host. Once derived, with presumably immediate though perhaps modest advantage, the STa progenitor apparently underwent further adaptive radiation and dissemination to other enteric pathogens. As noted above, STa is encoded upon a transposable element, greatly facilitating its distribution. It should be noted that, of the extant STa molecules, none is clearly primative in the evolutionary sense, yet it is interesting to note that, like guanylin, EAST-1 contains four cysteine residues, rather than the six present in STaH and STaP (137). Interestingly, EAST-1 is also encoded within a transposon (109). The evolutionary significance of the guanylin-like conotoxin from *Conus geographus* cannot be determined, though it could be derived independently or via a common lineage with guanylin.

The RTX Pore-Forming Toxins

The RTX toxins comprise a growing family of related factors from gram-negative bacteria (reviewed in references 105 and 167). The mature toxins, typically over 100 kDa in size, feature C-terminal aspartate and glycine-rich nonameric repeat signatures (hence the name repeats-in-toxin, or RTX family), which complex calcium cations. The RTX toxins are synthesized as inactive precursor molecules that become post-translationally activated, apparently outside the bacterium; at least two members of the toxin family are acylated. RTX toxins are exported via dedicated ATP-dependent systems, the so-called type I secretion apparatus (55, 56). The typical RTX toxin is encoded by a four gene operon comprising, in order, the modifying enzyme, the toxin structural gene, and the two components of the secretion system. The accessory genes are highly conserved among the RTX toxins, whereas there is substantial diversity among the toxin structural genes.

All RTX toxins are thought to execute their functions by inserting into eukaryotic plasma membranes, thereby resulting in the formation of a membrane pore (12, 104, 115, 132). The target cells differ for the various toxins, reflecting their various roles in pathogenesis. Most, if not all RTX toxins, however, are thought to act by poisoning leukocytes of various lineages, thereby facilitating immune evasion. The major RTX toxins are briefly considered below.

E. coli hemolysin is the prototype RTX toxin (104, 115, 122, 132). The hemolysin is produced by many strains of uropathogenic *E. coli,* but by certain other *E. coli* pathotypes as well. The hemolysin has been shown to act against a wide variety of cell types, effecting lysis of the plasma membrane by direct insertion and channel formation. The toxin acts against polymorphonuclear cells, monocytes, and T cells, thereby suppressing both innate and adaptive immune reponses (30, 167, 168). Sublethal cellular doses of toxin have milder effects, including induction of cytokine release and increase of cellular permeability (62–65).

The leukotoxin of *Pasteurella haemolytica* is an important virulence factor in bovine pneumonic pasteurellosis (32, 86, 90, 91, 144, 145, 164–166). The toxin has broad effects on bovine leukocytes, including cell lysis, the release of reactive oxygen intermediates, and induction of apoptosis (86, 91, 164). RTX toxins are also important in the pathogenesis of porcine pleuropneumonia caused by *Actinobacillus pleuropneumoniae* (13, 20, 22, 89, 121, 127, 155, 157). This organism secretes three different RTX leukotoxins: ApxI, II, and III; most strains produce more than one toxin type (28, 52). The human pathogen *Actinobacillus actinomycetemcomitans,* a cause of periodontal disease, produces a potent leukotoxin that is specifically lethal for human and primate polymorphonuclear cells, monocytes, and T lymphocytes (106). The adenylate cyclase toxin of *B. pertussis* is an unusually large (177-kDa) bifunctional RTX toxin (11, 41, 59, 79–83, 88, 120, 146, 172). The RTX domain of this toxin may function primarily to promote cell binding of an adenylate cyclase domain, which enters the target eukaryotic cell and catalyzes the formation of high levels of adenylate cyclase. The adenylate cyclase is an essential virulence factor in the early stages of *B. pertussis* infection, as it induces apoptosis of macrophages and may cause epithelial damage (94).

Analysis of the *V. cholerae* genome revealed the presence of an unusually large RTX-like toxin (53, 54, 102). The cholera RTX, with a molecular mass of over 500 kDa, is a cytoskeletal toxin that appears to act by a novel mechanism. The RTX domain does not effect hemolysis.

Comparison of RTX toxin-encoding genes suggests the presence of highly conserved accessory genes, accompanied by a highly divergent toxin structural gene. We speculate that the toxins evolved as a single progenitor that was subsequently disseminated to other bacterial hosts, and that the toxins were modified to fulfill the requirements of their new pathogenetic niche. The secretion apparatus comprises an ABC transporter protein, which has features conserved with other ABC exporter proteins of gram-positive and gram-negative bacteria. The transport system may be derived from transporter proteins involved in routine housekeeping functions of the bacterial cell.

The evolution of the mature toxins themselves is a matter of speculation. The bifunctional adenylate cyclase toxin of *B. pertussis* features a high G+C content (ca. 66%), which is similar to that of the *B. pertussis* chromosome. This observation suggests that the toxin is ancient in this context (or derived from an organism with similar G+C). Other RTX toxins (that of *V. cholerae* excepted), however, display consistently low (ca. 40%) G+C content regardless of host species. This observation, together with their generally higher conservation, suggests that these toxins evolved from more recent common ancestry. Which of these toxins is the oldest cannot be determined with certainty, although *Actinobacillus* and *Pasteurella* G+C content more closely approximate the content of the toxins (whereas *E. coli* is approximately 50% G+C, and is therefore unlikely to represent the ancestral toxin).

The leukotoxins of *Mannheimia* and *Pasteurella* have been subjected to thorough phylogenic inspection (31, 32). Interestingly, the *Pasteurella* leukotoxins are not only important virulence factors, but are also both target cell and host specific, comprising pathogens of both sheep and cows. Accordingly, the family presents an interesting target for testing evolutionary hypotheses. By sequencing the *lktA* locus (encoding the leukotoxin structural genes) from 31 ovine and bovine strains of *M. (P.) haemolytica,* and superimposing the data on a previously derived phylogram, Davies et al. found that the same allele could be localized in phylogenetically distinct branches of the species, indicative of (frequent) recombination events (Fig. 1A). Similarly, the serotype of an isolate did not predict the *lktA* allele: a specific serotype could have multiple *lktA* alleles, and conversely, several different serotypes could have the same allele, again indicative of horizontal transfer between strains. The alleles were highly variable, with variation resulting from both recombination events and single nucleotide mutations. The authors inferred recombination when two contiguous stretches of the DNA sequence had two different closest relatives; the N terminus of *lktA*10, for

example, matches the N terminus of *lktA*6, but the C terminus matches the C terminus of *lktA*1. Certain specific gene segments were found in multiple alleles, and often with perfect conservation (Fig. 1A). Such data suggest that these recombination events were recent in evolutionary terms. In addition, the rate of synonymous substitutions was higher in regions that had recombined and, as expected, the synonymous substitutions were more frequent than nonsynonymous ones. Remarkably, the rate of nonsynonymous substitutions varied by an order of magnitude, with some portions (typically the buried hydrophobic regions) constrained against variation. Moreover, using the known source of the isolates, the authors were able to infer a host-switching phenomenon, in which alleles from ovine strains became adapted to bovine hosts. These authors inferred

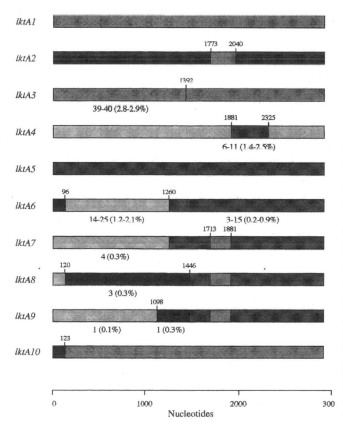

A

FIGURE 1 (A) Schematic representation of the mosaic structures of alleles representative of the major allelic groups of *lktA* leukotoxin in *Pasteurella*. The different colors indicate sequence identity and the likely origins of the recombinant segments. The number of sites different from those in the corresponding region of the likely donor allele(s) and the degree of divergence are indicated below certain recombinant segments; all other segments exhibited 100% sequence identity to the corresponding regions of the donor alleles. Numbers above the proposed recombination sites indicate the position of the last nucleotide at the downstream end of the recombination segment.

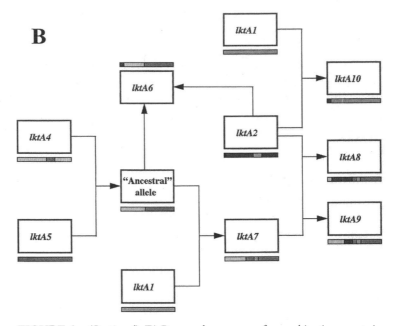

FIGURE 1 *(Continued)* (B) Proposed sequence of recombination events in the evolution of *lktA* to the formation of the *lktA8*- and *lktA10*-type alleles (see panel A) in the ovine-specific lineages of *Pasteurella* leukotoxins and the bovine-specific allele *lktA2*. This analysis suggests not only substantial mosaicism of the toxins, but also host-switching phenomena from ovine- to bovine- and back to ovine-specific alleles. Reprinted from reference 32 with permission.

a complex phylogenetic relationship among these toxins, illustrated in Figure 1B.

Following this analysis with further phylogenetic study of the complete leukotoxin gene clusters, Davies et al. not only corroborated their phylogenetic inferences, but also found that the frequency of substitution, especially nonsynonymous substitution, varied by gene as well as the region of the protein encoded (31). For example, the inner membrane protein LktB was found to be highly conserved, presumably due to the functional constraints of its membrane-spanning stretches. In contrast, the toxin gene was apparently subject to the diversifying selective pressure of the host immune system. Thus, the *Pasteurella* leukotoxin family illustrates each of the major of evolutionary phenomena: mutation, horizontal transmission, and selection for either conservation or diversity.

Shiga Toxins

The Shiga toxins are a family of enterotoxins produced by *Shigella dysenteriae* 1 and STEC (1, 87, 126, 154, 161). The toxins are lethal to Vero cells (as well as other epithelial and endothelial cells) and are therefore alternatively called Vero toxins. The toxins share an oligomeric structure comprising a single catalytic A subunit of 32 kDa, and five B subunits of 7.7 kDa each. The B subunit pentamer mediates binding to the plasma membrane via a glycolipid receptor, which is globotriaosylceramide (Gb3) in the majority of cases (and Gb4 in the case of one variant). Upon binding, the holotoxin is engulfed within a phagosome and undergoes retrograde transport through the Golgi apparatus, ultimately resulting in the delivery of the A1 subunit into the eukaryotic cytoplasm. Delivery is accompanied by an uncharacterized proteolytic event removing a ca. 4-kDa C-terminal moiety, called A2. The StxA subunit then acts as an *N*-glycosidase, depurinating an adenine residue in the 28S rRNA gene of the 60S ribosomal subunit. This event results in lethal inactivation of protein synthesis.

The Shiga toxin family can be assigned to two subgroups, Stx1 and Stx2, based on the sequence of the A subunit (1). The Stx1 group is very homogeneous and includes the Stx toxin of *S. dysenteriae* 1 and Stx1 of STEC, which differ by only a single amino acid residue. Finding these closely related toxins in phylogenetically distinct lineages is prima facie evidence for horizontal transfer of the toxin genes.

In contrast, the Stx2 subgroup is considerably more diverse, both serologically and functionally. Members of the Stx2 family display differences in potency in Vero cell intoxication and mouse lethality (103, 112, 114, 151). The B subunit of toxin variant Stx2e, which causes edema disease in pigs, shares 84% amino acid sequence identity with that of the prototype Stx2 toxin, but binds a different cellular receptor. Another fascinating anomaly within the Stx2 family is the case of Stx2d (97, 112, 113, 149). Alone among the Stx2 toxins, Stx2d requires activation by an elastase present in intestinal mucus. By analyzing a series of hybrid and deletion constructs, Melton-Celsa et al. showed that the A2 portion of Stx2d is required for toxin activation but that activation is abrogated if the Stx1 or Stx2e B subunit is substituted for the Stx2d B polypeptide (113). Furthermore, mass spectrometry of activated Stx2d revealed that its A2 peptide was 2 amino acids smaller than the A2 peptide from buffer-treated Stx2d. These data suggested that specificity of Stx2d activation by mucus requires both A2 and B pentamer sequences. Whereas the evolutionary significance of this unusual phenomenon among the Shiga toxins is unknown, it may represent an adaptation that permits the development of increased toxicity by restricting the activation of the toxin to the precise anatomical location at which it is needed for pathogenesis.

It should be noted that the precise evolutionary advantage of Shiga toxins themselves cannot be ascertained with certainty. The systemic sequelae of Stx intoxication, notably hemolytic-uremic syndrome, are unlikely to provide a benefit to the bacterium, and may result from a secondary host reaction. However, Stx production may exacerbate diarrheal illness (101), and therefore this toxin may have evolved to foster fecal dissemination of the bacteria. In addition, Stx has more recently been shown to induce immunologic dysregulation (84, 107), which may promote colonization by the pathogen, perhaps in a nonhuman host.

Most Stx toxin genes are encoded by toxinogenic phages; however, substantial diversity of these phages has been reported (159, 160). These data, along with the observation that Stx1 is also phage encoded, suggest that the acquisition of toxin genes by phages is a common event in evolutionary terms. Moreover, the promiscuity of these phages is documented by the not infrequent finding of Stx production by otherwise (presumably) avirulent *E. coli*. Nevertheless, not only are certain phages more prevalent, but virulent STEC clones have become common throughout the world, notably O157:H7, but also O111:H8 and O26:H11. Thus, toxin dissemination may be a frequent occurrence, but retention of toxin genes is the result of Darwinian selection favoring fit pathogenic clones.

Tetanus and Botulinum Toxins

The extracellular neurotoxins elaborated by *Clostridium botulinum* and *Clostridium tetani* are among the most potent poisons known (57). Intoxication with minute quantities is sufficient to cause the death of the patient from relentless descending paralysis (for botulinum neurotoxin [BoNT] intoxication) or intense global muscle spasm (in the case of tetanus neurotoxin [TeNT] intoxication). While only one form of TeNT has been identified, BoNT comprises a group of seven related toxins, types A through G, which can be defined serologically (58). BoNT and TeNT have similar proteolytic mechanisms (see below), yet attack different cellular targets, accounting for their dramatically different clinical manifestations. Phylogenetic analyses suggest that the BoNT group and TeNT share a common ancestor (133).

TeNT and BoNT toxins are zinc-dependent metalloproteinases that catalyze the cleavage of specific protein targets involved in the release of neurotransmitters (reviewed in reference 138). Intoxication of a neuron by just one molecule of botulinum toxin is sufficient to completely inactivate all of the synaptic vesicles involved in neurotransmitter release and block signaling from the presynaptic to the postsynaptic neuron. The release of neurotransmitters is a complex and highly regulated process mediated by synaptic vesicles, which become charged with neurotransmitter, dock with a presynaptic plasma membrane, and eventually fuse with the membrane to release neurotransmitter by exocytosis (50, 108, 138). The docking and fusion events involve specific recognition between a synaptic vesicle protein and two proteins anchored within the target plasma membrane. These docking/fusion proteins are called SNARE proteins; the vesicle-associated SNARE (v-SNARE) is called synaptobrevin (or VAMP) and the two target membrane proteins (t-SNAREs) are designated syntaxin and SNAP-25 (50). These three SNARE proteins are the targets of the TeNT and BoNT family: vesicular synaptobrevin is cleaved once by BoNT/B, BoNT/D, BoNT/F, BoNT/G, and TeNT, while BoNT/A, BoNT/C, and BoNT/E each cleave SNAP-25 once; BoNT/C also cleaves syntaxin once.

Clostridial TeNT and BoNT neurotoxins are intially synthesized as inactive ca. 150-kDa polypeptides, which undergo proteolytic activation to yield catalytic 50-kDa (L chain) and binding 100-kDa (H chain) fragments that remain covalently linked via a disulfide bond (7, 99, 100). The N terminus of the H chain mediates cellular translocation and the C terminus of the H chain (H_C) mediates cell binding, whereas the L chain comprises the proteolytic moiety. With solution of the BoNT/A and BoNT/B holotoxin crystal structures, alignment of the BoNT H_C domains with the crystal structure of TeNT H_C established that the H_C domains of BoNT/A, BoNT/B, and TeNT appear similar (99). These H_C domains consist of two further subdomains, of which that comprising the ultimate C terminus contains critical residues involved in binding to gangliosides of target neurons. Importantly, however, the clinical differences between TeNT and BoNT intoxication are in part due to the different routing of toxin mediated by the Hc fragments, as the TeNT Hc uniquely mediates the remarkable phenotype of retrograde axonal transport.

The seven serotypes of botulinum toxin are antigenically related to each other and to tetanus toxin, but neutralizing epitopes are unique to each serotype (7, 99). The overall amino acid identity of the neurotoxins ranges from 34 to 97%. Alignment of the amino acid sequences reveals invariant residues and regions that are highly conserved (e.g., the N termini of all family members), as well as regions with greater diversity. Conserved residues are either suspected or proven (e.g., catalytic residues) to contribute either to the maintenance of protein structure or the functions of the toxins.

A phylogenetic tree has been constructed based on amino acid sequences of the neurotoxin family (133) (Fig. 2). According to this analysis, TeNT occupies a separate branch from the BoNT family members. BoNT/A, the most potent BoNT serotype, also occupies its own branch. In contrast, BoNT toxins E and F, toxins C and D, and toxins B and G each fall within shared phylogenetic branches. BoNT serotypes C and D share 54% amino acid identity, whereas E/F and B/G are more conserved.

Closer analysis of the neurotoxin sequences provides evidence of mosaicism, indicative of recombination between toxin genes (133). Thus, BoNT C/D hybrids have been identified; the BoNT from strain Dsa comprises an N terminus highly related to the BoNT/D family, whereas the C terminus is related to BoNT/C (118).

The neurotoxin family displays diversity of

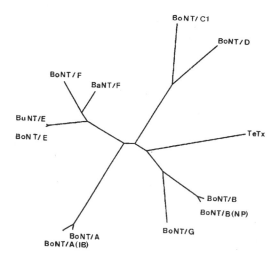

FIGURE 2 Phylogenic tree of the clostridial neurotoxins drawn with the Phylip program. Reprinted from reference 133 with permission.

genetic location (133). TeNT- and BoNT/G-encoding genes are located on mobilizable plasmids (44). BoNT/C and D toxins are encoded on a functional bacteriophage, which can transduce the genes to nontoxinogenic strains (42, 43, 45, 46). BoNT/A and F are encoded on the bacterial chromosome, but appear to reside on an integrated prophage, based on the presence of phagelike *lyc* genes close to the toxin genes (73). Indirect evidence for the role for transposable elements in neurotoxin phylogeny has been offered. The *bont/E* gene and flanking regions present in toxigenic *C. butyricum* are similar to those of BoNT/C-producing *C. botulinum*, but different from sequences of nontoxinogenic *C. butyricum*, suggesting the presence of a mobile DNA element. Clostridial exoenzyme C3 appears to be encoded by a Tn*1554*-like transposon carried within a bacteriophage (69–71). The general segregation of particular BoNT toxin types with distinct bacterial serotypes suggests that a single toxin progenitor, stably maintained in a single bacterial serotype, underwent evolution in the context of the rest of the bacterial genome. However, the additional plasticity provided by phage-, plasmid-, and transposon-mediated transfer suggests at least the possibility of considerably

greater complexity. The relative contributions of these two paradigms await further phylogenetic analysis of these important toxins.

Large Clostridial Toxins

Bacteria of the genus *Clostridium* produce a number of toxins in addition to the neurotoxins described above (10, 17, 21, 93, 152). These typically fall into one of two distinct groups, assigned according to pathophysiological mechanism. The ADP-ribosylating toxins include C3 exoenzyme and C2 of *C. botulinum*. These related toxins target different cellular proteins: Rho GTPase in the case of C3 and actin in the case of C2. Several other members of this family are found in other clostridia, and these affect either of these two targets.

A second family of toxins act as glycosyltransferases of Rho family GTPases (21). This family, of which toxins A and B of *C. difficile* are prototypical, has been adapted to glycosylate different GTPases in different cell lines in order to fulfill very specific pathogenetic functions.

Hofman et al. examined the structural basis for substrate specificity of the clostridial glycosyltransferases (85). These investigators constructed a series of fusions, deletions, and point mutations between the *C. sordellii* lethal toxin (LT; which glycosylates all Ras subfamily proteins) and *C. difficile* toxin B (TcdB, active only on Rho, Rac, and Cdc42). The studies were able to localize the region determining substrate specificity to between residues 364 and 516 of LT, yet other regions may make minor contributions. Importantly, LT and TcdB elicit quite different effects on target cells by virtue of their substrate specificities, as mediated by subtle molecular changes. Thus, the clostridial glycosyltransferases stand as an example of a toxin family in which the prototype toxin serves as a platform for the evolution of additional or modified functions.

This theme is also evident in the examination of the different effects of the paralogous genes for toxin A (TcdA) and toxin B (TcdB) from *C. difficile* (24, 25, 93, 152). TcdA has been suggested to be the major factor in intestinal pathogenesis, mediating a myriad of effects including apoptosis of colonocytes, release of cytokines, and Cl⁻secretion (92, 139). However, TcdA-negative strains are still implicated in colitis, though perhaps clinically milder (136). Despite their abilities to glycosylate the same Rho family GTPases, TcdA and TcdB (63% identical at the amino acid level) induce very different effects on tissue, with TcdB implicated in inhibition of interleukin-2 expression and apoptosis (134), and constituting a more potent in vitro cytotoxin than TcdA. Chaves-Olarte et al. addressed the molecular basis for the different effects of TcdA and TcdB (23). They reported that TcdA was more efficient at binding to an intestinal epithelial cell line (T84) than TcdB, but that TcdA was enzymatically less efficient than TcdB. At the same time, TcdA glycosylated two additional cellular targets, members of the Rap GTPase family. These investigators surmised that TcdA and TcdB play synergistic roles in *C. difficile* pathogenesis, with TcdB potentiating the effects of TcdA on the intestinal mucosa. Synergy by paralogous toxins could be a highly adaptive end point and may occur with other toxin pairs.

Autotransporter Toxins

Autotransporters are large proteins of gramnegative bacteria, which mediate their own passage through the outer membrane by virtue of a dedicated C-terminal β-barrel motif (74, 77, 78). A rapidly growing number of gramnegative virulence factors are found to belong to the autotransporter family (77), and recent genomic analyses have identified still more candidates by virtue of the highly conserved ca. 30-kDa β-barrel domain (77). A particular subfamily of autotransporter proteins can be assigned to a particular phylogenetic group. These proteins are ca. 100 to 110 kDa in size (when fully processed) and share a serine protease motif at a conserved N-terminal site. Those members present in *E. coli* and *Shigella* comprise the SPATEs (39). Members of the family share 40 to 55% amino acid identity. SPATEs include EspC from enteropathogenic *E. coli* (111), EspP from enterohemorrhagic *E. coli* (19), Pet from EAEC (47), Sat from

uropathogenic *E. coli* (68), Tsh from avian pathogenic *E. coli* (143), Pic from *Shigella flexneri* and EAEC (75), and SepA and SigA, also from *Shigella flexneri* (3, 14, 15). Recently, Fink et al. have localized the serine, aspartate, and histidine residues that apparently comprise the catalytic triad of the related Hap protease from *Haemophilus influenzae;* the proposed catalytic residues are conserved across the SPATE family (51).

Various functions have been proposed for the SPATE proteins. EspP cleaves both pepsin and human coagulation factor V (19), the latter effect potentially exacerbating hemorrhagic colitis; EspP may also act as a cytotoxin, causing disruption of the actin network when applied to Vero cells (37). Sat, located on a pathogenicity island in uropathogenic *E. coli* strain CFT073, elicits cytopathic effects on HEp-2 and Vero monkey kidney cells (68). Pic functions as a mucinase and is thought to inactivate the complement cascade (75). Benjelloun-Touimi and colleagues showed that SepA plays a role in causing intestinal inflammation and tissue invasion in *Shigella* (14). EspC has been shown to act as an enterotoxin on rat jejunal tissue mounted in Ussing chambers (111). Like EspC, Pet engenders rises in short circuit current in rabbit intestinal tissue mounted in an Ussing chamber (124), but unlike EspC, Pet also induces rounding and exfoliation of epithelial cells in culture (47) and is required for damage to the human intestinal mucosa induced by EAEC in an organ culture model (76). Pet has been shown to cleave the cytoskeletal protein spectrin (158), and this may be its fundamental mode of action. The various functions attributed to SPATE proteases are summarized in Table 2. Interestingly, although both Pet and EspC are able to cleave spectrin in vitro, only Pet is cytotoxic, and recent data suggest that the mechanism of this phenotypic divergence lies in the inability of EspC to enter eukaryotic cells (39).

We and others have studied the abilities of SPATE proteins to cleave a series of oligopeptides (15, 39). These studies demonstrated a wide variation in substrate preference for the

TABLE 2 Summary of SPATE functions

SPATE protein	Host organism[a]	Cleavage of biological substrates				Cytopathic to HEp-2 cells
		Mucin	Pepsin	Factor V	Spectrin	
EspC	EPEC	−	+	+	+	−
EspP	EHEC	−	+	+	−	−
Pet	EAEC	−	+	+	+	+
Sat	UPEC	−	−	+	+	+
SepA	*S. flexneri*	−	−	−	−	−
Tsh	APEC	+	−	+	−	−
Pic	*S. flexneri*, UPEC, EAEC	+	−	+	−	−
SigA	*S. flexneri*	−	−	−	−	+

[a] APEC, avian pathogenic *Escherichia coli;* EAEC, enteroaggregative *E. coli;* EHEC, enterohemorrhagic *E. coli;* EPEC, enteropathogenic *E. coli;* UPEC, uropathogenic *E. coli.*

various SPATEs. Correlation of substrate specificities and phylogenetic relationships has been reported (Fig. 3A) (39). When the complete protein sequences are considered, the SPATEs can be divided into two groups, with Pic and Pet as prototypes of the respective lineages. Interestingly, phylogenetic analysis of entire SPATE passenger domains did not reveal a correlation with the biological substrates, but did show evidence of homologous recombination among family members (Fig. 3A). Indeed, highly similar proteins, such as Pet and Sat (which are 53% identical overall at the amino acid level), do not share oligopeptide specificities, despite shared abilities to cleave spectrin and cause cytopathic effects in HEp-2 cells. In contrast, proteins that are less similar, such as Pic and Sat (30% identical), do share some specificities for oligopeptides, despite their being classified into different groups and cleaving different biological substrates.

In light of these data, we asked whether the SPATE protease domains would better predict cleavage profiles. Accordingly, split decomposition analysis was performed on the N-terminal third of each SPATE amino acid sequence, corresponding to the location of the predicted catalytic triad from Hap (51). The resulting phylogram is shown in Figure 3B. The original bifurcating phylogenetic pattern remains, with

EspC, EspP, Pet, and Sat comprising one group and Pic, Tsh, and SepA forming the other. The major difference in the second tree, however, is that EspC is now closer to Pet and Sat than in the original analysis. These data suggest that determinants of substrate specificity may largely reside within N-terminal protease domains.

However, the phylogenic groupings of the protease regions are not completely consistent with the oligopeptide cleavage profiles. For example, Pet, Sat, Pic, and Tsh show preferential cleavage of short chains of small, hydrophobic amino acids such as Ala-Ala-Pro-Ala, Ala-Ala-Pro-Abu (2-aminobutyric acid), and Ala-Ala-Pro-Val, thus indicating similarity to the elastase family of proteases. In contrast, both EspC and EspP, which the tree shows to be closely related, have a high affinity for the Arg-Arg oligopeptide. This observation indicates that the active site clefts of these proteases accommodate basic, positively charged amino acids, much like trypsin. SepA, on the other hand, is the most distantly related SPATE and uniquely cleaves large, hydrophobic amino acids (exemplified by cleavage of the oligopeptide Suc-Val-Pro-Phe). Of note, Hap has also been reported to accommodate bulky, hydrophobic residues in its active site (51).

Taken together, analyses of the SPATE family

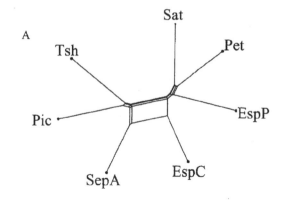

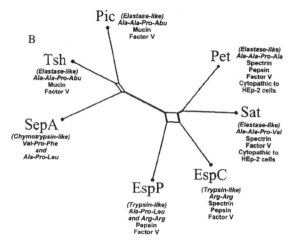

FIGURE 3 Phylogenetic trees of the SPATE proteins generated using ClustalX analysis of amino acid sequences from full-length SPATE passenger domains (A) or the N-terminal one-third (B) corresponding to amino acid 242 of the Pet toxin. Substrates subject to proteolysis are indicated in panel B. Reprinted from reference 39 with permission of the publisher.

suggest that their adaptive radiation within related but distinct pathotypes of *E. coli* and *Shigella* has included alteration in their abilities to interact with target cells, as well as modification of their substrate specificity, most likely as a result of both altered active site conformation and altered exosite structure. These adaptations may have arisen as a result of point mutation or recombination. Not only are autotransporters typically flanked by remnants of insertion sequences, suggesting a mechanism for their dissemination among the *Enterobacteriaceae,* but commonly there exist multiple SPATEs in a particular strain, providing a ready opportunity for recombination. In a separate analysis, we have shown that *Bordetella* autotransporters

(including pertactin, BrkA, and TcfA) display evidence of substantial recombination among themselves, further supporting the potential for intragenomic recombination events (I. R. Henderson, R. Cappello, P. Dutta, and J. P. Nataro, unpublished observations).

Similar evidence of mosaicism in the autotransporters was reported by Davis et al. (35), who described a *Haemophilus* autotransporter called Lav, which is related to the *E. coli* AIDA-adhesin. The *lav* gene was shown to be restricted to just a few pathogenic strains, including *H. influenzae* biotype aegyptius and Brazilian purpuric fever isolates. These investigators found that the *lav* DNA sequence was surprisingly similar to that of a gene previously described for *Neisseria meningitidis,* suggesting relatively recent transfer from *Haemophilus* to *Neisseria,* shortly before the divergence of *N. meningitidis* and *Neisseria gonorrhoeae.* In addition, segments of *lav* predicted to encode the autotransporter passenger and β domains differ significantly in G+C base content, supporting the idea that this gene evolved by fusing two domains that originated in different species.

CONCLUSION

The fundamental mechanisms of bacterial evolution operate on toxin genes as they do on all genetic loci. Toxin genes are subject to strong pressure favoring retention of pathogenic function. In addition, however, most toxins are exposed to host immune responses, introducing pressure toward antigenic diversification. Moreover, the opportunity for horizontal transmission of toxin genes presents the potential for toxins to be diversified as they fulfill different functions for pathogens occupying different niches. Understanding the interplay of these various forces provides a formidable challenge to evolutionary biologists and pathogenic microbiologists, and the field may yet see revolutionary advances that overturn current paradigms.

CHAPTER SUMMARY

- Bacterial toxins often can be assigned to groups or families that share a distant ancestor.
- Mosaicism is common in bacterial protein toxins.
- Toxin genes are commonly acquired by horizontal gene transfer using multiple mechanisms.
- Toxins acquired by a pathogen are subject to adaptive radiation.
- Toxins from the same lineage may exhibit shared function in multiple organisms, or functions may have diverged in different organisms.
- Toxins with similar functions can have diverse influences on pathogenesis in different microorganisms.
- Studying toxin families provides insight

into understanding the structure-function relationships of the toxin proteins.

ACKNOWLEDGMENTS

Work in the Nataro lab is funded by U.S. Public Health Service grants AI33096 and AI43615.

REFERENCES

1. **Acheson, D. W., A. V. Kane, and G. T. Keusch.** 2000. Shiga toxins. *Methods Mol. Biol.* **145:**41–63.
2. **Aimoto, S., T. Takao, Y. Shimonishi, S. Hara, T. Takeda, Y. Takeda, and T. Miwatani.** 1982. Amino-acid sequence of a heat-stable enterotoxin produced by human enterotoxigenic Escherichia coli. *Eur. J. Biochem.* **129:**257–263.
3. **Al-Hasani, K., I. R. Henderson, H. Sakellaris, K. Rajakumar, T. Grant, J. P. Nataro, R. Robins-Browne, and B. Adler.** 2000. The sigA gene which is borne on the she pathogenicity island of Shigella flexneri 2a encodes an exported cytopathic protease involved in intestinal fluid accumulation. *Infect. Immun.* **68:**2457–2463.
4. **Alonso, S., K. Pethe, N. Mielcarek, D. Raze, and C. Locht.** 2001. Role of ADP-ribosyltransferase activity of pertussis toxin in toxin-adhesin redundancy with filamentous hemagglutinin during Bordetella pertussis infection. *Infect. Immun.* **69:**6038–6043.
5. **Arita, M., T. Honda, T. Miwatani, K. Ohmori, T. Takao, and Y. Shimonishi.** 1991. Purification and characterization of a new heat-stable enterotoxin produced by Vibrio cholerae non-O1 serogroup Hakata. *Infect. Immun.* **59:**2186–2188.
6. **Arita, M., T. Honda, T. Miwatani, T. Takeda, T. Takao, and Y. Shimonishi.** 1991. Purification and characterization of a heat-stable enterotoxin of Vibrio mimicus. *FEMS Microbiol. Lett.* **63:**105–110.
7. **Atassi, M. Z., and M. Oshima.** 1999. Structure, activity, and immune (T and B cell) recognition of botulinum neurotoxins. *Crit. Rev. Immunol.* **19:**219–260.
8. **Bagley, K. C., S. F. Abdelwahab, R. G. Tuskan, T. R. Fouts, and G. K. Lewis.** 2002. Pertussis toxin and the adenylate cyclase toxin from Bordetella pertussis activate human monocyte-derived dendritic cells and dominantly inhibit cytokine production through a cAMP-dependent pathway. *J. Leukoc. Biol.* **72:**962–969.
9. **Balint, J. P., J. L. Kosiba, and M. B. Cohen.** 1997. The heat-stable enterotoxin-guanylin receptor is expressed in rat hepatocytes and in a rat hepatoma (H-35) cell line. *J. Recept. Signal Transduct. Res.* **17:**609–630.
10. **Barbieri, J. T., M. J. Riese, and K. Aktories.** 2002. Bacterial toxins that modify the actin

cytoskeleton. *Annu. Rev. Cell Dev. Biol.* **18:** 315–344.

11. **Barry, E. M., A. A. Weiss, I. E. Ehrmann, M. C. Gray, E. L. Hewlett, and M. S. Goodwin.** 1991. Bordetella pertussis adenylate cyclase toxin and hemolytic activities require a second gene, cyaC, for activation. *J. Bacteriol.* **173:**720–726.

12. **Bauer, M. E., and R. A. Welch.** 1996. Association of RTX toxins with erythrocytes. *Infect. Immun.* **64:**4665–4672.

13. **Beck, M., J. F. van den Bosch, I. M. Jongenelen, P. L. Loeffen, R. Nielsen, J. Nicolet, and J. Frey.** 1994. RTX toxin genotypes and phenotypes in Actinobacillus pleuropneumoniae field strains. *J. Clin. Microbiol.* **32:**2749–2754.

14. **Benjelloun-Touimi, Z., P. J. Sansonetti, and C. Parsot.** 1995. SepA, the major extracellular protein of Shigella flexneri: autonomous secretion and involvement in tissue invasion. *Mol. Microbiol.* **17:**123–135.

15. **Benjelloun-Touimi, Z., M. S. Tahar, C. Montecucco, P. J. Sansonetti, and C. Parsot.** 1998. SepA, the 110 kDa protein secreted by Shigella flexneri: two-domain structure and proteolytic activity. *Microbiology* **144:**1815–1822.

16. **Bhuiyan, N. A., M. Ansaruzzaman, M. Kamruzzaman, K. Alam, N. R. Chowdhury, M. Nishibuchi, S. M. Faruque, D. A. Sack, Y. Takeda, and G. B. Nair.** 2002. Prevalence of the pandemic genotype of Vibrio parahaemolyticus in Dhaka, Bangladesh, and significance of its distribution across different serotypes. *J. Clin. Microbiol.* **40:**284–286.

17. **Bobak, D. A.** 1999. Clostridial toxins: molecular probes of Rho-dependent signaling and apoptosis. *Mol. Cell. Biochem.* **193:**37–42.

18. **Bowman, C. C., and J. D. Clements.** 2001. Differential biological and adjuvant activities of cholera toxin and Escherichia coli heat-labile enterotoxin hybrids. *Infect. Immun.* **69:**1528–1535.

19. **Brunder, W., H. Schmidt, and H. Karch.** 1997. EspP, a novel extracellular serine protease of enterohaemorrhagic Escherichia coli O157:H7 cleaves human coagulation factor V. *Mol. Microbiol.* **24:**767–778.

20. **Burrows, L. L., and R. Y. Lo.** 1992. Molecular characterization of an RTX toxin determinant from Actinobacillus suis. *Infect. Immun.* **60:**2166–2173.

21. **Busch, C., and K. Aktories.** 2000. Microbial toxins and the glycosylation of rho family GTPases. *Curr. Opin. Struct. Biol.* **10:**528–535.

22. **Chang, Y. F., J. Shi, D. P. Ma, S. J. Shin, and D. H. Lein.** 1993. Molecular analysis of the Actinobacillus pleuropneumoniae RTX toxin-III gene cluster. *DNA Cell Biol.* **12:**351–362.

23. **Chaves-Olarte, E., E. Freer, A. Parra, C. Guzman-Verri, E. Moreno, and M. Thelestam.** 2002. R-Ras glucosylation and transient RhoA activation determine the cytopathic effect produced by toxin B variants from toxin A-negative strains of Clostridium difficile. *J. Biol. Chem.* **78:**7956–7963.

24. **Chaves-Olarte, E., M. Weidmann, C. Eichel-Streiber, and M. Thelestam.** 1997. Toxins A and B from Clostridium difficile differ with respect to enzymatic potencies, cellular substrate specificities, and surface binding to cultured cells. *J. Clin. Investig.* **100:**1734–1741.

25. **Ciesla, W. P., Jr., and D. A. Bobak.** 1998. Clostridium difficile toxins A and B are cation-dependent UDP-glucose hydrolases with differing catalytic activities. *J. Biol. Chem.* **273:**16021–16026.

26. **Cohen, M. B.** 1992. The heat-stable enterotoxin receptor: a probe for ligand hunting. *J. Pediatr. Gastroenterol. Nutr.* **15:**337–338.

27. **Crane, J. K., M. S. Wehner, E. J. Bolen, J. J. Sando, J. Linden, R. L. Guerrant, and C. L. Sears.** 1992. Regulation of intestinal guanylate cyclase by the heat-stable enterotoxin of Escherichia coli (STa) and protein kinase C. *Infect. Immun.* **60:**5004–5012.

28. **Cullen, J. M., and A. N. Rycroft.** 1994. Phagocytosis by pig alveolar macrophages of Actinobacillus pleuropneumoniae serotype 2 mutant strains defective in haemolysin II (ApxII) and pleurotoxin (ApxIII). *Microbiology* **140:**237–244.

29. **Currie, M. G., K. F. Fok, J. Kato, R. J. Moore, F. K. Hamra, K. L. Duffin, and C. E. Smith.** 1992. Guanylin: an endogenous activator of intestinal guanylate cyclase. *Proc. Natl. Acad. Sci. USA* **89:**947–951.

30. **Czuprynski, C. J., and R. A. Welch.** 1995. Biological effects of RTX toxins: the possible role of lipopolysaccharide. *Trends Microbiol.* **3:**480–483.

31. **Davies, R. L., S. Campbell, and T. S. Whittam.** 2002. Mosaic structure and molecular evolution of the leukotoxin operon (lktCABD) in Mannheimia (Pasteurella) haemolytica, Mannheimia glucosida, and Pasteurella trehalosi. *J. Bacteriol.* **184:**266–277.

32. **Davies, R. L., T. S. Whittam, and R. K. Selander.** 2001. Sequence diversity and molecular evolution of the leukotoxin (lktA) gene in bovine and ovine strains of Mannheimia (Pasteurella) haemolytica. *J. Bacteriol.* **183:**1394–1404.

33. **Davis, B. M., H. H. Kimsey, W. Chang, and M. K. Waldor.** 1999. The Vibrio cholerae O139 Calcutta bacteriophage CTXphi is infectious and encodes a novel repressor. *J. Bacteriol.* **181:**6779–6787.

34. **Davis, B. M., K. E. Moyer, E. F. Boyd, and M. K. Waldor.** 2000. CTX prophages in classical biotype Vibrio cholerae: functional phage genes but

dysfunctional phage genomes. *J. Bacteriol.* **182:** 6992–6998.

35. **Davis, J., A. L. Smith, W. R. Hughes, and M. Golomb.** 2001. Evolution of an autotransporter: domain shuffling and lateral transfer from pathogenic Haemophilus to Neisseria. *J. Bacteriol.* **183:**4626–4635.

36. **de Sauvage, F. J., R. Horuk, G. Bennett, C. Quan, J. P. Burnier, and D. V. Goeddel.** 1992. Characterization of the recombinant human receptor for Escherichia coli heat-stable enterotoxin. *J. Biol. Chem.* **267:**6479–6482.

37. **Djafari, S., F. Ebel, C. Deibel, S. Kramer, M. Hudel, and T. Chakraborty.** 1997. Characterization of an exported protease from Shiga toxin-producing Escherichia coli. *Mol. Microbiol.* **25:**771–784.

38. **Donnenberg, M. S., and T. S. Whittam.** 2001. Pathogenesis and evolution of virulence in enteropathogenic and enterohemorrhagic Escherichia coli. *J. Clin. Investig.* **107:**539–548.

39. **Dutta, P. R., R. Cappello, F. Navarro-Garcia, and J. P. Nataro.** 2002. Functional comparison of serine protease autotransporters of enterobacteriaceae. *Infect. Immun.* **70:**7105–7113.

40. **Dziejman, M., E. Balon, D. Boyd, C. M. Fraser, J. F. Heidelberg, and J. J. Mekalanos.** 2002. Comparative genomic analysis of Vibrio cholerae: genes that correlate with cholera endemic and pandemic disease. *Proc. Natl. Acad. Sci. USA* **99:**1556–1561.

41. **Ehrmann, I. E., M. C. Gray, V. M. Gordon, L. S. Gray, and E. L. Hewlett.** 1991. Hemolytic activity of adenylate cyclase toxin from Bordetella pertussis. *FEBS Lett.* **278:**79–83.

42. **Eklund, M. W., and F. T. Poysky.** 1974. Interconversion of type C and D strains of Clostridium botulinum by specific bacteriophages. *Appl. Microbiol.* **27:**251–258.

43. **Eklund, M. W., F. T. Poysky, J. A. Meyers, and G. A. Pelroy.** 1974. Interspecies conversion of Clostridium botulinum type C to Clostridium novyi type A by bacteriophage. *Science* **186:** 456–458.

44. **Eklund, M. W., F. T. Poysky, L. M. Mseitif, and M. S. Strom.** 1988. Evidence for plasmid-mediated toxin and bacteriocin production in Clostridium botulinum type G. *Appl. Environ. Microbiol.* **54:**1405–1408.

45. **Eklund, M. W., F. T. Poysky, and S. M. Reed.** 1972. Bacteriophage and the toxigenicity of Clostridium botulinum type D. *Nat. New Biol.* **235:**16–17.

46. **Eklund, M. W., F. T. Poysky, S. M. Reed, and C. A. Smith.** 1971. Bacteriophage and the toxigenicity of Clostridium botulinum type C. *Science* **172:**480–482.

47. **Eslava, C., F. Navarro-Garcia, J. R. Czeczulin,** I. R. Henderson, A. Cravioto, and J. P. Nataro. 1998. Pet, an autotransporter enterotoxin from enteroaggregative Escherichia coli. *Infect. Immun.* **66:**3155–3163.

48. **Faruque, S. M., Asadulghani, M. M. Rahman, M. K. Waldor, and D. A. Sack.** 2000. Sunlight-induced propagation of the lysogenic phage encoding cholera toxin. *Infect. Immun.* **68:**4795–4801.

49. **Faruque, S. M., J. Zhu, Asadulghani, M. Kamruzzaman, and J. J. Mekalanos.** 2003. Examination of diverse toxin-coregulated pilus-positive Vibrio cholerae strains fails to demonstrate evidence for Vibrio pathogenicity island phage. *Infect. Immun.* **71:**2993–2999.

50. **Fasshauer, D., R. B. Sutton, A. T. Brunger, and R. Jahn.** 1998. Conserved structural features of the synaptic fusion complex: SNARE proteins reclassified as Q- and R-SNAREs. *Proc. Natl. Acad. Sci. USA* **95:**15781–15786.

51. **Fink, D. L., L. D. Cope, E. J. Hansen, and J. W. Geme III.** 2001. The Haemophilus influenzae Hap autotransporter is a chymotrypsin clan serine protease and undergoes autoproteolysis via an intermolecular mechanism. *J. Biol. Chem.* **276:**39492–39500.

52. **Frey, J., J. T. Bosse, Y. F. Chang, J. M. Cullen, B. Fenwick, G. F. Gerlach, D. Gygi, F. Haesebrouck, T. J. Inzana, R. Jansen, et al.** 1993. Actinobacillus pleuropneumoniae RTX-toxins: uniform designation of haemolysins, cytolysins, pleurotoxin and their genes. *J. Gen. Microbiol.* **139**(Pt. 8):1723–1728.

53. **Fullner, K. J., J. C. Boucher, M. A. Hanes, G. K. Haines III, B. M. Meehan, C. Walchle, P. J. Sansonetti, and J. J. Mekalanos.** 2002. The contribution of accessory toxins of Vibrio cholerae O1 El Tor to the proinflammatory response in a murine pulmonary cholera model. *J. Exp. Med.* **195:**1455–1462.

54. **Fullner, K. J., W. I. Lencer, and J. J. Mekalanos.** 2001. Vibrio cholerae-induced cellular responses of polarized T84 intestinal epithelial cells are dependent on production of cholera toxin and the RTX toxin. *Infect. Immun.* **69:**6310–6317.

55. **Gentschev, I., G. Dietrich, and W. Goebel.** 2002. The E. coli alpha-hemolysin secretion system and its use in vaccine development. *Trends Microbiol.* **10:**39–45.

56. **Gentschev, I., G. Dietrich, H. J. Mollenkopf, Z. Sokolovic, J. Hess, S. H. Kaufmann, and W. Goebel.** 1997. The Escherichia coli hemolysin secretion apparatus—a versatile antigen delivery system in attenuated Salmonella. *Behring Inst. Mitt.***:**103–113.

57. **Gill, D. M.** 1982. Bacterial toxins: a table of lethal amounts. *Microbiol. Rev.* **46:**86–94.

58. **Gimenez, D. F.** 1976. Serological classification

and typing of Clostridium botulinum. *Dev. Biol. Stand.* **32:**175–183.

59. **Gray, M. C., W. Ross, K. Kim, and E. L. Hewlett.** 1999. Characterization of binding of adenylate cyclase toxin to target cells by flow cytometry. *Infect. Immun.* **67:**4393–4399.

60. **Gray, W. R., A. Luque, B. M. Olivera, J. Barrett, and L. J. Cruz.** 1981. Peptide toxins from Conus geographus venom. *J. Biol. Chem.* **256:**4734–4740.

61. **Greenberg, R. N., M. Hill, J. Crytzer, W. J. Krause, S. L. Eber, F. K. Hamra, and L. R. Forte.** 1997. Comparison of effects of uroguanylin, guanylin, and Escherichia coli heat-stable enterotoxin STa in mouse intestine and kidney: evidence that uroguanylin is an intestinal natriuretic hormone. *J. Investig. Med.* **45:**276–282.

62. **Grimminger, F., C. Scholz, S. Bhakdi, and W. Seeger.** 1991. Subhemolytic doses of Escherichia coli hemolysin evoke large quantities of lipoxygenase products in human neutrophils. *J. Biol. Chem.* **266:**14262–14269.

63. **Grimminger, F., U. Sibelius, S. Bhakdi, N. Suttorp, and W. Seeger.** 1991. Escherichia coli hemolysin is a potent inductor of phosphoinositide hydrolysis and related metabolic responses in human neutrophils. *J. Clin. Invest.* **88:**1531–1539.

64. **Grimminger, F., M. Thomas, R. Obernitz, D. Walmrath, S. Bhakdi, and W. Seeger.** 1990. Inflammatory lipid mediator generation elicited by viable hemolysin-forming Escherichia coli in lung vasculature. *J. Exp. Med.* **172:**1115–1125.

65. **Grimminger, F., D. Walmrath, R. G. Birkemeyer, S. Bhakdi, and W. Seeger.** 1990. Leukotriene and hydroxyeicosatetraenoic acid generation elicited by low doses of Escherichia coli hemolysin in rabbit lungs. *Infect. Immun.* **58:**2659–2663.

66. **Guarino, A., R. Giannella, and M. R. Thompson.** 1989. Citrobacter freundii produces an 18-amino-acid heat-stable enterotoxin identical to the 18-amino-acid Escherichia coli heat-stable enterotoxin (ST Ia). *Infect. Immun.* **57:**649–652.

67. **Gutell, R. R., B. Weiser, C. R. Woese, and H. F. Noller.** 1985. Comparative anatomy of 16-S-like ribosomal RNA. *Prog. Nucleic Acid Res. Mol. Biol.* **32:**155–216.

68. **Guyer, D. M., I. R. Henderson, J. P. Nataro, and H. L. Mobley.** 2000. Identification of sat, an autotransporter toxin produced by uropathogenic Escherichia coli. *Mol. Microbiol.* **38:**53–66.

69. **Hauser, D., M. W. Eklund, P. Boquet, and M. R. Popoff.** 1994. Organization of the botulinum neurotoxin C1 gene and its associated non-toxic protein genes in Clostridium botulinum C 468. *Mol. Gen. Genet.* **243:**631–640.

70. **Hauser, D., M. Gibert, M. W. Eklund, P. Boquet, and M. R. Popoff.** 1993. Comparative analysis of C3 and botulinal neurotoxin genes and their environment in Clostridium botulinum types C and D. *J. Bacteriol.* **175:**7260–7268.

71. **Hauser, D., M. Gibert, J. C. Marvaud, M. W. Eklund, and M. R. Popoff.** 1995. Botulinal neurotoxin C1 complex genes, clostridial neurotoxin homology and genetic transfer in Clostridium botulinum. *Toxicon* **33:**515–526.

72. **Heidelberg, J. F., J. A. Eisen, W. C. Nelson, R. A. Clayton, M. L. Gwinn, R. J. Dodson, D. H. Haft, E. K. Hickey, J. D. Peterson, L. Umayam, S. R. Gill, K. E. Nelson, T. D. Read, H. Tettelin, D. Richardson, M. D. Ermolaeva, J. Vamathevan, S. Bass, H. Qin, I. Dragoi, P. Sellers, L. McDonald, T. Utterback, R. D. Fleishmann, W. C. Nierman, and O. White.** 2000. DNA sequence of both chromosomes of the cholera pathogen Vibrio cholerae. *Nature* **406:**477–483.

73. **Henderson, I., S. M. Whelan, T. O. Davis, and N. P. Minton.** 1996. Genetic characterisation of the botulinum toxin complex of Clostridium botulinum strain NCTC 2916. *FEMS Microbiol. Lett.* **140:**151–158.

74. **Henderson, I. R., R. Cappello, and J. P. Nataro.** 2000. Autotransporter proteins, evolution and redefining protein secretion. *Trends Microbiol.* **8:**529–532.

75. **Henderson, I. R., J. Czeczulin, C. Eslava, F. Noriega, and J. P. Nataro.** 1999. Characterization of pic, a secreted protease of Shigella flexneri and enteroaggregative Escherichia coli. *Infect. Immun.* **67:**5587–5596.

76. **Henderson, I. R., S. Hicks, F. Navarro-Garcia, W. P. Elias, A. D. Philips, and J. P. Nataro.** 1999. Involvement of the enteroaggregative Escherichia coli plasmid-encoded toxin in causing human intestinal damage. *Infect. Immun.* **67:**5338–5344.

77. **Henderson, I. R., and J. P. Nataro.** 2001. Virulence functions of autotransporter proteins. *Infect. Immun.* **69:**1231–1243.

78. **Henderson, I. R., F. Navarro-Garcia, and J. P. Nataro.** 1998. The great escape: structure and function of the autotransporter proteins. *Trends Microbiol.* **6:**370–378.

79. **Hewlett, E., and J. Wolff.** 1976. Soluble adenylate cyclase from the culture medium of Bordetella pertussis: purification and characterization. *J. Bacteriol.* **127:**890–898.

80. **Hewlett, E. L., V. M. Gordon, J. D. McCaffery, W. M. Sutherland, and M. C. Gray.** 1989. Adenylate cyclase toxin from Bordetella pertussis. Identification and purification of the holotoxin molecule. *J. Biol. Chem.* **264:**19379–19384.

81. **Hewlett, E. L., L. Gray, M. Allietta, I. Ehrmann, V. M. Gordon, and M. C. Gray.**

1991. Adenylate cyclase toxin from Bordetella pertussis. Conformational change associated with toxin activity. *J. Biol. Chem.* **266:**17503–17508.

82. **Hewlett, E. L., K. J. Kim, S. J. Lee, and M. C. Gray.** 2000. Adenylate cyclase toxin from Bordetella pertussis: current concepts and problems in the study of toxin functions. *Int. J. Med. Microbiol.* **290:**333–335.

83. **Hewlett, E. L., M. A. Urban, C. R. Manclark, and J. Wolff.** 1976. Extracytoplasmic adenylate cyclase of Bordetella pertussis. *Proc. Natl. Acad. Sci. USA* **73:**1926–1930.

84. **Heyderman, R. S., M. Soriani, and T. R. Hirst.** 2001. Is immune cell activation the missing link in the pathogenesis of post-diarrhoeal HUS? *Trends Microbiol.* **9:**262–266.

85. **Hofmann, F., C. Busch, and K. Aktories.** 1998. Chimeric clostridial cytotoxins: identification of the N-terminal region involved in protein substrate recognition. *Infect. Immun.* **66:**1076–1081.

86. **Hsuan, S. L., M. S. Kannan, S. Jeyaseelan, Y. S. Prakash, C. Malazdrewich, M. S. Abrahamsen, G. C. Sieck, and S. K. Maheswaran.** 1999. Pasteurella haemolytica leukotoxin and endotoxin induced cytokine gene expression in bovine alveolar macrophages requires NF-kappaB activation and calcium elevation. *Microb. Pathog.* **26:**263–273.

87. **Jaeger, J. L., and D. W. Acheson.** 2000. Shiga toxin-producing Escherichia coli. *Curr. Infect. Dis. Rep.* **2:**61–67.

88. **Jansen, R., J. Briaire, E. M. Kamp, A. L. Gielkens, and M. A. Smits.** 1993. Cloning and characterization of the Actinobacillus pleuropneumoniae-RTX-toxin III (ApxIII) gene. *Infect. Immun.* **61:**947–954.

89. **Jansen, R., J. Briaire, A. B. van Geel, E. M. Kamp, A. L. Gielkens, and M. A. Smits.** 1994. Genetic map of the Actinobacillus pleuropneumoniae RTX-toxin (Apx) operons: characterization of the ApxIII operons. *Infect. Immun.* **62:**4411–4418.

90. **Jeyaseelan, S., S. L. Hsuan, M. S. Kannan, B. Walcheck, J. F. Wang, M. E. Kehrli, E. T. Lally, G. C. Sieck, and S. K. Maheswaran.** 2000. Lymphocyte function-associated antigen 1 is a receptor for Pasteurella haemolytica leukotoxin in bovine leukocytes. *Infect. Immun.* **68:**72–79.

91. **Jeyaseelan, S., M. S. Kannan, S. L. Hsuan, A. K. Singh, T. F. Walseth, and S. K. Maheswaran.** 2001. Pasteurella (Mannheimia) haemolytica leukotoxin-induced cytolysis of bovine leukocytes: role of arachidonic acid and its regulation. *Microb. Pathog.* **30:**59–69.

92. **Johnson, S., and D. N. Gerding.** 1998.

Clostridium difficile–associated diarrhea. *Clin. Infect. Dis.* **26:**1027–1034; quiz 1035–1036.

93. **Just, I., F. Hofmann, and K. Aktories.** 2000. Molecular mode of action of the large clostridial cytotoxins. *Curr. Top. Microbiol. Immunol.* **250:**55–83.

94. **Khelef, N., P. Gounon, and N. Guiso.** 2001. Internalization of Bordetella pertussis adenylate cyclase-haemolysin into endocytic vesicles contributes to macrophage cytotoxicity. *Cell Microbiol.* **3:**721–730.

95. **Kimsey, H. H., G. B. Nair, A. Ghosh, and M. K. Waldor.** 1998. Diverse CTXphis and evolution of new pathogenic Vibrio cholerae. *Lancet* **352:**457–458.

96. **Koehler, T. M.** 2002. Bacillus anthracis genetics and virulence gene regulation. *Curr. Top. Microbiol. Immunol.* **271:**143–164.

97. **Kokai-Kun, J. F., A. R. Melton-Celsa, and A. D. O'Brien.** 2000. Elastase in intestinal mucus enhances the cytotoxicity of Shiga toxin type 2d. *J. Biol. Chem.* **275:**3713–3721.

98. **Konig, B., A. Drynda, A. Ambrosch, and W. Konig.** 1999. Toxin-induced modulation of inflammatory processes, p. 637–656. *In* J. E. Alouf and J. H. Freer (ed.), *The Comprehensive Sourcebook of Bacterial Protein Toxins,* 2nd ed. Academic Press, London, United Kingdom.

99. **Lacy, D. B., and R. C. Stevens.** 1999. Sequence homology and structural analysis of the clostridial neurotoxins. *J. Mol. Biol.* **291:**1091–1104.

100. **Lacy, D. B., and R. C. Stevens.** 1998. Unraveling the structures and modes of action of bacterial toxins. *Curr. Opin. Struct. Biol.* **8:**778–784.

101. **Levine, M. M., H. L. DuPont, S. B. Formal, R. B. Hornick, A. Takeuchi, E. J. Gangarosa, M. J. Snyder, and J. P. Libonati.** 1973. Pathogenesis of Shigella dysenteriae 1 (Shiga) dysentery. *J. Infect. Dis.* **127:**261–270.

102. **Lin, W., K. J. Fullner, R. Clayton, J. A. Sexton, M. B. Rogers, K. E. Calia, S. D. Calderwood, C. Fraser, and J. J. Mekalanos.** 1999. Identification of a vibrio cholerae RTX toxin gene cluster that is tightly linked to the cholera toxin prophage. *Proc. Natl. Acad. Sci. USA* **96:**1071–1076.

103. **Lindgren, S. W., J. E. Samuel, C. K. Schmitt, and A. D. O'Brien.** 1994. The specific activities of Shiga-like toxin type II (SLT-II) and SLT-II-related toxins of enterohemorrhagic Escherichia coli differ when measured by Vero cell cytotoxicity but not by mouse lethality. *Infect. Immun.* **62:**623–631.

104. **Ludwig, A., and W. Goebel.** 2000. Dangerous signals from E. coli toxin. *Nat. Med.* **6:**741–742.

105. **Ludwig, A., and W. Goebel.** 1999. The family of the multigenic encoded RTX toxins,

p. 330–348. *In* J. E. Alouf and J. H. Freer (ed.), *The Comprehensive Sourcebook of Bacterial Protein Toxins,* 2nd ed. Academic Press, London, United Kingdom.

106. **Mangan, D. F., N. S. Taichman, E. T. Lally, and S. M. Wahl.** 1991. Lethal effects of Actinobacillus actinomycetemcomitans leukotoxin on human T lymphocytes. *Infect. Immun.* **59:**3267–3272.

107. **Marcato, P., G. Mulvey, and G. D. Armstrong.** 2002. Cloned Shiga toxin 2 B subunit induces apoptosis in Ramos Burkitt's lymphoma B cells. *Infect. Immun.* **70:**1279–1286.

108. **Matteoli, M., C. Verderio, O. Rossetto, N. Iezzi, S. Coco, G. Schiavo, and C. Montecucco.** 1996. Synaptic vesicle endocytosis mediates the entry of tetanus neurotoxin into hippocampal neurons. *Proc. Natl. Acad. Sci. USA* **93:**13310–13315.

109. **McVeigh, A., A. Fasano, D. A. Scott, S. Jelacic, S. L. Moseley, D. C. Robertson, and S. J. Savarino.** 2000. IS1414, an Escherichia coli insertion sequence with a heat-stable enterotoxin gene embedded in a transposase-like gene. *Infect. Immun.* **68:**5710–5715.

110. **Mekalanos, J. J., E. J. Rubin, and M. K. Waldor.** 1997. Cholera: molecular basis for emergence and pathogenesis. *FEMS Immunol. Med. Microbiol.* **18:**241–248.

111. **Mellies, J. L., F. Navarro-Garcia, I. Okeke, J. Frederickson, J. P. Nataro, and J. B. Kaper.** 2001. espC pathogenicity island of enteropathogenic Escherichia coli encodes an enterotoxin. *Infect. Immun.* **69:**315–324.

112. **Melton-Celsa, A. R., S. C. Darnell, and A. D. O'Brien.** 1996. Activation of Shiga-like toxins by mouse and human intestinal mucus correlates with virulence of enterohemorrhagic Escherichia coli O91:H21 isolates in orally infected, streptomycin-treated mice. *Infect. Immun.* **64:**1569–1576.

113. **Melton-Celsa, A. R., J. F. Kokai-Kun, and A. D. O'Brien.** 2002. Activation of Shiga toxin type 2d (Stx2d) by elastase involves cleavage of the C-terminal two amino acids of the A2 peptide in the context of the appropriate B pentamer. *Mol. Microbiol.* **43:**207–215.

114. **Melton-Celsa, A. R., J. E. Rogers, C. K. Schmitt, S. C. Darnell, and A. D. O'Brien.** 1998. Virulence of Shiga toxin-producing Escherichia coli (STEC) in orally-infected mice correlates with the type of toxin produced by the infecting strain. *Jpn. J. Med. Sci. Biol.* **51**(Suppl.):S108–S114.

115. **Menestrina, G., C. Moser, S. Pellet, and R. Welch.** 1994. Pore-formation by Escherichia coli hemolysin (HlyA) and other members of the RTX toxins family. *Toxicology* **87:**249–267.

116. **Mezoff, A. G., R. A. Giannella, M. N. Eade, and M. B. Cohen.** 1992. Escherichia coli enterotoxin (STa) binds to receptors, stimulates guanyl cyclase, and impairs absorption in rat colon. *Gastroenterology* **102:**816–822.

117. **Michel, J. L., R. Rappuoli, J. R. Murphy, and A. M. Pappenheimer, Jr.** 1982. Restriction endonuclease map of the nontoxigenic corynephage gamma c and its relationship to the toxigenic corynephage beta c. *J. Virol.* **42:**510–518.

118. **Moriishi, K., M. Koura, N. Abe, N. Fujii, Y. Fujinaga, K. Inoue, and K. Ogumad.** 1996. Mosaic structures of neurotoxins produced from Clostridium botulinum types C and D organisms. *Biochim. Biophys. Acta* **1307:**123–126.

119. **Morris, J. G., Jr., G. E. Losonsky, J. A. Johnson, C. O. Tacket, J. P. Nataro, P. Panigrahi, and M. M. Levin.** 1995. Clinical and immunologic characteristics of Vibrio cholerae O139 Bengal infection in North American volunteers. *J. Infect. Dis.* **171:**903–908.

120. **Moss, J., S. C. Tsai, P. Bruni, R. Adamik, Y. Kanaho, E. L. Hewlett, and M. Vaughan.** 1985. Pertussis toxin-catalyzed ADP-ribosylation of adenylate cyclase. Effects of guanyl nucleotides and rhodopsin. *Dev. Biol. Stand.* **61:**43–49.

121. **Nagai, S., T. Yagihashi, and A. Ishihama.** 1993. DNA sequence analysis of an allelic variant of the Actinobacillus pleuropneumoniae-RTX-toxin I (ApxIA) from serotype 10. *Microb. Pathog.* **15:**485–495.

122. **Nagy, G., U. Dobrindt, G. Blum-Oehler, L. Emody, W. Goebel, and J. Hacker.** 2000. Analysis of the hemolysin determinants of the uropathogenic Escherichia coli strain 536. *Adv. Exp. Med. Biol.* **485:**57–61.

123. **Nataro, J. P., and J. B. Kaper.** 1998. Diarrheagenic Escherichia coli. *Clin. Microbiol. Rev.* **11:**142–201.

124. **Navarro-Garcia, F., C. Eslava, J. M. Villaseca, R. Lopez-Revilla, J. R. Czeczulin, S. Srinivas, J. P. Nataro, and A. Cravioto.** 1998. In vitro effects of a high-molecular-weight heat-labile enterotoxin from enteroaggregative Escherichia coli. *Infect. Immun.* **66:**3149–3154.

125. **Nencioni, L., M. G. Pizza, G. Volpini, M. T. De Magistris, F. Giovannoni, and R. Rappuoli.** 1991. Properties of the B oligomer of pertussis toxin. *Infect. Immun.* **59:**4732–4734.

126. **O'Brien, A. D., V. L. Tesh, A. Donohue-Rolfe, M. P. Jackson, S. Olsnes, K. Sandvig, A. A. Lindberg, and G. T. Keusch.** 1992. Shiga toxin: biochemistry, genetics, mode of action, and role in pathogenesis. *Curr. Top. Microbiol. Immunol.* **180:**65–94.

127. **Ohta, H., A. Miyagi, K. Kato, and K. Fukui.** 1996. The relationships between leukotoxin pro-

duction, growth rate and the bicarbonate concentration in a toxin-production-variable strain of Actinobacillus actinomycetemcomitans. *Microbiology* **142**(Pt. 4):963–970.

128. **Okeke, I. N., A. Lamikanra, J. Czeczulin, F. Dubovsky, J. B. Kaper, and J. P. Nataro.** 2000. Heterogeneous virulence of enteroaggregative Escherichia coli strains isolated from children in Southwest Nigeria. *J. Infect. Dis.* **181:** 252–260.

129. **Okeke, I. N., and J. P. Nataro.** 2001. Enteroaggregative Escherichia coli. *Lancet Infect. Dis.* **1:**304–313.

130. **Ozaki, H., T. Sato, H. Kubota, Y. Hata, Y. Katsube, and Y. Shimonishi.** 1991. Molecular structure of the toxin domain of heat-stable enterotoxin produced by a pathogenic strain of Escherichia coli. A putative binding site for a binding protein on rat intestinal epithelial cell membranes. *J. Biol. Chem.* **266:**5934–5941.

131. **Pappenheimer, A. M., Jr., and J. R. Murphy.** 1983. Studies on the molecular epidemiology of diphtheria. *Lancet* **2:**923–926.

132. **Pellett, S., and R. A. Welch.** 1996. Escherichia coli hemolysin mutants with altered target cell specificity. *Infect. Immun.* **64:**3081–3087.

133. **Popoff, M. R., and J.-C. Marvaud.** 1999. Structural and genomic features of clostridial neurotoxins, p. 174–201. *In* J. E. Alouf and J. H. Freer (ed.), *The Comprehensive Sourcebook of Bacterial Protein Toxins*, 2nd ed. Academic Press, London, United Kingdom.

134. **Qa'Dan, M., M. Ramsey, J. Daniel, L. M. Spyres, B. Safiejko-Mroczka, W. Ortiz-Leduc, and J. D. Ballard.** 2002. Clostridium difficile toxin B activates dual caspase-dependent and caspase-independent apoptosis in intoxicated cells. *Cell Microbiol.* **4:**425–434.

135. **Rosoff, P. M., R. Walker, and L. Winberry.** 1987. Pertussis toxin triggers rapid second messenger production in human T lymphocytes. *J. Immunol.* **139:**2419–2423.

136. **Samra, Z., S. Talmor, and J. Bahar.** 2002. High prevalence of toxin A-negative toxin B-positive Clostridium difficile in hospitalized patients with gastrointestinal disease. *Diagn. Microbiol. Infect. Dis.* **43:**189–192.

137. **Savarino, S. J., A. Fasano, J. Watson, B. M. Martin, M. M. Levine, S. Guandalini, and P. Guerry.** 1993. Enteroaggregative Escherichia coli heat-stable enterotoxin 1 represents another subfamily of E. coli heat-stable toxin. *Proc. Natl. Acad. Sci. USA* **90:**3093–3097.

138. **Schiavo, G., M. Matteoli, and C. Montecucco.** 2000. Neurotoxins affecting neuroexocytosis. *Physiol. Rev.* **80:**717–766.

139. **Sears, C. L., and J. B. Kaper.** 1996. Enteric bacterial toxins: mechanisms of action and linkage to intestinal secretion. *Microbiol. Rev.* **60:** 167–215.

140. **So, M., R. Atchison, S. Falkow, S. Moseley, and B. J. McCarthy.** 1981. A study of the dissemination of Tn1681: a bacterial transposon encoding a heat-stable toxin among enterotoxigenic Escherichia coli isolates. *Cold Spring Harbor Symp. Quant. Biol.* **45**(Pt. 1):53–58.

141. **So, M., F. Heffron, and B. J. McCarthy.** 1979. The E. coli gene encoding heat stable toxin is a bacterial transposon flanked by inverted repeats of IS1. *Nature* **277:**453–456.

142. **So, M., and B. J. McCarthy.** 1980. Nucleotide sequence of the bacterial transposon Tn1681 encoding a heat-stable (ST) toxin and its identification in enterotoxigenic Escherichia coli strains. *Proc. Natl. Acad. Sci. USA* **77:**4011–4015.

143. **Stathopoulos, C., D. L. Provence, and R. Curtiss III.** 1999. Characterization of the avian pathogenic Escherichia coli hemagglutinin Tsh, a member of the immunoglobulin A protease-type family of autotransporters. *Infect. Immun.* **67:** 772–781.

144. **Sun, Y., K. D. Clinkenbeard, C. Clarke, L. Cudd, S. K. Highlander, and S. M. Dabo.** 1999. Pasteurella haemolytica leukotoxin induced apoptosis of bovine lymphocytes involves DNA fragmentation. *Vet. Microbiol.* **65:** 153–166.

145. **Sun, Y., K. D. Clinkenbeard, L. A. Cudd, C. R. Clarke, and P. A. Clinkenbeard.** 1999. Correlation of Pasteurella haemolytica leukotoxin binding with susceptibility to intoxication of lymphoid cells from various species. *Infect. Immun.* **67:**6264–6269.

146. **Szabo, G., M. C. Gray, and E. L. Hewlett.** 1994. Adenylate cyclase toxin from Bordetella pertussis produces ion conductance across artificial lipid bilayers in a calcium- and polarity-dependent manner. *J. Biol. Chem.* **269:**22496–22499.

147. **Takao, T., T. Hitouji, S. Aimoto, Y. Shimonishi, S. Hara, T. Takeda, Y. Takeda, and T. Miwatani.** 1983. Amino acid sequence of a heat-stable enterotoxin isolated from enterotoxigenic Escherichia coli strain 18D. *FEBS Lett.* **152:**1–5.

148. **Takao, T., N. Tominaga, S. Yoshimura, Y. Shimonishi, S. Hara, T. Inoue, and A. Miyama.** 1985. Isolation, primary structure and synthesis of heat-stable enterotoxin produced by Yersinia enterocolitica. *Eur. J. Biochem.* **152:** 199–206.

149. **Teel, L. D., A. R. Melton-Celsa, C. K. Schmitt, and A. D. O'Brien.** 2002. One of two copies of the gene for the activatable shiga toxin type 2d in Escherichia coli O91:H21 strain B2F1

is associated with an inducible bacteriophage. *Infect. Immun.* **70:**4282–4291.

150. **Tesh, V.** 1998. Cytokine response to Shiga toxins, p. 226–235. *In* J. B. Kaper and A. D. O'Brien (ed.), Escherichia coli *O157:H7 and Other Shiga Toxin-Producing* E. coli *Strains.* American Society for Microbiology Press, Washington, D.C.

151. **Tesh, V. L., J. A. Burris, J. W. Owens, V. M. Gordon, E. A. Wadolkowski, A. D. O'Brien, and J. E. Samuel.** 1993. Comparison of the relative toxicities of Shiga-like toxins type I and type II for mice. *Infect. Immun.* **61:**3392–3402.

152. **Thelestam, M., and E. Chaves-Olarte.** 2000. Cytotoxic effects of the Clostridium difficile toxins. *Curr. Top. Microbiol. Immunol.* **250:**85–96.

153. **Thom, R. E., and J. E. Casnellie.** 1989. Pertussis toxin activates protein kinase C and a tyrosine protein kinase in the human T cell line Jurkat. *FEBS Lett.* **244:**181–184.

154. **Thorpe, C. M., B. P. Hurley, and D. W. Acheson.** 2003. Shiga toxin interactions with the intestinal epithelium. *Methods Mol. Med.* **73:**263–273.

155. **Tu, A. H., C. Hausler, R. Young, and D. K. Struck.** 1994. Differential expression of the cytotoxic and hemolytic activities of the ApxIIA toxin from Actinobacillus pleuropneumoniae. *Infect. Immun.* **62:**2119–2121.

156. **van den Berg, B. M., H. Beekhuizen, R. J. Willems, F. R. Mooi, and R. van Furth.** 1999. Role of Bordetella pertussis virulence factors in adherence to epithelial cell lines derived from the human respiratory tract. *Infect. Immun.* **67:**1056–1062.

157. **Van Ostaaijen, J., J. Frey, S. Rosendal, and J. I. MacInnes.** 1997. Actinobacillus suis strains isolated from healthy and diseased swine are clonal and carry apxICABDvar. suis and apxIICAvar. suis toxin genes. *J. Clin. Microbiol.* **35:**1131–1137.

158. **Villaseca, J. M., F. Navarro-Garcia, G. Mendoza-Hernandez, J. P. Nataro, A. Cravioto, and C. Eslava.** 2000. Pet toxin from enteroaggregative Escherichia coli produces cellular damage associated with fodrin disruption. *Infect. Immun.* **68:**5920–5927.

159. **Wagner, P. L., D. W. Acheson, and M. K. Waldor.** 1999. Isogenic lysogens of diverse shiga toxin 2-encoding bacteriophages produce markedly different amounts of shiga toxin. *Infect. Immun.* **67:**6710–6714.

160. **Wagner, P. L., J. Livny, M. N. Neely, D. W. Acheson, D. I. Friedman, and M. K. Waldor.** 2002. Bacteriophage control of Shiga toxin 1 production and release by Escherichia coli. *Mol. Microbiol.* **44:**957–970.

161. **Wagner, P. L., and M. K. Waldor.** 2002. Bacteriophage control of bacterial virulence. *Infect. Immun.* **70:**3985–3993.

162. **Waldor, M. K.** 1998. Bacteriophage biology and bacterial virulence. *Trends Microbiol.* **6:**295–297.

163. **Waldor, M. K., and J. J. Mekalanos.** 1996. Lysogenic conversion by a filamentous phage encoding cholera toxin. *Science* **272:**1910–1914.

164. **Wang, J. F., I. R. Kieba, J. Korostoff, T. L. Guo, N. Yamaguchi, H. Rozmiarek, P. C. Billings, B. J. Shenker, and E. T. Lally.** 1998. Molecular and biochemical mechanisms of Pasteurella haemolytica leukotoxin-induced cell death. *Microb. Pathog.* **25:**317–331.

165. **Wang, Z., C. Clarke, and K. Clinkenbeard.** 1998. Pasteurella haemolytica leukotoxin-induced increase in phospholipase A2 activity in bovine neutrophils. *Infect. Immun.* **66:**1885–1890.

166. **Wang, Z., C. R. Clarke, and K. D. Clinkenbeard.** 1999. Role of phospholipase D in Pasteurella haemolytica leukotoxin-induced increase in phospholipase A(2) activity in bovine neutrophils. *Infect. Immun.* **67:**3768–3772.

167. **Welch, R. A.** 2001. RTX toxin structure and function: a story of numerous anomalies and few analogies in toxin biology. *Curr. Top. Microbiol. Immunol.* **257:**85–111.

168. **Welch, R. A., M. E. Bauer, A. D. Kent, J. A. Leeds, M. Moayeri, L. B. Regassa, and D. L. Swenson.** 1995. Battling against host phagocytes: the wherefore of the RTX family of toxins? *Infect Agents Dis.* **4:**254–272.

169. **Wiegand, R. C., J. Kato, M. D. Huang, K. F. Fok, J. F. Kachur, and M. G. Currie.** 1992. Human guanylin: cDNA isolation, structure, and activity. *FEBS Lett.* **311:**150–154.

170. **Woese, C. R., E. Stackebrandt, T. J. Macke, and G. E. Fox.** 1985. A phylogenetic definition of the major eubacterial taxa. *Syst. Appl. Microbiol.* **6:**143–151.

171. **Yoshimura, S., T. Takao, Y. Shimonishi, S. Hara, M. Arita, T. Takeda, H. Imaishi, T. Honda, and T. Miwatani.** 1986. A heat-stable enterotoxin of Vibrio cholerae non-O1: chemical synthesis, and biological and physicochemical properties. *Biopolymers* **25**(Suppl.):S69–S83.

172. **Zaretzky, F. R., M. C. Gray, and E. L. Hewlett.** 2002. Mechanism of association of adenylate cyclase toxin with the surface of Bordetella pertussis: a role for toxin–filamentous haemagglutinin interaction. *Mol. Microbiol.* **45:**1589–1598.

FUNCTION, EVOLUTION, AND CLASSIFICATION OF MACROMOLECULAR TRANSPORT SYSTEMS

Paul J. Planet, David H. Figurski, and Rob DeSalle

11

Nothing in biology makes sense except in the light of evolution.
> T. Dobzhansky (36)

Nothing in evolution makes sense except in the light of systematics.
> G. Nelson (120)

Transport of nucleic acids and proteins into and out of the cell is one of the major ways in which prokaryotes interact with their environments. These processes are so fundamental that many of the systems responsible for transport have origins before the most recent common ancestor of all known life. Transport systems are crucial for interactions, which include the passage of DNA between distant relatives, establishment of contacts and adherence, and mechanisms of defense and attack. All of these functions can be related directly or indirectly to disease, and transport systems are often involved in more than one of these processes.

To understand functional diversity, it is essential to study the evolutionary history of these systems. Phylogenetic techniques can be used as tools to study function and test evolutionary hypotheses about functional change.

One important objective of this endeavor is to understand the emergence and course of disease. Although the study of the evolution of transport systems is still in its infancy, it has already begun to confront some of the major ideas and controversies in modern evolutionary biology, including the role of horizontal gene transfer in microbial diversification and the nature of the universal ancestor of all life.

Inferences of evolutionary history provide a natural and universally applicable way to organize the world and predict the function of new genes and systems. Therefore, we propose a universal classification scheme for macromolecular transport systems based on the phylogeny of genes involved in transport and the sequence of events (associations between genes) that led to the construction of each system.

TYPES OF MACROMOLECULAR TRANSPORT SYSTEMS

Macromolecular transport in gram-negative bacteria occurs across two membranes—the inner and outer lipid bilayers. The additional obstacles presented by having a second membrane may well have led to the great diversity of systems for transport that exists in modern-day bacteria. This chapter will focus on the systems of gram-negative proteobacteria and their relatives in other prokaryotes and eukaryotes.

Paul J. Planet and Rob DeSalle, Molecular Biology Laboratory, American Museum of Natural History, Molecular Laboratories, Central Park West at 79th St., New York, NY 10024. *David H. Figurski,* Department of Microbiology, College of Physicians and Surgeons, Columbia University, 701 West 168th St., New York, NY 10032.

Evolution of Microbial Pathogens, Edited by H. S. Seifert and V. J. DiRita, © 2006 ASM Press, Washington, D.C.

Some systems transport macromolecules across both membranes. Others are considered to be terminal branches of the general secretory pathway or *sec* system, which delivers unfolded proteins to the periplasmic space for their subsequent secretion across the outer membrane. Proteins are targeted to the *sec* machinery for export if they possess a characteristic amino-terminal signal peptide, which is removed during translocation or very soon after. The *sec* system is one of the major systems for transport in gram-positive bacteria, archaea, and eukaryotes, in addition to transporting molecules across the inner membrane in gram-negative bacteria (141). In this chapter, we concentrate on the terminal branches of the *sec* system along with the *sec*-independent transporters. For in-depth treatments of the *sec* system itself, we refer the reader to several recent reviews (40, 42, 43, 141, 185).

With the growing number of recognized macromolecular transport systems in bacteria, there has been confusion and inconsistency about how many types of systems are known and which systems belong to which types. In this chapter, we lay out current functional models and discuss evolutionary evidence and hypotheses for eight overarching types, making note of classification disagreements where appropriate. We refer the reader to several excellent reviews for detailed discussion of functional and disease-causing aspects of each secretion system (20, 24, 25, 61, 73, 76, 79, 85, 123, 138, 150, 175, 179, 181).

Type I Secretion: the ATP-Binding Cassette Transporters

Type I secretion systems, which are typified by the α-hemolysin (HlyA) secretion system from uropathogenic *Escherichia coli,* can transport proteases, lipases, and toxins, including the repeat-in-toxin (RTX) proteins of gram-negative bacteria (61, 189). Secretion occurs in one step that does not require the *sec* system. The secretion apparatus is composed of three proteins that bridge the inner and outer membrane, allowing proteins to bypass an intermediate stage in the periplasm. The inner

membrane protein (e.g., HlyB) contains the ATP-binding cassette (ABC), from which the descriptive name of the system is derived, that couples secretion to the energy of ATP hydrolysis. The membrane-spanning portion of this molecule probably recognizes the protein that is about to be transported. Homologs (Box 1) of *hlyB* form a subgroup of the large ABC-ATPase superfamily. A second protein (e.g., HlyD) was originally thought to either create a tunnel for transport through the periplasm or pull the inner and outer membranes close together for direct secretion. This component belongs to the so-called membrane fusion protein (MFP) superfamily, suggestive of the latter model of periplasmic bridging (35). However, recent studies have suggested that a third integral outer membrane protein (e.g., TolC) may actually constitute the bulk of the periplasmic tunnel, leaving the function of the MFP protein in doubt (98, 109, 195). Genes for TolC and their homologs constitute the outer membrane factor (OMF) superfamily of membrane pores (196). The three secretion apparatus polypep-

---

■

BOX 1
Homology and Analogy, Synapomorphy and Homoplasy

The term "homology," which has been the subject of much debate in evolutionary biology, is often misused or used without an explicit definition. In this chapter, we use "homology" to mean "similarity because of common ancestry." Thus, homology is always based on a hypothesis of common ancestry. We use the word "similarity" to refer to the observation that two sequences share certain amino acids with similar chemical properties at equivalent positions. Two sequences with *similarity* may either be homologous or *analogous* (i.e., they may be similar without any underlying common ancestry).

The terms "synapomorphy" and "homoplasy" are derived from Hennigian systematics (75), and are comparable to "homology" and "analogy," respectively. A *synapomorphy* is a characteristic that is shared between organisms that arose in one specific event in the past. *Homoplasy* occurs when shared characteristics arose in different (parallel or convergent) events.

tides are also sometimes referred to as inner, outer, and periplasmic efflux proteins (87).

Type I protein secretion appears to be a relatively recent adaptation of a very old and diverse transport system that is involved in the export and import of heavy metals, oligosaccharides, amino acids, and antibiotics, among many other substrates (162). Phylogenetic analysis (Box 2) of this diversity is possible by focusing on the evolutionarily conserved genes for ABC-ATPases, which are found in systems throughout all three of the major domains of life—the *Archaea, Bacteria,* and *Eucarya* (78, 162).

On a large scale, phylogenies of the genes for ABC-ATPases have shown interesting correlations of phylogenetic topology with function (162). Export and import systems tend to segregate into two major clades (Box 2). The exporter clade includes genes from both eukaryotes and bacteria, while the importer clade is entirely bacterial. This topology led to the hypothesis that a primary divergence in function occurred a long time before the divergence of eukaryotes and bacteria. Thus, the most recent common ancestor of extant life must have had a number of different ABC transporters both importing and exporting very different substrates. Subsequently, all importers were lost in the eukaryotes. An alternative hypothesis is that the great diversity of transporters was generated more recently in bacteria, and some of the export systems were horizontally transferred into various eukaryotes. It is important to consider the possibility that the tree may not have its root between the exporters and importers (Box 3). Changing the root would alter ideas about an early divergence and may suggest that one of the functions, either import or export, preceded the other. Phylogenies that include archaeal genes and a broad sampling of other taxa will be required to explicitly test a root to distinguish between these hypotheses.

According to the ABC-ATPase phylogeny, protein secretion in gram-negative bacteria arose from one of the branches of the exporter lineage that also gave rise to many eukaryotic

---

BOX 2
Phylogenetic Inference: Trees, Clades, and Support

A *phylogenetic tree* is the graphical representation of the evolutionary relationships between entities called *taxa,* which can be genes, collections of genes, organisms, populations, or species. *Branches* in a phylogenetic tree describe the relationships between *nodes,* which represent both the taxa used in the analysis (the tips of the tree) and hypothetical ancestors of these taxa (the branching points in the tree). Thus, a tree can be thought of as a depiction of the evolutionary processes of lineage splitting and divergence between organisms or genes.

Any phylogenetic tree can be divided into nonarbitrary units called *clades* that are defined as a group of taxa that contains all the descendants of a particular ancestor. Clades are useful, natural units for evolutionary biology and classification because they are composed of taxa that are more closely related to each other than they are to any other taxa in the tree. Two clades or taxa that are more closely related to each other than any other taxa in the tree are said to be *sister* taxa.

Several different methods of tree building are used in phylogenetic analysis, and there is considerable debate about the relative merits and drawbacks of the different methods (47, 52, 97, 108). Many studies presented in this chapter use tree-building techniques such as neighbor joining, which base the branching pattern of tree topology on measurements of aggregate sequence similarities. Such methods can be misleading when the rates of sequence evolution differ. Other techniques, such as parsimony-based, maximum likelihood, and Bayesian analysis, are generally regarded as better at inferring evolutionary history than similarity-based techniques, and rigorous phylogenetic analysis may often include analysis using more than one of these techniques. A good inference of evolutionary history is critical to understanding functional change because even small topological changes can lead to very different interpretations of the order in which functions arose.

Another important aspect of phylogentic analysis is the calculation of confidence in tree topology. The most popular measure of confidence is the bootstrap value, which tests how often a random subset of the data gives the same phylogenetic structure seen in the overall analysis (51). Bremer decay indices (16) and jackknifing (49) are also widely used measures of support. Some inference techniques, such as Bayesian analysis, produce measures of support as they are building the tree (81).

■
BOX 3
Rooting

Without a root, the representation of the most ancient part of the tree, a phylogenetic tree loses much of its information because the direction of change of characters or functions on the tree is not known. Unrooted trees do not even allow definitive statements of how closely related two taxa are. Even if lineages branch from the same node in the tree, the root may be in one of the branches, such that the two lineages are not closest relatives.

For gene superfamilies, rooting the tree or defining the most ancient branching point is very problematic. This is especially true in superfamilies that have a history that can be traced back to or before the most recent common ancestor of all life. At this point, the traditional way of rooting phylogenies using an outgroup breaks down, because there is no outgroup when considering all known life. Reciprocal paralog rooting has been used to establish the root of known life by using two related gene families to root each other (63, 83). In this technique, two related genes (A and B) that exist in every organism and are assumed to have diverged in a very ancient duplication event before the most recent common ancestor are included in the same analysis. The branch in the phylogeny that separates all the As from all the Bs is then considered to be the root because it represents the initial duplication event that created the two families. This technique does not work when three or more paralogous groups exist in the same phylogeny. In these cases, or until some other technique becomes available, external criteria can be used to propose plausible roots.

three components have evolved together over long periods of time with little shuffling of components (Box 4). More sophisticated methods of alignment may help in this endeavor

■
BOX 4
Horizontal Gene Transfer and Phylogenetic Incongruence

Horizontal gene transfer has recently been an issue of much debate in evolutionary biology primarily because it severely rearranges our classification systems, methods for reconstructing evolutionary change, and the way that we conceive of organisms in general (38, 135, 194). However, the importance of gene transfer between distant relatives in the evolution of organisms and the extent to which it disrupts traditional evolutionary views has only begun to be examined in a systematic way.

One of the best ways to study horizontal transfer is through the study of incongruence between evolutionary histories. To understand horizontal transfer of secretion systems, one could compare the genes of the secretion system to a representative organismal phylogeny. To understand shuffling of genes between secretion systems, one could compare the phylogenies of genes within the same system.

Phylogenetic approaches to gene transfer usually take the form of comparisons of tree topology. Differences in tree topology should indicate different histories. However, different histories can also be caused by historical events other than horizontal transfer, such as gene duplication, lineage sorting or loss, and convergence. Therefore, efforts should be made to test the hypothesis of horizontal transfer against other hypotheses. Evidence might come from variations in sequence composition, such as G+C content or codon bias, that signal a foreign origin (105). Other evidence might include genes and sequences in the region that suggest that that the locus might be mobile (68). One technique, called tree reconciliation, treats genes as parasites in their host genomes and tries to find the scenario that best accounts for topological incongruencies between trees (23, 131). This type of analysis is important because hypotheses of horizontal transfer can often be as parsimoniously explained by gene duplication and subsequent loss.

Topological differences between trees can also be due to problems with sampling or just nonsignificant variation in the data. Several tests are available that can be used to test the overall significance of differences in topology (17, 31, 50, 80). Incongruence can also be assessed at specific nodes (184).

exporters, such as the TAP-like genes of major histocompatibility complex I (162). Again, this relationship either signals a very ancient origin for the protein secretion systems, before eukaryotes split from the bacteria, or more recent horizontal transfer. Phylogenies of genes for the MFP (periplasmic efflux protein) (35) and outer membrane factor (outer efflux protein) (196) families have also been done, but lower sequence conservation makes these less reliable and less broadly applicable for understanding the origin of these macromolecular transporters. It remains to be seen whether the phylogenies of these genes are phylogenetically (statistically) congruent with the ABC-ATPase phylogeny, which would signal that the

(87). Initial topological appraisals have suggested that there has been little horizontal transfer of the OMF components (196), but this hypothesis awaits further and more rigorous tests of congruence with robust organismal phylogenies.

Type II Secretion: the Main Terminal Branch

Like many other transport systems, type II systems are involved in the disease process in organisms ranging from plants to humans (160). These systems rely on the *sec* system to transport proteins to the periplasm, at which point the type II secretion system acts to secrete fully folded proteins across the outer membrane. Thus, classical type II secretion is often called the main terminal branch of the general secretory pathway or *sec* system, and standard nomenclature for the genes involved uses the designation *gsp*. The gene letter (A through O or S) indicates homology to the genes of the *pul* system of *Klebsiella oxytoca*.

The type II apparatus is composed of approximately 12 to 15 proteins that extend across both membranes and the periplasmic space at least transiently. An inner membrane-associated ATP binding protein (e.g., PulE or GspE) may be important for supplying energy for secretion by hydrolyzing ATP, in addition to the energy supplied by proton motive force (107, 161). An alternative model suggests that ATP binding and autophosphorylation by the GspE protein regulates secretion (161). GspE proteins are encoded by genes that belong to a large superfamily of genes for putative nucleoside triphosphatases (NTPases) that includes those from type II and IV secretion systems, often referred to as the *virB11/pulE* superfamily (136, 147). Another protein called GspD (e.g., PulD) is encoded by a gene that belongs to the widespread secretin superfamily, which is also found in type III secretion. GspD forms a ring-shaped complex in the outer membrane (9). Several other proteins (GspGHIJK) are called "pseudopilins" because they are similar in sequence and predicted structure to pilin subunits. These proteins may form a piston-like structure for pumping substrates out of the cell or may supply a channel or guide for secretion (159).

CLOSE RELATIVES OF TYPE II SECRETION

The type II secretion apparatus is very closely related to systems that perform functions as seemingly diverse as type IV pilus assembly, phage extrusion, and competence for DNA uptake (76, 133). Due to the high level of similarity and the fact that pilin subunits can be thought of as secreted protein substrates, one might argue that type IV pilus systems are indeed type II secretion systems. This idea is reinforced by recent studies that show that overexpression of a type II pseudopilin from *K. oxytoca* can produce a pilus-like structure (163), and that known pilus biogenesis systems are required for secretion of soluble proteins (94, 187).

Type IV pili are involved in attachment, active movement, and natural competence for uptake of DNA (117). They are found in a wide variety of bacteria, such as the pathogens *Neisseria gonorrhoeae* and *Pseudomonas aeruginosa* (117). More distantly related type IVb pili systems, such as the toxin-coregulated pilus of *Vibrio cholerae* and the bundle-forming pilus of entropathogenic *E. coli*, appear to be important for colonization of the host (8, 96).

Type IV pilin subunits (e.g., PilA) are processed by a prepilin peptidase (e.g., PilD [124]) that is similar to GspO (e.g., PulO), an enzyme that processes pseudopilins of the type II protein secretion apparatus (142). Genes of the *virB11/pulE* superfamily, which encode PilT, PilU, PilF, and PilB, are thought to energize the processes of pilus assembly (PilB, PilF) and pilus retraction (PilT PilU) that together form the basis for pilin-mediated movement called "twitching motility" (117, 169). A similar movement of a much shorter "pilus" has been invoked in the piston model for type II secretion (159). The outer membrane secretin, PilQ, which is similar to GspD, is thought to mediate passage of substrate through the outer membrane (115).

Many type IV pilus assembly genes are also involved in natural competence in gram-negative organisms (41). Closely related systems in gram-positive organisms also mediate DNA uptake, and they also contain the core components of type II secretion, including genes for NTPases encoded by *virB11/pulE* superfamily members (e.g., ComGA), pilin-like subunits (ComCDEG), a potential prepilin (ComC), and a GspF-like component (ComGB) (185). Gram-positive uptake systems, understandably, lack an outer membrane secretin superfamily homolog.

One example that illustrates the close functional connection between type II protein secretion relatives is the apparent evolutionary convergence of the *epsD* gene. It encodes an outer membrane secretin for secretion of chitinase, protease, and cholera toxin in *V. cholerae*, and also serves as a channel for extrusion of the filamentous phage CTXφ (34). CTXφ carries the cholera toxin gene, showing that the same protein is involved in horizontal transfer of a gene and the secretion of the protein it encodes. Many filamentous phages carry their own secretin homologs, such as the well-studied gene pIV. Others do not, and these phages may use host genomic secretins for extrusion through the outer membrane (34).

The evolution of classical type II secretion systems in relation to the closely related pathways of type IV pilus assembly and DNA uptake systems has not been studied in great detail. Existing phylogenies for the *virB11/pulE* NTPase superfamily (21, 133, 136) show a close relationship between *pilB* and *gspE* that excludes all examples of *pilT, pilU,* and genes for other putative NTPases involved in type IVb pilus assembly. This tree topology suggests that systems that secrete soluble proteins might have evolved from an ancient type IV pilus system that may already have had the ability to move bacteria by twitching motility.

OTHER TYPE II-RELATED SYSTEMS

Recently, a system dedicated to type IV-like pilus assembly was discovered in *Actinobacillus actinomycetemcomitans* (67, 82, 91, 92, 137), a periodontal pathogen, and *Caulobacter crescentus* (170), a nonpathogenic marine bacterium. In *A. actinomycetemcomitans* this system is required for nonspecific adherence, tight biofilm formation, and colonization of hosts (92, 137, 164). Genes in the region in *A. actinomycetemcomitans* are named *tad,* for the tight adherence phenotype, and those in *C. crescentus* are referred to as *cpa,* for caulobacter pilus assembly. The function of the pilus in *C. crescentus* is unknown, but it has been suggested that it is involved in initial colonization of surfaces in the environment (172). Strikingly similar regions are found in a broad array of archaea and bacteria (92), and some have been shown to be required in disease caused by other organisms (59, 122, 164, 174).

Many of the genes of this system are similar to the core component genes of type IV pilus assembly and type II secretion. The pilin subunits (e.g., Flp1 or PilA) are similar in structure and sequence to other type IV pilins, but they are shorter, have distinguishing sequence motifs, and form a monophyletic subfamily in phylogenetic analyses (93, 170). Tight adherence also requires a gene that is a truncated homolog of gspO (e.g., *tadV* or *cpaA*) (170). The *tad* genes are required for secretion and localization of the major pilus subunit (137). In addition, the system requires genes for an outer membrane protein belonging to the secretin superfamily (e.g., RcpA or CpaC) and an ATPase from the *virB11/pulE* superfamily (e.g., TadA or CpaF) (6). Curiously, *tadA, cpaF,* and their close homologs are much more closely related in phylogenetic analyses to genes for the NTPases of type IV secretion than to those of any of the type II secretion systems or previously known type IV pilus assembly systems (21, 136). This suggests that *tad* gene loci may originate from the fusion of a type IV secretion NTPase and a type II secretion system. Furthermore, at least six other genes that are unlike genes found in any other secretion system are required for pilus assembly, and it remains unclear whether these were part of the system before or after the hypothesized fusion event. The classification of this system is unresolved.

From an evolutionary standpoint, the *tad* locus provides clear evidence that very different systems can and did shuffle components and that horizontal transfer has probably been instrumental in the formation of new systems (Box 4). Horizontal transfer, duplication, and loss of the entire *tad* locus also appear to be surprisingly frequent in evolutionary history (137). This apparent mobility created situations in which multiple copies of this locus were in the same cell at the same time, allowing for recombination and shuffling of components (137). Gene shuffling has also been noted in type III secretion systems (18) and the chaperone/usher pathway (12, 18). Because of their apparent propensity to be mobilized as a cluster of genes, the *tad* gene regions can be considered as transferable "genomic islands" and were designated the widespread colonization island (WCI) (137).

Another tantalizing connection in the everincreasing type II web is the relationship of the archaeal flagellum to type IV pili (182). The archaeal flagellum has no established homology to the bacterial flagellum (182). Instead, flagellar subunits are structurally similar to type IV pilins (27, 45); the genes encoding FlaI, a putative NTPase, are members of the *virB11*/*pulE* superfamily; and FlaJ is similar to GspF and TadB (133). According to phylogenetic analysis, *flaI* is more closely related to *tadA* than to *pilT*, suggesting that the closest bacterial relative of the archaeal flagellar apparatus is the WCI-borne secretion system (133, 136).

Type III Secretion: Contact-Dependent Systems

Type III secretion occurs across both membranes in a process that is independent of the *sec* system. Many type III systems translocate proteins across the membrane of a eukaryotic cell upon contact, injecting an effector protein that subverts the host machinery for the benefit of the bacterium. Many effectors, with functions ranging from inducing apoptosis to inhibiting phagocytosis, have been described (79). Although such systems are mainly associated with disease and disease-causing organisms of both animals and plants, recent examples from symbiotic organisms suggest that type III

systems may be more broadly involved in a variety of bacterium-eukaryote interactions and may play an important role in the transition from pathogen to symbiont (32, 33, 57).

Striking similarity between type III secretion systems and the components of the bacterial flagellar apparatus leads to the natural inclusion of the flagellar apparatus as a kind of type III machine (112). While this classification is not universally accepted (121), functional evidence indicates that the flagellar apparatus can function as a secretion system (197).

Type III systems are composed of approximately 20 or more protein components. The gene designation *sct,* for secretion and cellular translocation, has been proposed as a unified nomenclature for these systems (79). Type III component proteins span both membranes in a complex architecture, with the majority of proteins located at the inner membrane. A membrane-associated cytoplasmic ATPase (YscN/SctN) is thought to energize the process of secretion and flagellum assembly (1). Genes for these ATPases have no established homology to genes for ATPases in other bacterial macromolecular transport systems, but are probably homologous to the genes for F_0F_1 proton-translocating ATPases. An outer membrane protein (YscC/SctC) is encoded by genes belonging to the *secretin* superfamily that is also found in type II-related systems. However, secretin proteins appear not to be involved in flagellar systems.

Nonflagellar type III systems, which are visible using electron microscopy, form a structure called an "injectisome," which is composed of a cytoplasmic base, a transmembrane/periplasmic channel, and an extracellular needlelike projection (10, 101). The flagellar apparatus has a similar structure consisting of a basal transmembrane/periplasmic portion with the hook and flagellum filament extending away from the cell surface (26).

Many type III secretion systems are encoded by genetic loci that appear to have been inherited by acquisition from distant relatives because of their anomalous G+C content compared to the rest of the genome (66, 68).

Two well-known examples are the *Salmonella enterica* pathogenicity islands SPI-1 and SPI-2. Many other type III secretion systems are located in potentially transferred or transferable loci (68, 79). Comparison of the phylogenies of the type III system genes with genes representing organismal evolution indicated an extraordinary amount of horizontal transfer of these gene clusters between species and subspecies (15, 56, 64, 69, 121, 126). Although topologies of individual gene genealogies in some studies indicated little or no shuffling of genes between different type III systems (121), other analyses revealed statistically significant phylogenetic incongruence within type III system gene clusters that is best explained by shuffling (18) (Box 4).

Interestingly, it has been postulated that flagellar assembly genes have been inherited mostly vertically because their phylogenetic branching patterns roughly track the most likely phylogeny of organisms (64, 121). Additionally, in unrooted phylogenies, flagellar assembly genes are almost always separated from nonflagellar genes by a single branch, which led to the conclusion that there was a very early divergence of flagellar and nonflagellar systems (64, 121). These analyses challenge the widely held position that type III secretion of proteins is a more recent adaptation of the ancient flagellum assembly machinery (112, 121) and have led to renewed debate in the literature despite the congruence between phylogenetic topologies from all studies (64, 121). If it is true that flagellar genes are inherited mostly vertically and the branching pattern in the flagellar clade is the same (with the same root) as the organismal phylogeny, then this pushes the hypothetical root for all injectisome genes at least to the base of the flagellar clade. Since this root would occupy the branch separating the flagellar systems from injectisome systems, this would mean that the two systems are equally old, which would support the idea that the injectisome is an ancient structure that evolved alongside flagella for competition with other bacteria, early eukaryotes, or even archaea (1). The long branch length separating injectisome genes from flagellar genes has also been used to support a more

ancient divergence (64), but this has been criticized by pointing out that differences in rates of evolution, represented by differing branch lengths, are common and not necessarily indicative of ancient origins (152).

The two hypotheses (ancient versus more recent origin) have been argued for and against, without clear resolution (64, 152), using assumptions about the probable direction of change of certain key functions. Evolutionary hypotheses of functional change can be tested using simple topological phylogenetic analysis. For type III secretion of proteins to be an adaptation of a vertically inherited gram-negative proteobacterial flagellar apparatus, the branch separating flagellar genes from injectisome genes must be closely allied with proteobacterial flagellar genes in the tree and not with bacteria that represent early bacterial divergences, such as *Aeropyrum pernix, Thermotoga maritima,* gram-positive bacteria, or the chlamydiae. Although existing phylogenetic analyses do not give an unambiguous answer in this regard, it appears that there is a tendency for proteobacterial injectisome genes to be separated from flagellar genes by several nonproteobacterial branches (64, 95, 121), which could signal that injectisomes and flagella are equally old. Alternative hypotheses that suggest that either injectisomes or flagella came first require ad hoc hypotheses of horizontal transfer, duplication, and/or loss. For instance, it has been suggested that the close phylogenetic alliance between chlamydial and proteobacterial systems may signal an origin for injectisomes in *Chlamydia* with a subsequent transfer to the proteobacteria (95). Additional phylogenetic analysis that includes broad taxonomic sampling, statistical assessment of gene tree topology, and serious consideration of the root of the tree of life may be able to resolutely provide a well-supported answer in this debate (Boxes 2, 3, and 4).

Type IV Secretion: Conjugation-Related Systems

Type IV transport systems are involved in both the secretion of proteins and conjugative transport of plasmid DNA between bacterial cells

(24). Recent studies indicate that some type IV systems are involved in DNA uptake or natural transformation by a process that resembles "inverse conjugation" (77, 171). In addition, there is a diverse collection of type IV systems that appear to function quite differently and are only beginning to be understood (104).

Type IV systems secrete several protein virulence factors that include the pertussis toxin of *Bordetella pertussis,* the cause of whooping cough, and the CagA effector protein of *Helicobacter pylori,* which causes peptic ulcer disease. Other important pathogens, such as *Legionella pneumophila* and *Brucella* spp., also carry likely protein transporters (24). However, type IV systems also appear to be present in several nonpathogens, such as *Wolbachia* spp., which are drosophilid symbionts (116).

Protein secretion of pertussis toxin appears to be a two-step process in which the toxin is first secreted to the periplasmic space by the *sec* system, where it is assembled and is then secreted (46). In contrast to this pathway, DNA conjugation and transport of other proteins appears to be independent of the *sec* system, yet also seems to occur in two distinct steps with an intermediate stage in the periplasm (132).

Much of the work on type IV secretion has been done in the *vir* system of *Agrobacterium tumefaciens,* a pathogen that causes crown gall tumors in dicotyledonous plants. The *vir* gene nomenclature is often used as a reference point. This system transports transfer DNA and several proteins into plant cells (24).

DNA transport is believed to proceed by covalent attachment to the 5′ end of the DNA of a protein called the relaxase (VirD2) to form a nucleoprotein complex. The protein portion of this complex is then probably recognized by a "coupling" protein (TraG or VirD4) that directs it to the secretion pore or apparatus, dragging the DNA passively behind. This has led to the conclusion that type IV systems are fundamentally—perhaps ancestrally—protein secretion systems in which the transported proteins have gained the ability to bind DNA (24). However, some models suggest that the coupling protein may also serve to actively transport the DNA itself after the protein has been transferred (110).

Type IV systems are involved in the production of a pilus called the T pilus in *A. tumefaciens* or the sex pilus of conjugative plasmids (102). This structure differs fundamentally from type IV pili assembled by type II–related systems. The T pilus is composed of pilin subunits (e.g., VirB2) that have N-terminal signal sequences and are cyclized in a head-to-tail (N-to-C) peptide bond in the periplasm (44). Although pilus assembly and DNA transport are tightly coupled genetically, requiring many of the same genes, it now appears that the two processes can be genetically decoupled (151). This finding suggests that the pilus probably does not act as a conduit for transfer of the nucleoprotein complex, and may be more important for initiating or stabilizing contact with the recipient. However, the extraordinarily close functional relationship between pilus assembly and substrate transfer deserves further examination.

Most type IV systems have three different putative ATPases. Genes for VirB11 and its close relatives are members of the *virB11/pulE* superfamily. Recent evidence has suggested that *virB11* is required for both pilus assembly and secretion (151). Several different functions have been proposed for VirB11, including a chaperone for transported substrates, an ATPase that couples the energy of hydrolysis to assembly and/or secretion, or an ATP-binding protein that induces a conformational change in the assembly apparatus. The second kind of putative ATPase, encoded by *virD4* and its homologs, is a member of the *traG* coupling superfamily that is named after the gene on the Ti plasmid of *A. tumefaciens.* The third ATPase is encoded by *virB4,* whose protein product may act as a structural transducer of information or as an energizer of secretion. Interestingly, while *virB11* and *virB4* are required for pilus assembly, *virD4* is not (102).

A core of genes including those for VirB7–10 appear to form the structural core of the secretion apparatus and may act together to bridge the periplasm and outer membrane (100, 188). Interestingly, TraK, a VirB9 homolog, has recently been shown to have low but significant sequence similarity members of the secretin superfamily (103, 104).

The evolutionary connection between conjugation and protein secretion is a currently unresolved issue. Both functions have been proposed to be the ancestral function at different times. Conjugation can be seen as the coupling of DNA replication to a preexisting protein secretion system (24, 110). Conversely, protein secretion can be thought of as a conjugation system that has lost its ability to bind DNA or has adapted to a new protein substrate (25, 192). Current reconstructions favor a "conjugation first" hypothesis (Fig. 2), but it remains possible that both transitions may have happened at different points in the evolutionary history of this large and ancient secretion type. More functional information combined with phylogenetic evidence is required to test the directionality of these hypotheses.

The issue has been made more complex by the finding that some type IV systems function in DNA uptake (77, 171). Genes for NTPases of type IV uptake systems are located near the base of the virB11/pulE family tree close to the main divergence between genes for NTPases from type II and type IV systems. Considering the role of type II-related systems in natural transformation, this new functional information allows for the formal possibility that the primordial function of type II and IV systems was DNA uptake. Although this idea is not currently supported by reconstruction on phylogenetic trees (Fig. 2), it is consistent with the hypothesis that the most recent common ancestor of extant life might be best described as a group of living things that primarily inherited traits from one another by horizontal transfer and not by descent (193). Natural transformation and conjugation may have been the most important functions in such an ancestor. An additional role for a primordial system may have been uptake of nucleic acids as a carbon source (53, 144). Teasing the order of these different processes apart will require combined efforts in functional and phylogenetic studies.

Topological phylogenetic comparison of each of the virB genes has suggested that there has been relatively little shuffling or even loss of constituents in type IV secretion and DNA transport (21). However, the fact that many of these systems exist today in the same cell and are plasmid-borne suggests that the potential for recombination is high and that the hypothesis of mostly vertical inheritance should be very rigorously tested.

Type V Secretion: the Autotransporters

The classical (or "linked") autotransporter family is composed of a single protein that encodes both the substrate (passenger domain) and the outer membrane pore (β domain) through which the passenger is exported. The system is typified by the IgA1 protease that helps to evade the immune response by cleaving immunoglobulin A antibodies in *N. gonorrheae* and other pathogens (139, 175). Transported substrates also include toxins, adhesins, invasins, and proteases (72, 74).

The single protein arrives in the periplasmic space generally via the *sec* system, though this may not be the universal route, and the β domain then inserts into the outer membrane, forming a channel (167). The passenger domain is then guided through the channel and either remains attached to the outside of the cell, in the case of adhesins (176), or is released into the environment by proteolysis (74, 140).

This system has been referred to as type IV secretion, a confusing classification that now seems to have been abandoned in favor of the descriptive term "autotransporter" or the more neutral designation "type V secretion" (73).

Adding to the confusion in taxonomy, potentially related systems composed of separately translated passenger and β domains have been alternately classified as a subset of type V secretion designated "unlinked" (72) or as their own independent system called the "two-partner" system or the "single-accessory" pathway (65, 85). Two-partner transport is typified by the secretion of filamentous hemagglutinin of *Bordetella* spp. and the high-molecular-weight proteins of *Haemophilus influenzae*. In this system, two proteins with the unified

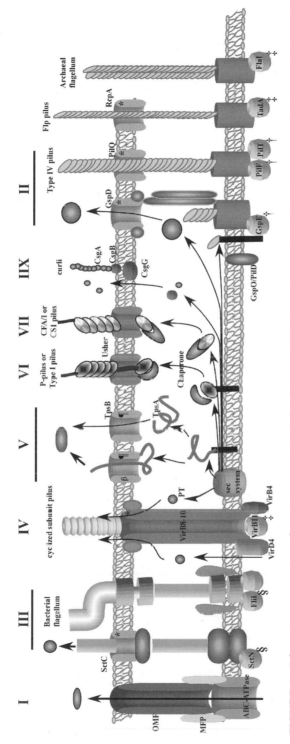

FIGURE 1 Schematic representations of secretion systems. Symbols indicate established homologous relationships between genes for the proteins pictured. Putative NTPases from the *pulE/virB11* superfamily are given single and double daggers. Single daggers indicate putative NTPases from the type II secretion family, and type IV secretion family NTPases are indicated by double daggers. Flagellar apparatuses and type IV pilus systems are grouped with their close relatives. See text for details.

nomenclature TpsA and TpsB are equivalent to the passenger and β domains of linked type V systems, respectively (85). The TpsA protein is probably transported to the periplasm via the *sec* system, where its signal peptide is removed. The TpsB protein recognizes a characteristic amino-proximal secretion sequence in TpsA and transports its partner across the membrane. This interaction seems to be highly specific such that each TpsA functions with exactly one TpsB and vice versa (85).

Some phylogenetic analyses have used separated data sets of the genes of linked and unlinked type V systems to construct trees (85, 196). Indeed, if sequence and structural similarities between the two systems simply represent convergent functions (84), the sequences should not be included in the same phylogenetic analysis because they would then not be homologous.

However, if the two systems do have a common ancestor, then they should be included in the same analysis. Phylogenies that include genes from linked and unlinked type V secretion systems may support combining these systems into same type. Although the two groups generally segregate into two major lineages, some important exceptions place unlinked versions as close relatives of linked systems and vice versa (73). This suggests that linking and/or unlinking has occurred more than once in the evolution of this family, and that the distinction between the two is not supported by phylogeny.

One problem with including genes from linked and unlinked systems in the same analysis is that they appear to have diverged to the point that they are difficult to align. Alignment problems can give very misleading results in phylogenetic inference (134, 190). Future phylogenetic analysis should include specific attention to primary statements of homology and tests of how alignment parameters affect reconstructions of evolutionary history. Additionally, known potential homologs, such as outer membrane pores from chloroplasts (146), should be considered for inclusion in any new analysis.

The Chaperone/Usher Pathway

The chaperone/usher pathway is often neglected in tallies of known secretion systems, even though much is known about both its function and evolution. Adhesins and pili secreted and assembled by this pathway are involved in diseases such as gastroenteritis, otitis media, and urinary tract infections (180).

The chaperone/usher pathway, typified by the P pilus and type 1 pilus assembly pathways, requires the *sec* system to transport substrates initially across the inner membrane. Only two active participant proteins are needed. A chaperone (e.g., PapD from the P pilus system) binds the substrate (e.g., PapG, the major pilin subunit), allowing it to dissociate from the inner membrane, and delivers it folded to the usher protein (e.g., PapC) (89). The usher forms a pore in the outer membrane that is rich in β sheets, suggesting a connection (either by analogy or homology) to the secretin superfamily of type II and III secretion; however, no significant sequence similarity has been found between these two superfamilies. The usher binds to the chaperone-substrate complex, and it can even distinguish between different substrates (subunits) bound to the chaperone depending on their position in the pilus (37). The interaction is quite stable, and a subsequent interaction with another chaperone-substrate complex, as it docks, may release the first chaperone, and allow subunit-subunit binding (19, 90). The growing pilus fiber is then threaded through the usher and assumes its coiled conformation as it exits the cell (181). Interestingly, the process does not appear to require ATP (86).

The presence of chaperone/usher systems in bacterial strains is correlated with the ability to cause disease (4, 13, 55, 88, 113). As with other virulence genes, the pattern of chaperone/usher systems is not easily explained by vertical inheritance from parent to daughter, but, instead, may be more parsimoniously explained by transfer of genes from distant relatives. Genes may have been exchanged in linked clusters called "pathogenicity islands," especially if signs suggest past or potential mobility (68). Such patterns reinforce current notions that horizontal transfer, rather than mutation, may be the major engine driving microbial diversity (127), and that diseases can be caused by groups of organisms that are not monophyletic (i.e., not every descendant of the common ancestor causes the disease) when different lineages acquire the same virulence determinants in separate, parallel events (143, 145, 191).

However, other processes such as duplications, losses, and positive and negative selection can also cause patterns that might seem to be caused by horizontal transfer, and although almost all reports suggest that there has been *some* horizontal transfer, there are different estimates of extent and frequency (Box 4) (4, 60, 88, 118).

As in other secretion systems, horizontal transfer may be occurring with different basic units consisting sometimes of single genes and sometimes of entire clusters of genes. Thus, a cluster of transferred genes can also be composed of genes that have radically different histories. Phylogenetic analysis and statistical tests of phylogenetic incongruence suggest that this may be true for at least one chaperone/usher system—the type I pilus *fim* gene cluster in *Salmonella* (12, 18).

Since the products of chaperone/usher secretion are required for disease in many instances, it would be expected that they would be under strong selection in the host. In fact, hypervariability of the chaperone/usher-secreted adhesin proteins from *E. coli* is best explained by these structures experiencing multiple, distinct selective regimes—a phenomenon called "diversifying selection" (14). However, it is difficult to completely rule out horizontal transfer/recombination as the source of the diversity in this system, especially as there is precedent for horizontal transfer in P pilus evolution (113). In general, distinguishing horizontal transfer (or duplication and loss) from homoplasy (Box 1) caused by selection is extremely difficult in bacteria. Bacteria are known to readily and naturally transfer genes to distant relatives, and therefore horizontal transfer can almost never be ruled out because it is "unlikely." Unfortunately, the problem becomes more complicated when studying virulence genes because of the expectation of a bizarre selective regime; virulence genes may be under selection that is strong in the host, different from host to host, and very weak when the pathogen is outside its host in the environment. Some authors have suggested that this pattern actually makes it more likely that sequences will develop ways of increasing the probability that they will be successfully horizontally transferred (106). It will be extremely important to establish the frequency of horizontal transfer among prokaryotes in the environment to begin to solve this problem.

Large-scale phylogenetic analysis of the components of the chaperone/usher pathway has given a preliminary view of the more ancient evolutionary history of these systems. In these studies, the distribution of chaperone/usher genes mostly appears to be restricted to the proteobacteria, especially the γ-proteobacteria, with a few exceptions suggesting that these systems have a more recent origin than some other secretion systems (196). As in other secretion types, phylogenetic groupings of these systems often correspond to functional and structural groupings, and certain discrete "signature sequences" can be used to define functional-phylogenetic subfamilies (11, 62).

The Alternate Chaperone/Usher Pathway

The alternate chaperone pathway (173) is encoded by genes that have no apparent (or established) sequence homology to the other chaperone/usher pathway (157). However, the mode of action is so strikingly similar that it has been suggested that the two chaperone/usher-based pathways are evolutionarily convergent (157). However, it is an equally legitimate conclusion to suggest that the two are functionally homologous and their sequences have diverged to the point that no obvious similarity remains at that level.

This pathway participates in the construction of a variety of pili (e.g., CS1, CS2, CS4, CS14, CS17, CS19, and CFA/I) in diarrhea-causing enterotoxigenic *E. coli* (157). Another related system assembles the cable type II pilus of *Burkholderia cepacia* (154). These pili are critical for colonization of the small intestine and initiation of disease, and are therefore the target of promising vaccine research (149).

The genes of this pathway, typified by the *coo* genes, are arranged in the same gene order as in all known systems, and anomalously low G+C content of the *coo* region suggests that the entire region may have been horizontally transferred as a pathogenicity island (58).

All of the required proteins for pilus assembly appear to be shuttled to the periplasm by the *sec* system. The major (e.g., CooA for CS1 pili) and minor (e.g., CooD) pilin subunits are both bound by the chaperone (e.g., CooB) in the periplasm. The chaperone delivers the subunits to a putative usher protein (e.g., CooC), which may act as a channel and nucleation point for the growing pilus. The minor pilin, which is weakly similar to the major pilin subunit, is associated with the tip of the pilus and has been shown, in at least one system, to be responsible for adhesion (156).

Interestingly, several genes from distinct alternate chaperone/usher pilus systems are able to substitute for (or "cross-complement") each other, which suggests a basic amount of functional conservation over time (58, 114). However, not all cross-complementations are mutual. For instance, though the major pilin subunit of the CFA/I pilus can complement a *cooA*-minus mutant, restoring its ability to make pili, the same is not true in the opposite direction (114). Asymmetrical complementation might just be the result of some trivial gene expression problem, but if a viable protein is expressed and unable to function in a new system, this might signal something interesting about the evolution of proteins in systems. Like organisms, proteins might be generalists or specialists. Some may be able to work in several different, distantly related systems. Perhaps these genes retain traits from a common ancestor. Some others may be so finely tuned to a specific cell environment or system that they may be unable to work in other contexts. Although this could be seen as just a curiosity of an artificial, genetically engineered system, it actually might tell us something about the likelihood of horizontal transfer of genes from one system to another. The prediction is that genes that are generalists are more likely to be horizontally transferred than specialist genes.

The Extracellular Nucleation-Precipitation Pathway

A class of bacterial appendages called curli, which are thin, aggregative, and irregular filaments, are exported by yet another transport system. Curli, which are sometimes called thin aggregative fibrils in *Salmonella* species, are amyloid fibrils (22) that are expressed in most enterohemolytic and enterotoxigenic *E. coli* (5, 128) and *Salmonella* spp. (28, 30, 148). Several other members of the *Enterobacteriaceae,* in the genera *Citrobacter, Klebsiella,* and *Enterobacter,* also express curli (39, 198). Interestingly, although curli genes seem to be widespread in the *E. coli/Salmonélla* clade (4, 29, 39), curli do not seem to be normally expressed in enteropathogenic *E. coli*, enteroinvasive *E. coli* (5, 128), and *Shigella* spp. (155). In fact, in *Shigella* species, the operons encoding curli are often multiply interrupted by insertion elements, suggesting that loss of curli is favored by strong "pathoadaptive" selection in the disease process of *Shigella* and enteroinvasive *E. coli* (155).

Expression of curli is associated with severe disease and sepsis (129), and they are known to bind to a multitude of human and host proteins, including major histocompatibility complex class I molecules (130). Curli have been implicated in autoaggregation of cells and biofilm formation (3, 148, 186).

The curli assembly system is encoded by two operons, *csgBA* and *csgDEFG,* which are transcribed in opposite directions. The major curlin subunit, CsgA (also called Agf in *S. enterica*), and its homologous protein, CsgB, are secreted to the periplasm by the *sec* system (71). CsgG is also secreted by the *sec* system, and is then bound to the outer membrane. CsgG may act as a channel for secretion of CsgA and CsgB or as a chaperone for protection from proteolytic degradation (111). Once outside of the cell, CsgB has been proposed to be the nucleus upon which soluble CsgA subunits precipitate and polymerize into fibrils (7). The presence of CsgB along the curlus may account for branching of curli (7). CsgD is a transcriptional regulator belonging to the LuxR/UhpA superfamily (70). CsgE may function as a chaperone and CsgF as a nucleator (22).

At the amino acid level, *csg/agf* genes appear to be very well conserved, with similarity scores that are mostly above the average usually seen between *Salmonella* spp. and *E. coli* (148). However, the nucleotide sequence varies much more, and in fact the sequences of *csgE* are almost completely saturated with synonymous substitutions (148). This pattern of sequence conservation suggests that curli genes have been under intense positive selection, but were present in a common ancestor of *Salmonella* spp. and *E. coli* and inherited vertically since then (4). This is an excellent example of a higher-than-expected similarity score due to something other than horizontal transfer.

SOLVING THE CHICKEN-AND-EGG DILEMMA: TRACING THE EVOLUTION OF FUNCTION USING PHYLOGENETIC TREES

The functional diversity of secretion systems and their relatives raises questions about how each of these functions evolved. To understand functional evolution, one must understand the direction (polarity) of evolutionary change: In what order did these functions arise? What was the function of the common ancestor?

One logical line of argument posits that functions that are used for interactions between bacteria and multicellular organisms (metazoans) cannot have evolved until both of the interacting partners existed. Therefore, widespread functions not based on metazoan-bacterial interactions must be more ancient. This argument has been used to suggest that flagella precede injectisomes (56, 79, 112, 121, 138, 152). Similarly, DNA conjugation was postulated to precede toxin secretion in type IV systems (25, 125, 158, 192). Unfortunately, the argument relies on hypotheses that may be hard

to test, especially with the poor fossil record that we have for microbial life, and more recent reappraisals have questioned both of these hypotheses (2, 24, 64, 136).

A good way to test hypotheses about the evolutionary polarity of function is to trace the most plausible scenario on a rooted phylogenetic tree. This type of evolutionary reconstruction can be done by using techniques that trace character changes on a tree (48, 54, 177). These techniques use the topology of the tree and the distribution of characteristics among taxa to reconstruct the most likely or most parsimonious characteristics of each ancestor in the tree (represented by each node). Reconstructing the characteristics of each ancestor carries with it the information about specific changes that happened in specific lineages with a clear polarity (direction) to the change. Therefore, given a reasonable inference of the phylogeny of a secretion system, one can often sort out which function came first.

Character reconstructions can test if functions evolved more than once in different lineages, suggesting parallel or convergent evolution, and if functional changes might be reversible. Importantly, character reconstruction can give an unresolved answer— there may be equally parsimonious explanations that describe different changes in function. In this case more data need to be collected, and one may want to evaluate the most parsimonious solutions under different models of change (177).

To illustrate this technique, we have reconstructed some basic functions of type II and IV secretion systems on the *virB11/pulE* superfamily phylogeny (Fig. 2). Several interesting conclusions emerge from these reconstructions. First, the common ancestor of both systems appears to have been a type IV pilus-like system that may have been involved in conjugative transfer of DNA. Second, natural competence seems to have arisen independently in the type IV and type II lineages. Third, the model suggests that (i) type II soluble protein secretion emerged relatively late from a type IV pilus system, perhaps in the proteobacteria; (ii) archaeal

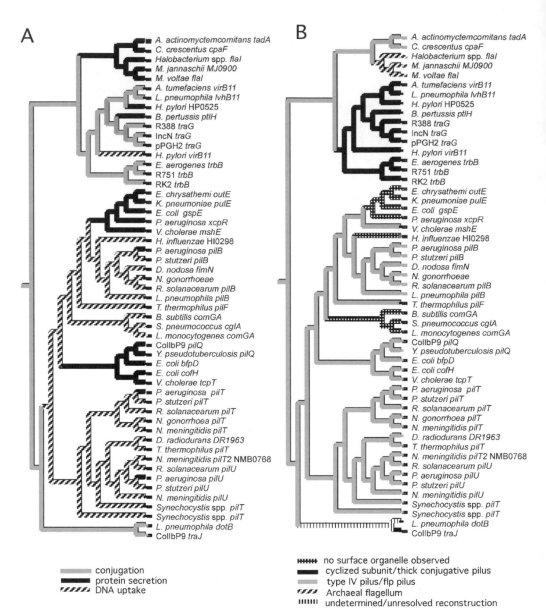

FIGURE 2 Functional reconstruction of type II and IV secretion using simple Fitch optimization and the *virB11/pulE* superfamily phylogeny. (A) Reconstruction of substrate evolution. Shades and patterns indicate conjugation (gray); DNA uptake (hatched); and protein secretion, including pilin and flagellar subunits (black). In cases in which two functions have been observed, DNA transport (either conjugation or uptake) is shown. (B) Evolutionary reconstruction of surface organelles: cyclized/thick conjugative pili (black), type IV pili (gray), archaeal flagella (hatched), or no surface structure observed (checked). Trees are derived from the NTPase phylogeny done in this study and are pruned to include better studied taxa. They are rooted with the uncharacterized archaeal NTPases as in reference 136.

flagella arose from a type IV pilus as well; and (iii) type IV systems are derived from an ancestor that was a conjugation system.

One other advantage of tree-based character

reconstruction is that it will reconstruct the most parsimonious function of some taxa for which functions are not known. For instance, Figure 2 predicts that a cyclized pilus may be important for the function of the *lvh* gene system of *L. pneumophila* and the *cag* pathogenicity island of *H. pylori*. The reconstructions also predict that *Yersinia pseudotuberculosis* may have a thin pilus that may help in gastrointestinal colonization.

It is important to stress that the reconstructions presented are the most parsimonious scenarios given available information, and further functional studies may cause drastic changes. It will be especially important to test the functions of transport systems in early branching prokaryotes such as the archaeal and bacterial thermophiles.

One interesting area of the tree that will greatly influence reconstructions is composed of the close relatives of the *dot/icm* system of *L. pneumophila*. These systems appear to be involved in both protein secretion and conjugation (165), and the functional interrelationship of these processes will be important in understanding the primordial function of both type II and IV secretion. Future sampling and functional testing from this branch and from other diverse type IV systems (eg., the F factor system) may lead to more reliable scenarios.

CLASSIFICATION

Classification of Genes in a Superfamily

With the recent flood of whole genome sequences, understanding and curating the diversity of related genes has become a bewildering task. Systematic classification and annotation of genes is only beginning to be explored. Methods such as the clusters of orthologous groups (COG) (178) or PROSITE signature motif patterns (168) can place sequences in broad family or superfamily categories. For more fine-tuned classification, genes are often named by searching public databases for the most similar gene—a technique called "best-hit" analysis. This technique is prone to error when rates of sequence evolution vary, and because it does not take phylogenetic hierarchy into account, it can falsely link genes that are in fact distant relatives (99, 119).

In addition, gene naming practices are not standardized. This has led to unfortunate situations in which totally unrelated genes are given exactly the same name. Examples of name overlap abound in the secretion system literature, especially for the *tra* and *pil* genes. With the high probability of horizontal transfer, this actually creates a situation in which two nonhomologous genes with the same name can be found in the same organism and perhaps in the same system.

Because genes have evolved in a pattern of lineage duplication followed by divergence that is equivalent to the way that populations of higher organisms speciate, gene family evolution can be traced using techniques developed for studying the patterns of organismal evolution (183). The best way to track the evolution of putative gene homologs is to build a new phylogenetic tree each time new sequences are discovered; however, this is very time and computationally intensive, especially with large gene superfamilies, and may be prohibitive. One available heuristic technique that closely approximates full-scale phylogenetic analysis—requiring only a tiny fraction of the time—uses existing published trees as templates upon which to classify a newly discovered gene (119, 136). This technique uses the presence of specific residues, called characteristic attributes, to classify genes according to the structure of a tree as a template or molecular key.

We have applied this technique to the NTPases of type II and IV secretion (*virB11/pulE* superfamily) and the outer membrane secretin superfamily of type II and III secretion. By searching public databases, we found 348 NTPases and 180 secretins and used these proteins to infer the phylogeny of each of these superfamilies using rigorous parsimony-based analysis. The resulting trees were then used as the templates to create classification keys for these two superfamilies, which can be found at www.genomecurator.org.

This type of classification should be especially useful because both of these superfamilies can be found in different secretion system types. In addition, they are involved in different functions from pilus assembly to phage extrusion. Thus, this technique not only allows for categorization of a newly found gene from one of these superfamilies into a secretion type but also allows a good first guess at the function of the new system. Additionally, classification keys can be used together to distinguish between systems. For instance, the co-occurrence of a gene for a type IV-related NTPase with a secretin most likely signals that the secretion system is related to systems carried on the WCI as opposed to the classical type II systems.

Classification of Systems

Confusion surrounding the classification of macromolecular transport systems is based on the lack of a standardized, logical, and systematic basis for nomenclature. Thus, disagreements in the literature about whether to lump or separate systems are categorically not resolvable, and might seem to be fruitless without some agreed-on standard for classification. Classification is an essential tool for both research and communicating ideas. Therefore, we suggest that an ideal classification scheme should seek to optimize both potential for learning and prediction. Thus, it should be the most unambiguous, easily used, logical, and natural way to organize and understand one's area of research, and it should be a good source for creating hypotheses about the possible functions of newly discovered systems. With these overall goals in mind, we assess different possible schemes for classification.

FUNCTIONAL CLASSIFICATION (SINGLE-CHARACTERISTIC CLASSIFICATION)

Most functional classification uses some set of discrete observed functions and properties to classify entities, but must arbitrarily emphasize certain functions over others to eliminate ambiguity and overlap. For secretion systems, all *sec*-dependent systems could be separated from *sec*-independent systems. Thus II, IV (pertussis toxin), V, and VI would form one group while I, III, and IV (all but pertussis toxin) would form another (Table 1; Fig. 1). Furthermore, each type could be defined by its descriptive name. Thus, any contact-dependent system would be included in type III secretion. Any molecule

that transported itself would be placed in type V. Obviously, this does not work for some types, as there is no good unifying descriptor (e.g., type II), and as can be seen in Table 1, this system of classification would result in a drastic reclassification of current types.

Functional classification is easy to understand and use, and it is unambiguous as long as a clear hierarchy of the importance of functions is established. However, it may not be a "natural" way to organize secretion systems. From an evolutionary perspective, this may be due to the phenomenon of convergence, in which systems with totally different ancestries come to perform the same function. Lumping contact-dependent systems with each other might be like lumping flying insects, birds, and bats together because they all fly.

Convergence affects the ability to make meaningful predictions about function or generate hypotheses. One could argue that functional classification is useful for making predictions because biological systems tend to solve problems in the same ways. Flight constrains bees, birds, and bats such that they have other factors in common as well. They might all need to be aerodynamic or they might not get very big. The result is that functional classification is probably best at making predictions about traits directly associated with the function that was used to classify initially. For instance, contact-dependent systems might all be associated with molecules that sense mechanical or chemical signals of the recipient for transport and so on.

Convergence causes functional classification to have less predictive value for unassociated factors. It would be better to make predictions about the metabolism of a bat using a mouse model than a bee model. It would be better to make predictions about type III injectisomes by looking at a flagellum model than a type IV conjugation (contact-dependent) model.

From a practical (operational) standpoint, functional classification requires that experiments be done to confirm that a system has a certain function. Therefore, formally, no predictions could be made until at least one function

TABLE 1 Properties of macromolecular transport systems[a]

System and name	Division	*sec* dependent	Location of secretion signal (N or C terminal)	NTP hydrolase or binding protein	Outer membrane pore	Contact dependent	No. of essential components	Substrate(s)[b]
I: ABC protein exporter		No	?	**Yes**	**Yes**	No	4	P
II: main terminal branch	classical and type IV pilus assembly	**Yes**	**N**	**Yes**	**Yes**	No[c]	~12–16	P,U
III: contact dependent		No	N[d]	**Yes**	**Yes**	**Yes**	~20	P
IV: conjugation related	Others	No	?	**Yes**	?	**Yes**	~11–12	P,U,C
	Pertussis toxin	**Yes**	**N**			No		
V: autotransporter	Linked	**Yes**	**N**	No	**Yes**	No	1	P
	Unlinked (two-partner)	**Yes**	N[e]	No	**Yes**	No	2–3	P
VI: chaperone/usher		**Yes**	N[f]	No	**Yes**	No	3	P
VII: alternate chaperone/usher		**Yes**	**N**	No	**Yes**	No	3	P
IIX: extracellular nucleation		**Yes**	**N**	No	?	No	6	P
Unclassified	*tad* locus	?	**N**	**Yes**	**Yes**	?	~9–14	P

[a] Properties in common in each column are in boldface type. Note that the descriptive names of several systems could apply to other systems as well.

[b] P, protein; C, DNA conjugation; U, uptake.

[c] Type IV pilus assembly may be regulated by contact-dependent mechanisms (192a).

[d] Two potential N-terminal secretion sequences are found in Yop proteins. There is disagreement about whether one of these resides in mRNA or protein.

[e] Once in the periplasm, an amino-proximal sequence targets these to the outer membrane pore.

[f] Once in the periplasm, a carboxy-terminal sequence interacts with the chaperone.

of the system is known. This would slow the process of making reasonable hypotheses about other functions and therefore might slow research.

HYBRID CLASSIFICATION (FUNCTION/HOMOLOGY)

In practice, most systems are not defined by function alone, but are defined using some combination of function and an inference of common ancestry (homology). This is often an informal classification scheme that relies partially on what researchers find as close gene database matches (reasonable BLAST scores) and partially on what is known about the system from experimental wet-lab experience. This type of classification relies on systems possessing readily identified and consistent differences in function and sequence comparisons such that all examples can be easily considered a different type. Such a system may lead to unclear classification boundaries when systems with subtle functional differences, similarities with more than one system, or significant but low sequence similarity are considered. However, several explicitly defined hybrid classification schemes do exist that differ in the emphasis that they place on function and homology.

One such scheme defines type IV secretion systems as those with homology (common ancestry) to conjugative DNA transfer systems (24, 158). Most applications of this approach use gene sequence similarity to infer basic common ancestry (primary homology) between the genes of systems (Box 1). Therefore, systems whose genes have sequence similarity to conjugation systems are classified as type IV secretion.

This approach is attractive because it allows classification of a newly discovered system as soon as it is shown to be similar to another system. However, this scheme is prone not only to lump convergent conjugation systems together, but also to lump relatives of these systems together. The argument for functional classification, which suggests that the same problem tends to be solved in similar ways, cannot be used when relatives of conjugation systems might have very different problems to solve. In fact, this method of classification has already been challenged with such a dilemma. The *dot/icm* system has been proposed to be a type IV secretion system because of its relationship to the conjugative transfer system of the ColIb plasmid (24), but the *dot/icm* system has only two genes that are similar to other type IV system genes (166). In fact, one of those putative homologs *(dotB)* is placed in the type II family of NTPases in phylogenetic analyses (133, 136). In this sense, this scheme of classification emphasizes relationship to conjugation systems and disregards other potentially interesting connections with type IV pili and type II secretion.

Another major problem with this approach is that systems might be classified as type IV even if conjugation arose in a distant but recognizable relative. The only functional connection between such systems, therefore, might be that an ancestor of the systems had the potential to one day become a conjugation system. This fact by itself may lead to very few, if any, commonalities between systems. In fact, as proposed by Christie and Vogel (25), a classification scheme based on having a common ancestor that is thought to have been a conjugation system might have more predictive value.

Other potential problems with this classification scheme include the following:

1. *Stability.* Any new conjugation system found would automatically drag all similar systems into type IV secretion. These may include other known and already classified systems.

2. *Extent of primary homology.* How many genes need to be similar to those of a conjugation system for a system to be considered "homologous"? If any similar gene provides an acceptable inference of homology, then this would lead to a reclassification of almost all type II systems as type IV systems because they share *virB11/pulE* superfamily genes.

3. *Applicability.* Using this scheme, secretion systems can only be grouped as related or unrelated to conjugation systems. Theoretically, other categories could be defined, such as "homology to bacterial flagellar apparatus" (type III) or "homology to type IV pilus assembly systems" (type II). However, such categories run the risk of conflicting with each other.

Another hybrid classification scheme has been proposed by Saier (153) that emphasizes homology based on phylogenetic analysis but includes functional data to delineate certain categories. In this system, called the transporter classification system (which applies to all transporters, not just macromolecular transporters), each transporter is designated by a unique combination of numbers and letters that denotes the overall functional category of energy use, the superfamily (family) and subfamily to which the system belongs—this is usually defined by the relationships of the major outer membrane protein for gram-negative secretion systems—and the category of substrate that is transported. This system is resistant to the problems of convergence, at least between types, because it emphasizes phylogeny first. If evolution is conservative of function at all, then a close relative will usually be a better overall predictor of function than a converged distant one. This scheme also allows immediate hypothesis generation as soon as new sequences are found because putative homology can usually be very quickly established by several different methods. However, this system does not, at present, allow for classification within a type below the subfamily level, and the system could benefit by explicit criteria for defining which nodes in phylogenetic trees represent subfamilies and subgroups.

If convergence is the major problem for functional classification, then horizontal transfer is the major confounder of systems that rely primarily on phylogenetic classification. The recent upheaval in evolutionary biology surrounding horizontal transfer is based on the fact that phylogenetic classification of organisms breaks down when confronted with widespread swapping of genes between distant relatives (38). This same concept applies to classification of any collection of genes, such as those that encode secretion systems. Systems can be misclassified when classification is based on single gene superfamilies that may have undergone horizontal transfer or shuffling events. This situation is equivalent to distrust of single gene phylogenies, such as small-subunit rRNA (e.g., 16S), as faithful indicators of organismal phylogenies (38, 193). There are differing estimations of the extent of horizontal tranfer within and among macromolecular transport systems. Where rigorous phylogenetic analysis has been applied, however, differences in evolutionary history abound, warranting further testing in other systems (12, 18, 137).

PHYLOGENETIC CLASSIFICATION

In a world dominated by vertical inheritance, a purely phylogenetic classification system for macromolecular transport systems would be easily implemented. Because it is based on the universally applicable principles of inheritance and divergence, phylogenetic classification is a natural way to organize and learn. In such a scheme, secretion systems would be placed in a type because they were related to other systems in that type, and in the absence of swapping of components, this would never leave any categories ambiguous. Subgroups based on discrete shared characteristics of sequence or function would allow precise classification of systems into subgroups. Such discrete changes could be loss or gain of a certain substrate specificity, or the utilization of the product of another gene in the secretion process.

Phylogenetic classification systems do not have to ignore function. In fact, functional characters are routinely included in phylogenetic analysis of organisms, and a phylogenetic tree is a good scaffold on which to reconstruct functional change because it can distinguish analogy from homology (Box 1). Since evolution usually conserves functions from one generation to the next, phylogenetic schemes are probably better predictors of overall function. Therefore, by taking a purely phylogenetic stance on classification, function might be better understood.

However, secretion systems share certain components, which is the first indication that horizontal transfer and recombination might be important forces shaping secretion systems. Type II and IV secretion systems share the *virB11/pulE* NTPase superfamily. Type II and III secretion systems share the secretin superfamily. WCI-borne systems convolute the situation even more because of the association of a gene for a type IV secretion family NTPase of the *virB11/pulE* superfamily with a secretin superfamily gene. This makes the phylogeny of the secretion systems appear more like a web than a hierarchical tree (Fig. 3).

A Hierarchical Phylogenetic Method for Classification of Systems: Historical Gene Associations.

If the model seen in Figure 3 is at all reasonable, then traditional hierarchical classification might be difficult. To account for potentially different histories of genes in transport systems, one solution is to link systems together in a type when they have genes in common and have been evolving together as a system for a long time.

We propose a system for classification based on the series of events that linked genes together to form a secretion system. Each of these events can be thought of as the first time that genes in a system interacted functionally with each other. In this classification system, a type is defined as the most ancient association of two or more genes that have evolved in association over time. This primary association would be the signifier for the type. The system could then be extended to include each new detectable association: the secondary association would be three or more genes that had evolved in concert over time, and the tertiary association would be composed of four or more, and so forth. This leads to a very precise method of classifying systems that can extend to individual systems and their closest relatives. It also has all the advantages of a phylogenetic classification system in that function can be mapped onto the hierarchy that it creates. It also would have easily identifiable events (gene associations) that would absolutely define subgroups, and probably represent biological changes. Although it is completely applicable to purely vertically inherited systems, it is also less sensitive to horizontal transfer, as a gene passing between systems would just be counted as new a gene association or dissociation. It would also have the benefit of preserving the most widely accepted types intact, as it appears that only single genes, usually not gene associations, are shared between types. Although this scheme is

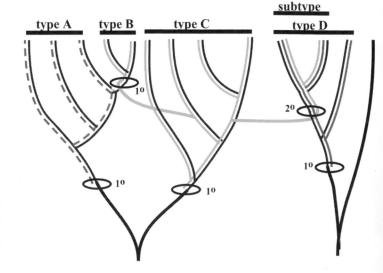

FIGURE 3 Hypothetical reticulogram for secretion systems. Each line represents a different gene phylogeny. Primary (1°) and secondary (2°) gene associations that could form the basis of a classification system are shown. Type B is defined by a new association between a light gray gene and a black gene after the loss of the dashed gene. Thus, this is defined as a new type independent of type C. Type D can be divided into two subgroups based on the presence or absence of a light gray gene.

not applicable to type V secretion, a simple one-gene phylogenetic scheme is applicable.

Historical gene associations provide explicit events for subdividing types that might encompass many different functions. For instance, flagellar apparatuses and injectisomes would be placed in the same type, as has been suggested (112), but the universal association with a secretin gene would probably place injectisomes in their own subgroup (121). This allows an appreciation of both differences and similarities between systems (123).

One possibility with the gene association classification scheme is the creation of chimeric types when at least two sets of associated genes can be shown to have fused into a single system. WCI-borne secretion systems may be the product of such an event (137). Chimeric classifications may inform functional studies more than placing a chimeric system in either one of the two progenitor types or in its own new type.

Of course, this classification scheme does entail serious phylogenetic analysis of multiple genes treated in a framework that allows shuffling and horizontal transfer. Techniques to assess the statistical significance of gene transfer and the ideas behind tree reconciliation can be used (Box 4). This type of analysis is required to test whether the gene associations seen in a newly found system are actually best explained as being inherited from a common ancestor with other members of a type (Box 4). For instance, a primary gene association for one system could re-form in a very distant and different situation, making a new type (Fig. 3) that without phylogenetic analysis probably would be lumped with unrelated systems. However, before rigorous phylogenetic analysis is done to test for this possibility, initial hypotheses can be based on similarity database searching or more complicated tree-based techniques.

CONCLUSIONS

The astounding functional diversity of secretion systems can only be understood with a two-pronged approach. The combination of functional studies with rigorous phylogenetic analysis allows reconstruction of functional diversification over time, and can test assumptions about the origins and primordial functions of different systems.

However, phylogenetic analysis is not useful only for understanding evolutionary patterns in time. Because evolution is the major organizing principle of life, phylogenetic approaches can have a central role in clarifying, aiding, and guiding functional studies. Phylogenetic models can be put to work for investigation as good predictors of function that allow reasonable hypotheses to be generated and tested. In addition, many classification disagreements could be clarified by using an explicit and systematic phylogenetic system.

CHAPTER SUMMARY

- Many pathogenic organisms use more than one secretion system in the disease process.
- Although many transport systems appear to be involved in virulence, close relatives are involved in symbiotic and other non-pathogenic processes, suggesting that "virulence" genes can have nonvirulent purposes in some organisms.
- In many cases there is a close connection between surface organelles and macromolecular secretion systems that transport soluble substrates. The links between these functions deserve further close phylogenetic and functional analysis.
- The role of horizontal gene transfer and shuffling in secretion systems, though not fully explored, is important to the evolution of secretion systems. Therefore, any phylogenetic classification scheme must allow for gene shuffling.
- Because evolution is mostly conservative of function, phylogeny can be used to predict function, and phylogenetic-based classification may be better at predicting function than other types of classification.

REFERENCES

1. **Aizawa, S. I.** 2001. Bacterial flagella and type III secretion systems. *FEMS Microbiol. Lett.* **202:** 157–164.
2. **Aizawa, S. I.** 1996. Flagellar assembly in Salmonella typhimurium. *Mol. Microbiol.* **19:**1–5.
3. **Austin, J. W., G. Sanders, W. W. Kay, and S. K. Collinson.** 1998. Thin aggregative fimbriae enhance Salmonella enteritidis biofilm formation. *FEMS Microbiol. Lett.* **162:**295–301.
4. **Baumler, A. J., A. J. Gilde, R. M. Tsolis, A. W. van der Velden, B. M. Ahmer, and F. Heffron.** 1997. Contribution of horizontal gene transfer and deletion events to development of distinctive patterns of fimbrial operons during evolution of *Salmonella* serotypes. *J. Bacteriol.* **179:**317–322.
5. **Ben Nasr, A., A. Olsen, U. Sjobring, W. Muller-Esterl, and L. Bjorck.** 1996. Assembly of human contact phase proteins and release of bradykinin at the surface of curli-expressing Escherichia coli. *Mol. Microbiol.* **20:**927–935.
6. **Bhattacharjee, M. K., S. C. Kachlany, D. H. Fine, and D. H. Figurski.** 2001. Nonspecific adherence and fibril biogenesis by *Actinobacillus actinomycetemcomitans:* TadA protein is an ATPase. *J. Bacteriol.* **183:**5927–5936.
7. **Bian, Z., and S. Normark.** 1997. Nucleator function of CsgB for the assembly of adhesive surface organelles in Escherichia coli. *EMBO J.* **16:**5827–5836.
8. **Bieber, D., S. W. Ramer, C. Y. Wu, W. J. Murray, T. Tobe, R. Fernandez, and G. K. Schoolnik.** 1998. Type IV pili, transient bacterial aggregates, and virulence of enteropathogenic Escherichia coli. *Science* **280:**2114–2118.
9. **Bitter, W., M. Koster, M. Latijnhouwers, H. de Cock, and J. Tommassen.** 1998. Formation of oligomeric rings by XcpQ and PilQ, which are involved in protein transport across the outer membrane of Pseudomonas aeruginosa. *Mol. Microbiol.* **27:**209–219.
10. **Blocker, A., N. Jouihri, E. Larquet, P. Gounon, F. Ebel, C. Parsot, P. Sansonetti, and A. Allaoui.** 2001. Structure and composition of the Shigella flexneri "needle complex", a part of its type III secretion. *Mol. Microbiol.* **39:**652–663.
11. **Bonci, A., A. Chiesurin, P. Muscas, and G. M. Rossolini.** 1997. Relatedness and phylogeny within the family of periplasmic chaperones involved in the assembly of pili or capsule-like structures of gram-negative bacteria. *J. Mol. Evol.* **44:**299–309.
12. **Boyd, E. F., and D. L. Hartl.** 1999. Analysis of the type 1 pilin gene cluster fim in *Salmonella:* its distinct evolutionary histories in the 5' and 3' regions. *J. Bacteriol.* **181:**1301–1308.
13. **Boyd, E. F., and D. L. Hartl.** 1998. Chromosomal regions specific to pathogenic isolates of *Escherichia coli* have a phylogenetically clustered distribution. *J. Bacteriol.* **180:**1159–1165.
14. **Boyd, E. F., and D. L. Hartl.** 1998. Diversifying selection governs sequence polymorphism in the major adhesin proteins fimA, papA, and sfaA of Escherichia coli. *J. Mol. Evol.* **47:**258–267.
15. **Boyd, E. F., and D. L. Hartl.** 1997. Recent horizontal transmission of plasmids between natural populations of *Escherichia coli* and *Salmonella enterica. J. Bacteriol.* **179:**1622–1627.
16. **Bremer, K.** 1995. Branch support and tree stability. *Cladistics* **10:**295–304.
17. **Brochier, C., E. Bapteste, D. Moreira, and H. Philippe.** 2002. Eubacterial phylogeny based on translational apparatus proteins. *Trends Genet.* **18:**1–5.
18. **Brown, E. W., M. L. Kotewicz, and T. A. Cebula.** 2002. Detection of recombination among Salmonella enterica strains using the incongruence length difference test. *Mol. Phylogenet. Evol.* **24:**102–120.
19. **Bullitt, E., C. H. Jones, R. Striker, G. Soto, F. Jacob-Dubuisson, J. Pinkner, M. J. Wick, L. Makowski, and S. J. Hultgren.** 1996. Development of pilus organelle subassemblies in vitro depends on chaperone uncapping of a beta zipper. *Proc. Natl. Acad. Sci. USA* **93:**12890–12895.
20. **Burns, D. L.** 1999. Biochemistry of type IV secretion. *Curr. Opin. Microbiol.* **2:**25–29.
21. **Cao, T. B., and M. H. Saier, Jr.** 2001. Conjugal type IV macromolecular transfer systems of gram-negative bacteria: organismal distribution, structural constraints and evolutionary conclusions. *Microbiology* **147:**3201–3214.
22. **Chapman, M. R., L. S. Robinson, J. S. Pinkner, R. Roth, J. Heuser, M. Hammar, S. Normark, and S. J. Hultgren.** 2002. Role of Escherichia coli curli operons in directing amyloid fiber formation. *Science* **295:**851–855.
23. **Charleston, M. A.** 1998. Jungles: a new solution to the host/parasite phylogeny reconciliation problem. *Math. Biosci.* **149:**191–223.
24. **Christie, P. J.** 2001. Type IV secretion: intercellular transfer of macromolecules by systems ancestrally related to conjugation machines. *Mol. Microbiol.* **40:**294–305.
25. **Christie, P. J., and J. P. Vogel.** 2000. Bacterial type IV secretion: conjugation systems adapted to deliver effector molecules to host cells. *Trends Microbiol.* **8:**354–360.
26. **Cohen-Bazire, G., and J. London.** 1967. Basal organelles of bacterial flagella. *J. Bacteriol.* **94:**458–465.
27. **Cohen-Krausz, S., and S. Trachtenberg.** 2002. The structure of the archaebacterial flagellar fila-

ment of the extreme halophile Halobacterium salinarum R1M1 and its relation to eubacterial flagellar filaments and type IV pili. *J. Mol. Biol.* **321**: 383–395.

28. **Collinson, S. K., S. C. Clouthier, J. L. Doran, P. A. Banser, and W. W. Kay.** 1996. *Salmonella enteritidis agfBAC* operon encoding thin, aggregative fimbriae. *J. Bacteriol.* **178**:662–667.

29. **Collinson, S. K., L. Emody, K. H. Muller, T. J. Trust, and W. W. Kay.** 1991. Purification and characterization of thin, aggregative fimbriae from *Salmonella enteritidis. J. Bacteriol.* **173**:4773–4781.

30. **Collinson, S. K., S. L. Liu, S. C. Clouthier, P. A. Banser, J. L. Doran, K. E. Sanderson, and W. W. Kay.** 1996. The location of four fimbrin-encoding genes, agfA, fimA, sefA and sefD, on the Salmonella enteritidis and/or S. typhimurium XbaI-BlnI genomic restriction maps. *Gene* **169**:75–80.

31. **Cunningham, C. W.** 1997. Can three incongruence tests predict when data should be combined? *Mol. Biol. Evol.* **14**:733–740.

32. **Dale, C., G. R. Plague, B. Wang, H. Ochman, and N. A. Moran.** 2002. Type III secretion systems and the evolution of mutualistic endosymbiosis. *Proc. Natl. Acad. Sci. USA* **99**:12397–12402.

33. **Dale, C., S. A. Young, D. T. Haydon, and S. C. Welburn.** 2001. The insect endosymbiont Sodalis glossinidius utilizes a type III secretion system for cell invasion. *Proc. Natl. Acad. Sci. USA* **98**: 1883–1888.

34. **Davis, B. M., E. H. Lawson, M. Sandkvist, A. Ali, S. Sozhamannan, and M. K. Waldor.** 2000. Convergence of the secretory pathways for cholera toxin and the filamentous phage, CTXphi. *Science* **288**:333–335.

35. **Dinh, T., I. T. Paulsen, and M. H. Saier, Jr.** 1994. A family of extracytoplasmic proteins that allow transport of large molecules across the outer membranes of gram-negative bacteria. *J. Bacteriol.* **176**:3825–3831.

36. **Dobzhansky, T.** 1948. Nothing in biology makes sense except in the light of evolution. *Am. Biol. Teacher* **35**:125–129.

37. **Dodson, K. W., F. Jacob-Dubuisson, R. T. Striker, and S. J. Hultgren.** 1993. Outer-membrane PapC molecular usher discriminately recognizes periplasmic chaperone-pilus subunit complexes. *Proc. Natl. Acad. Sci. USA* **90**: 3670–3674.

38. **Doolittle, W. F.** 1999. Phylogenetic classification and the universal tree [see comments]. *Science* **284**:2124–2129.

39. **Doran, J. L., S. K. Collinson, J. Burian, G. Sarlos, E. C. Todd, C. K. Munro, C. M. Kay, P. A. Banser, P. I. Peterkin, and W. W. Kay.** 1993. DNA-based diagnostic tests for Salmonella species targeting agfA, the structural gene for thin, aggregative fimbriae. *J. Clin. Microbiol.* **31**:2263–2273.

40. **Driessen, A. J., P. Fekkes, and J. P. van der Wolk.** 1998. The Sec system. *Curr. Opin. Microbiol.* **1**:216–222.

41. **Dubnau, D.** 1999. DNA uptake in bacteria. *Annu. Rev. Microbiol.* **53**:217–244.

42. **Economou, A.** 2000. Bacterial protein translocase: a unique molecular machine with an army of substrates. *FEBS Lett.* **476**:18–21.

43. **Economou, A.** 1999. Following the leader: bacterial protein export through the Sec pathway. *Trends Microbiol.* **7**:315–320.

44. **Eisenbrandt, R., M. Kalkum, E. M. Lai, R. Lurz, C. I. Kado, and E. Lanka.** 1999. Conjugative pili of IncP plasmids, and the Ti plasmid T pilus are composed of cyclic subunits. *J. Biol. Chem.* **274**:22548–22555.

45. **Faguy, D. M., K. F. Jarrell, J. Kuzio, and M. L. Kalmokoff.** 1994. Molecular analysis of archaeal flagellins: similarity to the type IV pilin-transport superfamily widespread in bacteria. *Can. J. Microbiol.* **40**:67–71.

46. **Farizo, K. M., T. Huang, and D. L. Burns.** 2000. Importance of holotoxin assembly in Ptl-mediated secretion of pertussis toxin from *Bordetella pertussis. Infect. Immun.* **68**:4049–4054.

47. **Farris, J. S.** 1982. Distance data in phylogenetic analysis. *Adv. Cladistics* **1**:3–23.

48. **Farris, J. S.** 1970. A method for computing Wagner trees. *Syst. Zool.* **19**:83–92.

49. **Farris, J. S., V. A. Albert, M. Kallersjo, D. Lipscomb, and A. G. Kluge.** 1996. Parsimony jackknifing outperforms neighbor-joining. *Cladistics* **12**:99–124.

50. **Farris, J. S., M. Kallersjo, A. G. Kluge, and C. Bult.** 1995. Constructing a significance test for incongruence. *Syst. Biol.* **44**:570–572.

51. **Felsenstein, J.** 1985. Confidence limits on phylogenies: an approach using the bootstrap. *Evolution* **39**:783–791.

52. **Felsenstein, J.** 1996. Inferring phylogenies from protein sequences by parsimony, distance, and likelihood methods. *Methods Enzymol.* **266**:418–427.

53. **Finkel, S. E., and R. Kolter.** 2001. DNA as a nutrient: novel role for bacterial competence gene homologs. *J. Bacteriol.* **183**:6288–6293.

54. **Fitch, W. M.** 1971. Toward defining the course of evolution: minimum change for a specific tree topology. *Syst. Zool.* **20**:406–416.

55. **Folkesson, A., A. Advani, S. Sukupolvi, J. D. Pfeifer, S. Normark, and S. Lofdahl.** 1999. Multiple insertions of fimbrial operons correlate with the evolution of Salmonella serovars responsible for human disease. *Mol. Microbiol.* **33**: 612–622.

56. **Foultier, B., P. Troisfontaines, S. Muller, F. R. Opperdoes, and G. R. Cornelis.** 2002. Characterization of the ysa pathogenicity locus in the chromosome of Yersinia enterocolitica and phylogeny analysis of type III secretion systems. *J. Mol. Evol.* **55:**37–51.

57. **Freiberg, C., R. Fellay, A. Bairoch, W. J. Broughton, A. Rosenthal, and X. Perret.** 1997. Molecular basis of symbiosis between Rhizobium and legumes. *Nature* **387:**394–401.

58. **Froehlich, B. J., A. Karakashian, H. Sakellaris, and J. R. Scott.** 1995. Genes for CS2 pili of enterotoxigenic *Escherichia coli* and their interchangeability with those for CS1 pili. *Infect. Immun.* **63:**4849–4856.

59. **Fuller, T. E., M. J. Kennedy, and D. E. Lowery.** 2000. Identification of Pasteurella multocida virulence genes in a septicemic mouse model using signature-tagged mutagenesis. *Microb. Pathog.* **29:**25–38.

60. **Geluk, F., P. P. Eijk, S. M. van Ham, H. M. Jansen, and L. van Alphen.** 1998. The fimbria gene cluster of nonencapsulated *Haemophilus influenzae*. *Infect. Immun.* **66:**406–417.

61. **Gentschev, I., G. Dietrich, and W. Goebel.** 2002. The E. coli alpha-hemolysin secretion system and its use in vaccine development. *Trends Microbiol.* **10:**39–45.

62. **Girardeau, J. P., Y. Bertin, and I. Callebaut.** 2000. Conserved structural features in class I major fimbrial subunits (Pilin) in gram-negative bacteria. Molecular basis of classification in seven subfamilies and identification of intrasubfamily sequence signature motifs which might be implicated in quaternary structure. *J. Mol. Evol.* **50:**424–442.

63. **Gogarten, J. P., H. Kibak, P. Dittrich, L. Taiz, E. J. Bowman, B. J. Bowman, M. F. Manolson, R. J. Poole, T. Date, T. Oshima, et al.** 1989. Evolution of the vacuolar H^+-ATPase: implications for the origin of eukaryotes. *Proc. Natl. Acad. Sci. USA* **86:**6661–6665.

64. **Gophna, U., E. Z. Ron, and D. Graur.** 2003. Bacterial type III secretion systems are ancient and evolved by multiple horizontal-transfer events. *Gene* **312:**151–163.

65. **Grass, S., and J. W. St. Geme III.** 2000. Maturation and secretion of the non-typable Haemophilus influenzae HMW1 adhesin: roles of the N-terminal and C-terminal domains. *Mol. Microbiol.* **36:**55–67.

66. **Groisman, E. A., and H. Ochman.** 1996. Pathogenicity islands: bacterial evolution in quantum leaps. *Cell* **87:**791–794.

67. **Haase, E. M., J. L. Zmuda, and F. A. Scannapieco.** 1999. Identification and molecular analysis of rough-colony-specific outer membrane proteins of *Actinobacillus actinomycetemcomitans*. *Infect. Immun.* **67:**2901–2908.

68. **Hacker, J., and J. B. Kaper.** 2000. Pathogenicity islands and the evolution of microbes. *Annu. Rev. Microbiol.* **54:**641–679.

69. **Hale, T. L.** 1991. Genetic basis of virulence in Shigella species. *Microbiol. Rev.* **55:**206–224.

70. **Hammar, M., A. Arnqvist, Z. Bian, A. Olsen, and S. Normark.** 1995. Expression of two csg operons is required for production of fibronectin- and congo red-binding curli polymers in Escherichia coli K-12. *Mol. Microbiol.* **18:**661–670.

71. **Hammar, M., Z. Bian, and S. Normark.** 1996. Nucleator-dependent intercellular assembly of adhesive curli organelles in Escherichia coli. *Proc. Natl. Acad. Sci. USA* **93:**6562–6566.

72. **Henderson, I. R., R. Cappello, and J. P. Nataro.** 2000. Autotransporter proteins, evolution and redefining protein secretion: response. *Trends Microbiol.* **8:**534–535.

73. **Henderson, I. R., J. P. Nataro, J. B. Kaper, T. F. Meyer, S. K. Farrand, D. L. Burns, B. B. Finlay, and J. W. St. Geme III.** 2000. Renaming protein secretion in the gram-negative bacteria. *Trends Microbiol.* **8:**352.

74. **Henderson, I. R., F. Navarro-Garcia, and J. P. Nataro.** 1998. The great escape: structure and function of the autotransporter proteins. *Trends Microbiol.* **6:**370–378.

75. **Hennig, W.** 1966. *Phylogenetic Systematics.* University of Illinois Press, Urbana.

76. **Hobbs, M., and J. S. Mattick.** 1993. Common components in the assembly of type 4 fimbriae, DNA transfer systems, filamentous phage and protein-secretion apparatus: a general system for the formation of surface-associated protein complexes [see comments]. *Mol. Microbiol.* **10:**233–243.

77. **Hofreuter, D., S. Odenbreit, and R. Haas.** 2001. Natural transformation competence in Helicobacter pylori is mediated by the basic components of a type IV secretion system. *Mol. Microbiol.* **41:**379–391.

78. **Holland, I. B., and M. A. Blight.** 1999. ABC-ATPases, adaptable energy generators fuelling transmembrane movement of a variety of molecules in organisms from bacteria to humans. *J. Mol. Biol.* **293:**381–399.

79. **Hueck, C. J.** 1998. Type III protein secretion systems in bacterial pathogens of animals and plants. *Microbiol. Mol. Biol. Rev.* **62:**379–433.

80. **Huelsenbeck, J. P., and J. J. Bull.** 1996. A likli-hood ratio test to detect conflicting phylogenetic signal. *Syst. Biol.* **45:**92–98.

81. **Huelsenbeck, J. P., F. Ronquist, R. Nielsen, and J. P. Bollback.** 2001. Bayesian inference of phylogeny and its impact on evolutionary biology. *Science* **294:**2310–2314.

82. **Inoue, T., I. Tanimoto, H. Ohta, K. Kato, Y. Murayama, and K. Fukui.** 1998. Molecular characterization of low-molecular-weight com-

ponent protein, Flp, in Actinobacillus actino-mycetemcomitans fimbriae. *Microbiol. Immunol.* **42:**253–258.

83. **Iwabe, N., K. Kuma, M. Hasegawa, S. Osawa, and T. Miyata.** 1989. Evolutionary relationship of archaebacteria, eubacteria, and eukaryotes inferred from phylogenetic trees of duplicated genes. *Proc. Natl. Acad. Sci. USA* **86:**9355–9359.

84. **Jacob-Dubuisson, F., R. Antoine, and C. Locht.** 2000. Autotransporter proteins, evolution and redefining protein secretion: response. *Trends Microbiol.* **8:**533–534.

85. **Jacob-Dubuisson, F., C. Locht, and R. Antoine.** 2001. Two-partner secretion in gram-negative bacteria: a thrifty, specific pathway for large virulence proteins. *Mol. Microbiol.* **40:**306–313.

86. **Jacob-Dubuisson, F., R. Striker, and S. J. Hultgren.** 1994. Chaperone-assisted self-assembly of pili independent of cellular energy. *J. Biol. Chem.* **269:**12447–12455.

87. **Johnson, J. M., and G. M. Church.** 1999. Alignment and structure prediction of divergent protein families: periplasmic and outer membrane proteins of bacterial efflux pumps. *J. Mol. Biol.* **287:**695–715.

88. **Johnson, J. R., T. T. O'Bryan, M. Kuskowski, and J. N. Maslow.** 2001. Ongoing horizontal and vertical transmission of virulence genes and *papA* alleles among *Escherichia coli* blood isolates from patients with diverse-source bacteremia. *Infect. Immun.* **69:**5363–5374.

89. **Jones, C. H., P. N. Danese, J. S. Pinkner, T. J. Silhavy, and S. J. Hultgren.** 1997. The chaperone-assisted membrane release and folding pathway is sensed by two signal transduction systems. *EMBO J.* **16:**6394–6406.

90. **Jones, C. H., J. S. Pinkner, R. Roth, J. Heuser, A. V. Nicholes, S. N. Abraham, and S. J. Hultgren.** 1995. FimH adhesin of type 1 pili is assembled into a fibrillar tip structure in the Enterobacteriaceae. *Proc. Natl. Acad. Sci. USA* **92:**2081–2085.

91. **Kachlany, S. C., P. J. Planet, M. K. Bhattacharjee, E. Kollia, R. DeSalle, D. H. Fine, and D. H. Figurski.** 2000. Nonspecific adherence by *Actinobacillus actinomycetemcomitans* requires genes widespread in *Bacteria* and *Archaea*. *J. Bacteriol.* **182:**6169–6176.

92. **Kachlany, S. C., P. J. Planet, R. DeSalle, D. H. Fine, and D. H. Figurski.** 2001. Genes for tight adherence of Actinobacillus actinomycetemcomitans: from plaque to plague to pond scum. *Trends Microbiol.* **9:**429–437.

93. **Kachlany, S. C., P. J. Planet, R. Desalle, D. H. Fine, D. H. Figurski, and J. B. Kaplan.** 2001. flp-1, the first representative of a new pilin gene subfamily, is required for non-specific adherence of

Actinobacillus actinomycetemcomitans. *Mol. Microbiol.* **40:**542–554.

94. **Kennan, R. M., O. P. Dhungyel, R. J. Whittington, J. R. Egerton, and J. I. Rood.** 2001. The type IV fimbrial subunit gene (*fimA*) of *Dichelobacter nodosus* is essential for virulence, protease secretion, and natural competence. *J. Bacteriol.* **183:**4451–4458.

95. **Kim, J. F.** 2001. Revisiting the chlamydial type III protein secretion system: clues to the origin of type III protein secretion. *Trends Genet.* **17:**65–69.

96. **Kirn, T. J., M. J. Lafferty, C. M. Sandoe, and R. K. Taylor.** 2000. Delineation of pilin domains required for bacterial association into microcolonies and intestinal colonization by Vibrio cholerae. *Mol. Microbiol.* **35:**896–910.

97. **Kolaczkowski, B., and J. W. Thornton.** 2004. Performance of maximum parsimony and likelihood phylogenetics when evolution is heterogeneous. *Nature* **431:**980–984.

98. **Koronakis, V., A. Sharff, E. Koronakis, B. Luisi, and C. Hughes.** 2000. Crystal structure of the bacterial membrane protein TolC central to multidrug efflux and protein export. *Nature* **405:**914–919.

99. **Koski, L. B., and G. B. Golding.** 2001. The closest BLAST hit is often not the nearest neighbor. *J. Mol. Evol.* **52:**540–542.

100. **Krall, L., U. Wiedemann, G. Unsin, S. Weiss, N. Domke, and C. Baron.** 2002. Detergent extraction identifies different VirB protein subassemblies of the type IV secretion machinery in the membranes of Agrobacterium tumefaciens. *Proc. Natl. Acad. Sci. USA* **99:**11405–11410.

101. **Kubori, T., A. Sukhan, S. I. Aizawa, and J. E. Galan.** 2000. Molecular characterization and assembly of the needle complex of the Salmonella typhimurium type III protein secretion system. *Proc. Natl. Acad. Sci. USA* **97:**10225–10230.

102. **Lai, E. M., and C. I. Kado.** 2000. The T-pilus of Agrobacterium tumefaciens. *Trends Microbiol.* **8:**361–369.

103. **Lawley, T. D., M. W. Gilmour, J. E. Gunton, D. M. Tracz, and D. E. Taylor.** 2003. Functional and mutational analysis of conjugative transfer region 2 (Tra2) from the IncHI1 plasmid R27. *J. Bacteriol.* **185:**581–591.

104. **Lawley, T. D., W. A. Klimke, M. J. Gubbins, and L. S. Frost.** 2003. F factor conjugation is a true type IV secretion system. *FEMS Microbiol. Lett.* **224:**1–15.

105. **Lawrence, J. G.** 1997. Selfish operons and speciation by gene transfer. *Trends Microbiol.* **5:**355–359.

106. **Lawrence, J. G., and J. R. Roth.** 1996. Selfish operons: horizontal transfer may drive the evolution of gene clusters. *Genetics* **143:**1843–1860.

107. **Letellier, L., S. P. Howard, and J. T. Buckley.** 1997. Studies on the energetics of proaerolysin secretion across the outer membrane of Aeromonas species. Evidence for a requirement for both the protonmotive force and ATP. *J. Biol. Chem.* **272:**11109–11113.

108. **Lewis, P. O.** 2001. Phylogenetic systematics turns over a new leaf. *Trends Ecol. Evol.* **16:**30–37.

109. **Li, X. Z., and K. Poole.** 2001. Mutational analysis of the OprM outer membrane component of the MexA-MexB-OprM multidrug efflux system of *Pseudomonas aeruginosa. J. Bacteriol.* **183:**12–27.

110. **Llosa, M., F. X. Gomis-Ruth, M. Coll, and F. F. de la Cruz.** 2002. Bacterial conjugation: a two-step mechanism for DNA transport. *Mol. Microbiol.* **45:**1–8.

111. **Loferer, H., M. Hammar, and S. Normark.** 1997. Availability of the fibre subunit CsgA and the nucleator protein CsgB during assembly of fibronectin-binding curli is limited by the intracellular concentration of the novel lipoprotein CsgG. *Mol. Microbiol.* **26:**11–23.

112. **Macnab, R. M.** 1999. The bacterial flagellum: reversible rotary propellor and type III export apparatus. *J. Bacteriol.* **181:**7149–7153.

113. **Marklund, B. I., J. M. Tennent, E. Garcia, A. Hamers, M. Baga, F. Lindberg, W. Gaastra, and S. Normark.** 1992. Horizontal gene transfer of the Escherichia coli pap and prs pili operons as a mechanism for the development of tissue-specific adhesive properties. *Mol. Microbiol.* **6:**2225–2242.

114. **Marron, M. B., and C. J. Smyth.** 1995. Molecular analysis of the cso operon of enterotoxigenic Escherichia coli reveals that CsoA is the adhesin of CS1 fimbriae and that the accessory genes are interchangeable with those of the cfa operon. *Microbiology* **141**(Pt. 11):2849–2859.

115. **Martin, P. R., M. Hobbs, P. D. Free, Y. Jeske, and J. S. Mattick.** 1993. Characterization of pilQ, a new gene required for the biogenesis of type 4 fimbriae in Pseudomonas aeruginosa. *Mol. Microbiol.* **9:**857–868.

116. **Masui, S., T. Sasaki, and H. Ishikawa.** 2000. Genes for the type IV secretion system in an intracellular symbiont, *Wolbachia,* a causative agent of various sexual alterations in arthropods. *J. Bacteriol.* **182:**6529–6531.

117. **Mattick, J. S.** 2002. Type IV pili and twitching motility. *Annu. Rev. Microbiol.* **56:**289–314.

118. **Mhlanga-Mutangadura, T., G. Morlin, A. L. Smith, A. Eisenstark, and M. Golomb.** 1998. Evolution of the major pilus gene cluster of *Haemophilus influenzae. J. Bacteriol.* **180:**4693–4703.

119. **Neil Sarkar, I., J. Thornton, P. Planet, D. Figurski, B. Schierwater, and R. DeSalle.** 2002. An automated phylogenetic key for classifying homeoboxes. *Mol. Phylogenet. Evol.* **24:**388.

120. **Nelson, G.** 1994. Homology and systematics, p. xvi, 483. *In* B. K. Hall (ed.), *Homology: The Hierarchical Basis of Comparative Biology.* Academic Press, San Diego, Calif.

121. **Nguyen, L., I. T. Paulsen, J. Tchieu, C. J. Hueck, and M. H. Saier, Jr.** 2000. Phylogenetic analyses of the constituents of type III protein secretion systems. *J. Mol. Microbiol. Biotechnol.* **2:**125–144.

122. **Nika, J. R., J. L. Latimer, C. K. Ward, R. J. Blick, N. J. Wagner, L. D. Cope, G. G. Mahairas, R. S. Munson, Jr., and E. J. Hansen.** 2002. *Haemophilus ducreyi* requires the *flp* gene cluster for microcolony formation in vitro. *Infect. Immun.* **70:**2965–2975.

123. **Nunn, D.** 1999. Bacterial type II protein export and pilus biogenesis: more than just homologies? *Trends Cell Biol.* **9:**402–408.

124. **Nunn, D. N., and S. Lory.** 1991. Product of the Pseudomonas aeruginosa gene pilD is a prepilin leader peptidase. *Proc. Natl. Acad. Sci. USA* **88:**3281–3285.

125. **O'Callaghan, D., C. Cazevieille, A. Allardet-Servent, M. L. Boschiroli, G. Bourg, V. Foulongne, P. Frutos, Y. Kulakov, and M. Ramuz.** 1999. A homologue of the Agrobacterium tumefaciens VirB and Bordetella pertussis Ptl type IV secretion systems is essential for intracellular survival of Brucella suis. *Mol. Microbiol.* **33:**1210–1220.

126. **Ochman, H., and E. A. Groisman.** 1995. The evolution of invasion by enteric bacteria. *Can. J. Microbiol.* **41:**555–561.

127. **Ochman, H., J. G. Lawrence, and E. A. Groisman.** 2000. Lateral gene transfer and the nature of bacterial innovation. *Nature* **405:**299–304.

128. **Olsen, A., A. Arnqvist, M. Hammar, and S. Normark.** 1993. Environmental regulation of curli production in Escherichia coli. *Infect. Agents Dis.* **2:**272–274.

129. **Olsen, A., H. Herwald, M. Wikstrom, K. Persson, E. Mattsson, and L. Bjorck.** 2002. Identification of two protein-binding and functional regions of curli, a surface organelle and virulence determinant of Escherichia coli. *J. Biol. Chem.* **277:**34568–34572.

130. **Olsen, A., M. J. Wick, M. Morgelin, and L. Bjorck.** 1998. Curli, fibrous surface proteins of *Escherichia coli,* interact with major histocompatibility complex class I molecules. *Infect. Immun.* **66:**944–949.

131. **Page, R. D., and M. A. Charleston.** 1997. From gene to organismal phylogeny: reconciled trees and the gene tree/species tree problem. *Mol. Phylogenet. Evol.* **7:**231–240.

132. **Pantoja, M., L. Chen, Y. Chen, and E. W. Nester.** 2002. Agrobacterium type IV secretion is a two-step process in which export substrates associate with the virulence protein VirJ in the periplasm. *Mol. Microbiol.* **45:**1325–1335.

133. **Peabody, C. R., Y. J. Chung, M. R. Yen, D. Vidal-Ingigliardi, A. P. Pugsley, and M. H. Saier, Jr.** 2003. Type II protein secretion and its relationship to bacterial type IV pili and archaeal flagella. *Microbiology* **149:**3051–3072.

134. **Phillips, A., D. Janies, and W. Wheeler.** 2000. Multiple sequence alignment in phylogenetic analysis. *Mol. Phylogenet. Evol.* **16:**317–330.

135. **Planet, P. J.** 2002. Reexamining microbial evolution through the lens of horizontal transfer. *EXS* (92):247–303.

136. **Planet, P. J., S. C. Kachlany, R. DeSalle, and D. H. Figurski.** 2001. Phylogeny of genes for secretion NTPases: identification of the widespread tadA subfamily and development of a diagnostic key for gene classification. *Proc. Natl. Acad. Sci. USA* **98:**2503–2508.

137. **Planet, P. J., S. C. Kachlany, D. H. Fine, R. DeSalle, and D. H. Figurski.** 2003. The Widespread Colonization Island of Actinobacillus actinomycetemcomitans. *Nat. Genet.* **34:**193–198.

138. **Plano, G. V., J. B. Day, and F. Ferracci.** 2001. Type III export: new uses for an old pathway. *Mol. Microbiol.* **40:**284–293.

139. **Plaut, A. G.** 1983. The IgA1 proteases of pathogenic bacteria. *Annu. Rev. Microbiol.* **37:**603–622.

140. **Pohlner, J., R. Halter, K. Beyreuther, and T. F. Meyer.** 1987. Gene structure and extracellular secretion of Neisseria gonorrhoeae IgA protease. *Nature* **325:**458–462.

141. **Pohlschroder, M., W. A. Prinz, E. Hartmann, and J. Beckwith.** 1997. Protein translocation in the three domains of life: variations on a theme. *Cell* **91:**563–566.

142. **Pugsley, A. P., and B. Dupuy.** 1992. An enzyme with type IV prepilin peptidase activity is required to process components of the general extracellular protein secretion pathway of Klebsiella oxytoca. *Mol. Microbiol.* **6:**751–760.

143. **Pupo, G. M., D. K. Karaolis, R. Lan, and P. R. Reeves.** 1997. Evolutionary relationships among pathogenic and nonpathogenic Escherichia coli strains inferred from multilocus enzyme electrophoresis and *mdh* sequence studies. *Infect. Immun.* **65:**2685–2692.

144. **Redfield, R. J.** 1993. Genes for breakfast: the have-your-cake-and-eat-it-too of bacterial transformation. *J. Hered.* **84:**400–404.

145. **Reid, S. D., C. J. Herbelin, A. C. Bumbaugh, R. K. Selander, and T. S. Whittam.** 2000. Parallel evolution of virulence in pathogenic Escherichia coli. *Nature* **406:**64–67.

146. **Reumann, S., J. Davila-Aponte, and K. Keegstra.** 1999. The evolutionary origin of the protein-translocating channel of chloroplastic envelope membranes: identification of a cyanobacterial homolog. *Proc. Natl. Acad. Sci. USA* **96:**784–789.

147. **Rivas, S., S. Bolland, E. Cabezon, F. M. Goni, and F. de la Cruz.** 1997. TrwD, a protein encoded by the IncW plasmid R388, displays an ATP hydrolase activity essential for bacterial conjugation. *J. Biol. Chem.* **272:**25583–25590.

148. **Romling, U., Z. Bian, M. Hammar, W. D. Sierralta, and S. Normark.** 1998. Curli fibers are highly conserved between *Salmonella typhimurium* and *Escherichia coli* with respect to operon structure and regulation. *J. Bacteriol.* **180:**722–731.

149. **Rudin, A., L. Olbe, and A. M. Svennerholm.** 1996. Monoclonal antibodies against fimbrial subunits of colonization factor antigen I (CFA/I) inhibit binding to human enterocytes and protect against enterotoxigenic Escherichia coli expressing heterologous colonization factors. *Microb. Pathog.* **21:**35–45.

150. **Russel, M.** 1998. Macromolecular assembly and secretion across the bacterial cell envelope: type II protein secretion systems. *J. Mol. Biol.* **279:**485–499.

151. **Sagulenko, E., V. Sagulenko, J. Chen, and P. J. Christie.** 2001. Role of Agrobacterium VirB11 ATPase in T-pilus assembly and substrate selection. *J. Bacteriol.* **183:**5813–5825.

152. **Saier, M. H., Jr.** 2004. Evolution of bacterial type III protein secretion systems. *Trends Microbiol.* **12:**113–115.

153. **Saier, M. H., Jr.** 2000. A functional-phylogenetic classification system for transmembrane solute transporters. *Microbiol. Mol. Biol. Rev.* **64:**354–411.

154. **Sajjan, U. S., L. Sun, R. Goldstein, and J. F. Forstner.** 1995. Cable (cbl) type II pili of cystic fibrosis-associated *Burkholderia (Pseudomonas) cepacia*: nucleotide sequence of the *cblA* major subunit pilin gene and novel morphology of the assembled appendage fibers. *J. Bacteriol.* **177:**1030–1038.

155. **Sakellaris, H., N. K. Hannink, K. Rajakumar, D. Bulach, M. Hunt, C. Sasakawa, and B. Adler.** 2000. Curli loci of *Shigella* spp. *Infect. Immun.* **68:**3780–3783.

156. **Sakellaris, H., G. P. Munson, and J. R. Scott.** 1999. A conserved residue in the tip proteins of CS1 and CFA/I pili of enterotoxigenic Escherichia coli that is essential for adherence. *Proc. Natl. Acad. Sci. USA* **96:**12828–12832.

157. **Sakellaris, H., and J. R. Scott.** 1998. New tools in an old trade: CS1 pilus morphogenesis. *Mol. Microbiol.* **30:**681–687.

158. **Salmond, G. P. C.** 1994. Secretion of extracellular virulence factors by plant pathogenic bacteria. *Annu. Rev. Phytopathol.* **32:**181–200.

159. **Sandkvist, M.** 2001. Biology of type II secretion. *Mol. Microbiol.* **40:**271–283.

160. **Sandkvist, M.** 2001. Type II secretion and pathogenesis. *Infect. Immun.* **69:**3523–3535.

161. **Sandkvist, M., M. Bagdasarian, S. P. Howard, and V. J. DiRita.** 1995. Interaction between the autokinase EpsE and EpsL in the cytoplasmic membrane is required for extracellular secretion in Vibrio cholerae. *EMBO J.* **14:**1664–1673.

162. **Saurin, W., M. Hofnung, and E. Dassa.** 1999. Getting in or out: early segregation between importers and exporters in the evolution of ATP-binding cassette (ABC) transporters. *J. Mol. Evol.* **48:**22–41.

163. **Sauvonnet, N., G. Vignon, A. P. Pugsley, and P. Gounon.** 2000. Pilus formation and protein secretion by the same machinery in Escherichia coli. *EMBO J.* **19:**2221–2228.

164. **Schreiner, H. C., K. Sinatra, J. B. Kaplan, D. Furgang, S. C. Kachlany, P. J. Planet, B. A. Perez, D. H. Figurski, and D. H. Fine.** 2003. Tight-adherence genes of Actinobacillus actinomycetemcomitans are required for virulence in a rat model. *Proc. Natl. Acad. Sci. USA* **100:**7295–7300.

165. **Segal, G., M. Purcell, and H. A. Shuman.** 1998. Host cell killing and bacterial conjugation require overlapping sets of genes within a 22-kb region of the Legionella pneumophila genome. *Proc. Natl. Acad. Sci. USA* **95:**1669–1674.

166. **Segal, G., J. J. Russo, and H. A. Shuman.** 1999. Relationships between a new type IV secretion system and the icm/dot virulence system of Legionella pneumophila. *Mol. Microbiol.* **34:**799–809.

167. **Shannon, J. L., and R. C. Fernandez.** 1999. The C-terminal domain of the *Bordetella pertussis* autotransporter BrkA forms a pore in lipid bilayer membranes. *J. Bacteriol.* **181:**5838–5842.

168. **Sigrist, C. J., L. Cerutti, N. Hulo, A. Gattiker, L. Falquet, M. Pagni, A. Bairoch, and P. Bucher.** 2002. PROSITE: a documented database using patterns and profiles as motif descriptors. *Brief Bioinform.* **3:**265–274.

169. **Skerker, J. M., and H. C. Berg.** 2001. Direct observation of extension and retraction of type IV pili. *Proc. Natl. Acad. Sci. USA* **98:**6901–6904.

170. **Skerker, J. M., and L. Shapiro.** 2000. Identification and cell cycle control of a novel pilus system in Caulobacter crescentus. *EMBO J.* **19:**3223–3234.

171. **Smeets, L. C., and J. G. Kusters.** 2002. Natural transformation in Helicobacter pylori: DNA transport in an unexpected way. *Trends Microbiol.* **10:**159–162; discussion, 162.

172. **Sommer, J. M., and A. Newton.** 1989. Turning off flagellum rotation requires the pleiotropic gene *pleD: pleA, pleC,* and *pleD* define two morphogenic pathways in *Caulobacter crescentus. J. Bacteriol.* **171:**392–401.

173. **Soto, G. E., and S. J. Hultgren.** 1999. Bacterial adhesins: common themes and variations in architecture and assembly. *J. Bacteriol.* **181:**1059–1071.

174. **Spinola, S. M., K. R. Fortney, B. P. Katz, J. L. Latimer, J. R. Mock, M. Vakevainen, and E. J. Hansen.** 2003. *Haemophilus ducreyi* requires an intact *flp* gene cluster for virulence in humans. *Infect. Immun.* **71:**7178–7182.

175. **St. Geme, J. W., III.** 2000. The pathogenesis of nontypable Haemophilus influenzae otitis media. *Vaccine* **19**(Suppl. 1):S41–S50.

176. **St. Geme, J. W., III, and D. Cutter.** 2000. The *Haemophilus influenzae* Hia adhesin is an autotransporter protein that remains uncleaved at the C terminus and fully cell associated. *J. Bacteriol.* **182:**6005–6013.

177. **Swofford, D. L., and W. P. Maddison.** 1987. Reconstructing ancestral character states under Wagner parsimony. *Math. Biosci.* **87:**199–229.

178. **Tatusov, R. L., E. V. Koonin, and D. J. Lipman.** 1997. A genomic perspective on protein families. *Science* **278:**631–637.

179. **Thanassi, D. G., and S. J. Hultgren.** 2000. Multiple pathways allow protein secretion across the bacterial outer membrane. *Curr. Opin. Cell Biol.* **12:**420–430.

180. **Thanassi, D. G., E. T. Saulino, and S. J. Hultgren.** 1998. The chaperone/usher pathway: a major terminal branch of the general secretory pathway. *Curr. Opin. Microbiol.* **1:**223–231.

181. **Thanassi, D. G., E. T. Saulino, M. J. Lombardo, R. Roth, J. Heuser, and S. J. Hultgren.** 1998. The PapC usher forms an oligomeric channel: implications for pilus biogenesis across the outer membrane. *Proc. Natl. Acad. Sci. USA* **95:**3146–3151.

182. **Thomas, N. A., S. L. Bardy, and K. F. Jarrell.** 2001. The archaeal flagellum: a different kind of prokaryotic motility structure. *FEMS Microbiol. Rev.* **25:**147–174.

183. **Thornton, J. W., and R. DeSalle.** 2000. Gene family evolution and homology: genomics meets phylogenetics. *Annu. Rev. Genomics Hum. Genet.* **1:**41–73.

184. **Thornton, J. W., and R. DeSalle.** 2000. A new method to localize and test the significance of incongruence: detecting domain shuffling in the nuclear receptor superfamily. *Syst. Biol.* **49:**183–201.

185. van Wely, K. H., J. Swaving, R. Freudl, and A. J. Driessen. 2001. Translocation of proteins across the cell envelope of Gram-positive bacteria. *FEMS Microbiol. Rev.* **25**:437–454.

186. Vidal, O., R. Longin, C. Prigent-Combaret, C. Dorel, M. Hooreman, and P. Lejeune. 1998. Isolation of an *Escherichia coli* K-12 mutant strain able to form biofilms on inert surfaces: involvement of a new *ompR* allele that increases curli expression. *J. Bacteriol.* **180**:2442–2449.

187. Wall, D., P. E. Kolenbrander, and D. Kaiser. 1999. The *Myxococcus xanthus pilQ (sglA)* gene encodes a secretin homolog required for type IV pilus biogenesis, social motility, and development. *J. Bacteriol.* **181**:24–33.

188. Ward, D.V., O. Draper, J. R. Zupan, and P. C. Zambryski. 2002. Peptide linkage mapping of the Agrobacterium tumefaciens vir-encoded type IV secretion system reveals protein subassemblies. *Proc. Natl. Acad. Sci. USA* **99**: 11493–11500.

189. Welch, R. A. 2001. RTX toxin structure and function: a story of numerous anomalies and few analogies in toxin biology. *Curr. Top. Microbiol. Immunol.* **257**:85–111.

190. Wheeler, W. C. 1990. Nucleic acid sequence phylogeny and random outgroups. *Cladistics* **6**:363–368.

191. Whittam, T. S., M. L. Wolfe, I. K. Wachsmuth, F. Orskov, I. Orskov, and R. A. Wilson. 1993. Clonal relationships among *Escherichia coli* strains that cause hemorrhagic colitis and infantile diarrhea. *Infect. Immun.* **61**:1619–1629.

192. Winans, S. C., D. L. Burns, and P. J. Christie. 1996. Adaptation of a conjugal transfer system for the export of pathogenic macromolecules. *Trends Microbiol.* **4**:64–68.

193. Woese, C. 1998. The universal ancestor. *Proc. Natl. Acad. Sci. USA* **95**:6854–6859.

194. Woese, C. R. 2000. Interpreting the universal phylogenetic tree. *Proc. Natl. Acad. Sci. USA* **97**: 8392–8396.

195. Wong, K. K., F. S. Brinkman, R. S. Benz, and R. E. Hancock. 2001. Evaluation of a structural model of *Pseudomonas aeruginosa* outer membrane protein OprM, an efflux component involved in intrinsic antibiotic resistance. *J. Bacteriol.* **183**:367–374.

196. Yen, M. R., C. R. Peabody, S. M. Partovi, Y. Zhai, Y. H. Tseng, and M. H. Saier. 2002. Protein-translocating outer membrane porins of gram-negative bacteria. *Biochim. Biophys. Acta* **1562**:6–31.

197. Young, G. M., D. H. Schmiel, and V. L. Miller. 1999. A new pathway for the secretion of virulence factors by bacteria: the flagellar export apparatus functions as a protein-secretion system. *Proc. Natl. Acad. Sci. USA* **96**:6456–6461.

198. Zogaj, X., W. Bokranz, M. Nimtz, and U. Romling. 2003. Production of cellulose and curli fimbriae by members of the family *Enterobacteriaceae* isolated from the human gastrointestinal tract. *Infect. Immun.* **71**:4151–4158.

THE EVOLUTION OF
ANTIBIOTIC RESISTANCE

Dean Rowe-Magnus and Didier Mazel

12

FROM THE BEGINNING TO THE PRESENT-DAY SITUATION

The discovery of antibiotics in the 1930s and their development for the treatment of infectious diseases represented a major advancement for medicine. This golden age of antibiotics allowed most of the major human diseases caused by bacteria to be controlled, at least in industrialized countries. This situation is now threatened by the rapid rise in antibiotic resistance. Keeping in mind the scope of this book—the evolution of pathogens—it is essential to stress the key difference that distinguishes pathogenesis from clinical resistance: the evolutionary time scale over which these processes developed. At first glance, the aptitude of human and animal pathogens to develop antimicrobial resistance or virulence can be viewed as an adaptive response to comparable selective pressures in the same ecological niche. Indeed, the hosts are identical, and bacterial colonization implies circumvention of their immune or chemical defenses. However, the evolutionary timescale of virulence and resistance development in bacterial pathogens is quite different. Contemporary pathogens can be seen as the outcome of a long-term coevolutionary race between the escape attempts of the hosts and bacterial innovation that has been on going for millions of years, whereas antimicrobial therapy is only a 6 decade-old phenomenon.

Resistance has been encountered as an impediment to antibiotic therapy for as long as antibiotics have been used. With only a few exceptions, antibiotic resistance in bacterial pathogens was identified soon after the introduction of antibiotics into clinical practice, illustrating the genetic flexibility of bacteria. This was first seen in the development of resistance to sulfonamides and penicillinase in pneumococci in the late 30s, and streptomycin resistance mutations in mycobacteria in 1946. Between 1949 and 1951 in Japan, sulfonamide resistance in *Shigella* isolates rose from 10% to almost 90%. The development of resistance to sulfonamides and penicillin in pneumococci led to warnings in the medical community against misuse and abusive prescription as sources of drug resistance. Multidrug resistance, nonetheless, was never anticipated since the coappearance of multiple mutations conferring such phenotypes was considered to be beyond the evolutionary potential of a given bacterial

Dean Rowe-Magnus, Department of Microbiology, Clinical Integrative Biology Division, Sunnybrook & Women's College Health Sciences Centre, 2075 Bayview Ave., S1-26A, Toronto, Ontario, Canada M4N 3N5. *Didier Mazel,* Unité Plasticité du Génome Bactérien, Institut Pasteur, 25 rue du Dr. Roux, 75724 Paris cedex 15, France.

Evolution of Microbial Pathogens, Edited by H. S. Seifert and V. J. DiRita, © 2006 ASM Press, Washington, D.C.

population. However, in 1955 in Japan, 5 years after the introduction of streptomycin, tetracycline, and chloramphenicol in general practice and the beginning of massive production of these antibiotics, the first cases of multiple resistance were reported (43) (Fig. 1). In 1956 in Japan, increasing numbers of *Shigella dysenteriae* strains were isolated that were resistant to up to four antibiotics simultaneously (tetracycline, chloramphenicol, streptomycin, and sulfonamides). The appearance of chloramphenicol resistance in this context was particularly surprising since isolates resistant to chloramphenicol alone had not been previously identified. Furthermore, both sensitive and resistant *Shigella* could be isolated from a single patient, and *Shigella* spp. and *Escherichia coli* obtained from the same patients often exhibited the same multiple resistance patterns (3, 69). It became clear that the emergence of multidrug-resistant strains could not be attributed to mutation. Studies to localize the resistance genes led to the discovery of the first mobile DNA ele-

ments, the resistance (R) plasmids (69), and *interspecies* conjugative transfer of these resistance genes was demonstrated. At the same time, the first insertion sequences were discovered (29, 56), and the link between such elements and the demonstrated mobility of several resistance determinants (13, 51) soon led to the first characterizations of resistance-encoding transposons (Tn), and with them integrons, in the mid-1970s (4, 26, 39, 47, 60, 61). However, it soon became apparent that the development of resistance was not limited to the spread of transposons. In many cases, depending on the antibiotics and/or on the species, mutation of an endogenous gene led to the development new resistant strains (see "A Function of the Pathogen: *M. tuberculosis*" below). Furthermore, in a number of naturally transformable species, resistance development also happened through gene acquisition but involved mechanisms dependent on homologous recombination rather than transposition (see "Origins of Antibiotic Resistance Genes" below).

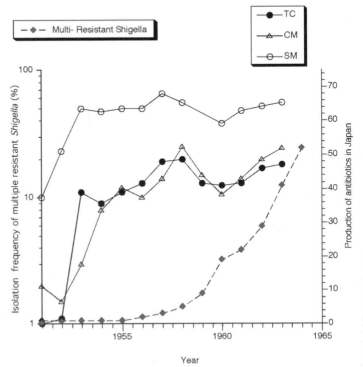

FIGURE 1 Production of antibiotics in Japan and isolation frequency of antibiotic-resistant *Shigella* strains. TC, tetracycline; CM, chloramphenicol; SM, streptomycin.

Conjugative plasmids (see "Conjugation" below) were common in enterobacteria isolated before the medical use of antibiotics. During the antibiotic era, R plasmids became common in bacteria of the same genera. This suggested that both the acquisition and the dissemination of antibiotic resistance genes in human pathogens and commensal strains occurred within a short time frame. Datta and Hughes examined the Murray Collection, a compilation of hundreds of mainly gram-negative pathogens (*Salmonella, Shigella, Klebsiella, Proteus,* and *Escherichia*) obtained from clinical specimens during the preantibiotic era, for their antibiotic resistance phenotype and conjugative plasmid content (14). They then assessed whether the "preantibiotic" plasmids belonged to the same compatibility groups as the modern R plasmids (i.e., shared replication functions). None of the strains isolated between 1917 and 1952 was resistant to any of the antibiotics in current use, yet 65 of the 84 plasmids identified belonged to the same compatibility groups as present R plasmids. This observation supported a recent invasion postulate, in which medically important bacteria rapidly developed antibiotic resistance through the insertion of new resistance genes into existing plasmids rather than by the spread of previously rare plasmids.

THE DEVELOPMENT OF ANTIBIOTIC RESISTANCE

There are several distinct biochemical mechanisms by which antibiotic resistance can arise (Table 1), and these will be discussed in the next paragraphs.

Reduced Permeability

This method of resistance involves modifying the composition of the bacterial envelope to reduce the permeability of the antimicrobial compound. Alterations in lipopolysaccharide composition and porin abundance correlating with increased resistance to a variety of antimicrobials (including polymyxin, moxalactam, chloramphenicol and some β-lactams) have been described for a number of gram-negative organisms. Lipopolysaccharide modification in gram-negative bacteria can also play a significant role in resistance to host antimicrobial

TABLE 1 Biochemical mechanisms of antibiotic resistance and their genetic determinants

Mechanism	Examples	Genetic determinants	
		Mutation	Gene acquisition
Reduced permeability	Aminoglycosides	+	+
Prodrug not activated	Isoniazid	+	+
Active efflux	Tetracycline, fluoroquinolones		+
Alteration of drug target	Erythromycin		+
	Fluoroquinolones	+	
	Rifampin	+	
	Tetracycline		+
Inactivation of drug	Aminoglycosides		+
	Chloramphenicol		+
	β-Lactams	+	+
	Rifampin	(+)	(+)
Bypass inhibited step	Sulfonamides		+
	Trimethoprim		+
Immunity protein	Bleomycin		+
	Fluoroquinolone		(+)
Amplification of target	Trimethoprim	+	
	Sulfonamides	+	
Sequestration of drug	β-Lactams	+	+

factors during infection. These modifications include the addition of fatty acids, phospho-ethanolamine, or 4-amino-4-deoxy-L-arabi-nose to the core and lipid A regions; acetylation of the O antigen; and possibly hydroxylation of fatty acids. Changes in the absolute number of pores or in qualitative function reduce the diffusion of antibiotics into the cell. This mechanism of reduced permeability can lead to cross-resistance to several families of antibiotics.

Active Efflux

In this instance, access of the antibiotic to its cellular target is impeded because the bacteria synthesize a membrane pump that expels the antibiotic. The intracellular concentration of the antibiotic is thus prevented from reaching levels that are sufficiently high to be toxic. Antibiotics that are rendered ineffective by this mechanism include tetracycline and the fluoro-quinolones.

Alteration of the Drug Target

In this mechanism, the bacteria modify the drug target to render it insensitive to the action of the drug. This type of mechanism is responsible for resistance to macrolides, lincosamides, and streptogramins (MLS) in gram-positive bacteria. For example, the cellular target of erythromycin is the 23S rRNA component of ribosomes. Erythromycin resistance can result from the production of a methylase that modifies the 23S rRNA component, markedly reducing its affinity for the antibiotic.

Inactivation of the Drug (Immunity Proteins)

Here, the drug is enzymatically altered to nullify its activity. Inactivation of drugs having cellular targets can take place after the antibiotic has traversed the bacterial membrane (intracellularly) or before the drug contacts the cell (extracellularly). An example of intracellular drug inactivation is provided by chloramphenicol, which is inactivated by the addition of an acetyl group by a cytosolic acetyltransferase enzyme. Conversely, the targets of the β-lactam antibiotics are extracellular. Hence, these drugs must be inactivated before they interact with the cell. Gram-negative bacteria direct β-lactamases to the periplasmic space, and gram-positive bacteria secrete these enzymes into the culture media to intercept and inactivate the antibiotic before it reaches its target. Bleomycin, produced by *Streptomyces verticillus,* is a glycopeptide antibiotic that induces DNA damage. Bleomycin-producing S. *verticillus* must be protected from the lethal effect of its own product. These organisms produce a bleomycin-binding protein and an N-acetyltransferase to inactivate the drug.

Bypass

In the bypass mechanism, the sensitive drug target is substituted with a metabolic equivalent that is resistant to the drug's action. This is commonly observed with resistance to trimethoprim and the sulfonamides. Both drugs affect bacterial folic acid production, an essential step in nucleic acid biosynthesis. Sulfonamides inhibit dihydropteroate synthetase (DHPS), which catalyzes the formation of dihydrofolate from *para*-aminobenzoic acid. In the subsequent step of the pathway, trimethoprim inhibits dihydrofolate reductase (DHFR), which catalyzes the formation of tetrahydrofolate from dihydrofolate. The most common mechanism of resistance to trimethoprim in enterobacteria is the production of an additional DHFR, which, unlike the wild-type enzyme, is less sensitive to inhibition by trimethoprim.

Target Amplification

Regulatory mutations that lead to the cellular overproduction of the drug target can induce very high levels of resistance. A clinical isolate of *E. coli* found to be highly resistant to trimethoprim (MIC, >1 g/liter) harbored several mutations in regulatory elements for the gene encoding the chromosomal DHFR (*folA*). These included a promoter up-mutation in the -35 region, a 1-bp increase in the distance between the -10 region and the start codon, several mutations leading to an optimal ribosome-binding site, and several mutations in the structural gene giving more frequently used codons (23). These changes collectively resulted in a several-hundredfold overproduction of a DHFR.

Prodrug Not Activated

Mycobacterium tuberculosis is the causative agent of tuberculosis, and antibiotics have been used to treat the infection since the 1940s. Although isoniazid (isonicotinic acid hydrazide, INH) is still one of the most effective antibiotics against tuberculosis, the number of INH- and other drug-resistant strains has increased dramatically. The mechanism of action of INH requires the catalase-peroxidase encoded by the *katG* gene for bacterial sensitivity to INH. INH is a prodrug that requires activation by KatG. The activated drug then disrupts mycolic acid biosynthesis, leading to cell death. Mutations in the *katG* gene are the major cause of INH resistance in clinical isolates of *M. tuberculosis.*

ORIGINS OF ANTIBIOTIC RESISTANCE GENES

In recent years, there has been considerable discussion about the role of pathogenicity islands (PAIs) in the increasing virulence of bacterial clinical isolates. Simply put, the difference between a pathogenic and a nonpathogenic strain is the presence of extra genes in the form of one or more PAIs in the pathogen (see chapter 5). PAIs are clusters of genes providing those components necessary for the establishment and survival of the pathogen in the hostile environment of the infected host. Likewise, antibiotic resistance genes are found in clusters that group different determinants of different origin (as shown by variations in overall G+C content and codon usage) at single sites on the bacterial chromosome. Such clustering has been recognized for some time and most likely reflects the roles of transposons, integrons, and plasmids as vehicles in the transport of resistance genes. The conclusion is that virulence and resistance genes are usually "foreign" to their bacterial

hosts, and an obvious question is, "Where do they come from?" A number of plausible sources of resistance determinants have been proposed and are described below.

Housekeeping Genes

Recruitment of general housekeeping genes is a means by which resistance determinants can evolve. Several examples of chromosomally encoded resistance homologues, whose functions are not related to antibiotic resistance, are known. These include aminoglycoside acetyltransferase (AAC) and β-lactamase genes in *Serratia marcescens, Providencia stuartii,* and *Streptomyces* and *Mycobacterium* spp. for which the level of resistance to the corresponding antibiotics could not be correlated with their universal presence in these organisms (1, 2, 10, 24, 53, 57, 70). Mutation of such genes could lead to new substrate recognition profiles and provide a potential source for the evolution of resistance. Furthermore, in some cases these genes, which may be quiescent with respect to antibiotic resistance, can confer resistance on certain strains when upregulated. In addition, VanX-like homologues have been described in *E. coli, Salmonella enterica,* and *Synechocystis* spp. Their presence in gram-negative bacteria suggests that these proteins have physiological roles not related to vancomycin resistance, as gram-negative bacteria are insensitive to vancomycin because their outer membrane prevents access of the drug to its target. The implication is that antibiotic-modifying enzymes may have been derived from general housekeeping genes that are normally involved in other cellular processes in other organisms.

Antibiotic-Producing Microbes

Although no single origin for an antibiotic resistance gene has been definitively identified, in a few cases a strong relationship can be established between the resistance gene(s) found in clinical isolates and their putative source organisms. Several antibiotics are known to be of bacterial origin, implying the existence of protective mechanisms in producer organisms and thus a potential source for resistance genes. Characterization studies of resistance to the glycopeptides provide an excellent example (or highlight an extraordinary coincidence) of the relationship between producer and clinical isolate (37). Glycopeptide resistance in the enterococci is due to a cluster of genes that encode the synthesis of a novel cell envelope component, D-Ala–D-Lac, that replaces the D-Ala–D-Ala moiety normally present (37). The replacement of D-Ala by D-Lac results in a 1,000-fold reduction in glycopeptide binding, which explains the consequent high level of resistance to the antibiotics vancomycin and teicoplanin. Three genes are required for the synthesis of D-Ala–D-Lac, and nucleotide sequence comparisons show a striking similarity between the *vanH, -A,* and *-X* genes of enterococci and the related clusters found in *Streptomyces toyocaensis* and *Amycolatopsis orientalis,* the two organisms producing glycopeptide antibiotics (Fig. 2). This

similarity extends to the structures of intergenic sequences in the various clusters, where the *vanH* and *vanA* genes and the actinomycete analogues are all translationally coupled through overlapping reading frames. The VanA and VanB proteins of the vancomycin-resistance gene cluster of enterococci *also* share significantly higher homology with the dipeptide ligases of the glycopeptide-producing organisms *S. toyocaensis* and *A. orientalis* than with other dipeptide ligases, including those of intrinsically resistant organisms (37). This supports the notion that antibiotic-producing organisms may be the source of resistance genes found in clinical isolates.

A novel rifampin resistance gene, *arr-2,* was identified within a typical integron structure in *Pseudomonas aeruginosa* (66). Rifampin, used extensively in the treatment of tuberculosis and leprosy, is a derivative of the naturally occurring product rifamycin produced by the

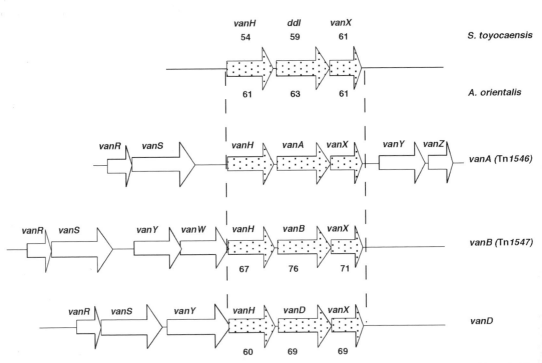

FIGURE 2 The *vanHAX* cluster of antibiotic-resistant enterococci compared with related clusters identified in glycopeptide-producing actinomycetes. The numbers between the clusters indicate percent amino acid identity to the *vanA* cluster.

soil bacterium *Amycolatopsis mediterranei*. Since rifampin has rarely been employed in the treatment of gram-negative bacterial infections, the presence of the *arr-2* gene in *P. aeruginosa*—and as a gene cassette, no less (see below)—clearly indicates its acquisition by a horizontal gene transfer event. Since *arr-2* and its lone homologue, the *arr* gene of *Mycobacterium smegmatis,* share only 54% amino acid identity, the *arr-2* gene may have been procured from an as-yet-unidentified bacterium with which *P. aeruginosa* might share a microbial habitat. Either a soil or mammalian host environment may have been conducive to the extension of the resistance gene pool from one bacterial species to another in a process promoted by rifampin within soil communities or the selective pressure of antibiotic therapy regimens.

Mosaic Genes

Resistance to the β-lactam antibiotics in *Neisseria* and *Streptococcus* spp. is due to the development of altered penicillin-binding proteins (PBPs) creating a decreased affinity for β-lactam antibiotics. Comparisons of the PBP genes from resistant and sensitive strains have shown that resistant PBPs have multiple gene segment replacements leading to mosaic structures. In most cases, the new gene segments were highly similar or identical to the corresponding part of the PBP gene from a closely related commensal species (6, 16–18, 38, 58). For example, in penicillin-resistant *Neisseria meningitidis,* the *penA* gene contained two segments that showed 22% divergence from the *penA* allele found in penicillin-sensitive strains, but that were identical to the corresponding regions from the *penA* gene of *Neisseria flavescens,* a commensal species (59).

Resistance to sulfonamide drugs is due to either the development or the acquisition of an altered DHPS with a decreased affinity for the inhibitor. In *N. meningitidis, Streptococcus pneumoniae,* and *Streptococcus pyogenes,* sulfonamide resistance is mediated by mutations in the chromosomal DHPS gene, *folP.* Comparisons of *folP* from resistant and sensitive strains have shown

that, in resistant isolates, the *folP* genes diverged by 8 to 14% from their counterparts in sensitive isolates, some of them having a mosaic structure (22, 41, 49). Notably, one *N. meningitidis*-resistant isolate had a mosaic *folP* gene whose central segment was identical to the corresponding segment of a *Neisseria gonorrhoeae* strain. As found for the mosaic *penA* genes, the number of different mosaic *folP* genes suggests that resistance has arisen independently on many occasions in these species.

However, in the majority of cases, the evidence permitting identification of antibiotic resistance genes is largely circumstantial and comes mostly from comparative biochemical and molecular studies; in several instances, the closeness of the nucleotide sequences indicates a strong relationship. One of the best examples is that of the gene cluster responsible for methicillin resistance (the *mec* cluster) found in *Staphylococcus aureus,* which was first identified in the early 1960s (shortly after the introduction of the new drug) and which has had a profound effect on the treatment of infection by this organism. Methicillin-resistant *S. aureus* is found worldwide and has been responsible for numerous serious hospital outbreaks that have proved difficult to treat. While they are known to possess methicillin resistance, it has been found that such strains often carry resistance determinants for other antibiotics. Work done by Wu et al. indicates that these determinants may have originated in *Staphylococcus sciuri* (71). Similarly, the aminoglycoside acetyltransferase *(aac)* genes found in the enteric bacteria appear to have evolved from the chromosomal genes of other species of gram-negative bacteria (30) as a result of horizontal gene transfer and mutation processes. Other AACs have significant primary sequence similarities to the acetyltransferases found in streptomycetes, and this is also the case for the aminoglycoside phosphotransferases (APHs), which are members of the protein kinase superfamily. In the latter case, the similarity extends to the three-dimensional structures of the APH proteins and other kinases (12).

An example of an antibiotic resistance gene of an unusual source is provided by mupirocin (pseudomonic acid), an antibiotic employed frequently in the treatment of topical infections caused by gram-positive bacteria. Resistance to mupirocin is due to the presence of an altered isoleucyl tRNA synthase that may have originated in eukaryotes and was only recently acquired and transferred within *S. aureus* strains (7). The molecular details of this unusual acquisition remain to be ascertained. It should be emphasized that in none of the cases described above has direct gene transfer been demonstrated between the source organism and the pathogen. However, as mentioned earlier, these are almost certainly multicomponent transfer processes that take place within mixed bacterial populations.

With respect to origins of resistance, it should be noted that, long before the use of antibiotics, a variety of mercury compounds were used as disinfectants (19, 21), as were quaternary ammonium compounds. The significance of the preantibiotic use of such agents is not easy to assess, but it has been observed that genetic determinants for resistance to a variety of metallic compounds and detergents are linked to genes for antibiotic resistance. For example, a screen for mercury-resistant (Hg^r) strains in the Murray Collection of preantibiotic enterobacteria led to the identification of three *mer* transposons that showed >99% identity with present-day Hg^r transposon sequences. Notably, one of these transposons, Tn*5075*, was 99.6% identical to Tn*21* but the integron, In*2*, was not present. This observation was consistent with the hypothesis that integrons were incorporated into preexisting Hg^r transposons during the antibiotic era.

In many instances, multiple antibiotic resistance in bacteria is caused exclusively by the combination of several resistance genes, each coding for resistance to a single drug. More recently, it has become clear that such phenotypes are often achieved by the activity of drug efflux pumps. Some of these efflux pumps exhibit an extremely wide specificity, covering practically all antibiotics, chemotherapeutic agents, detergents, dyes, and other inhibitors (46, 48).

RESISTANCE BY MUTATION

The appearance of antibiotic resistance in bacterial populations can occur in two ways: through mutation of an endogenous gene or acquisition of a resistance gene from an exogenous source. The evolution of resistance by mutation of an endogenous gene is more the exception than the rule, since the genetic basis of most antibiotic resistance among clinically significant bacteria is horizontal transfer. However, mutation does play an important role in this process. But why does mutation play an important role in some cases and not others? The answer to this question is difficult and may involve various factors, such as the nature of the pathogen, the treatment regimen, and the biochemical nature of antibiotic action.

A Function of the Pathogen: *M. tuberculosis*

Mutations appear spontaneously with a frequency on the order of 10^{-6} to 10^{-9}, depending on the bacterial type and the considered characteristic. The first significant resistant pathogen that influenced the use of a drug (streptomycin-resistant *M. tuberculosis*) developed resistance as the result of mutations affecting the target site of the antibiotic. A steady increase in the frequency of *M. tuberculosis* strains resistant to one or more agents commonly used as front-line antibiotics in treatment regimens has been reported. In light of the relatively few efficacious therapeutic agents available to treat tuberculosis, a renewed effort has been launched to define the molecular basis of antimicrobial resistance in mycobacteria. Despite the fact that mobile genetic elements such as insertion sequences are common in mycobacteria, no compound transposons are found in this pathogen. In fact, no exogenously acquired resistance genes have been identified, and plasmids have yet to be characterized in this species. Thus, the generation of the multidrug-resistant *Mycobacterium* strains that are so feared by physicians and patients alike requires a series of independent mutations (45). Genetic studies indicate that resistance to all the primary antituberculosis drugs currently in use has arisen by way of mutation. Rifampin resistance is due to mutations in the *rpoB* locus that codes for the β subunit of RNA polymerase. Streptomycin resistance is caused by mutations in the *rrs* and *rpsL* genes, coding for 16S rRNA and the ribosomal protein S12, respectively. Mutations in the *katG* gene, which encodes a catalase-peroxidase enzyme, or the *inhA* gene, which encodes a protein involved in fatty acid biosynthesis, confer resistance to isoniazid. Resistance to fluoroquinolones and clarithromycin can be traced to mutations in the *gyrA* (coding the DNA gyrase A subunit) and 23S rRNA genes, respectively. Since it has been shown that resistance arises in successive mutational steps, the frequency of appearance for a strain resistant to four drugs would be less than 1 in 10^{24}. Hence, combinatorial therapy for the treatment of drug-resistant *M. tuberculosis* strains remains an effective therapeutic approach.

Mutations also play an important role in the evolution of resistance enzymes in order to expand their recognition spectrum toward new derivatives produced by the pharmaceutical industry. The best example is certainly the development of extended-spectrum β-lactamases (which engender resistance to newer synthetic derivatives of penicillins and cephalosporins) that arose by in vivo protein engineering. Point mutations that change critical amino acids within the β-lactamases have been characterized; these lead to alterations in enzyme-substrate recognition and have generated a huge family of genetically engineered resistance genes. Thus a critical juxtaposition of mutation and gene transfer is well established in the evolution of extended-spectrum β-lactamases (9).

A Function of the Antibiotics: the Synthetic Quinolone, Trimethoprim, and Sulfonamide Drugs

Quinolones are potent antibacterial agents that specifically target bacterial DNA gyrase and topoisomerase IV. While the frequency of fluoroquinolone resistance in the laboratory is relatively low, in clinical practice resistant strains appear during the course of patient treatment. Since the fluoroquinolones are completely synthetic agents with no known natural counterparts, the acquisition of dominant plasmid-encoded resistance determinants would not be expected; mutation is therefore a predictable process for the clinical development of resistance to this class of antibiotics. In keeping with this initial hypothesis, early studies showed that the only known mechanisms for quinolone resistance arose by mutations in the chromosomal genes for type II topoisomerases (40), the targets of quinolone action, and by changes in expression of efflux pumps and porins that control the accumulation of these agents inside the bacterial cell. However, the fact that a drug is completely synthetic is not a guarantee for the absence of plasmid-encoded resistance determinants. Unexpectedly, plasmid-encoded low-level resistance to fluoroquinolones has been recently identified (65, 67, 68). A multidrug-resistant isolate of *Klebsiella pneumoniae* contained a broad host range plasmid that increased resistance to nalidixic acid and to ciprofloxacin in *E. coli* transconjugants. The resistance gene, *qnr*, from this plasmid was surrounded by a nucleotide sequence originally characterized in the integrons In6 from plasmid pSa and In7 from pDGO100. The *qnr* gene was cloned and sequenced, and the protein product purified. Qnr was shown to protect *E. coli* DNA gyrase, but not topoisomerase IV, from inhibition by ciprofloxacin. Gyrase protection did not involve quinolone inactivation or the activation of an independent gyrase activity. Qnr belongs to the pentapeptide repeat family. One member of this family is McbG, a component of the system that protects bacteria synthesizing microcin B17 (MccB17) from self-inhibition. MccB17 is a 3.1-kDa post-translationally modified peptide that blocks DNA replication and can, like ciprofloxacin, inhibit DNA gyrase supercoiling. It was proposed that Qnr could have evolved from an immunity protein designed to protect DNA gyrase from a naturally occurring inhibitor or from a chromosomal gene of unknown function encoding a protein in the pentapeptide repeat family.

Furthermore, acquired resistance to trimethoprim and sulfonamides, which are also synthetic drugs, is almost exclusively due to plasmid-encoded resistance genes. In these cases resistance occurs through a metabolic bypass mechanism that introduces a metabolic equivalent of the protein that is resistant to the drug's action.

The Price To Pay for Resistance: Compensatory Mutations

In the absence of selecting drugs, chromosomal resistance mutations commonly engender a cost in the fitness of microorganisms. This is because such mutations typically alter essential cellular factors such as the ribosome, DNA gyrase, RNA polymerase, or cell wall. Resistance mutation can often lead to reduced growth rate and virulence. Hence, once the transition is made to an antibiotic-free environment, resistant bacteria are expected to be at a disadvantage compared to sensitive strains because of their lowered fitness. However, in vivo and in vitro experimental studies of E. coli and S. enterica serovar Typhimurium found that mutation in the absence of drugs commonly resulted in mutations that restored fitness to wild-type levels without the loss of high-level resistance (34, 35, 55). For example, most S. enterica serovar Typhimurium mutants resistant to streptomycin, rifampicin, and nalidixic acid were avirulent in mice, which suggested that such mutants would be spontaneously eliminated from the host (5). Interestingly, a proportion of these avirulent mutants survived in the host and was found to have acquired compensatory mutations that restored virulence while not affecting the resistance phenotype. Although compensatory mutants can be readily selected under laboratory conditions, it is notable that such resistant mutants have not been encountered among clinical isolates of S. enterica serovar Typhimurium. Additional studies are required to see if such compensatory mutants are found in human infections with bacterial pathogens.

Mutator Phenotypes in Clinical Isolates and Their Impact

It is postulated that extensive tailoring and adaptation of resistance genes can take place during the passage of these genes from source organism to clinical isolates via intermediate transfer hosts with different G+C composition, codon usage, and gene expression systems. It is not known how these modifications occur, as only the resistant clinical isolate is identified by the clinical microbiologist. The rate of successful gene transfer between bacterial populations in nature depends on numerous factors such as ecological isolation, host range of genetic exchange vectors, activity of the recipient cell protective systems, DNA sequence divergence between recombining molecules, type and efficiency of the recipient cell recombination machinery, and, finally, the hybrid fitness. It is likely that hypermutable strains and mutator genes have a significant influence in the process of horizontal gene transfer. The fidelity of recombination is controlled by the methyl-directed mismatch repair (MMR) system. MMR proteins, such as *mutS, mutH,* and *mutL,* recognize mispaired and unpaired bases in the joint heteroduplex regions and block RecA-catalyzed strand transfer. Thus, MMR is a potent inhibitor of recombination between nonidentical DNA sequences (homeologous recombination). Recent studies have shown that many natural bacterial isolates, particularly pathogenic strains, may be hypermutagenic because they carry one or more mutator genes (33, 62). Inactivation of MMR genes increases mutation rates 10^2- to 10^3-fold. Although the incidence of mutator strains in environmental microbes and their possible roles in the tailoring of antibiotic resistance genes (or any horizontally transferred determinants, such as biodegradation clusters) is difficult to examine systematically in natural populations, their importance in the evolution of resistance should not be underestimated. Because inactivation of MMR greatly increases recombination rates between related strains and species (15), MMR-deficient strains might have contributed considerably to recombination that has given rise to the observed genomic sequence mosaicism of resistance genes such as *penA* and *folP*. In addition, the *mutT* mutator displays a unique and strict specificity: only A:T-to-C:G transversions are induced. The *mutY* mutator acts in a similar but reciprocal fashion, as it displays a specific G:C-to-A:T transversion activity. These activities could readily contribute to the adaptation of codon usage patterns to new cellular environments.

MECHANISMS OF RESISTANCE GENE ACQUISITION

As developed previously in this book, horizontal gene transfer differs from vertical gene transfer in that the acquisition of genetic material is not dependent on reproduction. There are three main mechanisms of horizontal gene transfer: transduction, transformation and conjugation.

Transformation: *Neisseria* and *Streptococcus*

Natural transformation is a physiological process characteristic of many bacterial species in which the cell takes up and expresses exogenous DNA (see "From the Beginning to the Present-Day Situation" above). There are a few examples for which transformation has been implicated in acquisition of antibiotic resistance, mainly for penicillin resistance in *S. pneumoniae*, *N. gonorrhoeae*, and *N. meningitidis*; for sulfonamide resistance in *N. meningitidis*, *S. pneumoniae*, and *S. pyogenes*; and recently for chloramphenicol resistance in *N. meningitidis*.

As mentioned earlier, β-lactam and sulfonamide resistance in *Neisseria* and *Streptococcus* is due to the development of mosaic *penA* and *folP* genes. The fact that more than 30 different mosaic *penA* genes have been found in 78 isolates of penicillin-resistant *N. meningitidis* and that a number of different *folP* mosaic genes have been found in *N. meningitidis*, *S. pneumoniae*, and *S. pyogenes* exemplifies how common a mechanism transformation followed by recombination is in naturally transformable species. As transformation is also suspected to play a role for other variable phenotypic traits

of *Streptococcus* species, it has to be considered as a general means of adaptation in these species.

Transformation is also very likely involved in the recent dissemination of a chloramphenicol acetyltransferase gene of exogenous origin among *N. meningitidis* strains. In a study of 12 chloramphenicol-resistant isolates of *N. meningitidis*, it has been observed that all carried a chromosomal *catP* gene (25). The nucleotide sequence of this gene and its flanking region was identical to an internal portion of transposon Tn*4451* characterized in *Clostridium perfringens*. In *Neisseria*, this truncated transposon corresponded almost exclusively to the *catP* gene and had lost its ability to transpose. The resistant isolates showed a high degree of diversity; however, the location of the *catP* gene was invariant, and the authors have demonstrated that this gene could be efficiently propagated to different susceptible strains through natural transformation with genomic DNA from chloramphenicol-resistant strains.

It is not always simple to prove that transformation is the mechanism of gene transfer that allowed a new resistance determinant to be acquired. For example, the propagation of the chromosomal nonconjugative TetB determinant among naturally transformable *Haemophilus* species and in *Moraxella catarrhalis* may have occurred by transformation. However, the data from molecular analysis required to substantiate the mechanism are still forthcoming, and another mechanism cannot be firmly ruled out.

Conjugation

Conjugative DNA transfer occurs during cell-to-cell contact. It is the principal mechanism for the dissemination of antibiotic resistance genes. First discovered in 1946 through genetic recombination experiments in *E. coli*, the impact of this type of antibiotic resistance gene movement soon became apparent. During an epidemic of dysentery in Japan in the late 1950s, increasing numbers of *S. dysenteriae* strains were isolated that were resistant to up to four antibiotics simultaneously. It became clear that the emergence of multiple resistant strains could not be attributed to mutation alone.

Furthermore, both sensitive and resistant *Shigella* could be isolated from a single patient, and *Shigella* spp. and *E. coli* obtained from the same patients often exhibited the same multiple resistance patterns. These findings led to the discovery of resistance transfer factors and were also an early indication of the contribution of conjugative transfer to the natural evolution of new bacterial phenotypes. The first conjugative elements identified were conjugative plasmids, which encode their own transfer functions. These studies also led to the discovery of mobilizable plasmids that do not specify the functions for their transfer, but could use the conjugative functions of other plasmids. These plasmids could either be transferred through cointegrate formation with a conjugative plasmid (a phenomenon also referred to as plasmid conduction) or, more commonly, by using the conjugation apparatus of a self-conjugative plasmid (if they carry an origin of transfer recognized by the conjugation machinery). In addition to plasmid-mediated conjugal transfer, another form of conjugation, conjugative transposition, has been reported in an increasing number of cases (see "Conjugative Transposons" below).

CONJUGATIVE PLASMIDS

Over the last 40 years, an extensive list has been compiled of plasmids carrying antibiotic resistance determinants. It contains more than 500 different plasmids that have been studied in enteric bacteria and pseudomonads, as well as about 60 plasmids characterized mainly in the gram-positive species *S. aureus* and *E. faecalis*. Most of these plasmids are conjugative. More than 25 different groups of plasmids have been defined on the basis of incompatibility (Inc) properties in gram-negative species. Among these, several (especially those from incompatibility groups N, P, Q, and W) are known to have a broad host range and, therefore, are able to transfer and replicate in remote bacterial species. The host range spectrum depends on many traits, including the replication and maintenance functions, the ability of plasmid-encoded markers to be expressed in the new host, and the specificity of the conjugative apparatus. The different types of conjugative plasmids use different and distinct transfer systems. They do, however, share two properties. First, conjugation always occurs through the transfer of a single-stranded DNA molecule after nicking at a specific site called *oriT*. Second, usually the expression of the plasmid-encoded genes needed for conjugative transfer is tightly regulated so as to minimize the burden on the host.

Three distinct bacteria-to-bacteria transfer systems have been the focus of study: those found in F and IncP plasmids of gram-negative bacteria, and the pheromone-regulated plasmids of the gram-positive bacterium *Enterococcus faecalis*. Broad host range plasmids found in streptococci and staphylococci have also been studied to a certain extent.

Gram-Negative Plasmids. The bacterial conjugation system encoded by the F sex factor was the first to be described and subjected to detailed analysis (28). F belongs to a large group of plasmids that encode a common transfer *(tra)* mechanism, which includes several Inc subgroups (31). Many of the F-like plasmids carry determinants for antibiotic resistance or for toxin and hemolysin production.

IncP plasmids, such as the R plasmids RK2 and RP4, have been studied widely because of their ability to transfer between and stably replicate themselves in almost all gram-negative bacterial species (63). In laboratory conditions, they can also promote conjugative transfer of DNA from gram-negative bacteria to gram-positive bacteria as well as to yeast. Furthermore, there is evidence of a genetic relationship between IncP conjugation and the bacteria-to-plant DNA transfer system of *Agrobacterium tumefaciens* (T-DNA transfer). Transfer frequencies of IncP plasmids are very high (upward of one per donor per hour).

Gram-Positive Plasmids. Several enterococcal plasmids encoding virulence factors and/or resistance genes have been shown to transfer very efficiently in liquid cultures among enterococci. As for the gram-negative plasmids described above, their transfer is tightly regulated, and a sex-pheromone recognition mechanism controls their dissemination. The most extensively studied plasmids from this group are pAD1, encoding hemolysin-bacteriocin production and UV resistance (11); pCF10, encoding tetracycline resistance (20); and pPD1, encoding bacteriocin production (36). Plasmid-free cells secrete multiple sex pheromones that trigger the donor cells to express transfer functions. Thus pheromone accumulation in the medium indicates to donors that recipients are in close vicinity. These pheromones are short, linear, hydrophobic peptides excreted in tiny amounts. As few as 1 to 10 molecules of a pheromone per donor is sufficient to initiate the mating process. A plasmid-free strain will secrete several pheromones (at least five) that are specific for the corresponding conjugative plasmid. When such a strain receives a conjugative plasmid, the production of the corresponding pheromone is stopped, whereas secretion of the remaining pheromones continues. Pheromones induce the coordinated expression of different genes and gene sets involved in mating and DNA transfer functions. This system of recipient recognition through a pheromone-mediated pathway is very sophisticated and unique among plasmids studied to date; however, this specialization may also be a factor that limits the host range of these plasmids.

The two most extensively studied examples of conjugative broad host range streptococcal plasmids are pIP501 (64) and pAMbeta-1 (32), which are both about 30 kb in size. pIP501 confers inducible resistance to MLS and chloramphenicol. pAM1beta-1 confers constitutively expressed MLS resistance. Both plasmids are able to transfer and replicate in many gram-positive species, and pAM1beta-1 conjugative functions have been demonstrated to work in gram-positive to gram-negative transfer.

Another type of broad host range plasmid found in gram-positive bacteria was identified after the emergence of gentamicin resistance among staphylococci in the mid-1970s, for which plasmid pGO1 is the prototype (44). pGO1 is a 52-kb plasmid that carries a gene for a bifunctional AAC (6') APH (2") enzyme that confers resistance to several aminoglycosides, a *qac* gene encoding resistance to quaternary ammonium compounds, and a DHFR gene conferring trimethoprim resistance. In laboratory experiments, pGO1 transfers at low frequency (10^4 to 10^6 transconjugants per donor), and the signals that modulate or trigger the conjugation are not known.

CONJUGATIVE TRANSPOSONS

Conjugative transposons were first found in gram-positive cocci but are now known to be present in a variety of clinically important groups of gram-positive and gram-negative bacteria (8). They were first identified when the transfer of antibiotic resistance determinants occurred in the absence of plasmids. Conjugative transposons are discrete elements that are normally integrated into a bacterial genome. Their transposition and transfer are thought to start by an excision event and the formation of a covalently closed circular intermediate, which can integrate either elsewhere in the same cell or into the genome of a recipient cell following self-transfer by conjugation. In contrast to conjugative plasmids, their propagation through integration in the host genome emancipates transposons from the constraint of a compatible replication system. This property certainly contributes to the broad host range that is observed for several of them, and led Salyers and collaborators to suggest that conjugative transposons may be as important as conjugative plasmids in broad host range gene transfer between some species of bacteria (54a).

Conjugative transposons are not considered typical transposons as they have a covalently closed circular transposition intermediate and they do not duplicate the target site when they integrate. At present, five different families of conjugative transposons have been established: (i) the Tn916 family (originally found in streptococci but now known also to occur in gram-negative bacteria such as *Campylobacter*); (ii) the *S. pneumoniae* family (Tn5253); (iii) the

Bacteroides family; (iv) Ctnscr94, a conjugative transposon found in enterobacteria; and (v) the SXT element found in *V. cholerae*. Two other mobile elements are also conjugative elements that integrate rather than replicate and behave like conjugative transposons. The sizes of the different conjugative transposons range from 15 to 150 kb, and all but the Ctnscr94 have been identified through their capacity to transfer resistance genes. Indeed, in, addition to other resistance genes, most encode tetracycline resistance determinants (e.g., Tn916 encodes the TetM determinant, and the TetQ determinant is found on the conjugative transposons from the *Bacteroides* group), while the SXT element encodes resistance to sulfamethoxazole, trimethoprim, chloramphenicol, and streptomycin. These transposons use an integration machinery similar to that of lambdoid phages, and all characterized elements carry an *int* gene. However, the target specificity for their integration varies considerably; Tn916 behaves more like a real transposon (i.e., with a poor specificity), while other elements behave more like lambdoid phages and have a higher specificity. For example, *Bacteroides* elements show a preference for three to seven sites, Ctnscr94 integration is restricted to two sites, and one unique site of integration has been identified for SXT.

By contrast to most conjugative plasmids, elements of the Tn916 or the *Bacteroides* family do not inhibit transfer of further copies or further transposition events. Thus, a strain can accumulate more than one conjugative transposon, the only limitation being their site specificity. Flannagan and Clewell have observed that the presence of two copies of Tn916 in the same strain results in a stimulation of transposition, a phenomenon termed "transactivation" (22a).

Where does conjugation take place in the environment? This is a difficult question to answer, but an ideal site for gene transfer is the warm, wet, nutrient-rich environment of the mammalian intestinal tract with its associated high concentration of bacteria. The resident microflora are believed to serve as a reservoir

for genes encoding antibiotic resistance that could be transferred not only to other members of this diverse bacterial population, but also to transient colonizers of the intestine, such as soil or water microbes or human pathogens. There is clear evidence that identical R plasmids can be identified in pathogen isolates of *Salmonella* as well as in native intestinal flora such as *E. coli*. Several sets of experiments have shown that transfer could occur efficiently even between distantly related bacteria in such an environment, for both conjugative plasmids and transposons. Using oligonucleotide probes having DNA sequence homology to the hypervariable regions of the TetQ determinant, Salyers and coworkers have provided evidence that gene transfer between species of *Bacteroides*, one of the predominant genera of the human intestine, and *Prevotella*, one of the predominant genera of livestock rumen, has taken place under physiological conditions.

MECHANISMS OF CAPTURE

Composite Transposons

As mentioned in the introductory section, bacteria isolated during the preantibiotic era did not carry antibiotic resistance determinants, yet they harbored conjugative plasmids from the same compatibility group as the R plasmids. Therefore, the multiple-resistance plasmids found in pathogens must have arisen within the past 5 decades. What really takes place when a new antimicrobial agent is introduced and plasmid-determined resistance develops within a few years? The most significant component in the process of antibiotic resistance flux in the microbial population is gene capture by way of transposons, which can move from replicon to replicon, be they chromosomes or episomes.

The crucial question is, "How do transposons acquire these resistance genes?" The answer has been found for two types of transposons: composite transposons, found in both gram-positive and gram-negative species, and transposons harboring an integron, which are mainly observed in *Enterobacteriaceae*. Composite transposons can be constructed when an insertion sequence inserts on either side of any gene or cluster of genes. Most of these mobile elements carry only one or two resistance loci (e.g., Tn9, Tn10, Tn903, Tn1546, Tn4001, Tn4003, Tn4351, and Tn4400) and rarely more (e.g., three in Tn5). Conversely, integrons do not rely on random processes and therefore offer more flexibility.

Integrons

Integrons were discovered in the late 1980s through the observation that transposons with different antibiotic resistance spectra shared the same backbone and differed only in the resistance genes they harbored. It is clear, however, that integrons were definitely part of the first multidrug resistance outbreaks in the 1950s, as attested to by the involvement of Tn21, an integron-containing transposon, in the very first events. Restriction mapping and heteroduplex analysis of various plasmids and transposons (such as Tn21) revealed that the different resistance genes were flanked by identical sequences with no obvious relationship to insertion sequences. Nucleotide sequence analysis confirmed that the resistance genes were integrated at a specific site. The mechanism has been dissected genetically and biochemically. Integrons are, in essence, natural gene cloning and expression systems. The functional integron platform consists of three key elements: a gene coding for an integrase (intI) of the tyrosine recombinase family, a proximal primary recombination site (attI), and a strong promoter. The integrase mediates recombination between the attI site and a secondary target called an attC site (or 59-base element [50]). The attC site is generally associated with a single open reading frame (ORF) in a circular structure termed a "gene cassette," and the gene cassette constitutes the mobile component of the system. Insertion of the gene cassette at the attI site places it downstream of a promoter, P_c, within the intI gene that drives expression of the encoded proteins. The most notable gene cassettes code for antibiotic resistance determinants, and the stockpiling and/or replacement of these cassettes can produce integrons con-

taining several antibiotic resistance genes in tandem (called "multiresistant integrons" [MRIs]). MRIs have contributed substantially to the current dilemma in the treatment of infectious disease, as MRIs containing up to eight resistance gene cassettes have been found in multiresistant clinical isolates. At present, more than 70 different resistance cassettes have been described that enable bacteria to resist most of the antibiotic classes used against gram-negative bacteria. Most of their associated attC sites are unique in length (from 53 to 141 bp) and sequence. Thus, contrary to integrases of the λ family, those from the integrons are able to efficiently recombine DNA sequences with little homology.

Five classes of MRIs have been defined based on the homology of the integrase genes, and they share between 45 and 58% amino acid identity (52). The common association of MRIs with mobile DNA elements facilitates the transit of the resistance genes that have been amassed by integrons across phylogenetic boundaries and augments the impact of integrons on bacterial evolution. The proficiency of this partnership is confirmed by the marked differences in codon usage among cassettes within the same MRI, indicating that the antibiotic resistance determinants are of diverse origins.

Integrase-catalyzed insertion of resistance gene cassettes into resident integrons has been demonstrated. In addition, site-specific deletion and rearrangement of the inserted resistance gene cassettes can result from integrase-catalyzed events. It has also been shown that the class 1 integrase can act on secondary target sites at significant frequencies; two R plasmids can be fused by interaction between the recombination hot spot of one plasmid and a secondary integrase target site on the other. However, even if the mechanisms of cassette acquisition and loss are well understood, many important details remain to be elucidated. For example, what are the origins of the integrons and their cassettes, and how are gene cassettes formed?

Until recently, integrons were thought to be dedicated to the capture and dissemination of antibiotic resistance genes. However, the divergence among the five classes of MRI inte-grases suggested that their evolutionary history extended over a much longer period than the 50 years of the antibiotic era. Examination of the relationship between MRI gene cassette arrays and a cluster of repeated sequences in the *V. cholerae* genome (the VCRs, for *V. cholerae* repeated sequences) revealed a striking struc-tural similarity (Fig. 3). Both the VCR cluster and antibiotic-resistance integrons possess spe-cific integrases that are responsible for the insertion of coding sequences (ORFs) into a unique chromosomal attachment site, leading to the formation of tandem arrays of genes. Further characterization of the VCR cluster led to the discovery of a distinct type of integron, designated a superintegron (SI), in the *V. cholerae* genome (42). The *V. cholerae* SI, clustered in one region of chromosome II, spanned 126 kb and harbored 214 ORFs in 179 cassettes (27). This corresponded to about 3% of the genome and dwarfed any previously described MRI. The VCRs (the cassette-associated *attC* sites of the *V. cholerae* SI) displayed a strikingly high degree of sequence relatedness, unlike their counterparts the MRIs, and the *V. cholerae* SI cassettes were substrates for the class 1 integrase of MRIs.

A systematic search for similar SI structures among vibrios and more distantly related gen-era revealed that SIs are ancient systems that are widespread among the proteobacteria (54). SIs in the *Vibrionaceae* (this includes *Vibrio, Listonella, Photobacteria,* and *Moritella* species), *Shewanella,* xanthomonads, pseudomonads, nitrosomonads, acidithiobacilli, *Geobacteraceae,* and treponemes share the same general charac-teristics as MRIs and the *V. cholerae* SI, with an integrase gene divergently transcribed from an upstream cluster of gene cassettes. SIs and MRIs possess specific and related integrases, and the integrases of the class 1, 2, and 3 MRIs as well as the *V. cholerae* and *Shewanella oneidensis* SIs have been shown to be active for cassette recombina-tion. Phylogenetic analysis of these SIs revealed that the extent of divergence between their *intI* genes largely adhered to the line of descent among the bacterial species in which they were

found, clearly demonstrating that integrons predate the antibiotic era. Furthermore, no evi-dence suggests that the SI platforms are mobile. Thus, SIs are ancient, sedentary structures that have been steering the evolution of bacterial genomes for hundreds of millions of years. The phylogenetic relationship between MRIs and SIs indicated that SIs are the likely ancestors of the MRIs found in clinical isolates and sug-gested that MRIs evolved from SIs through entrapment in highly mobile structures such as transposons. It therefore appears that, under the heavy selective pressure of liberal antibiotic use, evolutionarily old genetic recombination mechanisms for gene transfer have been adapted to the new antibiotic environment.

Several observations drawn from the struc-tural characteristics of SI cassette arrays may give some clues to enable us to decipher the mechanism of cassette genesis. SIs differ from MRIs in that (i) an almost identical *attC* site is associated with each ORF, (ii) the ORFs encode mostly unknown functions, (iii) a cer-tain number of ORFs possess their own pro-moter, and (iv) some are encoded in the inverse orientation compared to their recombination sequence. A model for the formation of cas-settes through a reverse transcription mecha-nism has been proposed to account for the lack of a promoter in most gene cassettes and the transcription termination characteristics of the *attC* sites. According to the G+C content and codon usage differences observed in the ORFs found in the cassettes of SIs, they must have many different origins, whereas their associated *attC* sites are highly homologous (about 85% sequence identity). This last characteristic sug-gests that the *attC* sites were added to the ORFs inside the bacterial cell. It is conceivable that a VCR could act as primer for a reverse tran-scriptase (RT), but the efficiency of transcrip-tion of DNA from a plethora of foreign sources is likely to be severely compromised, limiting the substrate for the RT enzyme. Furthermore, several integron cassettes have their own promoter and/or are in the opposite orienta-tion compared to the VCR, characteristics incongruent with a VCR primer/RT model. In

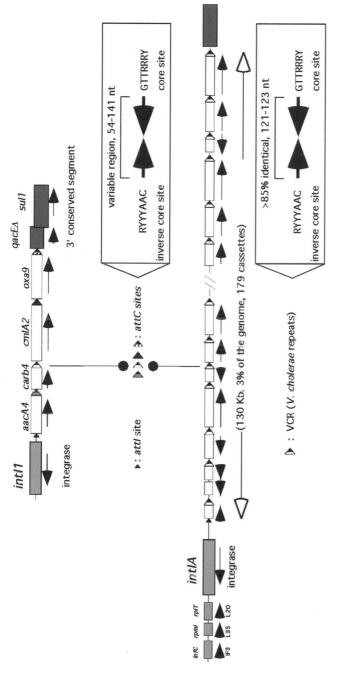

FIGURE 3 Structural comparison of a "classical" mult drug-resistant integron and the *V. cholerae* N16961 superintegron. (Top) Schematic representation of In*40*; the various resistance genes are associated with different *attC* sites (see text). Antibiotic resistance cassettes confer resistance to the following compounds: *aacA4*, aminoglycosides; *cmlA2*, chloramphenicol; *qac*, quarternary ammonium compounds; *oxa9*, β-lactams. The *sul* gene. which provides resistance to sulfonamides, is not a gene cassette. (Bottom) The ORFs are separated by highly homologous sequences, the VCRs.

237

conclusion, it is very likely that the capture process occurs inside the *Vibrio* cells, but its mechanism remains to be established.

Two cassettes in *V. cholerae* SIs code for virulence determinants (a heat-stable enterotoxin and a hemagglutinin), two code for antibiotic resistance genes (a chloramphenicol acetyltransferase and a carbenicillinase), and others code for various metabolic functions. The variety of cassettes within the caches of SIs suggests that virtually any gene has the potential to be structured as a gene cassette. If this is true, then the combined activities of SIs and MRIs may lead to the rapid and widespread dissemination of resistance and virulence genes among clinical and environmental bacterial populations. This notion is underscored by the demonstration that gene cassettes move between SIs and MRIs in vivo. The recruitment process is random, i.e., any gene cassette from the SI could be captured by the MRI. By then specifically applying a selective pressure for antibiotic resistance development, the evolution of an MRI was demonstrated by the recruitment of a novel chloramphenicol antibiotic resistance gene cassette from the SI by the MRI. This demonstrated that the cassettes that are retained within a particular integron are selected in response to the environmental conditions to which the bacterium is exposed.

Because virulence factors, antibiotic resistance, and metabolic genes are present as cassettes in SIs, the cassettes of a particular SI likely play specific roles in the adaptation of the bacterium to its particular niche. Just five *Vibrio* SIs contain a transferable genetic reservoir that is equivalent in size to a small genome. Since the genetic cache of SIs is presumably available to other bacterial species, the potential reservoir of virulence and resistance cassettes available to be propagated by MRIs may be substantial. It should be noted that tandem arrays of resistance genes have been characterized in gram-positive bacteria such as *Staphylococcus aureus*, although no associated intergenic structural element or integrase can be identified.

Analyses of the integron-type transposons provide a good model to understand (i) how antibiotic resistance genes from various unknown sources may be incorporated into an integron by recombination events; (ii) how integrons may subsequently become associated with mobile elements such as transposons, and (iii) how these determinants become relocated onto a plethora of bacterial replicons. The succession of events could produce the R plasmids that we know today. However, in bacterial pathogens a variety of transposable elements have been found that undergo different processes of recombinational excision and insertion. It is not known what evolutionary mechanisms are implicated or whether some form of integron-related structure is present in all cases. For the type of integron found in transposons, we have plausible models, supported by in vivo and in vitro studies, that provide a modus operandi for the cloning of antibiotic resistance genes in the evolution of R plasmids. A large number of transposable elements carrying virtually all possible combinations of antibiotic resistance genes have been identified, and nucleotide sequence analysis of MRIs shows that the inserted resistance gene cassettes differ markedly in codon usage and G+C content, indicating that the antibiotic resistance determinants are of diverse origins. The effect of integron-driven gene capture clearly extends beyond the dissemination of antibiotic resistance and pathogenicity determinants, and this phenomenon is likely to be an important factor in the more general process of horizontal (lateral) gene transfer in the evolution of bacterial genomes.

CHAPTER SUMMARY

- The evolution of antibiotic resistance has occurred over a much shorter time frame than the evolution of pathogenicity.
- The "antibiotic resistance phenomenon" is the rapid and widespread development of similar multiple-antibiotic resistance profiles among phylogenetically diverse clinical isolates during the antibiotic era.
- Resistance phenotypes can evolve through mutations in endogenous genes, which generally cause small and local-

ized changes in a cell. More frequently, the development of resistance is due to the acquisition of genes of exogenous origin, which gives rise to much broader changes and allows evolution to occur in quantum leaps. Because of this, the origin of most resistance genes is unknown.

• Bacteria can use several mechanisms simultaneously to attain high-level resistance to both natural and synthetic antibiotics.

REFERENCES

1. Ainsa, J. A., C. Martin, B. Gicquel, and R. Gomez-Lus. 1996. Characterization of the chromosomal aminoglycoside 2'-N-acetyltransferase gene from Mycobacterium fortuitum. *Antimicrob. Agents Chemother.* 40:2350–2355.

2. Ainsa, J. A., E. Perez, V. Pelicic, F. X. Berthet, B. Gicquel, and C. Martin. 1997. Aminoglycoside 2'-N-acetyltransferase genes are universally present in mycobacteria: characterization of the aac(2')-Ic gene from Mycobacterium tuberculosis and the aac(2')-Id gene from Mycobacterium smegmatis. *Mol. Microbiol.* 24:431–441.

3. Akido, T., K. Koyama, Y. Ishiki, S. Kimura, and T. Fukushima. 1960. On the mechanism of the development of multiple-drug-resistant clones of Shigella. *Jpn. J. Microbiol.* 4:219–227.

4. Berg, D. E., J. Davies, B. Allet, and J. D. Rochaix. 1975. Transposition of R factor genes to bacteriophage lambda. *Proc. Natl. Acad. Sci. USA* 72:3628–3632.

5. Bjorkman, J., D. Hughes, and D. I. Andersson. 1998. Virulence of antibiotic-resistant Salmonella typhimurium. *Proc. Natl. Acad. Sci. USA* 95:3949–3953.

6. Bowler, L. D., Q. Y. Zhang, J. Y. Riou, and B. G. Spratt. 1994. Interspecies recombination between the penA genes of Neisseria meningitidis and commensal Neisseria species during the emergence of penicillin resistance in N. meningitidis: natural events and laboratory simulation. *J. Bacteriol.* 176:333–337.

7. Brown, J. R., J. Z. Zhang, and J. E. Hodgson. 1998. A bacterial antibiotic resistance gene with eukaryotic origins. *Curr. Biol.* 8:R365–R367.

8. Burrus, V., G. Pavlovic, B. Decaris, and G. Guedon. 2002. Conjugative transposons: the tip of the iceberg. *Mol. Microbiol.* 46:601–610.

9. Bush, K., G. Jacoby, and A. Medeiros. 1995. A functional classification scheme for beta-lactamases and its correlation with molecular structure. *Antimicrob. Agents Chemother.* 39:1211–1233.

10. Choury, D., G. Aubert, M. F. Szajnert, K. Azibi, M. Delpech, and G. Paul. 1999. Characterization and nucleotide sequence of CARB-6, a new carbenicillin-hydrolyzing beta-lactamase from Vibrio cholerae. *Antimicrob. Agents Chemother.* 43:297–301.

11. Clewell, D. B., and K. E. Weaver. 1989. Sex pheromones and plasmid transfer in Enterococcus faecalis. *Plasmid* 21:175–184.

12. Daigle, D. M., G. A. McKay, P. R. Thompson, and G. D. Wright. 1999. Aminoglycoside antibiotic phosphotransferases are also serine protein kinases. *Chem. Biol.* 6:11–18.

13. Datta, N., R. W. Hedges, E. J. Shaw, R. B. Sykes, and M. H. Richmond. 1971. Properties of an R factor from Pseudomonas aeruginosa. *J. Bacteriol.* 108:1244–1249.

14. Datta, N., and V. Hughes. 1983. Plasmids of the same Inc groups in Enterobacteria before and after the medical use of antibiotics. *Nature* 306:616–617.

15. Denamur, E., G. Lecointre, P. Darlu, O. Tenaillon, C. Acquaviva, C. Sayada, I. Sunjevaric, R. Rothstein, J. Elion, F. Taddei, M. Radman, and I. Matic. 2000. Evolutionary implications of the frequent horizontal transfer of mismatch repair genes. *Cell* 103:711–721.

16. Dowson, C. G., T. J. Coffey, C. Kell, and R. A. Whiley. 1993. Evolution of penicillin resistance in Streptococcus pneumoniae; the role of Streptococcus mitis in the formation of a low affinity PBP2B in S. pneumoniae. *Mol. Microbiol.* 9:635–643.

17. Dowson, C. G., T. J. Coffey, and B. G. Spratt. 1994. Origin and molecular epidemiology of penicillin-binding-protein-mediated resistance to beta-lactam antibiotics. *Trends Microbiol.* 2:361–366.

18. Dowson, C. G., A. Hutchison, J. A. Brannigan, R. C. George, D. Hansman, J. Linares, A. Tomasz, J. M. Smith, and B. G. Spratt. 1989. Horizontal transfer of penicillin-binding protein genes in penicillin-resistant clinical isolates of Streptococcus pneumoniae. *Proc. Natl. Acad. Sci. USA* 86:8842–8846.

19. Dracobly, A. 2004. Theoretical change and therapeutic innovation in the treatment of syphilis in mid-nineteenth-century France. *J. Hist. Med. Allied Sci.* 59:522–554.

20. Dunny, G. M., M. H. Antiporta, and H. Hirt. 2001. Peptide pheromone induced transfer of plasmid pCF10 in Enterococcus faecalis: probing the genetic and molecular basis for specificity of the pheromone response. *Peptides* 22:1529–1539.

21. Essa, A. M., D. J. Julian, S. P. Kidd, N. L. Brown, and J. L. Hobman. 2003. Mercury resistance determinants related to tn21, tn1696, and tn5053 in enterobacteria from the preantibiotic era. *Antimicrob. Agents Chemother.* 47:1115–1119.

22. Fermer, C., B. E. Kristiansen, O. Skold, and

G. Swedberg. 1995. Sulfonamide resistance in *Neisseria meningitidis* as defined by site-directed mutagenesis could have its origin in other species. *J. Bacteriol.* **177:**4669–4675.

22a. Flannagan, S. E., and D. B. Clewell. 1991. Conjugative transfer of Tn916 in Enterococcus faecalis: trans activation of homologous transposons. *J. Bacteriol.* **173:**7136–7141.

23. Flensburg, J., and O. Skold. 1987. Massive overproduction of dihydrofolate reductase in bacteria as a response to the use of trimethoprim. *Eur. J. Biochem.* **162:**473–476.

24. Fournier, B., A. Gravel, D. C. Hooper, and P. H. Roy. 1999. Strength and regulation of the different promoters for chromosomal beta-lactamases of *Klebsiella oxytoca*. *Antimicrob. Agents Chemother.* **43:**850–855.

25. Galimand, M., G. Gerbaud, M. Guibourdenche, J. Y. Riou, and P. Courvalin. 1998. High-level chloramphenicol resistance in Neisseria meningitidis. *N. Engl. J. Med.* **339:**868–874.

26. Hedges, R. W., and A. E. Jacob. 1974. Transposition of ampicillin resistance from RP4 to other replicons. *Mol. Gen. Genet.* **132:**31–40.

27. Heidelberg, J. F., J. A. Eisen, W. C. Nelson, R. A. Clayton, M. L. Gwinn, R. J. Dodson, D. H. Haft, E. K. Hickey, J. D. Peterson, L. Umayam, S. R. Gill, K. E. Nelson, T. D. Read, H. Tettelin, D. Richardson, M. D. Ermolaeva, J. Vamathevan, S. Bass, H. Qin, I. Dragoi, P. Sellers, L. McDonald, T. Utterback, R. D. Fleishmann, W. C. Nierman, O. White, S. L. Salzberg, H. O. Smith, R. R. Colwell, J. J. Mekalanos, J. C. Venter, and C. M. Fraser. 2000. DNA sequence of both chromosomes of the cholera pathogen *Vibrio cholerae*. *Nature* **406:**477–483.

28. Ippen-Ihler, K. A., and E. G. Minkley, Jr. 1986. The conjugation system of F, the fertility factor of Escherichia coli. *Annu. Rev. Genet.* **20:**593–624.

29. Jordan, E., H. Saedler, and P. Starlinger. 1968. O^0 and strong-polar mutations in the gal operon are insertions. *Mol. Gen. Genet.* **102:**353–363.

30. Lambert, T., G. Gerbaud, and P. Courvalin. 1994. Characterization of the chromosomal aac(6')-Ij gene of *Acinetobacter* sp. 13 and the aac(6')-Ih plasmid gene of *Acinetobacter baumannii*. *Antimicrob. Agents Chemother.* **38:**1883–1889.

31. Lane, H. E. 1981. Replication and incompatibility of F and plasmids in the IncFI group. *Plasmid* **5:**100–126.

32. Leblanc, D. J., and L. N. Lee. 1984. Physical and genetic analyses of streptococcal plasmid pAM beta 1 and cloning of its replication region. *J. Bacteriol.* **157:**445–453.

33. LeClerc, J. E., B. Li, W. L. Payne, and T. A. Cebula. 1996. High mutation frequencies among Escherichia coli and Salmonella pathogens. *Science* **274:**1208–1211.

34. Levin, B. R., V. Perrot, and N. Walker. 2000. Compensatory mutations, antibiotic resistance and the population genetics of adaptive evolution in bacteria. *Genetics* **154:**985–997.

35. Maisnier-Patin, S., O. G. Berg, L. Liljas, and D. I. Andersson. 2002. Compensatory adaptation to the deleterious effect of antibiotic resistance in Salmonella typhimurium. *Mol. Microbiol.* **46:**355–366.

36. Maqueda, M., R. Quirants, I. Martin, A. Galvez, M. Martinez-Bueno, and E. Valdivia. 1997. Chemical signals in gram-positive bacteria: the sex-pheromone system in Enterococcus faecalis. *Microbiologia* **13:**23–36.

37. Marshall, C. G., G. Broadhead, B. K. Leskiw, and G. D. Wright. 1997. D-Ala–D-Ala ligases from glycopeptide antibiotic-producing organisms are highly homologous to the enterococcal vancomycin-resistance ligases VanA and VanB. *Proc. Natl. Acad. Sci. USA* **94:**6480–6483.

38. Martin, C., C. Sibold, and R. Hakenbeck. 1992. Relatedness of penicillin-binding protein 1a genes from different clones of penicillin-resistant Streptococcus pneumoniae isolated in South Africa and Spain. *EMBO J.* **11:**3831–3836.

39. Martinez, E., and F. de la Cruz. 1990. Genetic elements involved in Tn21 site-specific integration, a novel mechanism for the dissemination of antibiotic resistance genes. *EMBO J.* **9:**1275–1281.

40. Martinez, J. L., A. Alonso, J. M. Gomez-Gomez, and F. Baquero. 1998. Quinolone resistance by mutations in chromosomal gyrase genes. Just the tip of the iceberg? *J. Antimicrob. Chemother.* **42:**683–688.

41. Maskell, J. P., A. M. Sefton, and L. M. Hall. 1997. Mechanism of sulfonamide resistance in clinical isolates of *Streptococcus pneumoniae*. *Antimicrob. Agents Chemother.* **41:**2121–2126.

42. Mazel, D., B. Dychinco, V. A. Webb, and J. Davies. 1998. A distinctive class of integron in the *Vibrio cholerae* genome. *Science* **280:**605–608.

43. Mitsuhashi, S., K. Harada, H. Hashimoto, and R. Egawa. 1961. On the drug-resistance of enteric bacteria. *Jpn. J. Exp. Med.* **31:**47–52.

44. Morton, T. M., J. L. Johnston, J. Patterson, and G. L. Archer. 1995. Characterization of a conjugative staphylococcal mupirocin resistance plasmid. *Antimicrob. Agents Chemother.* **39:**1272–1280.

45. Musser, J. M. 1995. Antimicrobial agent resistance in mycobacteria: molecular genetic insights. *Clin. Microbiol. Rev.* **8:**496–514.

46. Nikaido, H. 1998. Multiple antibiotic resistance and efflux. *Curr. Opin. Microbiol.* **1:**516–523.

47. Ouellette, M., L. Bissonnette, and P. H. Roy. 1987. Precise insertion of antibiotic resistance

determinants into Tn21-like transposons: nucleotide sequence of the OXA-1 beta-lactamase gene. *Proc. Natl. Acad. Sci. USA* **84**:7378–7382.

48. **Poole, K.** 2002. Outer membranes and efflux: the path to multidrug resistance in Gram-negative bacteria. *Curr. Pharm. Biotechnol.* **3**:77–98.

49. **Radstrom, P., C. Fermer, B. E. Kristiansen, A. Jenkins, O. Skold, and G. Swedberg.** 1992. Transformational exchanges in the dihydropteroate synthase gene of *Neisseria meningitidis:* a novel mechanism for acquisition of sulfonamide resistance. *J. Bacteriol.* **174**:6386–6393.

50. **Recchia, G. D., H. W. Stokes, and R. M. Hall.** 1994. Characterisation of specific and secondary recombination sites recognised by the integron DNA integrase. *Nucleic Acids Res.* **22**:2071–2078.

51. **Richmond, M. H., and R. B. Sykes.** 1972. The chromosomal integration of a β-lactamase gene derived from the P-type R-factor RP1 in Escherichia coli. *Genet. Res.* **20**:231–237.

52. **Rowe-Magnus, D. A., J. Davies, and D. Mazel.** 2002. Impact of integrons and transposons on the evolution of resistance and virulence. *Curr. Top. Microbiol. Immunol.* **264**:167–188.

53. **Rowe-Magnus, D. A., A.-M. Guerout, and D. Mazel.** 1999. Super-integrons. *Res. Microbiol.* **150**:641–651.

54. **Rowe-Magnus, D. A., A. M. Guerout, P. Ploncard, B. Dychinco, J. Davies, and D. Mazel.** 2001. The evolutionary history of chromosomal super-integrons provides an ancestry for multiresistant integrons. *Proc. Natl. Acad. Sci. USA* **98**:652–657.

54a. **Salyers, A. A., N. B. Shoemaker, A. M. Stevens, and L. Y. Li.** 1995. Conjugative transposons: an unusual and diverse set of integrated gene transfer elements. *Microbiol. Rev.* **59**:579–590.

55. **Schrag, S. J., V. Perrot, and B. R. Levin.** 1997. Adaptation to the fitness costs of antibiotic resistance in *Escherichia coli*. *Proc. R. Soc. Lond. B* **264**:1287–1291.

56. **Shapiro, J. A.** 1969. Mutations caused by the insertion of genetic material into the galactose operon of Escherichia coli. *J. Mol. Biol.* **40**:93–105.

57. **Shaw, K. J., P. N. Rather, R. S. Hare, and G. H. Miller.** 1993. Molecular genetics of aminoglycoside resistance genes and familial relationships of the aminoglycoside-modifying enzymes. *Microbiol. Rev.* **57**:138–163.

58. **Spratt, B. G., L. D. Bowler, Q. Y. Zhang, J. Zhou, and J. M. Smith.** 1992. Role of interspecies transfer of chromosomal genes in the evolution of penicillin resistance in pathogenic and commensal Neisseria species. *J. Mol. Evol.* **34**:115–125.

59. **Spratt, B. G., Q. Y. Zhang, D. M. Jones, A. Hutchison, J. A. Brannigan, and C. G. Dowson.** 1989. Recruitment of a penicillin-binding protein gene from Neisseria flavescens during the emergence of penicillin resistance in Neisseria meningitidis. *Proc. Natl. Acad. Sci. USA* **86**:8988–8992.

60. **Stokes, H. W., and R. M. Hall.** 1989. A novel family of potentially mobile DNA elements encoding site-specific gene-integration functions: integrons. *Mol. Microbiol.* **3**:1669–1683.

61. **Sundström, L., P. Radström, G. Swedberg, and O. Sköld.** 1988. Site-specific recombination promotes linkage between trimethoprim- and sulfonamide resistance genes. Sequence characterization of dhfrV and sulI and a recombination active locus of Tn21. *Mol. Gen. Genet.* **213**:191–201.

62. **Taddei, F., I. Matic, B. Godelle, and M. Radman.** 1997. To be a mutator, or how pathogenic and commensal bacteria can evolve rapidly. *Trends Microbiol.* **5**:427–428, discussion 428–429.

63. **Thomas, C. M., and C. A. Smith.** 1987. Incompatibility group P plasmids: genetics, evolution, and use in genetic manipulation. *Annu. Rev. Microbiol.* **41**:77–101.

64. **Thompson, J. K., and M. A. Collins.** 2003. Completed sequence of plasmid pIP501 and origin of spontaneous deletion derivatives. *Plasmid* **50**:28–35.

65. **Tran, J. H., and G. A. Jacoby.** 2002. Mechanism of plasmid-mediated quinolone resistance. *Proc. Natl. Acad. Sci. USA* **99**:5638–5642.

66. **Tribuddharat, C., and M. Fennewald.** 1999. Integron-mediated rifampin resistance in *Pseudomonas aeruginosa*. *Antimicrob. Agents Chemother.* **43**:960–962.

67. **Wang, M., D. F. Sahm, G. A. Jacoby, and D. C. Hooper.** 2004. Emerging plasmid-mediated quinolone resistance associated with the *qnr* gene in *Klebsiella pneumoniae* clinical isolates in the United States. *Antimicrob. Agents Chemother.* **48**:1295–1299.

68. **Wang, M., J. H. Tran, G. A. Jacoby, Y. Zhang, F. Wang, and D. C. Hooper.** 2003. Plasmid-mediated quinolone resistance in clinical isolates of *Escherichia coli* from Shanghai, China. *Antimicrob. Agents Chemother.* **47**:2242–2248.

69. **Watanabe, T.** 1963. Infective heredity of multiple resistance in bacteria. *Bacteriol. Rev.* **27**:87–115.

70. **Weng, S. F., C. Y. Chen, Y. S. Lee, J. W. Lin, and Y. H. Tseng.** 1999. Identification of a novel beta-lactamase produced by *Xanthomonas campestris,* a phytopathogenic bacterium. *Antimicrob. Agents Chemother.* **43**:1792–1797.

71. **Wu, S., C. Piscitelli, H. de Lencastre, and A. Tomasz.** 1996. Tracking the evolutionary origin of the methicillin resistance gene: cloning and sequencing of a homologue of mecA from a methicillin susceptible strain of Staphylococcus sciuri. *Microb. Drug Resist.* **2**:435–441.

EVOLUTION OF SELECTED PATHOGENIC SPECIES AND MECHANISMS

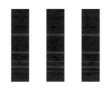

PART III OVERVIEW

James B. Kaper

13

The first two sections of this book deal with broad concepts of microbial evolution, experimental model systems, and the evolution of microbial systems found in a wide variety of organisms. The third and final section presents selected examples to illustrate how the broad concepts apply to specific pathogenic organisms. These examples are informative for similarities as well as differences that are seen among these organisms, and this summary will briefly highlight some interesting aspects of these pathogens.

In chapter 14, Reid and colleagues discuss the evolution of two major gram-positive pathogens, group A *Streptococcus* (GAS) and *Staphylococcus aureus*. Although GAS has always been an important cause of pharyngitis, it had waned as a cause of more serious infections in industrialized countries by the late 1980s. However, the mid-1980s and early 1990s saw a resurgence of serious GAS disease, such as streptococcal toxic shock syndrome, necrotizing fasciitis ("flesh-eating bacteria"), and other infections. The determination of the genome sequence of three GAS strains of different M types and subsequent DNA microarray analysis

of GAS strain collections revealed that bacteriophages account for the majority of variation in gene content among GAS strains. Of the 15 prophages in the three sequenced genomes, 13 encode at least one proven or putative virulence factor, most notably pyrogenic toxin superantigens. The sequence of a particularly virulent M3 strain associated with invasive soft tissue infections revealed the presence of six prophages. Analysis of M3 strains isolated from the 1920s to the present showed that strains with the full complement of phages and virulence factors were isolated only after 1985, which is coincident with the arrival of particularly severe M3 infections.

In contrast to GAS, whose only known reservoir is humans, *S. aureus* causes a wide range of infections in animals as well as humans. Notably, about 30% of healthy people are colonized with this organism, allowing it to evolve not only during the course of disease but also during asymptomatic colonization. Virulence factors in this species are encoded by phages, plasmids, pathogenicity islands (PAIs), and PAI-like elements called staphylococcal cassette chromosomes. One major event in the evolution of this pathogen was an epidemic of toxic shock syndrome (TSS) during the late 1970s associated with *S. aureus* strains expressing what subsequently became known as toxic shock

James B. Kaper, Center for Vaccine Development, Department of Microbiology and Immunology, University of Maryland School of Medicine, Baltimore, MD 21201.

Evolution of Microbial Pathogens, Edited by H. S. Seifert and V. J. DiRita, © 2006 ASM Press, Washington, D.C.

syndrome toxin-1 (TSST-1). Initially it was thought that a single, highly virulent clone was responsible for this epidemic, but microarray analysis revealed considerable variation in gene content among strains associated with TSS, indicating that they were not genetically identical. It therefore appears that the TSS epidemic was caused by a change in the host environment facilitated by technological advances, namely, the use of a new superabsorbent tampon that provided enhanced conditions for *S. aureus* growth and elevated production of TSST-1 by a number of different strains. Another major development in the evolution of *S. aureus* is the emergence of antibiotic resistance in this species. Methicillin-resistant *S. aureus* (MRSA) express a modified penicillin-binding protein encoded by the *mecA* gene, which is present on one of four major forms of staphylococcal cassette chromosomes. An initial theory held that all contemporary strains of MRSA arose from a single progenitor MRSA strain, but multilocus enzyme electrophoresis (MLEE) analysis revealed that MRSA strains have evolved multiple times through horizontal gene transfer of the *mecA* gene to a wide variety of methicillin-susceptible *S. aureus* strains. For years, the last line of treatment for MRSA strains was vancomycin, but in 2002, a strain of *S. aureus* with high-level vancomycin resistance was isolated. Genetic analysis demonstrated that this high-level resistance was encoded by a transposon, Tn*1546*, that was inserted into a conjugative plasmid that also encoded resistance to trimethoprim, beta-lactams, aminoglycosides, and disinfectants (6). The emergence of vancomycin-resistant *S. aureus* is just the latest example of a long series of evolutionary events leading to antibiotic resistance in a wide range of bacterial pathogens.

A much larger group of pathogens involved in intestinal rather than extraintestinal disease is discussed in chapter 15. Lan and Reeves describe the evolution of three important groups of enteric pathogens, *Salmonella enterica*, *Escherichia coli* (including *Shigella*), and *Yersinia* spp. At one time, the genus *Salmonella* was divided into more than 2,000 species based on surface and flagella antigens, but these are now considered to be one species, *S. enterica*, which is subdivided into seven subspecies and 2,501 serovars. The subspecies are well defined on the basis of MLEE and sequencing of housekeeping genes. The evolution of *Salmonella* as a pathogen is closely related to the phylogenetic lineages of these subspecies via the acquisition of PAIs called SPIs. Thus, SPI-1 contains genes for invasion of epithelial cells and is present in all *Salmonella* subspecies but not in its close relative *E. coli*. All subspecies then acquired SPI-2 except subspecies V (sometimes referred to as a distinct species, *Salmonella bongori*), which contains no significant pathogenic forms. Further acquisition of SPIs conferred additional pathogenic capabilities, as did acquisition of plasmids and lysogenic prophages (5). Host specificity also evolved, with some serovars being found only in certain hosts, e.g., Gallinarum (poultry) and Typhi (humans). Some serovars gained the ability to invade into the bloodstream and cause enteric fever (e.g., typhoid fever caused by serovar Typhi), while other serovars remain in the intestine and cause only enterocolitis. The adaptation to invasive disease also apparently involved gene decay, as the genome sequence of *S. enterica* serovar Typhi revealed more than 200 pseudogenes, many of which correspond to genes known to contribute to enterocolitis due to *S. enterica* serovar Typhimurium (4).

An enteric species that exhibits much greater diversity than *S. enterica* is *E. coli*. This species is an important member of the human intestinal commensal flora as well as a remarkably versatile pathogen of humans and animals. Different pathotypes of *E. coli* can cause a wide spectrum of disease ranging from diarrhea and dysentery to meningitis, urinary tract infections, and toxinogenic kidney failure (3). Although a distinction has historically been made between *Shigella* species and *E. coli*, a variety of techniques, including MLEE, ribotyping, and sequencing, have shown that *Shigella dysenteriae*, *S. sonnei*, *S. flexneri*, and *S. boydii*, along with enteroinvasive *E. coli*, constitute a single pathotype of the species *E. coli*. *Shigella* are restricted to human infections, in contrast to several other pathotypes of *E. coli* that can also infect animals, albeit with host-specific colonization factors. Pathogenicity islands were first described in uropathogenic *E. coli* (UPEC) and then recognized to occur in a wide variety of pathogenic bacteria (see chapter 5). Different PAIs in different *E. coli* pathotypes are frequently found in the same chromosomal location, suggesting "hot spots" for insertion of such elements. For example, PAI I of UPEC strain 536 is inserted at the *selC* tRNA gene, as is the locus of enterocyte effacement PAI of enteropathogenic *E. coli* strain E2348/69. In addition to PAIs, other mobile genetic elements encode *E. coli* virulence factors, including plasmids, bacteriophages, and transposons. Acquisition of these mobile genetic elements can usually but not always be correlated with phylogenetic lineages established by MLEE and other techniques.

Although the ability of *E. coli* to cause disease is not a new development (Theodor Escherich himself first suggested that the *Bacterium coli commune* organisms he had previously described as normal intestinal inhabitants of healthy individuals might also be associated with infections of the intestine and urinary tract), certain particularly virulent clones of pathogenic *E. coli* have emerged in the last quarter century. For example, enterohemorrhagic *E. coli* O157:H7 was first reported in 1983, and its emergence and spread have been aided by technological developments in the fast food industry. Although particularly virulent clones exist, an argument can be made that pathogenic *E. coli* represent a spectrum of pathogens with varying combinations of virulence factors encoded on mobile genetic elements, a situation that complicates our efforts to categorize the various subgroups into sharply delineated pathotypes. Genome sequence data indicate a mosaic genomic structure wherein different *E. coli* pathotypes share lower percentages of common genes than are seen in other pathogenic species. The available sequences for the UPEC (5.0 Mb), enterohemorrhagic *E. coli* (5.1 Mb), and nonpathogenic K-12 (4.3 Mb) strains predict a total of 7,638 unique proteins in one or more strains. However, only 39.2% of these proteins

are shared by all three strains. This figure is strikingly different from the situation in GAS, where 1.7 Mb of the 1.9-Mb genome is shared by all GAS strains (chapter 14).

The genus *Yersinia* contains three species that are pathogenic for humans: *Y. pseudotuberculosis* and *Y. enterocolitica,* which are food- and waterborne pathogens that cause enterocolitis, and *Y. pestis,* the causative agent of plague, which is transmitted primarily by fleas but also by aerosols. The first two species share a 70-kb virulence plasmid that encodes a number of proteins (e.g., Yops) that help the organisms evade host defenses plus several chromosomally encoded virulence factors, such as invasin, which mediates cell invasion. The other major virulence determinant is a PAI called HPI (for "high-pathogenicity island") that is present in some but not all strains of these species. Given its limited distribution in *Yersinia,* acquisition of HPI appears to be recent, and variants of HPI have also been found in *Klebsiella, Citrobacter,* and some *E. coli* strains. In contrast to *Y. enterocolitica,* which comprises seven biotypes and >70 serotypes, and *Y. pseudotuberculosis,* which contains 15 serogroups with 21 types, *Y. pestis* appears to be a phenotypically homogeneous species with only one serotype and three biovars. *Y. pestis* is a recently emerged clone that shares 99.7% identity in 16S ribosomal RNA with *Y. pseudotuberculosis* and might more properly called *Y. pseudotuberculosis* Pestis. This clone has acquired additional virulence factors such as *Yersinia* murine toxin (Ymt) and plasminogen activator (Pla) that allow it to colonize the flea gut, be transmitted to a new host via biting, and disseminate hematogenously from the infected site. Both Ymt and Pla are encoded on plasmids that are *Y. pestis* specific and not found in *Y. enterocolitica* or *Y. pseudotuberculosis.*

One other common theme of the enteric pathogens discussed in chapter 15 concerns the taxonomic status of pathogenic clones. Prior to recent molecular advances in our understanding of microbial evolution and systematics, many pathogens were seen as such distinct organisms that full species or even genus status was given to forms that can now be seen as clones of another species. The specific examples among the enterics are the Typhi serovar of *S. enterica,* the Pestis clone of *Y. pseudotuberculosis,* and the *Shigella* clones of *E. coli.* All three contain many pseudogenes, and the authors suggest that these pathogenic clones are losing many of their more general species properties as they become adapted to new niches. Other taxonomic anomalies are found outside the enterics, e.g., *Bordetella pertussis,* and as additional genomes are sequenced, other examples will undoubtedly be found.

Chapters 14 and 15 concern acute bacterial infections caused by *Streptococcus, Staphylococcus,* and the *Enterobacteriaceae.* In chapter 16, Pym and Small discuss the evolution of the organism responsible for chronic infections in approximately one-third of the world's population, *Mycobacterium tuberculosis.* An important distinction exists within the genus *Mycobacterium* with regard to growth rate, with the three obligate human pathogens *M. tuberculosis, M. leprae,* and *M. ulcerans* among the slow-growing species in this genus. Evolutionary studies indicate that fast growth was the ancestral phenotype in this genus, but the development of the slow-growth phenotype undoubtedly helps explain the success of these species in chronic infections lasting for decades. A notable observation from the genome sequences of several *Mycobacterium* species is the small genome size of the pathogenic mycobacterium (3.3 to 4.6 Mb) compared to the fast-growing environmental species *M. smegmatis* (ca. 7.0 Mb). This genomic downsizing is most pronounced with the obligate intracellular pathogen *M. leprae,* whose 3.3-Mb genome has undergone extensive gene deletion and decay. Less than half of the *M. leprae* genome (49.5%) contains functional genes, but 27% of the genome consists of pseudogenes that have intact counterparts in *M. tuberculosis* (1). Many important metabolic features necessary for extracellular growth have been eliminated in the genomic downsizing of *M. leprae.* Reduced genomes are common in obligate intracellular bacteria, but downsizing mechanisms differ among pathogenic species.

For example, in *M. leprae* and *Rickettisa prowazekii,* pseudogenes are numerous, whereas in *Mycoplasma,* few pseudogenes are found and outright gene deletion is more prevalent.

M. tuberculosis lacks plasmids and obvious PAIs, but other mobile genetic elements, specifically insertion sequences and bacteriophages, are present in the genome. However, these elements apparently do not encode virulence factors. There is little evidence that horizontal gene transfer has played a dominant role in the recent evolution of *M. tuberculosis* pathogenicity. A very low incidence of single nucleotide polymorphisms was found in more than 50 structural genes studied in a large collection of strains, and the synonymous substitution rate in *M. tuberculosis* is about 2 orders of magnitude less than that observed for other bacteria such as *E. coli, Helicobacter pylori,* and *Neisseria meningitidis.* The lack of sequence diversity indicates that this species has undergone clonal expansion after recently emerging from a bottleneck some 15,000 to 36,000 years ago. The low genetic heterogeneity of *M. tuberculosis* nonetheless does allow individual strains to be differentiated using a variety of approaches, and with these, clonal families have now been described. These studies have suggested a phylogeographical structure for *M. tuberculosis* in which segregated human populations have been colonized by specific clones. Clonal associations probably reflect the historical or prehistorical dissemination of *M. tuberculosis* with human migrations, similar to the associations that have been established for *H. pylori* (2).

In the final chapter of this section (chapter 17), Steenbergen and Casadevall discuss the evolution of human fungal pathogens, which did not emerge as major human pathogens until the late 20th century. The most important factor accounting for this emergence is not a change in the pathogens but rather a significant change in the host population, namely, the far greater numbers of immunocompromised individuals now present in the population. The increase in such individuals and in individuals in whom other nonspecific defenses have been diminished is due in large part to advances in medical technology, such as steroid therapies, chemotherapy for malignancies, broad-spectrum antibiotics, indwelling catheters, and new surgical procedures. In addition, the AIDS epidemic has had an enormous influence on the rate of symptomatic fungal infection. This is illustrated by the prevalence of cryptococcosis in the United States, which prior to the AIDS epidemic was estimated at 1 to 2 cases per million but by the 1990s approached 1 case per 100,000 in several cities. The low incidence of symptomatic disease among immunocompetent individuals sharply contrasts with the high frequency of infection in the general population, which for *Cryptococcus neoformans* exceeds 90% in New York City based on seroprevalence studies.

The great diversity of fungi, among which pathogenic species are dispersed across three phyla, plus the lack of information on virulence factors and the pathogenesis of fungal infections make the promulgation of generalized concepts for the evolution of fungal pathogens extremely difficult, if not impossible. One general theme that frequently appears, however, is the phylogenetic interspersal of nonpathogenic and pathogenic fungi, implying that the potential for human pathogenicity has independently arisen several times in the evolutionary history of fungi. Microevolution resulting from genetic rearrangements and point mutations can be responsible for the development of new strains and variants of a species. An important example of such a process is the development of fluconazole-resistant strains of *Candida* through selection of various point mutations during treatment. Macroevolution describes evolutionary changes occurring at the level of species and above. Although convincing evidence for horizontal gene transfer is so far lacking, macroevolution is aided in many human pathogenic fungi by their capacity to reproduce both sexually and clonally. Sexual reproduction results in a population structure in which all individuals are genetically different as a result of gene recombination and reassortment. Clonal

reproduction results in a population structure in which the individuals are each related to a common ancestor and diverge by the accumulation of mutation, gene gain and loss, duplication, and other processes. The capacity to undergo both types of reproduction can lead to mixed populations in which some members are clonally related and others have sexual origins. The great diversity of human fungal pathogens, the paucity of information about the pathogenic mechanisms, and the ever-increasing numbers of individuals susceptible to fungal infections ensure that this will be a fertile field of study for the foreseeable future.

Studying the evolution of microbial pathogens is unlike studying the evolution of any other organism. The incredibly short generation times of microorganisms mean that the evolutionary data set is not merely a static collection of ancient fossil records and sequence information on contemporary organisms. Rather, it is a dynamic chronicle of evolution occurring on a daily basis in a process that is influenced by host immune systems, technological advances, and other factors as described in these chapters. Because of this ongoing evolution, the field of infectious diseases is unlike any other area of medicine. Textbooks from 30 years ago in areas such as cardiology or gastroenterology would contain the same basic cardiovascular or gastroenterological diseases that are found in today's textbooks. Obviously there have been tremendous advances in the diagnosis, treatment, and understanding of these diseases over the last 30 years, but the basic disease syndromes remain the same. However, today's textbooks of medical microbiology and infectious diseases contain chapters on diseases that were unknown 30 years ago, such as AIDS, toxic shock syndrome, and Legionnaires' disease. In some cases, such as Legionnaires' disease, archived clinical specimens may reveal that the disease existed decades ago but appropriate diagnostic techniques did not yet exist. But in many other cases, new pathogens have emerged via the processes described in this book, and changes in technology, the environment, or sexual practices helped to amplify and enhance the transmission of these organisms. In the late 1960s, the U.S. Surgeon General declared that it was "time to close the book on infectious diseases" since vaccines and antibiotics had greatly diminished the threat of infectious diseases. As documented repeatedly in this volume, new chapters in the "book" on infectious diseases continue to be written as a result of the evolution of microbial pathogens.

REFERENCES

1. Cole, S. T., K. Eiglmeier, J. Parkhill, K. D. James, N. R. Thomson, P. R. Wheeler, N. Honore, T. Garnier, C. Churcher, D. Harris, K. Mungall, D. Basham, D. Brown, T. Chillingworth, R. Connor, R. M. Davies, K. Devlin, S. Duthoy, T. Feltwell, A. Fraser, N. Hamlin, S. Holroyd, T. Hornsby, K. Jagels, C. Lacroix, J. Maclean, S. Moule, L. Murphy, K. Oliver, M. A. Quail, M. A. Rajandream, K. M. Rutherford, S. Rutter, K. Seeger, S. Simon, M. Simmonds, J. Skelton, R. Squares, S. Squares, K. Stevens, K. Taylor, S. Whitehead, J. R. Woodward, and B. G. Barrell. 2001. Massive gene decay in the leprosy bacillus. *Nature* **409:**1007–1011.

2. Falush, D., T. Wirth, B. Linz, J. K. Pritchard, M. Stephens, M. Kidd, M. J. Blaser, D. Y. Graham, S. Vacher, G. I. Perez-Perez, Y. Yamaoka, F. Megraud, K. Otto, U. Reichard, E. Katzowitsch, X. Wang, M. Achtman, and S. Suerbaum. 2003. Traces of human migrations in *Helicobacter pylori* populations. *Science* **299:**1582–1585.

3. Kaper, J. B., J. P. Nataro, and H. L. Mobley. 2004. Pathogenic *Escherichia coli*. *Nat. Rev. Microbiol.* **2:**123–140.

4. Parkhill, J., G. Dougan, K. D. James, N. R. Thomson, D. Pickard, J. Wain, C. Churcher, K. L. Mungall, S. D. Bentley, M. T. Holden, M. Sebaihia, S. Baker, D. Basham, K. Brooks, T. Chillingworth, P. Connerton, A. Cronin, P. Davis, R. M. Davies, L. Dowd, N. White, J. Farrar, T. Feltwell, N. Hamlin, A. Haque, T. T. Hien, S. Holroyd, K. Jagels, A. Krogh, T. S. Larsen, S. Leather, S. Moule, P. O'Gaora, C. Parry, M. Quail, K. Rutherford, M. Simmonds, J. Skelton, K. Stevens, S. Whitehead, and B. G. Barrell. 2001. Complete genome sequence of a multiple drug resistant *Salmonella enterica* serovar Typhi CT18. *Nature* **413:**848–852.

5. Thomson, N., S. Baker, D. Pickard, M. Fookes, M. Anjum, N. Hamlin, J. Wain, D. House, Z. Bhutta, K. Chan, S. Falkow, J. Parkhill, M. Woodward, A. Ivens, and G. Dougan. 2004. The role of prophage-like elements in the diversity of *Salmonella enterica* serovars. *J. Mol. Biol.* **339:**279–300.

6. Weigel, L. M., D. B. Clewell, S. R. Gill, N. C. Clark, L. K. McDougal, S. E. Flannagan, J. F. Kolonay, J. Shetty, G. E. Killgore, and F. C. Tenover. 2003. Genetic analysis of a high-level vancomycin-resistant isolate of *Staphylococcus aureus*. *Science* **302:**1569–1571.

GROUP A *Streptococcus* AND *Staphylococcus aureus:* EVOLUTION, REEMERGENCE, AND STRAIN DIVERSIFICATION

Sean D. Reid, J. Ross Fitzgerald, Stephen B. Beres, Nicole M. Green, and James M. Musser

14

GROUP A STREPTOCOCCUS

Group A *Streptococcus* (GAS) is a Gram-positive pathogen that causes numerous human diseases, including pharyngitis, skin infections (impetigo, erysipelas, and cellulitis), necrotizing fasciitis, streptococcal toxic shock syndrome (TSS), and septicemia (18, 22, 73). This bacterium also is responsible for nonsuppurative sequelae such as acute rheumatic fever (ARF) and acute glomerulonephritis (18, 22, 73). The only known reservoir of GAS is humans, and the organism is generally disseminated by individuals with symptomatic infection of the mucous membranes or skin, although asymptomatic carriers also can transmit the pathogen (18, 22, 73). Approximately 15 million cases of streptococcal pharyngitis are estimated to occur annually in the United States, representing 15 to 30% of all childhood cases of acute pharyngitis and 5 to 10% of adult cases (17). The annual direct health care costs associated with pharyngitis are approximately 2 billion dollars (23). Globally,

GAS causes extensive human morbidity and mortality, and in the United States, ~11,000 cases of severe invasive disease (http://www.cdc.gov/ncidod/dbmd/abcs/default.htm) and ~220 cases of postpartum GAS infection occur each year.

GAS reemerged as a cause of serious human infections throughout the United States, Europe, and elsewhere in the mid-1980s and early 1990s (73). Disease resurgence, coupled with the lack of a licensed GAS vaccine and growing concerns about the acquisition of antibiotic resistance, has renewed interest in the molecular mechanisms of GAS pathogenesis and the development of new therapeutics. Importantly, the revival of GAS has underscored the need to understand the molecular basis of pathogen variation not solely as a means to discriminate between clinically important strains, but also to provide data relevant to pathogenesis, host adaptation, and the origin of new pathogenic forms (85). GAS is characterized by extensive chromosomal, allelic, and serologic diversity (11, 32, 38, 39, 84, 85, 90). In the first half of this chapter, we highlight key aspects of the genetic variation present in GAS, and relate this diversity to the evolution, reemergence, and strain diversification of this biomedically important human pathogen.

Sean D. Reid, Department of Microbiology and Immunology, Wake Forest University School of Medicine, Winston-Salem, NC 27157. *J. Ross Fitzgerald,* Centre for Infectious Diseases, Medical Microbiology, University of Edinburgh Medical School, Teviot Place, Edinburgh, Scotland, United Kingdom. *Stephen B. Beres, Nicole M. Green and James M. Musser,* Department of Pathology, Baylor College of Medicine, One Baylor Plaza, Houston, TX 77030.

Evolution of Microbial Pathogens, Edited by H. S. Seifert and V. J. DiRita, © 2006 ASM Press, Washington, D.C.

GAS Reemergence

Historically, GAS has been associated with outbreaks of puerperal sepsis, scarlet fever, pharyngitis, and rheumatic fever. In developed nations, improved public health measures and the use of antibiotics contributed to a sharp decline in the incidence of GAS disease between 1940 and 1980. However, epidemiological observations over the last 2 decades suggest a worldwide increase of severe GAS disease and postinfectious sequelae, including streptococcal TSS, invasive disease, soft tissue infections, ARF, and pharyngitis treatment failures (18, 22, 73). Moreover, the infections have not been limited to the extremely young, elderly, or immunocompromised populations, but included seemingly healthy adults.

Until relatively recently, our understanding of genetic variation in GAS was based largely on serologic differences in M protein, a virulence factor attached to the bacterial cell surface that has antiphagocytic properties (33, 34, 60, 61, 88). Recently this serotype scheme of strain classification has been supplanted by sequencing of the hypervariable part of the gene *(emm)* encoding the amino terminus of M protein; >125 *emm* types are currently recognized (8–10, 28–30). This classification scheme

has been useful in many epidemiological investigations. For example, over the past 2 decades, strains expressing certain M protein serotypes have been increasingly associated with specific GAS disease types and resistance to antibiotics (13, 14, 16, 27, 69, 73, 86). Invasive infections are commonly caused by serotype M1 and M3 strains (73), whereas rheumatic fever has been associated with serotypes M1, M3, M5, M6, and especially M18 in the United States (47, 51, 52, 65, 81, 90, 91, 97). Furthermore, resistance to erythromycin, an antibiotic used as an alternative to penicillin, has been repeatedly associated with isolates of serotypes M4, M6, and M12 (6, 7, 86, 96). However, the convention of classifying isolates on the basis of a single surface antigen does not permit study of genetic variation in natural populations occurring in connection with temporal changes in the frequency or character of GAS disease. Use of this single method of typing led many to the incorrect notion that strains of the same serotype were genetically identical or nearly so. It is now known that the population structure of GAS is highly diverse, with strains differing in allelic content, phage content, and complement of virulence factors (Fig. 1) (11). Moreover, it is clear that several mechanisms contribute to

FIGURE 1 Variation in the number, integration site, and virulence gene complement of GAS prophage. The core GAS genome is shown (~1.7 Mb), and phage integration sites are indicated by triangles. The recipient strain is indicated within each triangle. The prophages of each strain are numbered clockwise from the origin of replication (Ori). Stacked triangles indicate that the phages share the same chromosomal integration site. Strain-to-strain variation in phage content and phage-encoded virulence factors may substantially alter strain virulence, resistance to the host innate immune response, and the landscape of the GAS cell surface. This variation may complicate development of novel therapeutics and vaccination strategies. Modified from reference 11.

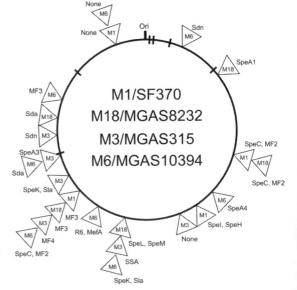

GAS diversity, including point mutations, assortive recombination, and phage acquisition and loss (5, 6, 11, 32, 39, 73, 85, 90).

Extensive chromosome-wide allelic variation in GAS was first revealed by a multilocus enzyme electrophoresis (MLEE) study of genetic diversity and clonal relationships among 108 GAS isolates obtained from patients with invasive disease (70). MLEE indexes allelic variation by assessing differences in the electrophoretic mobility of a set of randomly selected cellular enzymes. Amino acid substitutions that alter protein migration in an electrical field generate mobility variants that can be directly equated with alleles at the corresponding gene locus. The resultant profiles correspond to multilocus genotypes referred to as electrophoretic types (ET). Thirty-two distinct ETs were identified, but more than half of the isolates belonged to only two types, designated ET1 and ET2 (70). These ETs comprised serotypes M1 and M3, respectively. To provide additional information related to strain virulence, the 108 isolates also were examined for the presence of the genes encoding the streptococcal pyrogenic exotoxins A, B, and C (*speA*, *speB*, and *speC*, respectively) (70). The analysis indicated that a statistically significant number of isolates obtained from patients with streptococcal TSS possessed the *speA* gene (70). Hence, study of genetic variation in GAS recovered from clinically relevant human infections provided new insight into host-pathogen relationships.

Extensive Allelic Variation in GAS Structural Genes: Selected Examples

speA VARIANTS AND THE RESURGENCE OF GAS DISEASE

SpeA is one of many pyrogenic toxin superantigens (PTSags) produced by GAS. PTSags such as SpeA simultaneously bind to class II major histocompatibility complex (MHC) and T-cell receptors, resulting in the proliferation of host T cells, massive cytokine production, shock, and sometimes death (56). The identification of streptococcal TSS, and the significant association of SpeA production with organisms causing this syndrome (70), led to study of *speA* allelic diversity. Comparative sequencing of the gene in isolates representing a broad range of ETs identified four alleles, *speA1* through *speA4* (78). The *speA1* allele was found in strains with many distinct chromosomal backgrounds, suggesting that it is the ancestral allele (78). SpeA2 and SpeA3 each differed from the SpeA1 variant by single amino acid replacements in two closely related positions (78). Importantly, strains of ET1 and ET2 recovered before 1950 contained the ancestral *speA1* allele; however, contemporary strains such as M1/ET1 and M3/ET2 had the *speA2* and *speA3* alleles, respectively (72). The association of two variant *speA* alleles with two widely disseminated clones that have caused the majority of invasive disease episodes over the last 2 decades suggested that SpeA2 and SpeA3 differ functionally. The amino acid replacements in SpeA2 and SpeA3 are located near a zinc-binding site believed to be involved in class II MHC recognition. Of note, the SpeA3 variant is more mitogenic and has higher affinity for class II MHC compared to the SpeA1 variant (54). Although the role of SpeA in GAS infections and streptococcal toxic shock is still unclear, these results indicate that these two *speA* allelic variants are genetic markers for very successful clones, and their expression may lead to increased virulence in some forms of GAS infection.

EXTENSIVE STRUCTURAL VARIATION IN THE STREPTOCOCCAL INHIBITOR OF COMPLEMENT

M1 strains of GAS are the most common serotype recovered from invasive disease episodes (73). Heretofore, epidemics of M1 disease were thought to be mono- or pauciclonal. However, investigations into molecular mechanisms responsible for the abundance of M1 organisms in invasive disease led to an analysis of allelic variation in the streptococcal inhibitor of complement (*sic*), a virulence gene primarily found in M1 organisms (42, 44, 92). Sic is an extracellular protein that inhibits the complement C5b-C9 membrane attack complex in vitro by preventing target cell lysis (1). In addition, Sic colocalized with ezrin, a human protein involved in linking the cytoskeleton to the plasma membrane, inside epithelial cells (43). Through interaction with the F-actin-binding site of ezrin, Sic enhances bacterial survival by interrupting cellular processes necessary for GAS internalization and killing (43). Analysis of allelic variation in the *sic* gene in 1,673 M1 GAS isolates obtained from comprehensive, population-based surveillance studies of invasive disease discovered a strikingly high level of diversity among organisms that are otherwise closely related genetically (42, 44, 92). Almost all polymorphisms in the *sic* gene resulted in structural variation due to in-frame insertions and deletions and nonsynonymous substitutions, suggesting that strong positive selective pressure is acting on *sic* (42, 44, 92). Hence, M1 epidemic waves are composed of related strains expressing a remarkably heterogeneous array of Sic variants. A 37-month population-based study found that the majority of GAS isolated from cases of invasive disease were present in a pool of organisms causing pharyngitis in the same geographical location (45). New Sic variants identified among pharyngitis isolates were found an average of 9.8 months earlier than variants among isolates collected from invasive disease episodes in the same location (45). This evidence unambiguously demonstrates rapid mucosal selection of Sic variants and suggests that the abundance of M1 organisms in human infections involves a mechanism in which Sic enhances GAS persistence in the host upper respiratory tract (45). Interestingly, analysis of allelic variation in the *emm1* gene encoding M1 protein revealed no allelic variation, ruling out the idea that diversity at this locus contributes to epidemic waves (45). Very recently, a study by Matsumoto et al. of serotype M1 GAS isolates obtained from 20 patients with acute pharyngitis found that 25% of the patients were infected with a GAS population expressing two Sic variants (67). Thus, Sic variation occurs in vivo at a frequency that results in mixed infections and may contribute to pathogen survival.

MGA REGULON AND THE FIBRONECTIN-COLLAGEN–T ANTIGEN REGION

Two additional loci of the GAS genome, the Mga regulon and the fibronectin-collagen–T antigen (FCT) region, warrant mention because they encode multiple proteins mediating interactions with the host. The Mga regulon includes the global gene regulator *mga* (multigene activator), the *emm* gene, the *scpA* gene encoding C5a peptidase, and, depending on the strain, a varying complement of additional genes encoding secreted proteins implicated in host adherence and invasion (such as Sic and a laminin-binding protein homologue) (11, 32, 90). Similarly, the FCT region includes one of two global regulators *(nra or rofA)*, various genes encoding fibronectin-binding proteins and collagen-binding proteins involved in adherence and invasion, and an allele of the T antigen that is the basis of another serologic typing method (15, 82).

The Mga regulon and the FCT region are composed of segments of DNA with different phylogenetic histories that have been brought together by horizontal transfer and recombination (evidenced by their mosaic structure) (11, 15, 32, 82, 90). For example, the Mga regulons of the sequenced serotype M3 and M18 genomes are identical in gene content (although they have different alleles), with each region encoding six proteins (11, 90). However, they differ from the Mga region present in the genome of the sequenced serotype M1 strain, which has three additional genes (11, 32, 90). Transposons also are present within the Mga region and the FCT region in certain M protein serotypes, but the molecular mechanisms mediating variation at these loci are unknown. It is likely that some of the protein products of the Mga and FCT regions that are ultimately secreted or bound to the GAS cell surface encounter selective pressure from the host immune system. Unique alleles and combinations of genes at these loci may help GAS to escape the host immune system and colonize diverse anatomical sites.

Recombination and Its Impact on GAS Species Diversity and Evolution

Studies of individual GAS genes have shown repeatedly that horizontal gene transfer and recombination contribute substantially to the population diversity and evolution of GAS (11, 15, 32, 82, 90). In the absence of recombination, one would expect the topology of phylogenetic trees generated for individual genes to be similar. A lack of congruency between gene trees is an indicator of past horizontal gene transfer resulting in the interruption of the clonal frame (relic of the ancestral genome) by recombined segments. Multilocus sequence analysis of 12 GAS genes (encoding 11 putative extracellular virulence proteins and one putative regulator) from 37 genetically diverse strains identified low levels of diversity (<7.0% polymorphic nucleotide sites), a relatively unexpected trait for proteins that presumably encounter selective pressure from the host immune system (83). Phylogenetic analysis revealed that the topologies of individual gene trees were not congruent, suggesting the occurrence of recombination (83). In light of these findings, split decomposition analysis was used to determine the extent to which recombination had contributed to chromosomal diversification (Fig. 2). Unlike many other tree-building algorithms, this method does not force the data into a bifurcating tree; rather, in cases of high frequencies of interstrain gene transfer, split decomposition results in a weblike network highlighting each of the different evolutionary pathways that may have led to the extant state. Several alternate evolutionary pathways were identified for each strain representing the 12 M types studied (Fig. 2) (83). These results, together with the restricted allelic variation, suggested that recombination had occurred recently and insufficient time has elapsed for nucleotide polymorphisms to accumulate by other mechanisms (83). The primary discovery of the lack of congruence between gene trees was confirmed by multilocus sequence typing of seven housekeeping genes (83).

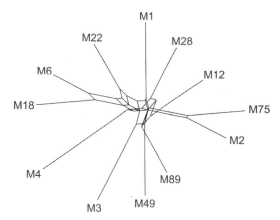

FIGURE 2 Split decomposition analysis of 12 genes from 12 GAS strains representing different M serotypes. The advantage of split decomposition analysis is that it allows us to visualize the extent of past recombination depicted by the number of separate evolutionary branches. Each branch represents one possible pathway to explain the extant state. The more weblike the pathways, the greater the contribution of recombination. In this case, a large number of alternate evolutionary pathways are predicted, underscoring the importance of genetic exchange in the evolution of GAS. Modified from reference 83.

Insights Gained from Comparative Genomics

Complete genome sequences have been published for five GAS strains—serotypes M1 (strain SF370), M3 (strains MGAS315 and SSI1), M6 (strain MGAS10394), and M18 (strain MGAS8232)—with more on the way (6, 11, 32, 77, 90). These serotypes are of particular biomedical interest due to their prevalence in human infections. As noted, serotype M1 strains are the most common cause of pharyngitis and invasive disease episodes in humans, and are often implicated in GAS epidemics (73). Serotype M3 strains cause a disproportionate number of severe invasive infections, such as necrotizing fasciitis and streptococcal TSS (11, 12). A recent study by Sharkawy et al. of GAS soft tissue infections over a 4-year period (1992 to 1996) in Ontario, Canada, found that patients infected with a serotype M3 organism were more likely to develop necrotizing fasciitis (22/40 patients, 55%) (89). Similarly, patients infected with an M3 organism were more likely to die (11/40 patients, 28%) (89). In addition, a recent large population-based study in the United States found serotype M1 and M3 strains to cause a higher rate of lethal infections compared to other serotypes (51). Serotype M6 was recently associated with an outbreak of erythromycin-resistant GAS pharyngitis in Pittsburgh, Pennsylvania (64). Subsequent population genetic analysis indicated that 24% of serotype M6 strains encoded some form of antibiotic resistance. M18 GAS strains have been repeatedly associated with ARF episodes in the United States, including outbreaks of ARF in several localities during the 1980s (90, 91).

The serotype M1, M3, M6, and M18 genomes have much in common, including size (~1.9 Mb), G+C content (~38.6%), and highly conserved rRNA operons (6, 11, 32, 77, 90). Protein coding sequences account for ~87% of each genome, with the majority of coding sequences oriented in the direction of DNA replication. The aligned genomes are collinear in structure (i.e., open reading frames [ORFs] occur in the same order), lack large chromosomal rearrangements, and share ~1.7 Mb (~90%). This conserved sequence constitutes a "core" genome encoding many well-studied proven and putative virulence factors, including pore-forming toxins (streptolysin O and streptolysin S), secreted proteases (streptococcal cysteine protease and C5a peptidase), antiphagocytic surface molecules (M protein, hyaluronic acid capsule, and Mac protein), and PTSags such as streptococcal mitogenic exotoxin Z and streptococcal pyrogenic exotoxin G. This core genetic content is likely responsible for much of what is common to GAS pathogenesis in general.

Interspersed in the core genome of these strains are several regions of inserted sequence that vary in size from 8.3 to 58.8 kb and disrupt the collinear alignment. These regions correspond to prophages. (For simplicity, elements that appear to be prophages or the remnants of such will be referred to as "prophages" with the full understanding of the limitations of this nomenclature.) Each of the five sequenced GAS strains are polylysogenic, that is, they have four to eight largely intact prophages that constitute ~10% of the genome (6, 11, 32, 77, 90). Importantly, the distinct prophages identified thus far by genome sequencing account for the great majority of variation in gene content (up to 74%) between the sequenced strains (Table 1; Fig. 1).

Elements resembling insertion sequences (IS), and numerous smaller insertions, deletions, and regions of variant sequence (the majority of which are <20 bp in size), also contribute to genome-to-genome variation. Although each of the sequenced GAS genomes has many IS-like elements, they rarely disrupt protein

TABLE 1 BLAST comparisons of sequenced GAS genomes' protein coding sequences reveal that phage genes account for the majority of variation in gene content[a]

Coding sequences	M3 vs M1 (TBLASTN)	M1 vs M3 (BLASTP)	M3 vs M18 (TBLASTN)	M18 vs M3 (BLASTP)
Common[b]	1,652/1,894 (87.2%)	1,607/1,752 91.7%	1,753/1,894 92.6%	1,761/1,889 93.2%
Unique[c]	242/1,894 12.8%	145/1,752 8.3%	141/1,894 7.4%	128/1,889 6.8%
Phage and unique	216/242 89.3%	71/145 49.0%	112/141 79.4%	71/128 55.5%

[a] Modified from reference 11.

[b] A protein coding sequence was defined "common" if it had a homologue in the comparison genome sharing greater than 50% positive (identical plus similar) amino acids across its complete sequence.

[c] A protein coding sequence was defined "unique" if it lacked a homologue in the comparison genome sharing greater than 50% positive (identical plus similar) amino acids across its complete sequence.

coding sequences. Finally, the strains differ at the level of single nucleotide polymorphisms (SNPs). SNPs are the most common form of genetic variation and occur once every 100 to 300 nucleotides. A pairwise comparison (MUMmer, www.tigr.org) of MGAS5005, MGAS315, and MGAS8232 indicates that the three genomes differ from each other on average by ~6,672 SNPs, or ~3.5 SNPs per every 1,000 nucleotides of sequence (11). Thus, GAS genome diversification has occurred through multiple processes, with prophages and other mobile genetic elements responsible for the great majority of the variation in gene content.

The availability of genome sequences for five GAS strains facilitates examination of variation in gene content among strains of the same serotype. Whole-genome comparison of 30 serotype M1 strains by DNA microarray revealed unexpectedly high genome differentiation between the sequenced M1 strain SF370 and the majority of strains responsible for contemporary episodes of pharyngitis and invasive disease (94). Strain SF370 differs from abundant M1 GAS strains by ~7% in gene content (94). The majority of test strains examined ($n = 25$) lacked protein coding sequences from three of the four prophages present in SF370 (94). Specifically, 27 of 30 strains lacked prophage SF370.1, the phage containing the virulence factors pyrogenic exotoxin C and a homologue of mitogenic factor. Twenty-seven of 30 strains lacked prophage SF370.2, encoding streptococcal superantigens H and I. All 30 strains had one of three variants of prophage SF370.3. Each of the test strains examined lacked prophage SF370.4, a prophage devoid of virulence factors. Moreover, microarray analysis of strains using the strain SF370 reference gene array supplemented with unique sequences identified in the M3 and M18 genomes revealed that additional prophages were present in M1 strains responsible for abundant contemporary disease episodes (94). These phages contain additional putative virulence factors, including the *speA* gene, which is associated with two widely disseminated clones causing the majority of invasive disease episodes over

the last 2 decades. This analysis indicates that gene content differences among serotype M1 strains are due predominantly to variation in phage content. An analogous conclusion was reached for serotype M18 strains. Moreover, the data provide additional evidence that strain SF370 is genetically divergent relative to M1 strains responsible for most contemporary cases of human morbidity and mortality caused by GAS (94).

Phage and Phage-Encoded Toxins

Perhaps the most important discovery to derive from the comparison of the available GAS genomes is the extent to which prophages contribute to variation in gene content between strains, including genes likely to contribute to GAS pathogenesis. The five sequenced GAS genomes differ in the number of prophages, the composition of one or more prophages, and the position of chromosomal integration (Fig. 1). These prophages are all members of the *Siphoviridae* family of double-stranded DNA (dsDNA) phages, and have similar genome organization, and most share lengthy regions of sequence homology. Phylogenetic analysis of full-length GAS prophage sequences results in phylogenetic topologies that are different from those based on individual phage genes such as integrase or hyaluronidase. This lack of congruency is consistent with the notion that dsDNA bacteriophage genomes are mosaic in structure as a result of lateral transfer of DNA segments from a large common genetic pool (nearly 4,500 dsDNA phages capable of infecting a diverse array of bacterial hosts have been described).

Importantly, the vast majority of prophages present in the five sequenced GAS genomes encode at least one proven or putative virulence factor, many of which were unknown prior to the determination of the genome sequences (6, 11, 32, 77, 90). These factors can be separated into two functional groups, the first composed of PTSags SpeA, SpeC, SpeH, SpeI, SpeK, SpeL, SpeM, and SSA, and the second composed of degradative enzymes, including DNases and a phospholipase A_2. Antibodies against many of these proteins are present in convalescent sera from human patients, indicating that these prophage-encoded molecules are produced during the course of human infection (18, 76, 93). These genes are located adjacent to the phage chromosomal integration site, and some have a G+C content that is not characteristic of the GAS genome or resident prophage. This suggests that some of these putative or proven virulence factor genes were acquired from another organism by lateral gene transfer. To summarize, bacteriophages are a major source of variation in GAS virulence determinant content, and provide a mechanism for assorting virulence factors into new combinations, from which more fit clones can arise rapidly and become abundant (see below, Fig. 3).

Analysis of strain prophage content can provide valuable insight into strain virulence and reemergence. For example, a population-based surveillance study in Ontario, Canada, of invasive soft tissue infections due to GAS revealed that patients infected with serotype M3 organisms were more likely to develop necrotizing fasciitis and were more likely to die from the

infection (89). The genome sequence of a strain representative of M3 organisms isolated from patients with invasive disease revealed the presence of six prophages (11). Included among the putative or proven virulence determinants encoded by these prophages were PTSags SpeA3 and SpeK, streptococcal superantigen, and Sla (a phospholipase A_2 homologue) (11). Importantly, only contemporary M3 isolates (ca. 1985) contained all four of these genes, suggesting the recent emergence and widespread dissemination of an M3 subclone that expresses a unique combination of phage-encoded virulence factors (Fig. 3) (5).

Recombination processes involving phages are expected to occur most often when phage genomes are present within the same cell, such as when two phages coinfect the same cell, or when a phage infects a cell already harboring one or more prophages. Therefore, genetic recombination is likely to occur most commonly between phages with the same host range (i.e., among GAS phages). However, phage host ranges often are broader than a single bacterial species. For example, phage from GAS have been reported to form plaques on

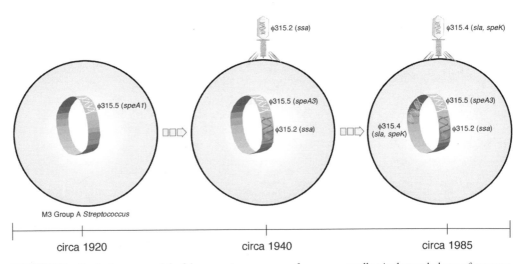

FIGURE 3 Evolutionary model of the recent emergence of a new, unusually virulent subclone of serotype M3 GAS. A single amino acid change in streptococcal pyrogenic exotoxin A (SpeA) and the stepwise acquisition of the bacteriophage-encoded virulence factors streptococcal superantigen (SSA), streptococcal phospholipase A_2 (Sla), and streptococcal pyrogenic exotoxin K (SpeK) have led to the emergence and widespread dissemination of this M3 subclone. Modified from references 5 and 11.

Lancefield group C, G, H, and L streptococci. Consistent with this observation, homologues of the GAS phage-encoded PTSAgs SpeI and SpeH have been identified in the genome of *Streptococcus equi,* a group C *Streptococcus* horse pathogen. These homologues, SePE-I and SePE-H, have 98% amino acid similarity with SpeI and SpeH, respectively, and are located at the end of a prophage in the *S. equi* genome (3). SePE-I and SePE-H may participate in the pathogenesis of strangles, an important disease of young horses (3). Acquisition of the phage encoding these genes is thought to have contributed to the evolution of virulent *S. equi* from its closely related but benign putative ancestor, *Streptococcus zooepidemicus* (3). Similarly, an overlap in the phage host range between GAS and *Staphylococcus aureus* (or recombination between phages infecting these bacteria) has been suggested, given that both organisms produce multiple PTSags with extensive sequence and structural homology. Moreover, many of the *S. aureus* PTSags are encoded by prophages or pathogenicity islands with phage-like elements such as integrases (see below). In fact, the GAS PTSags SpeA and SSA have greater homology with the PTSags of *S. aureus* than with the other PTSags of GAS, suggesting either a cross-species transfer or independent acquisition from a common origin (68). Additionally, comparative genomics has revealed that GAS phages share up to 70% sequence identity across several contiguous genes with phages of *Lactococcus lactis* and *Streptococcus thermophilus* (24). Therefore, given that there are more than 150 GAS *emm* types, and multiple, previously unrecognized prophage-encoded putative virulence factors have been found in each newly sequenced GAS genome, it appears that our current understanding of the breadth of GAS virulence factor diversity represents only a small portion of the genetic population. The results also suggest that the acquisition of bacteriophages confers increased fitness to GAS, and likely contributes to differences in phenotype and pathogen-host interactions in a strain-specific fashion.

STAPHYLOCOCCUS AUREUS

S. aureus causes a wide range of infection types in humans and animals. *S. aureus* infections usually are preceded by colonization, which occurs asymptomatically in about 30% of healthy people (55). *S. aureus* is the most common organism isolated from wound, soft tissue, and bloodstream infections. Common superficial infections include carbuncles, impetigo, cellulitis, and folliculitis. Community-acquired infections such as bacteremia, endocarditis, osteomyelitis, pneumonia, and wound infections are less common. Primary bloodstream infections, pneumonia, and wound infections caused by *S. aureus* are the predominant hospital-acquired infections, responsible for approximately 12% of all nosocomial infections. *S. aureus* also causes economically important mastitis in cows, sheep, and goats.

Population genetic analysis of *S. aureus* has demonstrated that a limited number of clonal lineages are responsible for the majority of infections (75). Moreover, there is very limited cross-species transfer of pathogenic *S. aureus* strains. For example, *S. aureus* clones have evolved the ability to infect specific niches in a variety of host species, including humans, cows, and sheep (53, 75).

A major problem in the treatment of nosocomial infections due to *S. aureus* has been the emergence of strains that are resistant to methicillin and related antimicrobial agents. The first methicillin-resistant *S. aureus* (MRSA) strain was identified in the United Kingdom in 1961, shortly after the introduction of the drug into therapeutic use in humans (50). MRSA strains are now ubiquitous worldwide and are a very significant health care problem. The recent identification of a strain of MRSA that is completely resistant to vancomycin treatment is a very worrisome development because this drug is the only effective treatment for many infections caused by MRSA (95). Discovery of alternative treatments for MRSA-associated infections is now an extremely critical public health goal.

Important advances in our understanding of

the evolution of *S. aureus* have been made in recent years. Genetic analysis of natural populations of *S. aureus* in the late 1980s/early1990s provided the first estimates of the degree of genetic variation among strains associated with disease and resulted in novel insights about the evolutionary relationships of strains (53, 75). More recently, complete genome sequence data for seven *S. aureus* strains, along with DNA microarray and multilocus sequence typing analysis of a large number of strains, has transformed our understanding of genome diversity and evolutionary mechanisms within the species (26, 31). Overall, the population genetic structure of this organism is largely clonal, with no significant differences between populations associated with disease or asymptomatic carriage (31). Diversification within the *S. aureus* population occurs through a combination of mutation, recombination, and horizontal gene transfer.

Historical Review of Population Genetic Analysis of *S. aureus*

Over the years, medical microbiologists have employed many different methods for differentiating among strains of *S. aureus*. Serologic, biochemical, and phage lytic patterns have been used to type pathogenic *S. aureus* strains from diverse sources. However, these methods fail to provide a basis for elucidating the genetic structure of natural populations of *S. aureus* and consequently provide limited information about evolutionary relationships among strains. Phage typing, serotyping, and protein profiling are useful methods for subtyping *S. aureus* into distinct phenotypic groups, but strains of the same phenotype may differ greatly in genetic composition and clonal origin. In the late 1980s, methods were developed that discriminated between strains on the basis of genetic polymorphisms. Such molecular methods allowed the grouping of strains by clonal lineage and the prediction of *S. aureus* evolutionary relationships. These population genetic frameworks are now being used to help guide investigations into microbial virulence and pathogenesis.

HOST SPECIFICITY OF LINEAGES

MLEE has been employed to construct a very detailed population genetic framework for *S. aureus* strains isolated from human and animal infections. Musser and Selander analyzed 2,077 isolates of *S. aureus* recovered from cases of human disease (wound infection, sepsis, endocarditis, TSS, furunculosis, scalded skin syndrome, and food poisoning) and strains of bovine and ovine mastitis origin (75). A total of 252 distinctive multilocus genotypes were identified, among which 14 major lineages were found. Thirty-three sublineages diverged from one another at genetic distances greater than 0.25. The majority of isolates were assigned to 3 of the 14 major lineages, and only 6 of the 33 distinct sublineages were shared between cows and humans. Hence, isolates of the great majority of multilocus enzyme genotypes are associated with only one host species, implying that successful cross-species transfer is rare in nature. The bovine host specialization phenotype is distributed narrowly throughout the dendrogram, indicating that the ability to specialize on cows arose relatively few times in the course of *S. aureus* evolution (75).

Kapur et al. used MLEE to perform a comprehensive population genetic analysis of *S. aureus* strains isolated from episodes of bovine mastitis (53). Almost 90% of isolates examined were assigned to one of eight multilocus enzyme genotypes, indicating that the majority of bovine *S. aureus* isolates belong to a small number of extant clones and that these clones have broad geographical distribution. Furthermore, 29% of all isolates were of a single genotype, designated ET3. The overall genetic diversity among bovine isolates is less than that found among human isolates, indicating that only a small subset of extant *S. aureus* clones commonly causes infections of the bovine udder. The limited cross infection of strains between different host species suggests that these clones have evolved the mechanisms required to survive preferentially in the bovine intramammary milieu (53). The genome of an *S. aureus* strain (RF122) representative of the common bovine MLEE genotype, ET3, has been recently sequenced (40). Several genetic loci have been identified in RF122 that are not present in genomes of the human *S. aureus* strains that have been sequenced. Further analysis of these loci may provide important insights into the host specificity of *S. aureus*.

PREDOMINANCE OF A SINGLE CLONE IN MOST CASES OF FEMALE UROGENITAL TSS

MLEE also has been used to analyze chromosomal relationships among *S. aureus* strains expressing toxic shock syndrome toxin-1 (TSST-1), recovered mainly from cases of TSS that occurred during the TSS epidemic of the late 1970s (74). The *tst* gene was identified among strains from several different clonal lineages, suggesting that horizontal gene transfer has contributed to the distribution of the *tst* gene among *S. aureus* strains. However, a single clone (ET234) accounted for 88% of cases of TSS with a female urogenital focus. This observation led to two plausible theories for the occurrence of the TSS epidemic. A single mutation may have produced a strain of *S. aureus* that is highly adapted to the female urogenital tract and that subsequently spread very rapidly among the human population. Alternatively, a change in the host environment led to conditions favorable for infection and disease caused by an extant TSST-1-producing organism. To address this question, an *S. aureus* DNA microarray was used to compare strains of the common female urogenital TSS clone ET234 (37). Phylogenetic analysis based on variation in gene content of the strains examined showed that ET234 strains were indeed closely related and had a common ancestor (Fig. 4). However, there was considerable variation in gene content among the strains, indicating that they were not genetically identical and that the last common ancestor has not been very recent in evolutionary time. Thus, the TSS epidemic was caused by a change in the host environment

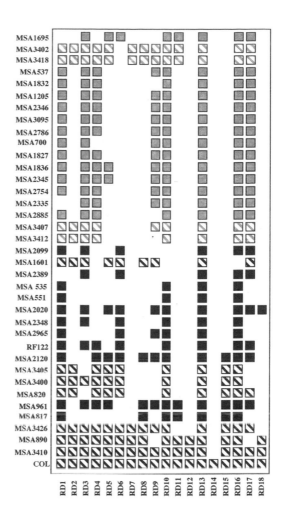

FIGURE 4 Presence or absence of large chromosomal regions of difference (RDs) in 36 *S. aureus* isolates examined by whole-genome DNA microarray analysis. A square symbol denotes presence of an RD and an empty space its absence. Hatched squares indicate presence of RDs in MRSA strains. Gray signifies ET234 strains. Modified from reference 37.

rather than by rapid spread of a single new hypervirulent clone (37). The change in the host environment was linked to the use of a new superabsorbent tampon that may have provided enhanced conditions for *S. aureus* growth and elevated production of TSST-1, the toxin responsible for many of the symptoms of TSS.

Comparative Genomic Analysis of *S. aureus*

EVOLUTION OF MRSA

In the early 1950s, plasmids encoding resistance to penicillin spread rapidly among *S. aureus* populations, rendering them resistant to this drug. In 1959, a modified synthetic penicillin known as methicillin was introduced as an alternative treatment for infections caused by penicillin-resistant strains. However, as stated previously, resistant strains emerged very rapidly. It was shown subsequently that MRSA strains had acquired a gene *(mecA)*, encoding a modified penicillin-binding protein (PBP2') responsible for methicillin resistance (66). This novel PBP has significantly reduced binding affinity for β-lactam antibiotics. Production of PBP2' permits continued cell wall synthesis by *S. aureus*, even when exposed to otherwise inhibitory concentrations of β-lactams. The *mecA* gene is contained within a chromosomal segment of DNA known as the staphylococcal cassette chromosome *mec* (SCC*mec*) (see "Mobile Genetic Elements of *S. aureus*" below). The origin of the *mecA* gene has been the subject of much investigation. A homologue of the *mecA* gene has been found in 13 different staphylococcal species (20) and also in *Enterococcus hirae* (2), and it has been speculated that *mecA* originated in *E. hirae*. In addition, *Staphylococcus sciuri* has a *mecA* homologue that encodes a protein with 88% similarity with PBP2', suggesting that the *S. sciuri mecA* homologue represents the evolutionary origin of the *mecA* gene (20).

There has been much speculation and controversy for many years concerning the evolutionary origin of MRSA strains. The existence of SCC*mec* elements with characteristics of mobile elements suggested that horizontal transfer may contribute to the spread of methicillin resistance among *S. aureus* strains. However, until recently the possibility that broad dissemination of a single clone of MRSA had occurred could not be ruled out.

The Single Clone Theory. In 1973, Lacey and Grinsted proposed the single clone origin theory for MRSA strains based on the phenotypic similarities of the strains they examined (59). This "monoclonal theory" postulated that all contemporary strains of MRSA arose from a single progenitor MRSA strain that had acquired the *mecA* determinant. Under this idea, the newly formed MRSA strain expanded by clonal dissemination, giving rise to all MRSA strains that exist today. Kreiswirth and colleagues carried out restriction fragment length polymorphism analysis of MRSA strains by Southern blot analysis with two DNA probes (57). The probes identified polymorphisms around the *mecA* gene and Tn*554* regions. Each of the Tn*554* profiles occurred in association with only one *mecA* pattern. The investigators reasoned that, if acquisition of *mecA* and Tn*554* were independent events, then association of patterns could only occur by clone microevolution, not horizontal gene transfer. They concluded that *mecA* was acquired only once by *S. aureus* and attributed the observed genetic variation in MRSA strains to subsequent acquisition and rearrangement of DNA within the *mecA* locus (57).

The Multiclone Theory. In the early 1990s, Musser and Kapur used MLEE to estimate chromosomal relationships among MRSA isolates from four continents (71). Among 254 isolates, 15 distinct ETs were identified, indicating the existence of multiple distinct clones of MRSA. The *mecA* gene occurred in association with chromosomal backgrounds representing the entire breadth of genetic differentiation among isolates of the species *S. aureus*. These data provided strong evidence that horizontal transfer of the *mecA* gene had contributed to the evolution of MRSA, and effectively ruled out the monoclonal theory. Other strain analysis methods have confirmed the multiclone theory of MRSA evolution, including multilocus sequence typing, ribotyping, and pulsed-field gel electrophoresis. Moreover, a whole-genome DNA microarray was used to investigate evolutionary relationships among MRSA and methicillin-susceptible *S. aureus* (MSSA) strains (37). Based on the pattern of variation in gene content among the strains examined, the MRSA strains represent at least five major chromosomal genotypic groups that differ in some cases by several hundred genes. Hence, MRSA strains have evolved multiple times through horizontal gene transfer of the *mecA* gene to MSSA strains that represent the breadth of diversity in the species (37).

Recent comparison of the sequence of an MSSA strain (476) with that of a very closely related MRSA strain (MW2) by Holden et al. indicated that at least five horizontal gene transfer events, including transfer of SCC*mec,* had occurred since separation from a common ancestor (46). These data highlight the critical role that horizontal gene transfer plays in the rapid evolution of *S. aureus* in response to a changing environment.

MOBILE GENETIC ELEMENTS OF *S. AUREUS*

It has been long known that *S. aureus* contains mobile genetic elements such as transposons, bacteriophages, and plasmids. Several recent studies have described members of a pathogenicity island family encoding virulence factors and a family of staphylococcal cassette chromosomes (SCCs) that encode resistance to antibiotics, including methicillin and related drugs, the antibiotics of choice for treatment of many staphylococcal infections (80). However, it was not until the sequences of the entire genome of several *S. aureus* strains became available that the full extent of the number and variety of discrete genetic elements present in the genome became apparent (4, 46, 58). Some of these genetic elements are actively mobile, while others are stably integrated but show evidence of being horizontally acquired at some stage in the evolution of *S. aureus.* Considering the large number of virulence factors, such as superantigens, other toxins, and capsular polysaccharide, that are encoded by mobile elements, along with genes encoding antibiotic

resistance, it is evident that these elements have been central to the evolution and success of pathogenic *S. aureus.*

Plasmids, Insertion Elements, and Transposons. *S. aureus* plasmids can encode resistance to antibiotics such as penicillin and erythromycin, and heavy metals such as cadmium. Some plasmids also contain genes for virulence factors such as staphylococcal enterotoxins D and J and exfoliative toxin B (99, 101). These plasmids are variably present among *S. aureus* strains in natural populations.

Many *S. aureus* transposons and ISs have been described. However, complete genome sequences for *S. aureus* strains have defined the copy number and insertion sites for the transposons and ISs present in those strains. Several transposonlike elements were identified in the complete genome sequences of strains Mu50 and N315 (58). For example, two copies of Tn*554* are present in strain N315 and five copies of this element are present in strain Mu50. Tn*554* encodes resistance to spectinomycin and macrolide-lincosamide-streptogramin B antibiotics. Mu50 and N315 contain 10 and 8 copies, respectively, of the IS*1181* insertion element. The genome of strain Mu50 contains a previously undescribed 25.8-kb element designated Tn*5801*, which has features of a conjugative transposon and encodes resistance to tetracycline and minocycline.

Although clearly some transposons may encode resistance to antibiotics, the integration of transposons and ISs at multiple and apparently random sites in the genome by illegitimate recombination suggests a more fundamental role for these elements in the evolution of *S. aureus* genomes. It is possible that the presence of multiple copies of identical elements scattered around the genome facilitates recombination and shuffling of genome architecture. These processes would ensure that the chromosome is a dynamic structure that can readily adapt to changing environmental conditions, thereby assisting survival.

Bacteriophages. Most strains of *S. aureus* contain integrated bacteriophages, and many of these elements have genes encoding known virulence factors such as staphylococcal enterotoxin A, Panton-Valentine leukocidin, staphylokinase, and exfoliative toxin A. For example, staphylococcal scalded skin syndrome affecting neonates and young children is caused by exfoliative toxins that can be phage (exfoliative toxin A) or plasmid (exfoliative toxin B) encoded (98). The 45-kb φ13 bacteriophage encodes the gene for staphylokinase, an enzyme that activates plasminogen to plasmin and has been implicated as a virulence factor by virtue of its ability to assist dissemination of staphylococci in host tissues (49). Genomic integration of φ13 results in the interruption of the β-toxin gene and concomitant conversion to staphylokinase production (19).

Recent genome sequencing efforts have allowed the examination of the phage content of several strains of *S. aureus*. The Panton-Valentine leukocidin genes are present on a bacteriophage (φSa2) that is present in strain MW2, an abundant MRSA strain isolated from a community-acquired infection (4). The *lukF-Panton-Valentine* and *lukS-Panton-Valentine* genes are present in only a small percentage of human clinical strains, but the toxin is associated with severe forms of pneumonia caused by community-acquired *S. aureus* strains (25).

With the exception of strain COL, all sequenced strains have φSa3. Alignment of the Sa3 prophages from different strains reveals a highly mosaic structure that is probably the result of recombination between different phages. Strain MW has a φSa3 phage that contains genes encoding enterotoxins homologous to SEK and SEG (4). These genes are not present in φSa3 phages found in other strains.

Staphylococcal Cassette Chromosomes. Five major forms of SCC*mec* have been identified that vary in size from 21 to 67 kb. All variants are integrated at an identical site in the chromosome close to the origin of replication,

but contain considerable variation in gene content. SCC*mec* I, II, and III are 39, 52, and 67 kb in size, respectively, and 34 of 38 MRSA strains examined contained one of these three types (41). Two related subtypes (20.9 kb and 24.3 kb) of SCC*mec* type IV have been identified among recently emerged community-acquired MRSA strains, including strain MW2 (41). These two SCC*mec* type IV elements do not contain genes encoding resistance to additional antibiotics, a characteristic of SCC*mec* types I through III. A novel SCC type V was recently identified in a community-acquired MRSA isolate from Australia. It is 28 kb in size and contains a distinct cassette chromosome recombinase *(ccr)* (48). All SCC*mec* variants have conserved terminal inverted repeats, direct repeats located at the chromosomal integration sites, genes for cassette chromosome recombinases that direct chromosomal integration and excision events of SCC*mec*, and conserved organization around the *mecA* gene. Although SCC*mec* II has an overall G+C content (33%) similar to that of the *S. aureus* genome (32 to 36%), several regions within SCC*mec* deviate significantly in G+C content, suggesting relatively recent horizontal acquisition (41). Of note, an SCC variant has been identified recently that encodes genes for synthesis of type I capsular polysaccharide, a structure involved in evasion of the host immune response (63). This indicates a role for SCC elements other than transfer and encoding of antibiotic resistance.

Staphylococcal Pathogenicity Islands. In recent years, *S. aureus* chromosomal segments have been described that together belong to the family of staphylococcal pathogenicity islands (SaPIs). Virtually all SaPIs contain genes encoding superantigens (79). In addition, SaPIbov2, an element present in a small number of bovine strains, has a gene *(bap)* encoding a protein involved in biofilm formation (21).

The best characterized of the SaPIs is SaPI1, which is 15.2 kb in length and encodes TSST-1 and SEK. SaPI1 is flanked by 17-bp direct repeats and contains a gene encoding an integrase (62). SaPI1 can integrate into the chromosome in a site-specific manner without the use of host RecA for recombination. A related element (SaPIbov) encodes TSST-1, SEC, and SEL (35). SaPIbov contains 74-nucleotide direct repeats flanking the integrated genetic element and an integrase gene, and is inserted into the chromosome upstream of the GMP synthase gene *(guaA)* (35). SaPI3 is 15.9 kb in size and encodes staphylococcal enterotoxins B, K, and Q. There are 24 ORFs encoding proteins of 50 amino acids, including an integrase gene. Expression of 22 of these 24 ORFs was detected in vitro or in vivo in a rabbit model of endocarditis (100).

Genome sequencing of *S. aureus* strains has revealed additional pathogenicity island variants, some of which have been shown to excise spontaneously from the genome and to replicate autonomously. Although there are large regions of conservation between the SaPIs, there is considerable variation in their virulence gene content (37). Recombination events involving insertion, deletion, or recombination of shorter regions of DNA outside of the conserved central core have likely contributed to the variation among SaPIs.

Other Genomic "Islands." Two other genomic islands (vSaα and vSaβ) have been identified in all *S. aureus* strains examined and appear to be stably integrated. However, there has been extensive recombination within these regions, resulting in large variation in virulence gene content in different strains (37). Both islands have nonfunctional transposase genes, suggesting that these elements were acquired horizontally in the past, and have since been stably inherited by all contemporary strains of *S. aureus*. Both islands also contain genes for a restriction modification system. vSaα has between 7 and 11 genes, depending on the strain, encoding variants of SET proteins that may be involved in host-pathogen interactions (see "Localized Molecular Processes of Evolution" below) (36). vSaβ has different combina-

tions of genes encoding a protease family, a bacteriocin production system, leukotoxins D and E, and a gene cluster encoding staphylococcal enterotoxins G, I, M, N, and O (37).

It is clear that recombination has contributed to extensive variation in virulence gene content in pathogenicity islands and genomic islands of *S. aureus*. Through horizontal gene transfer and recombination, *S. aureus* can share genetic material, which may facilitate survival in different environmental niches. In addition, reassortive recombination results in different combinations of virulence factor genes, which may result in variable levels of virulence. Rarely, very large chromosomal fragments may undergo recombination, resulting in replacements of up to 20% of the genome with genetic information from another strain, as demonstrated recently by Robinson and Enright (87). This may contribute to the rapid generation of new pathogenic clones of *S. aureus*. The repertoire of pathogenicity and genomic islands of a strain is a major contributor to *S. aureus* virulence factor complement, and the different combinations of these traits influence the pathogenic potential of strains. Overall, mobile genetic elements of *S. aureus* have been fundamental in the evolution of such a versatile bacterium, which is constantly adapting to different environmental challenges.

LOCALIZED MOLECULAR
PROCESSES OF EVOLUTION
DNA microarray comparison of the gene content of strains representing the major lineages of *S. aureus* associated with human and animal infections identified 17 large chromosomal regions that were variably present or contained considerable variation in gene content between strains (37). One such region (RD13) was 12 to 17 kb in size, depending on the strain, and contained between 7 and 11 genes that would encode SET proteins (Fig. 5A). SET proteins contain homology with the classical superantigens of staphylococci and streptococci, including two superantigen consensus sequences. However, SET proteins do not have

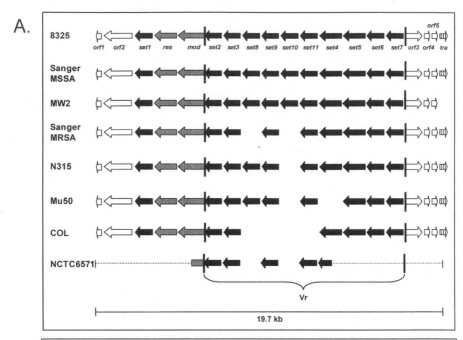

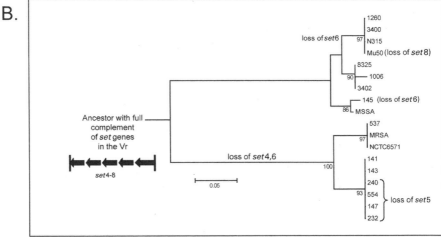

FIGURE 5 (A) Variation in gene content of chromosomal region RD13 in eight *S. aureus* strains: 8325, Sanger MSSA, MW2, Sanger MRSA, N315, Mu50, COL, and NCTC6571. The proteins encoded by the genes designated are as follows: *orf1* through *orf5* (white), hypothetical proteins; *set1* through *set11* (black), staphylococcal exotoxin-like proteins; *res, mod* (gray), restriction/modification subunits; *tra* (striped), transposase. Dashed lines represent DNA of unknown sequence. The central variable region (Vr) is indicated. (B) Model for the diversification of the chromosomal region RD13. The proposed ancestral state of the Vr is indicated at the hypothetical root. The loss of *set* genes necessary to explain the extant state of each strain is indicated in red. This model is supported by the observation that the proportion of silent mutations (synonymous substitution) within each *set* gene is the same. If the *set* genes of the Vr were gained at different times during the evolution of RD13, one would expect the number of silent mutations to differ between genes. The trees were constructed by the neighbor-joining algorithm based on the number of synonymous substitutions per synonymous site *(dS)*. A comparison of phylogenetic trees constructed from individual *set* gene nucleotide data and a concatenated sequence representing the conserved genes of RD13 indicated that the topologies were cognate. Thus, the extent of recombination present was insufficient to disrupt the underlying phylogenetic signal. The *set5* gene tree is shown. Bootstrap confidence limits are shown under the major nodes. Modified from reference 36.

the classical properties of superantigens, such as mitogenicity and fever induction, and hence their role in pathogenesis is not clear.

Polymerase chain reaction amplification was used to determine the size of a central variable region (Vr) among 63 strains of divergent genetic background (36). Three strains had a Vr of 7 kb, 5 strains had a Vr of 8 kb, 19 strains had a Vr of 9 kb, 17 strains had a Vr of 10 kb, and 19 strains had a Vr of 11 kb. Based on the *set* gene content of Vr in six *S. aureus* strains for which the genome has been completed, the results are consistent with the presence of 6, 7, 8, 9, or 10 *set* genes in this region in *S. aureus* strains. The variation in *set* gene content is remarkable and raises questions as to the evolutionary processes responsible for variation in this region. The presence of RD13 in all strains, and a G+C content equivalent to that of the *S. aureus* genome, suggest that RD13 is an ancient feature of the chromosome. To investigate the evolution of RD13 and the Vr, phylogenetic trees were constructed based on DNA sequence of the conserved region of RD13 and the variable *set* genes (36). The analysis revealed that the most likely evolutionary scenario is that an ancestral strain with a full complement of *set* genes in Vr underwent multiple independent losses of *set* genes in parallel, in separate lineages (Fig. 5B). These losses were confined to *set* genes *4* through *8*. The loss of *set* genes from different lineages without an apparent loss of virulence may indicate some redundancy in SET variant function (36).

While the biological function of the family of SET proteins remains unclear, the distinctive molecular processes shaping the architecture of this chromosomal region are intriguing. The ubiquity of this locus throughout the species and the detection of in vivo expression of SET proteins suggest an important role in host-pathogen interactions.

CONCLUDING COMMENTS

The revival of GAS disease and the endemic nature of *S. aureus* emphasize the resilience of these two organisms. Genome-scale investigation of allelic variation, population genetics, and host interactions has provided answers to long-

standing controversies, such as the evolution of methicillin-resistant strains of *S. aureus* and the emergence of TSS, and provided substrates for new testable hypotheses. For instance, it will be critical to understand how GAS interstrain differences mediated by phage transduction affect host-pathogen interactions and disease outcome. Importantly, genome-scale investigations are broadly applicable, and will provide new avenues to study bacterial variation, host adaptation, and the origin of new pathogenic forms.

CHAPTER SUMMARY

- Genome-scale investigation of allelic variation, population genetics, and host interactions has provided answers to long-standing controversies, such as the evolution of methicillin-resistant strains of *S. aureus* and the emergence of TSS.
- Multiple processes, including phage transduction, horizontal gene transfer, recombination, deletion, and mutation, have contributed to the extensive genetic variation found in natural populations of *S. aureus* and group A *Streptococcus*.
- It will be critical to understand how interstrain differences within *S. aureus* and group A *Streptococcus* populations affect host-pathogen interactions and disease outcome.
- Genome-scale investigations are broadly applicable, and will provide new avenues to study bacterial variation, host adaptation, and the origin of new pathogenic forms.

REFERENCES

1. **Akesson, P., A. G. Sjoholm, and L. Bjorck.** 1996. Protein SIC, a novel extracellular protein of *Streptococcus pyogenes* interfering with complement function. *J. Biol. Chem.* **271:**1081–1088.
2. **Archer, G. L., J. A. Thanassi, D. M. Niemeyer, and M. J. Pucci.** 1996. Characterization of IS1272, an insertion sequence-like element from *Staphylococcus haemolyticus. Antimicrob. Agents Chemother.* **40:**924–929.
3. **Artiushin, S. C., J. F. Timoney, A. S. Sheoran, and S. K. Muthupalani.** 2002. Characterization

and immunogenicity of pyrogenic mitogens SePE-H and SePE-I of *Streptococcus equi*. *Microb. Pathog.* **32:**71–85.

4. **Baba, T., F. Takeuchi, M. Kuroda, H. Yuzawa, K. Aoki, A. Oguchi, Y. Nagai, N. Iwama, K. Asano, T. Naimi, H. Kuroda, L. Cui, K. Yamamoto, and K. Hiramatsu.** 2002. Genome and virulence determinants of high virulence community-acquired MRSA. *Lancet* **359:**1819–1827.

5. **Banks, D. J., S. B. Beres, and J. M. Musser.** 2002. The fundamental contribution of phages to GAS evolution, genome diversification and strain emergence. *Trends Microbiol.* **10:**515–521.

6. **Banks, D. J., S. F. Porcella, K. D. Barbian, S. B. Beres, L. E. Philips, J. M. Voyich, F. R. DeLeo, J. M. Martin, G. A. Somerville, and J. M. Musser.** 2004. Progress toward characterization of the group A *Streptococcus* metagenome: complete genome sequence of a macrolide-resistant serotype M6 strain. *J. Infect. Dis.* **190:**727–738.

7. **Banks, D. J., S. F. Porcella, K. D. Barbian, J. M. Martin, and J. M. Musser.** 2003. Structure and distribution of an unusual chimeric genetic element encoding macrolide resistance in phylogenetically diverse clones of group A *Streptococcus*. *J. Infect. Dis.* **188:**1898–1908.

8. **Beall, B., R. Facklam, T. Hoenes, and B. Schwartz.** 1997. Application of *emm* gene sequencing and T antigen serology for typing group A streptococcal systemic isolates. Survey of random and outbreak-related isolates. *Adv. Exp. Med. Biol.* **418:**307–311.

9. **Beall, B., R. Facklam, T. Hoenes, and B. Schwartz.** 1997. Survey of *emm* gene sequences and T-antigen types from systemic *Streptococcus pyogenes* infection isolates collected in San Francisco, California; Atlanta, Georgia; and Connecticut in 1994 and 1995. *J. Clin. Microbiol.* **35:**1231–1235.

10. **Beall, B., R. Facklam, and T. Thompson.** 1996. Sequencing *emm*-specific PCR products for routine and accurate typing of group A streptococci. *J. Clin. Microbiol.* **34:**953–958.

11. **Beres, S. B., G. L. Sylva, K. D. Barbian, B. Lei, J. S. Hoff, N. D. Mammarella, M. Y. Liu, J. C. Smoot, S. F. Porcella, L. D. Parkins, D. S. Campbell, T. M. Smith, J. K. McCormick, D. Y. Leung, P. M. Schlievert, and J. M. Musser.** 2002. Genome sequence of a serotype M3 strain of group A *Streptococcus*: phage-encoded toxins, the high-virulence phenotype, and clone emergence. *Proc. Natl. Acad. Sci. USA* **99:**10078–10083.

12. **Beres, S. B., G. L. Sylva, D. E. Sturdevant, C. N. Granville, M. Liu, S. M. Ricklefs, A. R. Whitney, L. D. Parkins, N. P. Hoe, G. J. Adams, D. E. Low, F. R. DeLeo, A. McGeer, and J. M. Musser.** 2004. Genome-wide molecular dissection of serotype M3 group A *Streptococcus*

strains causing two epidemics of invasive infections. *Proc. Natl. Acad. Sci. USA* **101:**11833–11838.

13. **Bessen, D., K. F. Jones, and V. A. Fischetti.** 1989. Evidence for two distinct classes of streptococcal M protein and their relationship to rheumatic fever. *J. Exp. Med.* **169:**269–283.

14. **Bessen, D. E., M. W. Izzo, T. R. Fiorentino, R. M. Caringal, S. K. Hollingshead, and B. Beall.** 1999. Genetic linkage of exotoxin alleles and *emm* gene markers for tissue tropism in group A streptococci. *J. Infect. Dis.* **179:**627–636.

15. **Bessen, D. E., and A. Kalia.** 2002. Genomic localization of a T serotype locus to a recombinatorial zone encoding extracellular matrix-binding proteins in *Streptococcus pyogenes*. *Infect. Immun.* **70:**1159–1167.

16. **Bessen, D. E., C. M. Sotir, T. L. Readdy, and S. K. Hollingshead.** 1996. Genetic correlates of throat and skin isolates of group A streptococci. *J. Infect. Dis.* **173:**896–900.

17. **Bisno, A. L.** 2001. Primary care: acute pharyngitis. N Engl J Med **344:**205–211.

18. **Bisno, A. L., M. O. Brito, and C. M. Collins.** 2003. Molecular basis of group A streptococcal virulence. *Lancet Infect. Dis.* **3:**191–200.

19. **Coleman, D. C., D. J. Sullivan, R. J. Russell, J. P. Arbuthnott, B. F. Carey, and H. M. Pomeroy.** 1989. *Staphylococcus aureus* bacteriophages mediating the simultaneous lysogenic conversion of beta-lysin, staphylokinase and enterotoxin A: molecular mechanism of triple conversion. *J. Gen. Microbiol.* **135:**1679–1697.

20. **Couto, I., H. de Lencastre, E. Severina, W. Kloos, J. A. Webster, R. J. Hubner, I. S. Sanches, and A. Tomasz.** 1996. Ubiquitous presence of a *mecA* homologue in natural isolates of *Staphylococcus sciuri*. *Microb. Drug Resist.* **2:**377–391.

21. **Cucarella, C., C. Solano, J. Valle, B. Amorena, I. Lasa, and J. R. Penades.** 2001. Bap, a *Staphylococcus aureus* surface protein involved in biofilm formation. *J. Bacteriol.* **183:**2888–2896.

22. **Cunningham, M. W.** 2000. Pathogenesis of group A streptococcal infections. *Clin. Microbiol. Rev.* **13:**470–511.

23. **Dale, J. B.** 1999. Group A streptococcal vaccines. *Infect. Dis. Clin. N. Am.* **13:**227–43, viii.

24. **Desiere, F., W. M. McShan, D. van Sinderen, J. J. Ferretti, and H. Brussow.** 2001. Comparative genomics reveals close genetic relationships between phages from dairy bacteria and pathogenic streptococci: evolutionary implications for prophage-host interactions. *Virology* **288:**325–341.

25. **Diep, B. A., G. F. Sensabaugh, N. S. Somboona, H. A. Carleton, and F. Perdreau-Remington.** 2004. Widespread skin and soft-tissue infections due to two methicillin-resistant

Staphylococcus aureus strains harboring the genes for Panton-Valentine leucocidin. *J. Clin. Microbiol.* **42:**2080–2084.

26. **Enright, M. C., D. A. Robinson, G. Randle, E. J. Feil, H. Grundmann, and B. G. Spratt.** 2002. The evolutionary history of methicillin-resistant *Staphylococcus aureus* (MRSA). *Proc. Natl. Acad. Sci. USA* **99:**7687–7692.

27. **Enright, M. C., B. G. Spratt, A. Kalia, J. H. Cross, and D. E. Bessen.** 2001. Multilocus sequence typing of *Streptococcus pyogenes* and the relationships between *emm* type and clone. *Infect. Immun.* **69:**2416–2427.

28. **Facklam, R., and B. Beall.** 1997. Anomalies in *emm* typing of group A streptococci. *Adv. Exp. Med. Biol.* **418:**335–337.

29. **Facklam, R., B. Beall, A. Efstratiou, V. Fischetti, D. Johnson, E. Kaplan, P. Kriz, M. Lovgren, D. Martin, B. Schwartz, A. Totolian, D. Bessen, S. Hollingshead, F. Rubin, J. Scott, and G. Tyrrell.** 1999. *emm* typing and validation of provisional M types for group A streptococci. *Emerg. Infect. Dis.* **5:**247–253.

30. **Facklam, R. F., D. R. Martin, M. Lovgren, D. R. Johnson, A. Efstratiou, T. A. Thompson, S. Gowan, P. Kriz, G. J. Tyrrell, E. Kaplan, and B. Beall.** 2002. Extension of the Lancefield classification for group A streptococci by addition of 22 new M protein gene sequence types from clinical isolates: *emm*103 to *emm*124. *Clin. Infect. Dis.* **34:**28–38.

31. **Feil, E. J., J. E. Cooper, H. Grundmann, D. A. Robinson, M. C. Enright, T. Berendt, S. J. Peacock, J. M. Smith, M. Murphy, B. G. Spratt, C. E. Moore, and N. P. Day.** 2003. How clonal is *Staphylococcus aureus*? *J. Bacteriol.* **185:**3307–3316.

32. **Ferretti, J. J., W. M. McShan, D. Ajdic, D. J. Savic, G. Savic, K. Lyon, C. Primeaux, S. Sezate, A. N. Suvorov, S. Kenton, H. S. Lai, S. P. Lin, Y. Qian, H. G. Jia, F. Z. Najar, Q. Ren, H. Zhu, L. Song, J. White, X. Yuan, S. W. Clifton, B. A. Roe, and R. McLaughlin.** 2001. Complete genome sequence of an M1 strain of *Streptococcus pyogenes*. *Proc. Natl. Acad. Sci. USA* **98:**4658–4663.

33. **Fischetti, V. A.** 1989. Streptococcal M protein: molecular design and biological behavior. *Clin. Microbiol. Rev.* **2:**285–314.

34. **Fischetti, V. A., E. C. Gotschlich, G. Siviglia, and J. B. Zabriskie.** 1977. Streptococcal M protein: an antiphagocytic molecule assembled on the cell wall. *J. Infect. Dis.* **136**(Suppl.):S222–S233.

35. **Fitzgerald, J. R., S. R. Monday, T. J. Foster, G. A. Bohach, P. J. Hartigan, W. J. Meaney, and C. J. Smyth.** 2001. Characterization of a putative pathogenicity island from bovine *Staphylococcus*

aureus encoding multiple superantigens. *J. Bacteriol.* **183:**63–70.

36. **Fitzgerald, J. R., S. D. Reid, E. Ruotsalainen, T. J. Tripp, M. Liu, R. Cole, P. Kuusela, P. M. Schlievert, A. Jarvinen, and J. M. Musser.** 2003. Genome diversification in *Staphylococcus aureus*: molecular evolution of a highly variable chromosomal region encoding the staphylococcal exotoxin-like family of proteins. *Infect. Immun.* **71:**2827–2838.

37. **Fitzgerald, J. R., D. E. Sturdevant, S. M. Mackie, S. R. Gill, and J. M. Musser.** 2001. Evolutionary genomics of *Staphylococcus aureus*: insights into the origin of methicillin-resistant strains and the toxic shock syndrome epidemic. *Proc. Natl. Acad. Sci. USA* **98:**8821–8826.

38. **Green, N. M., S. B. Beres, E. A. Graviss, J. E. Allison, A. J. McGeer, J. Vuopio-Varkila, R. B. Lefebvre, and J. M. Musser.** 2005. Genetic diversity among type *emm*28 group A *Streptococcus* strains causing invasive infections and pharyngitis. *J. Clin. Microbiol.* **43:**4083–4091.

39. **Green, N. M., S. Zhang, S. F. Porcella, M. J. Nagiec, K. D. Barbian, S. B. Beres, R. B. Lefebvre, and J. M. Musser.** 2005. Genome sequence of a serotype M28 strain of group A *Streptococcus*: potential new insights into puerperal sepsis and bacterial disease specificity. *J. Infect. Dis.* **192:**760–770.

40. **Herron, L. L., R. Chakravarty, C. Dwan, J. R. Fitzgerald, J. M. Musser, E. Retzel, and V. Kapur.** 2002. Genome sequence survey identifies unique sequences and key virulence genes with unusual rates of amino acid substitution in bovine *Staphylococcus aureus*. *Infect. Immun.* **70:**3978–3981.

41. **Hiramatsu, K., L. Cui, M. Kuroda, and T. Ito.** 2001. The emergence and evolution of methicillin-resistant *Staphylococcus aureus*. *Trends Microbiol.* **9:**486–493.

42. **Hoe, N., K. Nakashima, D. Grigsby, X. Pan, S. J. Dou, S. Naidich, M. Garcia, E. Kahn, D. Bergmire-Sweat, and J. M. Musser.** 1999. Rapid molecular genetic subtyping of serotype M1 group A *Streptococcus* strains. *Emerg. Infect. Dis.* **5:**254–263.

43. **Hoe, N. P., R. M. Ireland, F. R. DeLeo, B. B. Gowen, D. W. Dorward, J. M. Voyich, M. Liu, E. H. Burns, Jr., D. M. Culnan, A. Bretscher, and J. M. Musser.** 2002. Insight into the molecular basis of pathogen abundance: group A *Streptococcus* inhibitor of complement inhibits bacterial adherence and internalization into human cells. *Proc. Natl. Acad. Sci. USA* **99:**7646–7651.

44. **Hoe, N. P., K. Nakashima, S. Lukomski, D. Grigsby, M. Liu, P. Kordari, S. J. Dou, X. Pan, J. Vuopio-Varkila, S. Salmelinna, A. McGeer, D. E. Low, B. Schwartz, A. Schuchat, S.**

Naidich, D. De Lorenzo, Y. X. Fu, and J. M. Musser. 1999. Rapid selection of complement-inhibiting protein variants in group A *Streptococcus* epidemic waves. *Nat. Med.* **5:**924–929.

45. Hoe, N. P., J. Vuopio-Varkila, M. Vaara, D. Grigsby, D. De Lorenzo, Y. X. Fu, S. J. Dou, X. Pan, K. Nakashima, and J. M. Musser. 2001. Distribution of streptococcal inhibitor of complement variants in pharyngitis and invasive isolates in an epidemic of serotype M1 group A *Streptococcus* infection. *J. Infect. Dis.* **183:**633–639.

46. Holden, M. T., E. J. Feil, J. A. Lindsay, S. J. Peacock, N. P. Day, M. C. Enright, T. J. Foster, C. E. Moore, L. Hurst, R. Atkin, A. Barron, N. Bason, S. D. Bentley, C. Chillingworth, T. Chillingworth, C. Churcher, L. Clark, C. Corton, A. Cronin, J. Doggett, L. Dowd, T. Feltwell, Z. Hance, B. Harris, H. Hauser, S. Holroyd, K. Jagels, K. D. James, N. Lennard, A. Line, R. Mayes, S. Moule, K. Mungall, D. Ormond, M. A. Quail, E. Rabbinowitsch, K. Rutherford, M. Sanders, S. Sharp, M. Simmonds, K. Stevens, S. Whitehead, B. G. Barrell, B. G. Spratt, and J. Parkhill. 2004. Complete genomes of two clinical *Staphylococcus aureus* strains: evidence for the rapid evolution of virulence and drug resistance. *Proc. Natl. Acad. Sci. USA* **101:**9786–9791.

47. Hosier, D. M., J. M. Craenen, D. W. Teske, and J. J. Wheller. 1987. Resurgence of acute rheumatic fever. *Am. J. Dis. Child.* **141:**730–733.

48. Ito, T., X. X. Ma, F. Takeuchi, K. Okuma, H. Yuzawa, and K. Hiramatsu. 2004. Novel type V staphylococcal cassette chromosome *mec* driven by a novel cassette chromosome recombinase, *ccrC*. *Antimicrob. Agents Chemother.* **48:**2637–2651.

49. Jespers, L., S. Vanwetswinkel, H. R. Lijnen, N. Van Herzeele, B. Van Hoef, E. Demarsin, D. Collen, and M. De Maeyer. 1999. Structural and functional basis of plasminogen activation by staphylokinase. *Thromb. Haemost.* **81:**479–485.

50. Jevons, M. P., A. W. Coe, and M. T. Parker. 1963. Methicillin resistance in staphylococci. *Lancet* **i:**904–907.

51. Johnson, D. R., D. L. Stevens, and E. L. Kaplan. 1992. Epidemiologic analysis of group A streptococcal serotypes associated with severe systemic infections, rheumatic fever, or uncomplicated pharyngitis. *J. Infect. Dis.* **166:**374–382.

52. Jones, K. F., S. S. Whitehead, M. W. Cunningham, and V. A. Fischetti. 2000. Reactivity of rheumatic fever and scarlet fever patients' sera with group A streptococcal M protein, cardiac myosin, and cardiac tropomyosin: a retrospective study. *Infect. Immun.* **68:**7132–7136.

53. Kapur, V., W. M. Sischo, R. S. Greer, T. S. Whittam, and J. M. Musser. 1995. Molecular

population genetic analysis of *Staphylococcus aureus* recovered from cows. *J. Clin. Microbiol.* **33:** 376–380.

54. Kline, J. B., and C. M. Collins. 1996. Analysis of the superantigenic activity of mutant and allelic forms of streptococcal pyrogenic exotoxin A. *Infect. Immun.* **64:**861–869.

55. Kluytmans, J., A. van Belkum, and H. Verbrugh. 1997. Nasal carriage of *Staphylococcus aureus:* epidemiology, underlying mechanisms and associated risks. *Clin. Microbiol. Rev.* **10:** 505–520.

56. Kotb, M. 1995. Bacterial pyrogenic exotoxins as superantigens. *Clin. Microbiol. Rev.* **8:**411–426.

57. Kreiswirth, B., J. Kornblum, R. D. Arbeit, W. Eisner, J. N. Maslow, A. McGeer, D. E. Low, and R. P. Novick. 1993. Evidence for a clonal origin of methicillin resistance in *Staphylococcus aureus. Science* **259:**227–230.

58. Kuroda, M., T. Ohta, I. Uchiyama, T. Baba, H. Yuzawa, I. Kobayashi, L. Cui, A. Oguchi, K. Aoki, Y. Nagai, J. Lian, T. Ito, M. Kanamori, H. Matsumaru, A. Maruyama, H. Murakami, A. Hosoyama, Y. Mizutani-Ui, N. K. Takahashi, T. Sawano, R. Inoue, C. Kaito, K. Sekimizu, H. Hirakawa, S. Kuhara, S. Goto, J. Yabuzaki, M. Kanehisa, A. Yamashita, K. Oshima, K. Furuya, C. Yoshino, T. Shiba, M. Hattori, N. Ogasawara, H. Hayashi, and K. Hiramatsu. 2001. Whole genome sequencing of methicillin-resistant *Staphylococcus aureus. Lancet* **357:**1225–1240.

59. Lacey, R. W., and J. Grinsted. 1973. Genetic analysis of methicillin-resistant strains of *Staphylococcus aureus;* evidence for their evolution from a single clone. *J. Med. Microbiol.* **6:**511–526.

60. Lancefield, R. C. 1962. Current knowledge of type-specific M antigens of group A streptococci. *J. Immunol.* **89:**307–313.

61. Lancefield, R. C., and G. E. Perlmann. 1952. Preparation and properties of type-specific M antigen isolated from a group A, type 1 hemolytic *Streptococcus. J. Exp. Med.* **96:**71–82.

62. Lindsay, J. A., A. Ruzin, H. F. Ross, N. Kurepina, and R. P. Novick. 1998. The gene for toxic shock toxin is carried by a family of mobile pathogenicity islands in *Staphylococcus aureus. Mol. Microbiol.* **29:**527–543.

63. Luong, T. T., S. Ouyang, K. Bush, and C. Y. Lee. 2002. Type 1 capsule genes of *Staphylococcus aureus* are carried in a staphylococcal cassette chromosome genetic element. *J. Bacteriol.* **184:** 3623–3629.

64. Martin, J. M., M. Green, K. A. Barbadora, and E. R. Wald. 2002. Erythromycin-resistant group A streptococci in schoolchildren in Pittsburgh. *N. Engl. J. Med.* **346:**1200–1206.

65. **Massell, B. F.** 1997. *Rheumatic Fever and Streptococcal Infection.* Harvard University Press, Boston, Mass.

66. **Matsuhashi, M., M. D. Song, F. Ishino, M. Wachi, M. Doi, M. Inoue, K. Ubukata, N. Yamashita, and M. Konno.** 1986. Molecular cloning of the gene of a penicillin-binding protein supposed to cause high resistance to beta-lactam antibiotics in *Staphylococcus aureus. J. Bacteriol.* **167:**975–980.

67. **Matsumoto, M., N. P. Hoe, M. Liu, S. B. Beres, G. L. Sylva, C. M. Brandt, G. Haase, and J. M. Musser.** 2003. Intrahost sequence variation in the streptococcal inhibitor of complement gene in patients with human pharyngitis. *J. Infect. Dis.* **187:**604–612.

68. **McCormick, J. K., J. M. Yarwood, and P. M. Schlievert.** 2001. Toxic shock syndrome and bacterial superantigens: an update. *Annu. Rev. Microbiol.* **55:**77–104.

69. **McGregor, K. F., B. G. Spratt, A. Kalia, A. Bennett, N. Bilek, B. Beall, and D. E. Bessen.** 2004. Multilocus sequence typing of *Streptococcus pyogenes* representing most known *emm* types and distinctions among subpopulation genetic structures. *J. Bacteriol.* **186:**4285–4294.

70. **Musser, J. M., A. R. Hauser, M. H. Kim, P. M. Schlievert, K. Nelson, and R. K. Selander.** 1991. *Streptococcus pyogenes* causing toxic-shock-like syndrome and other invasive diseases: clonal diversity and pyrogenic exotoxin expression. *Proc. Natl. Acad. Sci. USA* **88:**2668–2672.

71. **Musser, J. M., and V. Kapur.** 1992. Clonal analysis of methicillin-resistant *Staphylococcus aureus* strains from intercontinental sources: association of the *mec* gene with divergent phylogenetic lineages implies dissemination by horizontal transfer and recombination. *J. Clin. Microbiol.* **30:**2058–2063.

72. **Musser, J. M., V. Kapur, S. Kanjilal, U. Shah, D. M. Musher, N. L. Barg, K. H. Johnston, P. M. Schlievert, J. Henrichsen, D. Gerlach, et al.** 1993. Geographic and temporal distribution and molecular characterization of two highly pathogenic clones of *Streptococcus pyogenes* expressing allelic variants of pyrogenic exotoxin A (scarlet fever toxin). *J. Infect. Dis.* **167:**337–346.

73. **Musser, J. M., and R. M. Krause.** 1998. The revival of group A streptococcal diseases, with a commentary on staphylococcal toxic shock syndrome, p. 185–218. *In* R. M. Krause (ed.), *Emerging Infections.* Academic Press, New York, N.Y.

74. **Musser, J. M., P. M. Schlievert, A. W. Chow, P. Ewan, B. N. Kreiswirth, V. T. Rosdahl, A. S. Naidu, W. Witte, and R. K. Selander.** 1990. A single clone of *Staphylococcus aureus* causes the majority of cases of toxic shock syndrome. *Proc. Natl. Acad. Sci. USA* **87:**225–229.

75. **Musser, J. M., and R. K. Selander.** 1990. Genetic analysis of natural populations of *Staphylococcus aureus*, p. 59–68. *In* R. P. Novick (ed.), *Molecular Biology of the Staphylococci.* VCH, New York, N.Y.

76. **Nagiec, M. J., B. Lei, S. K. Parker, M. L. Vasil, M. Matsumoto, R. M. Ireland, S. B. Beres, N. P. Hoe, and J. M. Musser.** 2004. Analysis of a novel prophage-encoded group A *Streptococcus* extracellular phospholipase A(2). *J. Biol. Chem.* **279:**45909–45918.

77. **Nakagawa, I., K. Kurokawa, A. Yamashita, M. Nakata, Y. Tomiyasu, N. Okahashi, S. Kawabata, K. Yamazaki, T. Shiba, T. Yasunaga, H. Hayashi, M. Hattori, and S. Hamada.** 2003. Genome sequence of an M3 strain of *Streptococcus pyogenes* reveals a large-scale genomic rearrangement in invasive strains and new insights into phage evolution. *Genome Res.* **13:**1042–1055.

78. **Nelson, K., P. M. Schlievert, R. K. Selander, and J. M. Musser.** 1991. Characterization and clonal distribution of four alleles of the *speA* gene encoding pyrogenic exotoxin A (scarlet fever toxin) in *Streptococcus pyogenes. J. Exp. Med.* **174:**1271–1274.

79. **Novick, R. P.** 2003. Mobile genetic elements and bacterial toxinoses: the superantigen-encoding pathogenicity islands of *Staphylococcus aureus. Plasmid* **49:**93–105.

80. **Novick, R. P., P. Schlievert, and A. Ruzin.** 2001. Pathogenicity and resistance islands of staphylococci. *Microbes Infect.* **3:**585–594.

81. **Olivier, C.** 2000. Rheumatic fever—is it still a problem? *J. Antimicrob. Chemother.* **45**(Suppl.):13–21.

82. **Ramachandran, V., J. D. McArthur, C. E. Behm, C. Gutzeit, M. Dowton, P. K. Fagan, R. Towers, B. Currie, K. S. Sriprakash, and M. J. Walker.** 2004. Two distinct genotypes of *prtF2*, encoding a fibronectin binding protein, and evolution of the gene family in *Streptococcus pyogenes. J. Bacteriol.* **186:**7601–7609.

83. **Reid, S. D., N. M. Green, J. K. Buss, B. Lei, and J. M. Musser.** 2001. Multilocus analysis of extracellular putative virulence proteins made by group A *Streptococcus*: population genetics, human serologic response, and gene transcription. *Proc. Natl. Acad. Sci. USA* **98:**7552–7557.

84. **Reid, S. D., N. M. Green, G. L. Sylva, J. M. Voyich, E. T. Stenseth, F. R. DeLeo, T. Palzkill, D. E. Low, H. R. Hill, and J. M. Musser.** 2002. Postgenomic analysis of four novel antigens of group A *Streptococcus*: growth phase-dependent gene transcription and human serologic response. *J. Bacteriol.* **184:**6316–6324.

85. **Reid, S. D., N. P. Hoe, L. M. Smoot, and J. M.**

Musser. 2001. Group A *Streptococcus:* allelic variation, population genetics, and host-pathogen interactions. *J. Clin. Investig.* **107:**393–399.

86. **Richter, S. S., K. P. Heilmann, S. E. Beekmann, N. J. Miller, A. L. Miller, C. L. Rice, C. D. Doern, S. D. Reid, and G. V. Doern.** 2005. Macrolide-resistant *Streptococcus pyogenes* in the United States, 2002–03. *Clin. Infect. Dis.* **41:**599–608.

87. **Robinson, D. A., and M. C. Enright.** 2004. Evolution of *Staphylococcus aureus* by large chromosomal replacements. *J. Bacteriol.* **186:** 1060–1064.

88. **Rotta, J., R. M. Krause, R. C. Lancefield, W. Everly, and H. Lackland.** 1971. New approaches for the laboratory recognition of M types of group A streptococci. *J. Exp. Med.* **134:**1298–1315.

89. **Sharkawy, A., D. E. Low, R. Saginur, D. Gregson, B. Schwartz, P. Jessamine, K. Green, and A. McGeer.** 2002. Severe group A streptococcal soft-tissue infections in Ontario: 1992–1996. *Clin. Infect. Dis.* **34:**454–460.

90. **Smoot, J. C., K. D. Barbian, J. J. Van Gompel, L. M. Smoot, M. S. Chaussee, G. L. Sylva, D. E. Sturdevant, S. M. Ricklefs, S. F. Porcella, L. D. Parkins, S. B. Beres, D. S. Campbell, T. M. Smith, Q. Zhang, V. Kapur, J. A. Daly, L. G. Veasy, and J. M. Musser.** 2002. Genome sequence and comparative microarray analysis of serotype M18 group A *Streptococcus* strains associated with acute rheumatic fever outbreaks. *Proc. Natl. Acad. Sci. USA* **99:**4668–4673.

91. **Smoot, J. C., E. K. Korgenski, J. A. Daly, L. G. Veasy, and J. M. Musser.** 2002. Molecular analysis of group A *Streptococcus* type *emm*18 isolates temporally associated with acute rheumatic fever outbreaks in Salt Lake City, Utah. *J. Clin. Microbiol.* **40:**1805–1810.

92. **Stockbauer, K. E., D. Grigsby, X. Pan, Y. X. Fu, L. M. Mejia, A. Cravioto, and J. M. Musser.** 1998. Hypervariability generated by natural selection in an extracellular complement-inhibiting protein of serotype M1 strains of group A *Streptococcus*. *Proc. Natl. Acad. Sci. USA* **95:**3128–3133.

93. **Sumby, P., K. D. Barbian, D. J. Gardner, A. R. Whitney, D. M. Welty, R. D. Long, J. R. Bailey, M. J. Parnell, N. P. Hoe, G. G. Adams, F. R. Deleo, and J. M. Musser.** 2005. Extracellular deoxyribonuclease made by group A *Streptococcus* assists pathogenesis by enhancing evasion of the innate immune response. *Proc. Natl. Acad. Sci. USA* **102:**1679–1684.

94. **Sumby, P., S. F. Porcella, A. G. Madrigal, K. D. Barbian, K. Virtaneva, S. M. Ricklefs, D. E. Sturdevant, M. R. Graham, J. Vuopio-Varkila, N. P. Hoe, and J. M. Musser.** 2005. Evolutionary origin and emergence of a highly successful clone of serotype M1 group A *Streptococcus* involved multiple horizontal gene transfer events. *J. Infect. Dis.* **192:**771–782.

95. **Tenover, F. C., L. M. Weigel, P. C. Appelbaum, L. K. McDougal, J. Chaitram, S. McAllister, N. Clark, G. Killgore, C. M. O'Hara, L. Jevitt, J. B. Patel, and B. Bozdogan.** 2004. Vancomycin-resistant *Staphylococcus aureus* isolate from a patient in Pennsylvania. *Antimicrob. Agents Chemother.* **48:**275–280.

96. **Urbanek, K., M. Kolar, and L. Cekanova.** 2005. Utilisation of macrolides and the development of *Streptococcus pyogenes* resistance to erythromycin. *Pharm. World Sci.* **27:**104–107.

97. **Veasy, L. G., L. Y. Tani, and H. R. Hill.** 1994. Persistence of acute rheumatic fever in the intermountain area of the United States. *J. Pediatr.* **124:**9–16.

98. **Yamaguchi, T., T. Hayashi, H. Takami, K. Nakasone, M. Ohnishi, K. Nakayama, S. Yamada, H. Komatsuzawa, and M. Sugai.** 2000. Phage conversion of exfoliative toxin A production in *Staphylococcus aureus*. *Mol. Microbiol.* **38:**694–705.

99. **Yamaguchi, T., T. Hayashi, H. Takami, M. Ohnishi, T. Murata, K. Nakayama, K. Asakawa, M. Ohara, H. Komatsuzawa, and M. Sugai.** 2001. Complete nucleotide sequence of a *Staphylococcus aureus* exfoliative toxin B plasmid and identification of a novel ADP-ribosyltransferase, EDIN-C. *Infect. Immun.* **69:**7760–7771.

100. **Yarwood, J. M., J. K. McCormick, M. L. Paustian, P. M. Orwin, V. Kapur, and P. M. Schlievert.** 2002. Characterization and expression analysis of *Staphylococcus aureus* pathogenicity island 3. Implications for the evolution of staphylococcal pathogenicity islands. *J. Biol. Chem.* **277:**13138–13147.

101. **Zhang, S., J. J. Iandolo, and G. C. Stewart.** 1998. The enterotoxin D plasmid of *Staphylococcus aureus* encodes a second enterotoxin determinant *(sej)*. *FEMS Microbiol Lett.* **168:**227–233.

EVOLUTION OF ENTERIC PATHOGENS

Ruiting Lan and Peter R. Reeves

15

In this chapter we will focus on three significant human pathogens in the family *Enterobacteriaceae: Salmonella enterica, Escherichia coli* (including Shigella), and *Yersinia* spp. The *Enterobacteriaceae,* a large family of gram-negative bacteria commonly but not invariably inhabiting animal intestines, vary greatly in frequency of pathogenic forms. To complicate matters, some members of other families, such as *Vibrio cholerae,* resemble members of the *Enterobacteriaceae,* in this case enterotoxigenic *E. coli* (ETEC), in mode of pathogenesis, and are often included under the banner of enteric pathogens.

Most pathogenic members of the *Enterobacteriaceae* also at least initiate infection from the intestine, and can be divided into three categories: noninvasive, invasive, and systemic pathogens. A wide range of virulence mechanisms is used, but invasive enterics generally include type III secretory systems as part of their mechanism for interaction with host cells, with the gene clusters for invasion in *S. enterica,* Shigella forms of *E. coli,* and *Yersinia* having considerable homology (46). A common char-

acteristic of the invasive pathogens is the ability to avoid destruction by macrophages and leukocytes, but the strategies used differ (3, 49, 53).

EVOLUTION AND PATHOGENESIS OF SPECIFIC PATHOGENS

Evolution and Pathogenesis in *S. enterica*

POPULATION STRUCTURE, SUBSPECIES RELATIONSHIPS, AND SURFACE ANTIGENS

S. enterica has been assigned to serovars based on the combination of antigenic properties of the polysaccharide O antigen and flagellar H1 and H2 antigens. Each serovar was originally considered a distinct species, although this does not apply to forms that were only later incorporated into the genus *Salmonella,* but on usual criteria all serovars are clearly in one or at most two species (see below). The name *Salmonella enterica* is used to cover all salmonellae (with the possible exception of subspecies V [see below]). The original species names, where given, are retained and other serovars are indicated by antigenic formula alone (81). Thus the old *Salmonella typhimurium* is referred to as *S. enterica* serovar Typhimurium or, more simply, as Typhimurium. Unfortunately, both nomenclatures are still in use, but we will use *S. enterica* as

Ruiting Lan, School of Biotechnology and Biomolecular Sciences, University of New South Wales, Sydney, New South Wales 2052, Australia. *Peter Reeves,* School of Molecular and Microbial Biosciences, University of Sydney, Sydney, New South Wales 2006, Australia.

Evolution of Microbial Pathogens, Edited by H. S. Seifert and V. J. DiRita, © 2006 ASM Press, Washington, D.C.

the species name, which is consistent with the terminology used for *E. coli*. Currently 2,501 serovars are recognized (101). Many are sufficiently homogeneous to be treated as clones, such as serovar Typhi. However 11 serovars— Choleraesuis, Derby, Dublin, Enteritidis, Infantis, Muenchen, Newport, Paratyphi B, Paratyphi C, Saintpaul, and Typhisuis—were found to be polyphyletic using multilocus enzyme electrophoresis (MLEE) (14).

S. *enterica* has a well-defined subspecies structure. Seven subspecies, designated as I, II, IIIa, IIIb, IV,V, and VI, were recognized by biotyping, with 60% of the serovars belonging to subspecies I, which includes those responsible for greater than 99% of human infections (101) . The subspecies structure is confirmed by MLEE data and sequencing of housekeeping genes (6, 15, 92, 93, 110, 119–121, 123, 124) (Fig. 1). MLEE analysis also brought to light

another subspecies (VII), but as it is based on sequence only with no reported phenotypic distinction, only the two serovars used in that study, originally in subspecies IV, have been allocated to subspecies VII. Subspecies V has been elevated to species status as S. *bongori* (110), but this is not universally accepted and of no relevance here as it includes no significant pathogenic forms. DNA sequence divergence of S. *bongori* averages about 8%, and it is much closer to other subspecies than to any other species. There are very few isolates, and we prefer to treat it as a subspecies of S. *enterica*.

In S. *enterica,* the gene trees for different housekeeping genes are generally congruent (15), and also have the characteristic of long branch lengths for each subspecies. This indicates low levels of recombination, which allowed formation of subspecies that can be consistently differentiated by biotyping, MLEE, or multilocus sequence typing (MLST). This allows us to derive a phylogenetic tree for the subspecies and to relate the gain of virulence factors to nodes in the evolutionary tree with reasonable confidence, as they will appear in all derivatives after acquisition (Fig. 1) (see below).

It should also be mentioned that three S. *enterica* strain collections, named SARA, SARB, and SARC (7, 14, 15), were established by R. K. Selander, comprising strains used in much of the work emanating from his group, and now more widely used.

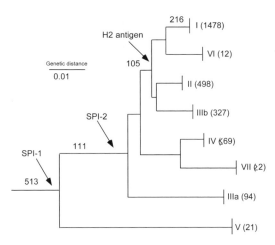

FIGURE 1 Evolutionary tree of *Salmonella enterica*. The tree shows phylogenetic relationships of the subspecies as determined by sequences of five housekeeping genes by Selander et al. (123), with the external edge and strain names removed. After the subspecies number is the number of serotypes reported for each subspecies (101), given in parentheses. Two subspecies IV serotypes were allocated to subspecies VII by genetic means (see text), and some of the remaining 69 subspecies IV serotypes may belong to subspecies VII. Major events are indicated, including the gain of SPI-1, SPI-2, and H2 antigen genes. The numbers at each node indicate the numbers of genes gained as determined by microarray analysis of LT2 genes (103).

PATHOGENICITY

S. *enterica* is found in reptiles and warm-blooded vertebrates. Most subspecies are generally isolated from reptiles and are often not disease associated, but subspecies 1 has far more serovars than the others and these are generally isolated from mammals or birds and known best as pathogens. The most common diseases caused by subspecies 1 serovars are acute enterocolitis and enteric fever. Enterocolitis occurs when the bacterium invades the epithelium of the small intestine and multiplies within mucosal cells, stimulating fluid secretion and diarrhea. Enteric fever is caused by only a few serovars as a result of extensive systemic infection. However, in their natural hosts, it seems quite common for *S. enterica* to behave more like a commensal with no obvious signs of disease, but occasionally causing disease in other species. The well-known example is food poisoning, in which food contaminated with *Salmonella* from one of the domestic animals causes a usually short-term enterocolitis. We will meet a similar situation in *E. coli* with hemolytic-uremic syndrome (HUS) strains. Other forms of *S. enterica* are characteristically pathogenic, generally host specific, or confined to a small number of hosts. Thus Typhi, Paratyphi A, Paratyphi B, and Paratyphi C are human specific. Some forms, such as Typhimurium, infect a range of hosts, but even here it seems that we are dealing with variation appearing within the serovar, in effect development of different specialized clones without change of antigens (107).

Virulence factors in *S. enterica* are commonly in pathogenicity islands (PAIs). Five PAIs, SPI1 through SPI5, were discovered by genetic analysis (54) and five more have been revealed by genome sequencing (98). The distribution of the known PAIs among subspecies indicates the order of acquisition by *S. enterica* (5) (Fig. 1). SPI1 contains genes for invasion of epithelial cells (88, 89) and is present in all subspecies but absent in the close relative *E. coli* (95). (The functions of SPI1 genes and associated functions in cell invasion have been particularly well dissected and reviewed recently [48], and will not be discussed here.) Thus all extant *S. enterica* are capable of invading intestinal epithelium and multiplying within gut-associated lymphoid tissue, effectively occupying a niche different from that in the gut lumen occupied by their closest relative, *E. coli*. We have, of course, no knowledge of the status of *S. enterica* prior to the radiation into the current subspecies, so it is not possible to be confident, although it is often said, that SPI1 has been present in *S. enterica* since divergence from *E. coli;* however, cell invasion does seem to have been a characteristic of *S. enterica* for a long time. Acquisition of additional PAIs after the divergence of subspecies V probably allowed *S. enterica* to spread from the intestinal tissue into the bloodstream

and multiply within macrophages, and thus expand the niche to intracellular locations. SPI2 is required for systemic infection and is present in all but subspecies V (60, 95). SPI3 (9) and possibly SPI4 (144) are required for survival within macrophages. SPI3 is variably present in all subspecies and must have a complex history involving lateral transfer or frequent loss (9). SPI5 (145) carries genes required for enteropathogenicity. Recent microarray analysis confirmed the distribution of SPI1, SPI2, and SPI3 and showed that SPI4 is absent in subspecies IIIa and IIIb, and that two of the eight SPI5 genes are absent in subspecies II and VI (103). There are different interpretations of the data for relationships of the subspecies (17), and this needs to be resolved before we can draw conclusions regarding the history of SPI 4 and SPI5. With SPI1 and SPI2 present in all but subspecies V (Fig. 1), *S. enterica* is clearly well adapted to invasion of host cells. However, many serovars do not seem to be strongly associated with disease in their natural hosts, and some seem never to cause food poisoning. Serovar Sofia is commonly found in chickens in Australia and not only seems not to cause disease in chickens, but is also not implicated in human food poisoning in Australia (58).

The most apparent but least understood feature of *Salmonella* pathogenesis is adaptation beyond the general invasion properties. A number of serovars cause enteric fever in humans: Paratyphi A, Paratyphi B, Paratyphi C, Sendai, and Typhi (123). Of these, Paratyphi A and Sendai are closely related but the others are not, indicating that the capacity to cause enteric fever was independently acquired several times. Paratyphi C is closely related to the swine-adapted Choleraesuis. Paratyphi B is a large heterogeneous group, and ability to cause enteric fever in humans is found only in the globally distributed clone PB1. Typhi is a distinctive and homogeneous serovar with two electrophoretic types, one of which is dominant. The two ETs are confirmed by MLST, which also identified an additional two sequence types (STs) (69). Chan et al. (26) identified genes that are common among the enteric fever-causing serovars using an LT2 genome-based microarray, and more light should be shed by a microarray analysis of Typhi-specific genes.

A common adaptation is to host specificity. Several serovars are host adapted (123). These include Gallinarum and Pullorum, adapted to poultry and causing fowl typhoid and pullorum disease; Choleraesuis, adapted to pigs and causing pig paratyphoid; Dublin, adapted to cattle and causing bacteremia; and, as discussed above, Typhi and Paratyphi A, C, and B (PB1 clone only), adapted to humans and causing typhoid fever. Within a serovar, subtypes may adapt to different hosts, with epidemiological evidence that Typhimurium phage types DT2 and DT99 are adapted to pigeons, DT8 and DT46 to ducks, and DT40 to wild birds (107). Very little is known of the mechanisms of host adaptation (70, 71).

Evolution and Pathogenesis in *E. coli*

E. coli is a diverse species. It is generally present in the large intestine and lower end of the small intestine of many mammals. It is perhaps the major species using the oxygen that diffuses into the intestine from the well-vascularized intestinal wall. The large intestine is occupied predominantly by anaerobic bacteria, but it is the presence of bacteria such as *E. coli* that maintains the anaerobic status of this region, where bacterial processes make some of the less digestible materials available to the host. *E. coli* is well known for its ability to ferment a range of sugars, but will grow faster in the presence of oxygen and, like other *Enterobacteriaceae,* seems ideally adapted to the role of oxygen scavenger.

The *E. coli* of interest here are the pathogenic forms, and this is an appropriate time to say that these include all Shigella, with the minor exception of Boydii serotype 13. It is clear that, in evolutionary terms, the various Shigella serotypes fit within *E. coli,* and as we are emphasizing evolution, we will refer to them as *E. coli.* However, it is important to retain the name Shigella and the Shigella species and serotype names in this discussion as they are familiar to many of us, so we will refer to *Shigella sonnei,* for example, as *E. coli* Sonnei (or just Sonnei).

POPULATION STRUCTURE OF COMMENSAL *E. COLI* AND THE ECOR SET

Early studies on evolution and population genetics of the species were centered on isolates from healthy humans and animals. These studies revealed the population structure of the species and initiated the study of bacterial population genetics. A key outcome was establishment of the *E. coli* reference (ECOR) set of 72 strains, selected to encompass the range of genetic variation observed in those studies (96). The ECOR set has now been used in many studies on population genetics and evolution of *E. coli* (87, 130). The use of one set of strains for a range of studies has greatly simplified interpretation, and it is hard to overemphasize the importance of this set of strains. However, one needs to keep in mind that there is more diversity in the species than found in the ECOR set (e.g., in intestines of wild animals [106, 128]), but this has not been added to the collection to expand its representation. The ECOR set strains were divided into four major subgroups (A, B1, B2, and D) by MLEE (61, 122), and many studies have confirmed the groupings. Group B2 includes many uropathogenic isolates. Group B1 is most heterogeneous, and group D is most divergent from other groups. Several laboratories have sequenced housekeeping genes from a number of ECOR set strains (80, 141), but an evolutionary tree based on housekeeping gene sequences for all ECOR strains is still lacking.

MULTIPLE PATHOGENIC FORMS OF *E. COLI*

The first pathogenic form of *E. coli* to be discovered has since become known as *Shigella dysenteriae,* or *E. coli* Dysenteriae 1 to us, and this was followed by a range of forms that were eventually put into four species of Shigella. Pathogenic forms considered at the time to be *E. coli* were not recognized until the 1940s. At least eight forms of pathogenic *E. coli* are now recognized (37, 91), and those discovered in the 1940s are now known as enteropathogenic *E. coli* (EPEC). Other forms include enterohemorrhagic (EHEC), ETEC, enteroaggregative, and enteroinvasive *E. coli* (EIEC). The pathogenic forms are often identified by serotyping, and serotypes frequently associated with major forms are shown in Table 1. The total number of serotypes involved is far greater, as shown by an extensive list compiled for ETEC (143), and the hundreds of Shiga toxin *E. coli* serotypes reported, with a proportion already reported in HUS cases (http://www.microbionet.com.au/frames/feature/vtec/intro.htm). Serotype identification is a good indication of the diversity of pathogenic forms, but it should be noted that serogroups, based on O antigen only, in many cases are not a reflection of clonal relatedness.

The major virulence factors for these pathogenic forms are all on mobile elements. EPEC strains carry the locus of enterocyte effacement (LEE) PAI encoding a type III secretion system, with proteins for effacing and attachment (86), and the EAF plasmid with genes for adherence (91). EHEC strains also carry LEE but with two crucial additional elements, Shiga toxin phage and an EHEC plasmid (91). ETEC strains contain plasmid-borne genes for enterotoxins (91) and specific pili with adhesins, and are perhaps the only pathogenic *E. coli* that are generally not invasive but remain in the gut lumen. EIEC and *Shigella* strains carry the same pINV invasion plasmid (57, 91) and they should be treated as one pathogenic form as both have the same mode of cell invasion, albeit with varying levels of virulence. There may be many other virulence factors, but these are the major factors that contribute to a particular pathogenic form. It should be noted that only for very few isolates carrying the virulence factors has pathogenicity been confirmed. This has led to alternative names for EHEC strains, which are often called Shiga toxin *E. coli* where there is no clinical evidence for HUS.

The pathogenic forms, in particular EPEC, EHEC, and *Shigella*/EIEC, have been extensively studied by MLEE and sequencing (37, 104, 105, 112, 140). Current studies show that there are two major groups of EPEC and EHEC, respectively. EPEC 1 and EHEC 1 have LEE inserted at *selC*, while EPEC 2 and EHEC

TABLE 1 Serotypes associated with pathogenic *E. coli* categories[a]

Category[b]	O antigen	H antigen(s)
ETEC	O6	H16
	O8	H9
	O11	H27
	O15	H11
	O20	NM
	O25	H42, NM
	O27	H7
	O78	H11, H12
	O128	H7
	O148	H28
	O149	H10
	O159	H20
	O173	NM
EPEC	O55	H6, NM
	O86	H34, NM
	O111	H2, H12, NM
	O119	H6, NM
	O125ac	H21
	O126	H27, NM
	O127	H6, NM
	O128	H2, H12
	O142	H6
EHEC	O26	H11, H32, NM
	O55	H7
	O111ab	H8, NM
	O113	H21
	O117	H14
	O157	H7
EAEC	O3	H2
	O15	H18
	O44	H18
	O86	NM
	O77	H18
	O111	H21
	O127	H2
EIEC	O28ac	NM
	O29	NM
	O112ac	NM
	O124	H30, NM
	O136	NM
	O143	NM
	O144	NM
	O152	NM
	O159	H2, NM
	O164	NM
	O167	H4, H5, NM

[a] Adapted from reference 91.

[b] EAEC, enteroaggregative *E. coli*; EHEC, enterohemorrhagic *E. coli*; EIEC, enteroinvasive *E. coli*; EPEC, enteropathogenic *E. coli*; ETEC, enterotoxigenic *E. coli*.

2 have LEE at *pheU.* EPEC 1 includes serotypes O55:H6, O119:H6, O125:H6, O127:H6, and O142:H6 (37, 112), and EPEC 2 includes O111:H2, O114:H2, O126:H2, and O128:H2. Of the two major EHEC groups, EHEC 1 consists of the O157:H7 clone only and was derived from the atypical (lacks EAF plasmid) EPEC O55:H7 strain, not related to the two major EPEC groups, while EHEC 2 includes O111:H8, O111:H–, O26:H11, O26:H–, and other serotypes. The situation, however, may be more complex as the studies did not include many commensal *E. coli,* so that it is not possible to see if commensal strains also group with the pathogenic strains. Some pathogenic strains are closely related, but the MLEE tree of pathogenic forms is deep and it is not excluded that it is interdigitated with commensal forms.

In a different analysis of the relationships between nonpathogenic *E. coli,* as represented by the complete ECOR set, and a variety of pathogenic strains of *E. coli* using MLEE and *mdh* gene (malate dehydrogenase) sequences, the EPEC, ETEC, EIEC, and EHEC strains were distributed among the ECOR subgroups (Fig. 2) (104).

EVOLUTION OF SHIGELLA CLONES AND ENTEROINVASIVE *E. COLI*

Various studies have shown that Shigella strains fall within *E. coli,* including studies using MLEE (97), ribotyping (116), or a combination of MLEE and sequencing (104). The evolutionary relationships of all 46 serotypes of Shigella were elucidated recently by analysis of sequence variation in eight housekeeping genes (105), showing that most fall into three clusters within *E. coli* (Fig. 3), each cluster representing a group of related *E. coli* clones. Interestingly, each cluster includes strains from different Shigella "species." (Note that Shigella serotype names are designated here with the first letter of the "species name" plus the serotype number, e.g., D1 is Dysenteriae serotype 1.) Cluster 1 contains one Flexneri and the majority of Boydii and Dysenteriae strains (B1 to B4, B6, B8, B10, B14, B18, D3 to D7, D9, D11 to D13, and F6).

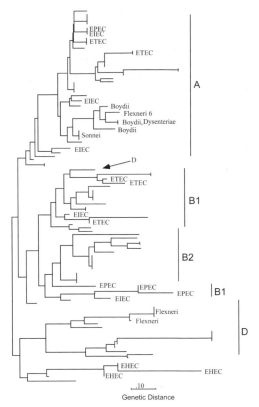

FIGURE 2 Genetic relationships of commensal *E. coli* strains represented by the ECOR set strains and representative pathogenic *E. coli* strains as resolved by MLEE (104). For clarity, all strain names were removed from the tree (see original paper for details). External branches, where pathogenic *E. coli* strains are represented or the sole member, are marked with the pathogenic form, while other branches without names are ECOR set strains.

Cluster 2 contains one Dysenteriae and seven Boydii strains (B5, B7, B9, B11, B15, B16, B17, and D2). Cluster 3 contains one Boydii strain (B12) and the Flexneri serotypes 1 through 5. Sonnei and three Dysenteriae strains (D1, D8, and D10) are outside of the three main clusters, but nonetheless clearly within *E. coli,* while B13 is distantly related to *E. coli* and represents an unnamed species.

EIEC has the same mode of pathogenesis as Shigella, carries the same pINV plasmid, and has similar metabolic deficiencies. They are only differentiated by a limited number of bio-

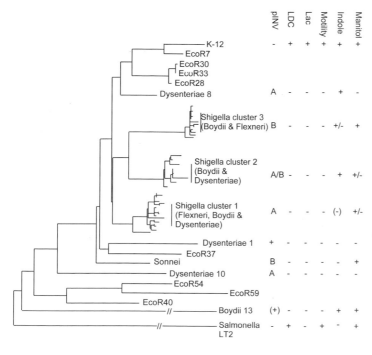

	pINV	LDC	Lac	Motility	Indole	Manitol
K-12	-	+	+	+	+	+
EcoR7						
EcoR30						
EcoR33						
EcoR28						
Dysenteriae 8	A	-	-	-	+	-
Shigella cluster 3 (Boydii & Flexneri)	B	-	-	-	+/-	+
Shigella cluster 2 (Boydii & Dysenteriae)	A/B	-	-	-	+	+/-
Shigella cluster 1 (Flexneri, Boydii & Dysenteriae)	A	-	-	-	(-)	+/-
Dysenteriae 1	+	-	-	-	-	-
EcoR37						
Sonnei	B	-	-	-	-	+
Dysenteriae 10	A	-	-	-	-	-
EcoR54						
EcoR59						
EcoR40						
Boydii 13	(+)	-	-	-	+	+
Salmonella LT2	-	+	-	+	-	+

FIGURE 3 The evolutionary tree of Shigella and other *E. coli* based on housekeeping genes (105), with distribution of key characteristics of *E. coli* and Shigella (adapted from reference 75). The pINV form is indicated as A or B (74), or as a "+" if not known to be A or B, or non-A/non-B. The common properties of commensal *E. coli* are represented by K-12 (top row). Other rows correspond to the cluster or strain on the left. The Shigella strains in the three clusters are shown in the original paper. It can be clearly seen that Shigella, with the exception of Boydii 13, are clones of *E. coli*.

chemical properties (44). Analysis of 32 EIEC strains representing 10 of the 14 known serotypes, using the same set of genes used for the study of Shigella strains, revealed that the EIEC strains are not grouped with Shigella strains, with the exception of one EIEC strain that falls into Shigella cluster 2 (73). The remaining 31 EIEC strains fall into four clusters with one outlier strain, mirroring the situation in Shigella with several independent derivations. The EIEC clusters are numbered from 4 to 7 following on from the three Shigella clusters. There are 11 strains in cluster 4 with five O antigens (O28, O29, O124, O136, and O164), 10 strains in cluster 5 with four O antigens (O124, O135, O152, and O164), and 6 strains in cluster 6 with two O antigens (O143 and O167). Cluster 7 has three strains and all are O144. The EIEC clusters are smaller in size relative to Shigella clusters in terms of the number of different O antigens, but this may reflect the level of attention given to them. The level of variation within a cluster is also lower in the EIEC clusters than Shigella clusters. These differences suggest that the EIEC clusters arose

later. It is not clear whether current EIEC strains would eventually lose all of the commensal *E. coli* properties absent in Shigella clones, to become "Shigella," as adaptation to the intestinal epithelial niche continues (see "Clone Specialization and Gene Decay" below). Escobar-Paramo et al. (43) undertook similar studies and concluded that the Shigella/EIEC pathovar arose once only, before divergence from the ECOR group A strains. The study had 10 non ECOR group A strains. The monophyletic picture of the Shigella and EIEC may be a result of insufficient representation of the commensal *E. coli*, but the matter is expected to be resolved in the MLST scheme being developed for *E. coli*, which has typed the 72 ECOR strains and a large number of other *E. coli* strains, including Shigella and EIEC (T. Wirth et al., unpublished data).

Evolutionary relationships of the pINV plasmids of Shigella and EIEC strains have also been determined (73, 74). Using *ipgD, mxiC,* and *mxiA* sequences of the invasion locus on the pINV plasmid, two closely related forms (pINV A and pINV B) of the plasmid were found. The phylogenetic relationships of plasmid and chromosomal genes of Shigella strains are largely consistent. The cluster 1 and cluster 3 strains tested have pINV A and pINV B plasmids, respectively. However, of the three cluster 2 strains, two have pINV A and one has a pINV B plasmid. D1 has a distinct pINV sequence, but the other Shigella strains (D8, D10, and Sonnei), which do not group with the main body of Shigella strains on the tree based on chromosomal gene sequences, were all found to have one or the other of the two major plasmid sequence forms. These strains must have obtained the plasmid relatively recently, after the divergence of the two pINV forms. All but 2 of the 32 EIEC strains studied were found to have pINV A, which seems to transfer more frequently to other *E. coli* than pINV B. Both chromosomal gene and plasmid gene sequences unequivocally support EIEC and Shigella as a single pathovar of *E. coli,* driving home the message that the demarcation of the two forms is rather arbitrary. It is true that the major health problem with this pathovar relates to a few Shigella forms (Sonnei, D1, and some of the Flexneri group) but one may question the long-standing perception that Shigella generally is more virulent than EIEC.

EVOLUTION OF THE EHEC O157:H7 *E. COLI* Clone

The EHEC O157:H7 clone was discovered in the early 1980s when several outbreaks of hemorrhagic colitis were associated with the serotype O157:H7 (114), and has since been implicated worldwide in outbreaks of food- and waterborne disease (52, 132). The clone is widely found in cattle, where it exists essentially as a commensal as disease is uncommon (12, 127). There is no reason to believe that the clone has not been in cattle for a long time, and even been causing human disease for some time despite its reputation as an emerging disease. It was first reported in 1983 but came to prominence after a 1993 outbreak on the U.S. West Coast, caused by contaminated hamburger meat. The clone could conceivably have gone undetected before it received its cur-

rent level of attention, as the infection rate is often low.

The O157:H7 clone carries the LEE PAI, *stx,* and EHEC plasmid as the major virulence factors. Only *stx* and EHEC plasmid are possibly of recent origin. The clone has accumulated little mutational variation (94) but much variation through genomic changes (72). O157:H7 does not ferment sorbital or exhibit glucuronidase (GUD) activity, although there is a nonmotile sorbital-positive variant (45). Feng et al. (45) proposed a stepwise model for the evolution of this clone. The closest ancestral strain is O55:H7. The O157:H7 clone seems to have first gained its O157 O antigen by recombination (133). It then developed into two lineages: a major sorbital-negative and GUD-negative form, and a minor variant that lost motility but retained the ancestral properties of Sob$^+$ and GUD$^+$. The minor variant carries only one (presumably ancestral) *stx* gene (*stx2*), while the major form has two *stx* genes (*stx1* and *stx2*) on separate phages. Recent analysis of *stx1* and *stx2* integration sites, showing truncation of *stx1* and movement of *stx2* to another locus, gave further insight into the evolution of this clone (125).

Evolution and Pathogenesis in *Yersinia* spp.

The genus *Yersinia* contains 11 species. Three are significant pathogens for mammals, including humans, while the others, generally treated as nonpathogenic, do have some pathogenic potential (131). *Yersinia pseudotuberculosis* and *Yersinia enterocolitica* are food- and waterborne pathogens that cause enterocolitis in humans (19). *Yersinia pestis,* the causative agent of plague, is transmitted primarily by fleas, and has been responsible for devastating epidemics throughout history (38). *Y. pestis* is clearly a clone of *Y. pseudotuberculosis* (1), but otherwise not enough sequence data are available to properly establish the relationships of the two diversified pathogenic species to each other and to the nonpathogenic species. However, the two species are no closer to each other than to other *Yersinia* spp. on a 16S rRNA tree (65) or DNA hybridization (16).

Y. ENTEROCOLITICA AND Y. PSEUDOTUBERCULOSIS

Y. enterocolitica and Y. pseudotuberculosis are not primarily human pathogens, and the major reservoirs are domestic animals and rodents, with human infections resulting from contact or contaminated foods. The two species share essential virulence factors (13, 19, 30, 113) not present in the nonpathogenic species, so if the 16S tree is correct, they must have independently acquired similar virulence factors. Both species evade the host immune system through proteins called Yersinia outer membrane proteins, which are encoded on a 70-kb virulence plasmid (pYV) (29, 31, 32). The other major virulence determinant is the high-pathogenicity island (HPI), which is present in biotype 1B of Y. enterocolitica (23) and in some Y. pseudotuberculosis, predominantly in serotypes O1 and O3 (13). HPI confers hypervirulence and contains genes for biosynthesis, regulation, and transport of the siderophore yersiniabactin. The acquisition of HPI is probably recent since it has limited distribution in the genus. However, HPI is mobile across Enterobacteriaceae, being present in some E. coli isolates, Klebsiella (five species), and Citrobacter diversus (4, 118). A number of chromosomally encoded virulence factors are also present, such as invasin, which promotes the uptake of bacteria by a variety of cells, and Ail, which promotes bacterial attachment to and invasion of epithelial cells in vitro and contributes to resistance to complement-mediated killing. These genes are present in both species (108).

Y. enterocolitica is widely distributed in nature in aquatic and animal reservoirs, with swine serving as a major reservoir for human pathogenic strains. There are seven biotypes (1A, 1B, 2, 3, 4, 5, and 6) and more than 70 serotypes (126, 137). All except biotype 1A are traditionally associated with human infections (13), but even 1A has been isolated from human feces and has been increasingly recognized as an etiological agent of gastroenteritis. Biotype 1A strains generally lack the chromosomally encoded invasin and Ail and the 70-kb pYV virulence plasmid. MLEE analysis showed that biotype 1 isolates were separated from the other biotypes as two major clusters (24, 36). It is not clear whether biotype 1B isolates cluster together, away from biotype 1A isolates, since the study by Caugant et al. (24) only had biotype 1B isolates, while the study by Dolina and Peduzzi (36) did not differentiate biotype 1 into 1A and 1B.

Y. pseudotuberculosis is divided into 15 serogroups with 21 types (11, 134). Serogroups O1 to O5 have been isolated in Europe and the Far East, and most are pathogenic to humans. Serogroups O6 to O14 have been isolated from animals and the environment but not from clinical samples. Fukushima et al. (47) conducted an extensive survey of three virulence factors (HPI, pYV, and the superantigenic toxin Y. pseudotuberculosis-derived mitogen [YPM]) in Y. pseudotuberculosis isolates from a variety of sources worldwide. The distribution was investigated by PCR of 2,235 isolates that fell into six subgroups. Subgroup 1 is positive for all three factors and was only seen in Far East isolates. Subgroup 2 lacks the toxin but has high pathogenicity ($HPI^+ YPM^- pYV^+$). It has been predominant in Europe as serotypes 1a and 1b, and also isolated in the Far East as serotypes 1a, 3, 5b, 13, and 14. Subgroup 3 lacks the HPI but has the toxin ($HPI^- YPM^+ pYV^+$) and is found in 11 serotypes causing systemic infections in the Far East. Subgroup 4 is nonpathogenic since it has neither HPI nor pYV ($YPM^+ HIP^- pYV^-$). There were 93 isolates from nine serotypes in this subgroup. Subgroup 5 has a partial HPI (partial $HPI^+ YPM^+ pYV^+$) and was found in serotype 3 isolates only. Subgroup 6 has neither HPI nor toxin ($HPI^- YPM^- pYV^+$). This subgroup is distributed worldwide with a large number of serotypes. It should be noted that, for all subgroups except subgroup 4, pYV is present in 50 to 89% of isolates. As pYV is essential for pathogenicity, it is not clear whether those isolates without pYV have lost the plasmid during culture or indeed have no pYV and hence are nonpathogenic. It would require phylogenetic analysis of these isolates to understand the heterogeneity of virulence factors and clonal distribution of these properties.

YERSINIA PESTIS, A CLONE OF Y. PSEUDOTUBERCULOSIS WITH A VERY DIFFERENT MODE OF PATHOGENESIS

Y. pestis, the flea-transmitted agent of plague, was long recognized to be very closely related to Y. pseudotuberculosis. The two are nearly identical genetically, being indistinguishable by standard DNA hybridization methods and 99.7% identical in 16S ribosomal RNA. Y. pestis is a phenotypically homogeneous species with only one serotype and three biovars, and has been shown to be a clone of the food-borne pathogen Y. pseudotuberculosis (1). There was no variation in the sequence of six housekeeping genes over 36 isolates of Y. pestis. The sequences were much closer to Y. pseudotuberculosis than Y. enterocolitica genes, and all were within the range of variation for Y. pseudotuberculosis isolates for the six housekeeping genes. Y. pestis is clearly a homogeneous clone that arose recently. It seems preferable to call it Pestis, as a Y. pseudotuberculosis clone, to clarify its real status as a recently established niche-adapted clone and not a low-variation species, and we do so in places to draw attention to its being a part of Y. pseudotuberculosis, although we recognize that this is not common practice.

How did Pestis evolve its different pathogenesis strategy? The infection cycle has three key elements: colonization of the flea gut, transmission to a new host through biting, and hematogenous dissemination from the infected site. Two of the three elements involve plasmids. The gut colonization factor, which is also known as Yersinia murine toxin, is determined by the ymt gene on the pFra plasmid, while the gene encoding a plasminogen activator, involved in dissemination, is on the pPla plasmid (22, 62).

Transmission from flea to host is achieved through reverse flow of blood during biting due to partial blockage of the flea proventriculus, leading to regurgitation of a blood meal. This ability is determined by the hms (hemin storage) genes (63), which allow the bacterium to accumulate around the proventriculus and block it. Interestingly, the hms genes are located together with HPI in the pgm locus in Pestis, and are found in the same locus in Y. pseudotuberculosis (20). The adaptation to fleas as a new host seem to be an accidental consequence as the hms genes were acquired by Y. pseudotuberculosis presumably for a different purpose. Transmission to fleas must have occurred infrequently before the acquisition of pFra, as mutants cured of the pFra plasmid infected and caused blockage in only a small number of fleas (64). This very inefficient process was then greatly enhanced by the acquisition of pFra, giving the bacterium the ability to survive and colonize the flea gut. The acquisition of pPla is another major step in gaining the capacity to cause pandemic-level disease as the dissemination of the bacterium from the biting site is greatly enhanced (22).

POPULATION GENETICS OF ENTERIC PATHOGENS

Clonal Structure in Enteric Bacteria

Bacteria reproduce by binary fission, and as a result, all bacterial populations are clonal to some extent. However, most and perhaps all species undergo recombination, which seems always to involve transfer of DNA fragments from one cell to another. The frequency varies greatly among species, but it is always very low relative to reproduction by binary fission. This circumstance allows clones to become specialized because members of the same species in different circumstances can adapt to local circumstances, whereas in most eukaryotes genetic recombination means that the population adapts as a whole. For bacteria, one can refer to the species niche, which is broad, and clonal niches within the broad niche to which clones adapt. The clones that we are discussing are clearly functionally different and adapted to their specific niche—we refer to them as niche adapted. It is the balance between the forces of mutation and recombination that determines the general population structure of a bacterial species. The spectrum ranges from species such as Neisseria spp., in which recombination occurs relatively freely, to those such as *S. enterica*, in which recombination is infrequent (84, 129).

Many studies indicate that *S. enterica* is more clonal than *E. coli* (40, 55, 84, 129). In *S. enterica*, there is a robust subspecies structure established by biotyping but easily detected by sequencing (123). The gene trees of the SARC strains representing the subspecies are generally congruent, although some recombination is detectable (17). However, a recent study looking at the *mutS* gene indicates that recombination is quite frequent in the SARB strains representing subspecies I (18). Our unpublished data also suggest that, within a subspecies, *Salmonella* may be less clonal than previously thought (S. Octavia and R. Lan, unpublished data).

In *E. coli*, the sequence variation at the tips of the branches, ie, among closely related clones, was shown to be largely due to recombination rather than mutation in the genes involved (55). This also seems to apply at deeper levels, with the major groups having extremely low bootstrap values, probably due to the impact of recombination. The effect of a higher level of recombination is that we do not get such consistent patterns of relationships among housekeeping genes and as a consequence can be far less confident about the relationships of *E. coli* isolates than those of *S. enterica*. Nonetheless *E. coli*, with many recognized forms, is clearly clonal. The *E. coli* clones that we recognize differ in adaptive traits, in this case traits related to mode of pathogenesis, and are generally homogeneous in sequence of housekeeping genes. It is only when clones are closely related (as, e.g., O55:H7 and O157:H7) that we can draw conclusions about details of relationships, at least with current levels of available data. If we pursue that example, we can expect that, over time, the O157:H7 and O55:H7 clones will suffer recombinational changes in their housekeeping genes, and eventually it will not be easy or perhaps even possible to establish their relatedness. But it is still quite possible that each clone could persist for a very long time, with selection for adaptation to a specific mode of pathogenicity ensuring that those genes that in combination

are adaptive in a niche remain associated despite pressure of recombination to break that combination.

In the case of *S. enterica*, the consistency of the different gene trees allows us to relate the level of divergence of subspecies to that of species divergence. The difference between subspecies V, the most divergent, and other subspecies is about 8% compared to 15% between *E. coli* and *S. enterica*, suggesting that subspecies V diverged from the others about 65 to 75 million years ago, if the estimate of 120 to 140 million years for *E. coli* and *S. enterica* is correct. However, one cannot attempt such analysis for the major groups of *E. coli*, at least with the number of housekeeping gene sequences available.

Diversity in Enteric Species

The diversity of *S. enterica* and *E. coli* has been extensively studied. However, genetic diversity of a species can only be fully appreciated when the entire living space of the species is sampled. This need is illustrated by recent sampling of *E. coli* from a variety of environments (106, 128), which has revealed more diversity than previous sampling largely from humans and human-associated animals. An appropriate sampling from a bacterial population is usually not easily achieved, but multiple isolates representing the known phenotypic diversity of the species will reduce bias. This aspect is not well addressed in many studies of variation and evolution of pathogens, and it is not clear how close we are to understanding the diversity of even the better known species, in particular those such as *E. coli* with both commensal and pathogenic forms.

Distinguishing Clones and Species

There has long been debate on the validity of the species concept in bacteria. However, it certainly seems to work, and for well-studied groups the boundaries are generally clear—clear enough indeed to see with hindsight that some errors have been made. We recently drew attention to the fact that several pathogenic "species" are in fact clones of other species, and to the need to properly define the clones and species in light of molecular data (78). It is the availability of sequences that allows easy identification of clones (42). This applies across many species, but it is of urgency for enteric pathogens as niche-adapted pathogenic clones are so often encountered.

We referred above to the desirability of treating *Y. pestis* as a clone of *Y. pseudotuberculosis.* This would follow the custom developed for *S. enterica,* in which all previously recognized species are referred to as *S. enterica.* In the case of Shigella, seven major clones are readily identifiable by sequence variation (excluding Boydii 13, a representative of an unnamed species), but only Sonnei corresponds to one of the originally named species (105).

Clones are a reality, and where they differ in pathogenicity, it is sensible to distinguish them by giving them names. And as species boundaries become clearer, if we are to follow the long-standing convention in biology, the names have to change to fit the new picture. However, it does seem to cause difficulty when names change for well-known organisms such as *Y. pestis* and Shigella spp., and the original names can be retained as clone or subspecies names as appropriate to minimize this. Also, if we are to use a more natural classification, it is important that the public and regulatory agencies recognize that changing a name does not change the nature of an organism. It is already generally accepted that there are good and bad *E. coli,* and the widespread change to treating all *Salmonella* as *S. enterica* has not stopped Typhi getting special treatment. We should be able to extend that to treating Shigella strains as forms of *E. coli* and *Y. pestis* as a form of *Y. pseudotuberculosis.*

NICHE ADAPTATION AND CLONE SPECIALIZATION

Polymorphism and Lateral Gene Transfer

One of the great advances in microbiology in recent years has been the recognition that the differences between forms of a species can be correlated with presence or absence of blocks of genes, often called islands or, in our case, PAIs (56). It has now become a major paradigm of

evolution of pathogenesis, and of course has a chapter in this book (see chapter 5).

Bacterial clones are clearly niche adapted, and at least for the species we are discussing, many of the differences observed lie in the presence or absence of specific PAIs, plasmids, or phages. PAIs often have clear indications of being mobile elements, and plasmids and phages certainly are. These elements as seen by us are probably quite mature and adapted to the species they inhabit and to their role in enhancing the fitness of the host strain. In effect, they are part of the genetic diversity of that species, and their movement from one cell to another can be treated either as a form of lateral transfer or as genetic recombination. Certainly PAIs or lysogenic phages could move by conjugation, followed by homologous chromosomal recombination or by transduction, or even by element-encoded excision and insertion mechanisms. As they move from one clone to another, they will continue to adapt to the species they are in. Lateral transfer in the more traditional sense refers to transfer between species, and this clearly does bring new capacity to a species. Movement within a species by homologous recombination should leave evidence in the sequence of adjacent genes that can be seen if we have sequences of related strains. This is currently not widely available, but as the number of full genome sequences grows, we can expect to make that distinction. In many ways, the blocks of genes that we call PAIs resemble the blocks of genes observed for metabolic pathways, often under coordinated expression and called "operons." These also may be present or absent in specific isolates and are generally treated as polymorphisms subject to reassortment by recombination.

Surface Antigen Polymorphisms and Pathogenicity

The loci for surface antigens provide an interesting comparison with PAIs. These loci are generally present in all strains but occur in many different forms. The best studied are the liposaccharides, capsules, and flagella, with the antigens often known as O, K, and H antigens, respectively. The O and H antigens are generally present in the *Enterobacteriaceae*. The number of O antigen forms varies in different species but is often very high, with 54 and 190 known O antigen forms recognized in *S. enterica* and *E. coli*, respectively. The genes for O, H1, and H2 antigens in *S. enterica* are not distributed according to subspecies, as most are found in two or more subspecies (101), the inference being that the genes for these antigens have undergone considerable lateral transfer.

The O antigen appears to be a major target of both the immune system and bacteriophages, both of which must apply intense selection, and are probably major factors in the origin and maintenance of the high level of variation, and in driving the lateral transfer. Other selection pressures such as protozoan predation may exist (142), but here we are only concerned with adaptation to a pathogenic niche. Each strain expresses only one O antigen form, and the variation is thought to allow the various clones of a species to each present a surface that offers a selective advantage in the niche occupied by that clone. It has been estimated that a selective advantage of only 0.1% for one O antigen over another in a given niche is more than sufficient to maintain different alleles in different clones (111), so the basis for advantage may be difficult to determine. Some O antigen forms are disproportionately represented in pathogenic clones, and O antigen specificity may be important in determining pathogenicity, although there are rather few data. The chain length is also controlled, and there is evidence of association between O polysaccharide chain length and pathogenicity in *E. coli* (Shigella) (90).

The Shigella clones provide a good example of O antigen variation. The 46 O antigens described for Shigella strains comprise 33 unique O antigen forms if the *E. coli* and *S. enterica* guidelines are followed (75), of which 12 are identical to other known *E. coli* O antigens and 21 are unique to Shigella clones (105). If the unique forms were gained in Shigella rather than lost by other *E. coli* strains, the 21 new O antigens gained by Shigella clones rep-resent 11% of the known *E. coli* forms. Most Shigella strains were estimated to have diverged over 50,000 to 270,000 years within *E. coli*, compared with the divergence of *E. coli* from *S. enterica* 120 to 140 million years ago. Considering this short time frame, the expansion of O antigen forms is extraordinarily rapid.

The H antigen is again highly variable and, as for the O antigen, it may be simply that there is ongoing selection by the immune system and perhaps other factors for novel forms; it may also be that this contributes to the maintenance of *E. coli* in any specific niche, but we are not aware of any data on this. In *E. coli*, there are several alternative loci for the flagellar protein gene (109), but 43 of the 53 recognized antigenic forms are at the *fliC* locus, all of which have been sequenced and are remarkably divergent (136). Variation is due to divergence affecting the part of the protein exposed on the outside of the flagellum (68). There are several forms that are distinguished by electron microscopy (79), and this accounts for much of the sequence divergence (136). This may be important in pathogenicity but does not appear to have been studied. There are also some strains for which flagella seem to be selected against, as discussed below.

In *S. enterica*, most serovars have two alternative flagellar forms, carrying the H1 and H2 antigens (also called phase 1 and phase 2), encoded by *fliC* and *fljB*, respectively. There is a regulatory system to ensure that they are not expressed simultaneously. Most serovars are diphasic, but many are monophasic. Interestingly, most serovars in subspecies I, II, IIIb, and VI are diphasic, while those in subspecies IIIa, IV, V, and VII are monophasic. As seen in Figure 1, the monophasic serovars are ancestral to the diphasic form. The basis for the diphasic condition is presumably to further evade the host immune system, and it is likely to have assisted in the exploitation of birds and mammals as hosts (82, 123). However, 10% of the serovars of subspecies I and II have reverted to the monophasic condition; also, as for *E. coli*, some *S. enterica* no longer make flagellae, indicating that they are not advantageous in these strains.

Clone Specialization and Gene Decay

During the course of evolution, genes may become redundant and will be lost by accumulation of mutations and deletions, undergoing what we call "decay" (77). Shigella strains provide a good example as they are generally less biochemically active than other *E. coli* strains, indicating loss of gene functions. In particular, Shigella strains lack catabolic pathways otherwise widely present in the species (44). With few or no exceptions, lactose and mucate are not utilized, and lysine is not decarboxylated. Shigella strains are also nonmotile. Other *E. coli* strains are usually positive for these properties. The loss of these catabolic functions is attributed to niche adaptation as Shigella occupies a very different niche from the commensal *E. coli*.

Gene decay is nicely explained by experimental data from chemostat studies. In an experimental population, *E. coli* adapting to live in an environment where a single carbon source (usually glucose) is used, the diet breadth of the population decayed as a trade-off for optimal fitness (28; also see chapter 4). This trade-off is clearly seen in *Shigella*, with several independently derived clones adapted for life inside a eukaryotic cell. The common phenotypic properties are due to loss of functions and have been shown to be due to different genetic changes in each clone. This includes motility (2), lactose fermentation (66), and lysine decarboxylation (33, 83).

In the case of lysine decarboxylation, it has been shown that the property is very deleterious for Shigella such that there would be strong selection against its presence (33, 83; also see chapter 6). One can understand that utilization of lactose is important for commensal *E. coli*. The organism is commonly found in the mammalian intestines, where lactose would be abundant in infant animals, lactose being the sugar present at high levels in mammalian milk. However, the trait is of little use for intracellular life. Similarly, since Shigella uses actin-assisted motility to move intracellularly, flagella-based motility becomes redundant for much of its life cycle. A large number of genes are involved in production of the flagellum and associated machinery, and turning it off would conserve significant resources. Also, because the number of genes involved is larger, there is a higher chance for inactivation by a mutation arising in any one of the genes. There is also the possibility that inactivating the immunogenic flagellum helps circumvent mucosal defenses (50).

EVOLUTIONARY GENOMICS OF ENTERIC BACTERIA

There are six published genome sequences of *E. coli* (including Shigella), three of *S. enterica,* and three of *Y. pseudotuberculosis,* including two Pestis genomes. The overall picture is of colinearity for most genes but with many blocks of genes found in only one or some of the genomes. We will attempt to summarize the major conclusions that can be drawn from studies based on these genomes. This first taste of the use of whole genomes makes it clear that we will gain a much clearer view of the population structures and clonal origins as more such data appear, and that will not take long as several other genomes have been completed but not yet published. Comparison of multiple genomes within a species will also give an appreciation of the size of a species genome, which we proposed (77) to consist of core genes present in all or most strains of a species and auxiliary genes present in some strains only.

Genome Comparison in *E. coli*

The six *E. coli* genome sequences (10, 59, 67, 100, 138, 139) have been used for direct comparisons and also as a basis for further experimental work using arrays or other techniques.

The two O157:H7 genomes were published at about the same time, and each was compared to the K-12 (strain MG1655) genome (10) but not with the other (59, 100). Comparison of the K-12 and O157:H7 strain EDL933 genomes showed that 4.1 Mb of sequence (3,574 genes) are shared with 1.6% nucleotide difference, and that K-12 and EDL933 have 0.53 Mb (528 genes) and 1.34 Mb (1,387 genes) of strain-specific sequence, respectively (100). Most of these strain-specific genes are localized in "islands." There are 108 islands larger than 1 kb in O157:H7, with many known and candidate virulence factors present, although 60% of the genes are of unknown function. The findings from the second O157:H7 genome sequence are similar but there are a larger number of genes, although some may be a result of differences in annotation. Of the 5,361 genes identified, 3,729 genes are shared with K-12, with 1,632 genes O157:H7 specific (59).

The fourth *E. coli* genome is from a uropathogenic strain, CFT073 (139). The CFT073 genome is 590,209 bp longer than K-12 and similar in size to EDL933. The genome contains 5,533 genes, of which 3,190 are also present in K-12. There are 2,004 CFT073-specific genes located on 247 islands, of which 204 are shared by O157:H7 EDL933. Analysis of proteins in the three genomes gives a picture of the species genome and strain gene content. A total of 7,638 proteins were identified in the three genomes (there were some exclusions). Only 2,996 (39.2%) genes are in all three (Fig. 4), and this will be an overestimate of the core genes in *E. coli* as the number is certain to go down as more genomes are sequenced. It seems clear that, for *E. coli* and probably for many bacteria, the majority of genes in the species are present in only some strains. Also, the core genes based

on three genomes are already only 60 to 70% of genes in a given strain, so it is clearly possible that, with addition of further genomes, the core genes will be less than 50% in at least the larger genomes of this species.

The other two *E. coli* genomes are from Flexneri 2a strains 301(67) and 2457T (138). Both have been compared with K-12 and EDL933 but neither with CFT073. The Flexneri genomes are slightly smaller than the K-12 genome, with 2,881 genes common to 2457T, K-12, and EDL933. 2457T shares 149 and 30 additional genes with K-12 and EDL933, respectively, with 175 genes 2457T specific. One of the remarkable features of the Flexneri genome is the large number of insertion sequence (IS) elements. There are 314 IS elements in the 301 genome compared with 39 and 40 in K-12 and EDL933, respectively. The virulence plasmid also contains a large number of IS elements that comprise 40% of its genes (21, 135). The two Flexneri genomes have also been compared (138). The 301 genome is slightly larger, accounted for largely by IS sequences. Both genomes have many pseudogenes relative to other *E. coli* genomes, with 254 and 372 in 301 and 2457T, respectively, although some of the differences are due to annotation criteria (138). Other differences include genome rearrangements, unique sets of

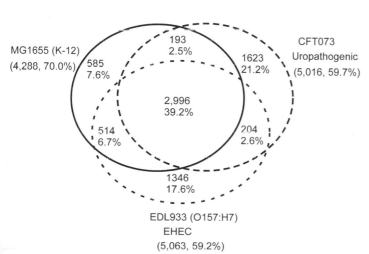

FIGURE 4 Distribution of *E. coli* proteins: core and unique genes among *E. coli* K-12, O157:H7 (EDL933), and uropathogenic *E. coli* CFT073 (adapted from reference 139). Areas represent categories of genes but are not proportional to the number of genes. The percentage within a category is based on the total of 7,638 proteins. The number of proteins used for comparison in each strain is indicated under the strain name, together with the percentage of core genes.

pseudogenes in each strain, and >1,400 single nucleotide differences. We used the sequences of the relevant genes to compare the two genome sequence strains to the F2a strain used for a dendrogram of Shigella strains (105), and found the three F2a strains to be near identical, with three differences in total. By MLST, they would be in very closely related STs, and the variation in pseudogenes indicates that loss of function is continuing in this clone.

We must bear in mind that *E. coli* is a high-recombination species (see "Clonal Structure in Enteric Bacteria" above) with pathogenic forms intermingled with commensals in phylogenetic trees. The strain-specific genes of the pathogenic strains are therefore not necessarily associated with pathogenicity. It is likely that many strain-specific genes (relative to K-12) play a role not in virulence but in other aspects of adaptation or survival. For example, genes specific to O157:H7, relative to K-12, include candidate genes for transporting diverse carbohydrates, aromatic compound degradation, tellurite resistance, and glutamate fermentation. There is no reason to assume that the large number of such genes results from acquisition of genes to become a pathogen. Many of the genes may be present in commensal strains that share recent common ancestry with the O157:H7 clone, and relate to the niche occupied by a predecessor. The genome studies bring home the need for better information on the relationships of pathogenic and commensal *E. coli* strains so that genomes of closely related strains can be sequenced and compared. The O157:H7 clone is related to ECOR 37 (104), which is known to have a similar genome size (8) and was isolated from a marmoset in the Washington Zoo with no suggestion that it was involved in disease. It would be interesting to determine how many O157:H7-specific genes (relative to K-12) are present in other strains.

Genome size variation in *E. coli* genomes has also been analyzed using pulsed-field gel electrophoresis, by which chromosome size of 35 ECOR set strains ranged from 4.5 to 5.5 Mb in length (8). The size variation is phylogenetically clustered, with isolates from certain subgroups having consistently larger chromosomes, suggesting that much of the additional DNA in larger chromosomes is shared through common ancestry (8). Note that, in their affinity with ECOR groups, K-12 is from group A and CFT073 is probably from group B2, based on the Clermont test (27), as it has both *chuA* and *yjaA* in its genome.

It is usual to treat the presence or absence of blocks of genes as insertions or deletions, and that is reasonable when considering their origins. However, when comparing two strains of a species, we have to consider the possibility of recombinational transfer for presence or absence of a block of genes. The data on *E. coli* discussed above make it clear that whole housekeeping genes can transfer by recombination, and one would expect the same to apply to niche-adaptive genes involved in pathogenesis. Thus, when we compare *E. coli* strains K-12, EDL933, and CFT073, the differences may well have arisen by recombination of preexisting variation, rather than by insertion or deletion. In effect, we have polymorphisms consisting of the presence or absence of genes or sets of genes. Of course, the differences must have arisen originally by insertion or deletion, but that may have occurred a long time ago, and the edges may have been cleaned up since then to account for the rather sharp junctions commonly observed. It is even possible for such a polymorphism to survive speciation, as is proposed for the O antigen forms found in both *E. coli* and *S. enterica* (117).

Genome Comparison in *S. enterica*

Complete genome sequences have been published for *S. enterica* serovar Typhimurium LT2 (85) and two serovar Typhi isolates, CT18 (98) and Ty2 (35), and genomes of several other serovars are being completed.

TWO SEROVAR TYPHI GENOMES

Two Typhi genome sequences are available, one of Ty2, isolated in 1918 well before the emergence of drug resistance in the 1970s (35), and

CT18, isolated in 1993 in Vietnam (98). The two isolates belong to different sequence types as defined by MLST (69). Ty2 has no plasmids while CT18 has two, one of them a large plasmid with multiple drug resistance cassettes. There are 4,599 and 4,545 genes on the chromosome (scored as coding sequences including pseudogenes [CDS]), with 84 and 29 unique to CT18 and Ty2, respectively, many of them in phagelike regions. It is not clear if any of the strain-specific genes are of any functional significance, or simply due to chance infection by phages or some other event. The most interesting differences are in the approximately 4,500 shared genes. The two Typhi strains have 4,195 identical CDS, and 282 differ by single base changes, which together comprise 97% of the total (35).

Both Typhi strains carry a significant number of pseudogenes. CT18 and Ty2 have, respectively, 204 and 206 pseudogenes, while LT2 has only 39. It is clear that Typhi has far more than LT2, and this is taken to be a reflection of its host specificity and adaptation. Of the pseudogenes, 195 are common to both Typhi strains, and the additional 9 and 11 in the two isolates presumably represent the increase since their last common ancestor. Of the 204 pseudogenes in CT18, 27 were remnants of ISs or other mobile elements; of the other 177, 124 (70%) were inactivated by a single frameshift or stop codon, suggesting a recent origin for Typhi, which was estimated to be about 50,000 years ago (69).

GENOME COMPARISON BETWEEN SEROVARS

The differences in *Salmonella* genomes were studied by genomic subtraction in the pre-genome sequencing era (76), with 6.4 to 13.1% of Typhimurium DNA estimated to be absent in Typhi and 16.2 to 26.8% absent in subspecies V. Complete genome sequences confirm the observation on Typhi and give us a detailed picture of the Typhimurium-Typhi comparison. There are 601 genes (13.1%) in 82 blocks that are unique to Typhi and 479 genes (10.9%) in

80 blocks that are unique to Typhimurium (85, 98). Comparison of the partly sequenced genomes of Dublin, Enteritidis, and Paratyphi A indicated a similar level of difference (41). The genome size variation seems smaller than seen in *E. coli* genomes, but it should be noted that all are human pathogens from subspecies I, whereas the *E. coli* genomes are more representative of the species diversity.

The presence of Typhimurium and Typhi genes in other *S. enterica* isolates has been assessed by microarray analysis using the SARC and SARB sets, covering different subspecies and subspecies I, respectively, and other strains (102, 103). In the first study, 1,424 (32%) of the 4,483 LT2 genes examined were absent or diverged beyond hybridization in at least one of the other genomes. A phylogenetic analysis based on homologue content relative to LT2 is largely concordant with previous studies based on housekeeping gene sequences. A total of 513 genes were acquired by *S. enterica*, 105 by diphasic *Salmonella* (subspecies I, II, IIIb, and VI), and 216 by subspecies I (Fig. 1).

One interesting observation is that 935 genes of LT2 were identified as *S. enterica* specific from comparisons with *E. coli* and *Y. tuberculosis Pestis* genomes. However, only 56 of these specific genes were consistently detected in all *Salmonella* isolates. The *Salmonella*-specific genes include the previously known SPI1 genes. Other genes include a DNA helicase gene and genes allowing *Salmonella* to use tetrathionate as an electron acceptor during anaerobic respiration, reducing it to hydrogen sulfide, the significance of which is not clear. Of these 56 genes, 34 have no assigned function, which indicates how little we know in terms of biology of *Salmonella*. The second study on subspecies I included multiple isolates of many of the serotypes studied (102). Even within the subspecies, 215 genes were absent or diverged beyond hybridization in at least one of the other genomes. Several serotypes included more than one genotype, confirming earlier observations based on MLEE but adding much detail. The term "genovar" was coined to describe groups of strains that share a similar profile of gene content.

Genome Comparison in *Y. pseudotuberculosis*

The Pestis strain CO92 genome was published in 2001 (99), followed by that of strain KIM (34) in 2002. It was immediately apparent that there were a large number of pseudogenes in the Pestis strains, and comparison of the two genomes also revealed a remarkable amount of genome rearrangement (34), the differences appearing to result from inversions of genome segments at insertion sequences. However, a much clearer view emerged with the publication of the genome of IP32935, a typical *Y. pseudotuberculosis* strain (25). IP32935 has 3,974 predicted genes and 62 pseudogenes, of which 43 are also pseudogenes in one or both of the Pestis genomes. With the availability of the genome of a strain that has not undergone extensive pseudogene formation, the number of pseudogenes detected in the Pestis strains was approximately doubled, to 398 in the case of CO92. This was because having a closely related strain with normal gene number provides a much higher number of good homologues for comparisons, and illustrates very clearly the benefits of comparative studies of pathogens with close relatives. Substantial differences were also seen in the number of IS elements, with 20 in IP32935, but 117 in KIM and 138 in CO92, with 12 integration locations common to all three. It can be seen that, as for Shigella strains, there has been a substantial expansion of IS elements and loss of gene function, some of which was due to IS insertion.

There are 317 genes unique to IP32953 and 112 unique to the two Pestis strains. Chain et al. (25) also looked at panels of *Y. pseudotuberculosis, Y. pestis,* and *Y. enterocolitica,* using PCR and sometimes sequencing to study the wider distribution of some of the genes in the three genomes. In this way, they were able to identify 32 genes present in all *Y. pestis* and no *Y. pseudotuberculosis* among the strains studied, comprising the only genes potentially gained during development of the Pestis mode of virulence, apart from the previously identified plasmids. Some of the 317 genes seen as IP32953 specific could have been due to loss in the Pestis strains, increasing the number of functions lost in the Pestis strains. It seems that about 10% of the Pestis genome has lost function during adaptation to its unique niche. Indeed, the major change observed in Pestis is the loss of gene function. It is not possible to say how much of this is adaptive to the new niche, as much or even all of it may be due to removal of selection for maintenance of functions no longer needed. However, the newly identified genes unique to Pestis may well be important in adaptation to the new niche, and this opens up new opportunities for analysis of the functional changes in the evolution of Pestis.

There were many differences in the details of pseudogene sequences and IS elements in the two Pestis genomes (not all discussed above), which is interesting as comparison of housekeeping gene sequences suggests that both would be in the same ST in an MLST scheme, whereas there is considerable variation within *Y. pseudotuberculosis* (1). The changes in Pestis must be ongoing and occurring at a much faster rate than accumulation of MLST variation.

Genome-Level Species Comparisons

The genetic maps of *E. coli* K-12 and *S. enterica* LT2 have long been studied by classical genetic means (115). The complete genome sequences allow a detailed comparison of the two species. Two *S. enterica* genomes have been compared with that of *E. coli* K-12. There are 1,106 LT2 genes not in K-12 (85) and 945 K-12 genes not in LT2. In the case of Typhi, there are 1,505 genes (32.7%) in 290 blocks that are unique to Typhi relative to K-12 and 1,220 genes (28.4%) in 268 blocks unique to K-12. Single gene insertions account for 128 of the unique genes in Typhi, and 456 genes are in islands of 5 genes or fewer (98). Approximately 3,000 genes are present in both *E. coli* K-12 and *S. enterica* LT2, representing about 70% of genes in either species for a given strain. This is similar to the situation within *E. coli* as discussed above. We look forward to genome sequences and microarray studies for more strains from both species, representing the species diversity, to give a clear picture of the genes shared in the two species, and any genes that are consistently present in one or the other species.

Yersinia is quite distant from *E. coli* and *S. enterica* (16), and comparison of the Pestis KIM and *E. coli* K-12 genome proteins showed a locally colinear "backbone," or synteny. Only 54% of KIM open reading frames are significantly similar to *E. coli* K-12 proteins, with conserved housekeeping functions (34). This is a big drop from the 70% of genes shared by *E. coli* and *S. enterica,* reflecting evolutionary distance as well as bigger differences in lifestyle between them.

PERSPECTIVES AND CONCLUSIONS

The Major Role of Pathogenicity Islands and Other Mobile Elements

The *Enterobacteriaceae* are generally commensal, with some pathogenic species and other species with pathogenic clones. It is striking that most of the major virulence factors are on plasmids, phages, or PAIs. We have focused on *S. enterica, E. coli* (including *Shigella*), and *Yersinia* spp., which differ in their general pattern of pathogenicity, but in each case gain of virulence factors led to expansion of niche space occupied by the species, although adaptation to some niches may lead to the clone losing ability to live in the general niche. There are perhaps generalists and specialists in a species. The focus of research on pathogenicity has been on these mobile elements. They clearly entered into the species in question by lateral gene transfer, but in general the donor species is not known, although other elements may have related components. We have learned a lot about these virulence factors but have yet to learn much about the origins of these most interesting elements. The detailed microarray studies of gene distribution in *S. enterica* in particular are adding great detail to our knowledge of islands of

genes and their distribution within the species. While these islands will not all be PAIs in the usual sense, they may well be important in the adaptation of the many forms of the species to particular hosts or other aspects of their niche.

The Possible Role of Adaptation without Adding Genes

It is important to remind ourselves that the focus of research on PAIs and other mobile elements does not mean that they are the only determinants of pathogenicity. It is natural that the focus has been on the most obvious components of pathogenesis because of their clear relationship to the disease and its symptoms. However, one would expect adaptation to involve not only gain of new genes but also changes in genes already present, as the pathogen is generally in a rather different environment than its commensal relatives. It is much harder to look at such adaptations, and we are not aware of any such studies. It is nonetheless very important to know how virulent are commensal *E. coli* strains after transfer of PAIs or virulence plasmids, as this would indicate the level of risk of new pathogenic clones arising in this way. It is often assumed that the presence of strains with virulence factors indicates a risk of transfer to generate new pathogenic forms, but the level of risk may be very low if other less easily observed factors are critical to pathogenesis. It is interesting in this regard to note that *E. coli* carrying Shiga-like toxin are commonly found in food samples, but only a few strains cause HUS, and the presence of *stx* genes alone is not a good predictor of risk. This indicates that there are factors not understood that determine the ability to cause HUS, and the same will apply to most infections by enteric organisms.

The Need for Good Data on Population Structures

We have not discussed population structures in much detail because more detailed work is being done on other groups of organisms, for which MLST schemes have been widely adopted. However, it is most important that the matter be addressed for the enteric pathogens. The large, well-maintained databases for *Neisseria* and *Sreptococcus pneumoniae* (http://www.mlst.net) have greatly facilitated study of the evolution of pathogenic clones in these species. We are aware that such schemes are under development for *E. coli* and *S. enterica* (see http://www.mlst.net and http://www.shiga-tox.net), and one (or more) is certainly needed for *Yersinia* spp. If we are to study the origins of pathogenicity in these species, we need to compare pathogenic strains with strains that on good grounds can be treated as closely related to the ancestor. In this way we can hope to learn about the adaptive changes that occurred across the genome, which is interesting in its own right and has major practical implications. We noted above the use of closely related strains to identify genes that are of interest for study of the pathogenesis of Pestis. We need both MLST schemes and good support for them to make the databases representative in order to get better value from genome sequences.

Pseudogenes in Pathogens

Genes that for some reason become deleterious or no longer beneficial to a clone will be lost by accumulation of mutations and deletions. Such losses occur at all levels, but when observed within a species, the evidence in the form of remnant genes (pseudogenes) and evidence of the role of transposable elements, etc., may still be clear, whereas older events are often seen only by the presence or absence of genes.

The Shigella clones of *E. coli,* the Pestis clone of *Y. pseudotuberculosis,* and serovar Typhi of *S. enterica* all have many pseudogenes, and are clearly losing many of their more general species properties as they become adapted to what appears to be in all three cases a new niche. The scale of gene decay only came to light with genome sequencing showing the large number of pseudogenes in these clones. There are two genome sequences for Pestis, Typhi and Flexneri 2a. In each case, the varia-

tion in housekeeping genes would place them in the same ST or very closely related STs, whereas there are substantial differences in the details of the pseudogenes, indicating that this is an ongoing process.

The Taxonomic Status of Pathogenic Clones

Many human and some animal pathogens were seen as so distinctive that full species or even genus status was given to forms that can now be seen to be clones of another species. The source of the problem is the enormous diversity of some bacterial species. The examples included in this chapter are Shigella clones of *E. coli* and the Pestis clone of *Y. pseudotuberculosis.* A third example is Typhi, which for a long time held species status as *S. typhi* but is now widely treated as a clone of *S. enterica.* In the case of Shigella, we have four species that do not correspond to natural groupings within *E. coli,* so that substantial revision is needed in any case. It is surely better to treat the Shigella forms of *E. coli* in the same way as the ETEC and other pathogenic forms of this rather well-defined species. In the case of *Y. pestis,* we have only a single clone, and one can argue that it has evolved to full species status over a very short time (39). It may be that, over a longer time, it will develop good separation from its parent species, *Y. pseudutoberculosis,* and not remain in genetic contact by recombination among the many genes common to both. However, it is too early to know that, and now that we have the data that clarified the relationship, it seems preferable to treat it as a clone, making the species definition more consistent with that used in *E. coli,* for example. There are other such cases, for example, *Bordetella pertussis* and *B. parapertussis,* which are clearly host-specific clones of *B. bronchiseptica* (78), and the latest addition of *Burkholderia mallei,* the causative agent of glanders, as a horse-adapted clone of *Burkholderia pseudomallei* (51). It is likely that many more cases will be found, and it may be sensible to face up to the growing anomaly in the taxonomy of such pathogens and formally treat Shigella and Pestis as clones of the "mother" species, as is done for Typhi as a clone of *S. enterica*.

CHAPTER SUMMARY

- Most enteric pathogens initiate infection from the intestine, and can be divided into three categories: noninvasive, invasive, and systemic pathogens. *Y. pestis* is an exception that developed an entirely different strategy, with acquisition of two plasmids from its ancestor in *Y. pseudotuberculosis*.

- *S. enterica* has a well-defined subspecies structure, with more than 2,000 serovars. Major steps in the evolution of *S. enterica* are sequential acquisitions of PAIs, and many genes have been gained during the development of subspecies and clones; presumably this is balanced by gene loss.

- *S. enterica* as a species has lower levels of recombination and hence is more clonal than *E. coli*. Little is known of the population structures of *Y. pseudotuberculosis* and *Y. enterocolitica*.

- *E. coli* is a diverse species with many pathogenic forms. Shigella strains, despite the genus status, are clones of *E. coli*.

- Surface antigens, exemplified by O antigens, are subjected to higher levels of lateral transfer between and within a species and exist as polymorphisms within a species.

- Gene decay in specialized clones is evident from genome sequencing, with a large number of pseudogenes in the genomes of *S. enterica* serovar Typhi, *E. coli* clone (Shigella) Flexneri 2a, and *Y. pestis*, in reality a clone of *Y. pseudotuberculosis*.

- The genomes of enteric bacteria are mosaics, composed of colinear regions interspersed with insertions or "islands" unique to a given genome. Only half of the genes present in any given genome are conserved among the enteric genomes.

ACKNOWLEDGMENTS

Research in our laboratories is supported by the National Health and Medical Research Council of Australia and the Australian Research Council.

REFERENCES

1. **Achtman, M., K. Zurth, G. Morelli, G. Torrea, A. Guiyoule, and E. Carniel.** 1999. *Yersinia pestis,* the cause of plague, is a recently emerged clone of *Yersinia pseudotuberculosis. Proc. Natl. Acad. Sci. USA* **96:**14043–14048.

2. **Al Mamun, A. A. M., A. Tominaga, and M. Enomoto.** 1997. Cloning and characterization of the region III flagellar operons of the four *Shigella* subgroups: genetic defects that cause loss of flagella of *Shigella boydii* and *Shigella sonnei. J. Bacteriol.* **179:** 4493–4500.

3. **Alpuche-Aranda, C. M., E. P. Berthiaume, B. Mock, J. A. Swanson, and S. I. Miller.** 1995. Spacious phagosome formation within mouse macrophages correlates with Salmonella serotype pathogenicity and host susceptibility. *Infect. Immun.* **63:**4456–4462.

4. **Bach, S., A. de Almeida, and E. Carniel.** 2000. The *Yersinia* high-pathogenicity island is present in different members of the family *Enterobacteriaceae. FEMS Microbiol. Lett.* **183:**289–294.

5. **Baumler, A. J.** 1997. The record of horizontal gene transfer in *Salmonella. Trends Microbiol.* **5:** 318–322.

6. **Beltran, P., J. M. Musser, R. Helmuth, J. J. Farmer, W. M. Frerichs, I. K. Wachsmuth, K. Ferris, A. C. M. Whorter, J. G. Wells, A. Cravioto, and R. K. Selander.** 1988. Toward a population genetic analysis of *Salmonella:* genetic diversity and relationships among strains of serotypes *S. choleraesuis, S. derby, S. dublin, S. enteritidis, S. heidelberg, S. infantis, S. newport,* and *S. typhimurium. Proc. Natl. Acad. Sci. USA* **85:**7753–7757.

7. **Beltran, P., S. A. Plock, N. H. Smith, T. S. Whittam, D. C. Old, and R. K. Selander.** 1991. Reference collection of strains of the *Salmonella typhimurium* complex from natural populations. *J. Gen. Microbiol.* **137:**601–606.

8. **Bergthorsson, U., and H. Ochman.** 1998. Distribution of chromosome length variation in natural isolates of *Escherichia coli. Mol. Biol. Evol.* **15:**6–16.

9. **Blanc-Potard, A. B., F. Solomon, J. Kayser, and E. A. Groisman.** 1999. The SPI-3 pathogenicity island of *Salmonella enterica. J. Bacteriol.* **181:**998–1004.

10. **Blattner, F. R., G. I. Plunkett III, C. A. Bloch, N. T. Perna, V. Burland, M. Riley, J. Collado-Vides, J. D. Glasner, C. K. Rode, G. F. Mayhew, J. Gregor, N. W. Davis, H. A.**

Kirkpatrick, M. A. Goeden, D. J. Rose, B. Mau, and Y. Shao. 1997. The complete genome sequence of *Escherichia coli* K-12. *Science* **277:**1453–1474.

11. Bogdanovich, T., E. Carniel, H. Fukushima, and M. Skurnik. 2003. Use of O-antigen gene cluster-specific PCRs for the identification and O-genotyping of *Yersinia pseudotuberculosis* and *Yersinia pestis. J. Clin. Microbiol.* **41:**5103–5112.

12. Borczyk, A. A., M. A. Karmali, H. Lior, and L. M. C. Duncan. 1987. Bovine reservoir for verotoxin-producing *Escherichia coli* O157:H7. *Lancet* **i:** 98.

13. Bottone, E. J. 1997. *Yersinia enterocolitica:* the charisma continues. *Clin. Microbiol. Rev.* **10:**257–276.

14. Boyd, E. F., F.-S. Wang, P. Beltran, S. A. Plock, K. Nelson, and R. K. Selander. 1993. Salmonella reference collection B (SARB): strains of 37 serovars of subspecies 1. *J. Gen. Microbiol.* **139:**1125–1132.

15. Boyd, E. F., F. S. Wang, T. S. Whittam, and R. K. Selander. 1996. Molecular genetic relationships of the *Salmonellae. Appl. Environ. Microbiol.* **62:**804–808.

16. Brenner, D. J. 1984. *Enterobacteriaceae,* p. 408–428. *In* N. R. Krieg and J. G. Holt (ed.), *Bergey's Manual of Systematic Bacteriology,* vol. 1. Williams & Wilkins, Baltimore, Md.

17. Brown, E. W., M. L. Kotewicz, and T. A. Cebula. 2002. Detection of recombination among *Salmonella enterica* strains using the incongruence length difference test. *Mol. Phylogenet. Evol.* **24:**102–120.

18. Brown, E. W., M. K. Mammel, J. E. LeClerc, and T. A. Cebula. 2003. Limited boundaries for extensive horizontal gene transfer among *Salmonella* pathogens. *Proc. Natl. Acad. Sci. USA* **100:**15676–15681.

19. Brubaker, R. R. 1991. Factors promoting acute and chronic diseases caused by yersiniae. *Clin. Microbiol. Rev.* **4:**309–324.

20. Buchrieser, C., R. Brosch, S. Bach, A. Guiyoule, and E. Carniel. 1998. The high-pathogenicity island of *Yersinia pseudotuberculosis* can be inserted into any of the three chromosomal *asn* tRNA genes. *Mol. Microbiol.* **30:**965–978.

21. Buchrieser, C., P. Glaser, C. Rusniok, H. Nedjari, H. D'Hauteville, F. Kunst, P. Sansonetti, and C. Parsot. 2000. The virulence plasmid pWR100 and the repertoire of proteins secreted by the type III secretion apparatus of *Shigella flexneri. Mol. Microbiol.* **38:**760–771.

22. Carniel, E. 2003. Evolution of pathogenic *Yersinia,* some lights in the dark, p. 3–12. *In* M. Skurnik, J. A. Bengoechea, and K. Granfors (ed.), *The Genus* Yersinia: *Entering the Functional Genomics Era.* Kluwer Academic/Plenum Publishers, New York.

23. Carniel, E., I. Guilvout, and M. Prentice. 1996. Characterization of a large chromosomal "high-pathogenicity island" in biotype 1B *Yersinia enterocolitica. J. Bacteriol.* **178:**6743–6751.

24. Caugant, D. A., S. Aleksic, H. H. Mollaret, R. K. Selander, and G. Kapperud. 1989. Clonal diversity and relationships among strains of *Yersinia enterocolitica. J. Clin. Microbiol.* **27:**2678–2683.

25. Chain, P. S., E. Carniel, F. W. Larimer, J. Lamerdin, P. O. Stoutland, W. M. Regala, A. M. Georgescu, L. M. Vergez, M. L. Land, V. L. Motin, R. R. Brubaker, J. Fowler, J. Hinnebusch, M. Marceau, C. Medigue, M. Simonet, V. Chenal-Francisque, B. Souza, D. Dacheux, J. M. Elliott, A. Derbise, L. J. Hauser, and E. Garcia. 2004. Insights into the evolution of *Yersinia pestis* through whole-genome comparison with *Yersinia pseudotuberculosis. Proc. Natl. Acad. Sci. USA* **101:**13826–13831.

26. Chan, K., S. Baker, C. C. Kim, C. S. Detweiler, G. Dougan, and S. Falkow. 2003. Genomic comparison of *Salmonella* enterica serovars and *Salmonella bongori* by use of an *S. enterica* serovar typhimurium DNA microarray. *J. Bacteriol.* **185:**553–563.

27. Clermont, O., S. Bonacorsi, and E. Bingen. 2000. Rapid and simple determination of the *Escherichia coli* phylogenetic group. *Appl. Environ. Microbiol.* **66:**4555–4558.

28. Cooper, V. S., and R. E. Lenski. 2000. The population genetics of ecological specialization in evolving *Escherichia coli* populations. *Nature* **407:**736–739.

29. Cornelis, G. R. 2000. Molecular and cell biology aspects of plague. *Proc. Natl. Acad. Sci. USA* **97:**8778–8783.

30. Cornelis, G. R. 1994. Yersinia pathogenicity factors. *Curr. Top. Microbiol. Immunol.* **192:**243–263.

31. Cornelis, G. R., T. Biot, C. Lambert de Rouvroit, T. Michiels, B. Mulder, C. Sluiters, M. P. Sory, M. Van Bouchaute, and J. C. Vanooteghem. 1989. The Yersinia yop regulon. *Mol. Microbiol.* **3:**1455–1459.

32. Cornelis, G. R., A. Boland, A. P. Boyd, C. Geuijen, M. Iriarte, C. Neyt, M. P. Sory, and I. Stainier. 1998. The virulence plasmid of *Yersinia,* an antihost genome. *Microbiol. Mol. Biol. Rev.* **62:**1315–1352.

33. Day, W. A., R. E. Fernandez, and A. T. Maurelli. 2001. Pathoadaptive mutations that enhance virulence: genetic organization of the *cadA* regions of *Shigella* spp. *Infect. Immun.* **69:**7471–7480.

34. Deng, W., V. Burland, G. Plunkett III, A. Boutin, G. F. Mayhew, P. Liss, N. T. Perna, D. J. Rose, B. Mau, S. Zhou, D. C. Schwartz, J. D. Fetherston, L. E. Lindler, R. R. Brubaker, G. V. Plano, S. C. Straley, K. A. McDonough,

M. L. Nilles, J. S. Matson, F. R. Blattner, and R. D. Perry. 2002. Genome sequence of *Yersinia pestis* KIM. *J. Bacteriol.* **184**:4601–4611.

35. Deng, W., S. R. Liou, G. Plunkett III, G. F. Mayhew, D. J. Rose, V. Burland, V. Kodoyianni, D. C. Schwartz, and F. R. Blattner. 2003. Comparative genomics of *Salmonella enterica* serovar Typhi strains Ty2 and CT18. *J. Bacteriol.* **185**:2330–2337.

36. Dolina, M., and R. Peduzzi. 1993. Population genetics of human, animal, and environmental *Yersinia* strains. *Appl. Environ. Microbiol.* **59**:442–450.

37. Donnenberg, M. S., and T. S. Whittam. 2001. Pathogenesis and evolution of virulence in enteropathogenic and enterohemorrhagic *Escherichia coli*. *J. Clin. Invest.* **107**:539–548.

38. Drancourt, M., and D. Raoult. 2002. Molecular insights into the history of plague. *Microbes Infect.* **4**:105–109.

39. Dykhuizen, D. E. 2000. *Yersinia pestis*: an instant species? *Trends Microbiol.* **8**:296–298.

40. Dykhuizen, D. E., and L. Green. 1991. Recombination in *Escherichia coli* and the definition of biological species. *J. Bacteriol.* **173**:7257–7268.

41. Edwards, R. A., G. J. Olsen, and S. R. Maloy. 2002. Comparative genomics of closely related salmonellae. *Trends Microbiol.* **10**:94–99.

42. Enright, M. C., and B. G. Spratt. 1999. Multilocus sequence typing. *Trends Microbiol.* **7**: 482–487.

43. Escobar-Paramo, P., C. Giudicelli, C. Parsot, and E. Denamur. 2003. The evolutionary history of *Shigella* and enteroinvasive *Escherichia coli* revised. *J. Mol. Evol.* **57**:140–148.

44. Ewing, W. H. 1986. *Edwards and Ewing's Identification of the* Enterobacteriaceae, 4th ed. Elsevier Science Publishers, Amsterdam, The Netherlands.

45. Feng, P., K. A. Lampel, H. Karch, and T. S. Whittam. 1998. Genotypic and phenotypic changes in the emergence of *Escherichia coli* O157:H7. *J. Infect. Dis.* **177**:1750–1753.

46. Foultier, B., P. Troisfontaines, S. Muller, F. R. Opperdoes, and G. R. Cornelis. 2002. Characterization of the *ysa* pathogenicity locus in the chromosome of *Yersinia enterocolitica* and phylogeny analysis of type III secretion systems. *J. Mol. Evol.* **55**:37–51.

47. Fukushima, H., Y. Matsuda, R. Seki, M. Tsubokura, N. Takeda, F. N. Shubin, I. K. Paik, and X. B. Zheng. 2001. Geographical heterogeneity between Far Eastern and Western countries in prevalence of the virulence plasmid, the superantigen *Yersinia pseudotuberculosis*-derived mitogen, and the high-pathogenicity island among *Yersinia pseudotuberculosis* strains. *J. Clin. Microbiol.* **39**:3541–3547.

48. Galan, J. E. 2001. *Salmonella* interactions with host cells: type III secretion at work. *Annu. Rev. Cell Dev. Biol.* **17**:53–86.

49. Galan, J. E., and P. J. Sansonetti. 1996. Molecular and cellular bases of *Salmonella* and *Shigella* interactions with host cells, p. 2757–2773. In F. C. Neidhardt, R. Curtiss III, J. L. Ingraham, E. C. C. Lin, K. B. Low, B. Magasanik, W. S. Reznikoff, M. Riley, M. Schaechter, and H. E. Umbarger (ed.), *Escherichia coli and Salmonella typhimurium: Cellular and Molecular Biology*, 2nd ed., vol. 2. ASM Press, Washington, D.C.

50. Giron, J. A. 1995. Expression of flagella and motility by *Shigella*. *Mol. Microbiol.* **18**:63–75.

51. Godoy, D., G. Randle, A. J. Simpson, D. M. Aanensen, T. L. Pitt, R. Kinoshita, and B. G. Spratt. 2003. Multilocus sequence typing and evolutionary relationships among the causative agents of melioidosis and glanders, *Burkholderia pseudomallei* and *Burkholderia mallei*. *J. Clin. Microbiol.* **41**:2068–2079.

52. Goldwater, P. N., and K. A. Bettelheim. 1998. New perspectives on the role of *Escherichia coli* O157:H7 and other enterohaemorrhagic *E. coli* serotypes in human disease. *J. Med. Microbiol.* **47**:1039–1045.

53. Grant, T., V. Bennett-Wood, and R. M. Robins-Browne. 1999. Characterization of the interaction between *Yersinia enterocolitica* biotype 1A and phagocytes and epithelial cells in vitro. *Infect. Immun.* **67**:4367–4375.

54. Groisman, E. A., A. Blanc-Potard, and K. Uchiya. 1999. Pathogenicity islands and the evolution of *Salmonella* virulence, p. 127–150. In J. B. Kaper and J. Hacker (ed.), *Pathogenicity Islands and Other Mobile Virulence Elements*. ASM Press, Washington, D.C.

55. Guttman, D. S., and D. E. Dykhuizen. 1994. Clonal divergence in *Escherichia coli* as a result of recombination, not mutation. *Science* **266**: 1380–1383.

56. Hacker, J., G. Blum-Oehler, I. Muhldorfer, and H. Tschape. 1997. Pathogenicity islands of virulent bacteria: structure, function and impact on microbial evolution. *Mol. Microbiol.* **23**: 1089–1097.

57. Hale, T. L. 1991. Genetic basis of virulence in *Shigella* species. *Microbiol. Rev.* **55**:206–224.

58. Harrington, C. S., J. A. Lanser, P. A. Manning, and C. J. Murray. 1991. Epidemiology of *Salmonella sofia* in Australia. *Appl. Environ. Microbiol.* **57**:223–227.

59. Hayashi, T., K. Makino, M. Ohnishi, K. Kurokawa, K. Ishii, K. Yokoyama, C. G. Han, E. Ohtsubo, K. Nakayama, T. Murata, M. Tanaka, T. Tobe, T. Iida, H. Takami, T. Honda, C. Sasakawa, N. Ogasawara, T. Yasunaga, S. Kuhara, T. Shiba, M. Hattori, and H.

Shinagawa. 2001. Complete genome sequence of enterohemorrhagic *Escherichia coli* O157:H7 and genomic comparison with a laboratory strain K-12. *DNA Res.* **8:**11–22.

60. **Hensel, M., J. E. Shea, A. J. Baumler, C. Gleeson, F. Blattner, and D. W. Holden.** 1997. Analysis of the boundaries of *Salmonella* pathogenicity island 2 and the corresponding chromosomal region of *Escherichia coli* K-12. *J. Bacteriol.* **179:**1105–1111.

61. **Herzer, P. J., S. Inouye, M. Inouye, and T. S. Whittam.** 1990. Phylogenetic distribution of branch RNA-linked multicopy single-stranded DNA among natural isolates of *Escherichia coli*. *J. Bacteriol.* **172:**6175–6181.

62. **Hinnebusch, B. J.** 2003. Transmission factors: *Yersinia pestis* genes required to infect the flea vector of plague, p. 55–62. *In* M. Skurnik, J. A. Bengoechea, and K. Granfors (ed.), *The Genus Yersinia: Entering the Functional Genomics Era.* Kluwer Academic/Plenum Publishers, New York.

63. **Hinnebusch, B. J., R. D. Perry, and T. G. Schwan.** 1996. Role of the *Yersinia pestis* hemin storage *(hms)* locus in the transmission of plague by fleas. *Science* **273:**367–370.

64. **Hinnebusch, B. J., A. E. Rudolph, P. Cherepanov, J. E. Dixon, T. G. Schwan, and A. Forsberg.** 2002. Role of *Yersinia murine* toxin in survival of *Yersinia pestis* in the midgut of the flea vector. *Science* **296:**733–735.

65. **Ibrahim, A., B. M. Goebel, W. Liesack, M. Griffiths, and E. Stackebrandt.** 1993. The phylogeny of the genus *Yersinia* based on 16S rDNA sequences. *FEMS Microbiol. Lett.* **114:**173–177.

66. **Ito, H., N. Kido, Y. Arakawa, M. Ohta, T. Sugiyama, and N. Kato.** 1991. Possible mechanisms underlying the slow lactose fermentation phenotype in *Shigella* spp. *Appl. Environ. Microbiol.* **57:**2912–2917.

67. **Jin, Q., Z. Yuan, J. Xu, Y. Wang, Y. Shen, W. Lu, J. Wang, H. Liu, J. Yang, F. Yang, X. Zhang, J. Zhang, G. Yang, H. Wu, D. Qu, J. Dong, et al.** 2002. Genome sequence of *Shigella flexneri* 2a: insights into pathogenicity through comparison with genomes of *Escherichia coli* K12 and O157. *Nucl. Acids Res.* **30:**4432–4441.

68. **Joys, T. M.** 1988. The flagellar filament protein. *Can. J. Microbiol.* **34:**452–458.

69. **Kidgell, C., U. Reichard, J. Wain, B. Linz, M. Torpdahl, G. Dougan, and M. Achtman.** 2002. *Salmonella typhi,* the causative agent of typhoid fever, is approximately 50,000 years old. *Infect. Genet. Evol.* **2:**39–45.

70. **Kingsley, R. A., and A. J. Baumler.** 2000. Host adaptation and the emergence of infectious disease: the *Salmonella* paradigm. *Mol. Microbiol.* **36:**1006–1014.

71. **Kingsley, R. A., and A. J. Baumler.** 2002. Pathogenicity islands and host adaptation of *Salmonella* serovars. *Curr. Top. Microbiol. Immunol.* **264:**67–87.

72. **Kudva, I. T., P. S. Evans, N. T. Perna, T. J. Barrett, F. M. Ausubel, F. R. Blattner, and S. B. Calderwood.** 2002. Strains of *Escherichia coli* O157:H7 differ primarily by insertions or deletions, not single-nucleotide polymorphisms. *J. Bacteriol.* **184:**1873–1879.

73. **Lan, R., M. C. Alles, K. Donohoe, M. B. Martinez, and P. R. Reeves.** 2004. Molecular evolutionary relationships of enteroinvasive *Escherichia coli* and *Shigella* spp. *Infect. Immun.* **72:**5080–5088.

74. **Lan, R., B. Lumb, D. Ryan, and P. R. Reeves.** 2001. Molecular evolution of the large virulence plasmid in Shigella clones and enteroinvasive *Escherichia coli*. *Infect. Immun.* **69:**6303–6309.

75. **Lan, R., and P. R. Reeves.** 2002. *Eschericheria coli* in disguise: molecular origins of Shigella. *Microbes Infect.* **4:**1125–1132.

76. **Lan, R., and P. R. Reeves.** 1996. Gene transfer is a major factor in bacterial evolution. *Mol. Biol. Evol.* **13:**47–55.

77. **Lan, R., and P. R. Reeves.** 2000. Intraspecies variation in bacterial genomes: the need for a species genome concept. *Trends Microbiol.* **8:**396–401.

78. **Lan, R., and P. R. Reeves.** 2001. When does a clone deserve a name: a perspective on bacterial species based on population genetics. *Trends Microbiol.* **9:**419–424.

79. **Lawn, A. M., I. Orskov, and F. Orskov.** 1977. Morphological distinction between different H serotypes of *Escherichia coli*. *J. Gen. Microbiol.* **101:**111–119.

80. **Lecointre, G., L. Rachdi, P. Darlu, and E. Denamur.** 1998. *Escherichia coli* molecular phylogeny using the incongruence length difference test. *Mol. Biol. Evol.* **15:**1685–1695.

81. **Le Minor, L., and M. Y. Popoff.** 1987. Designation of *Salmonella enterica* sp. nov., nom. rev., as the type and only species of the genus *Salmonella*. *Int. J. Syst. Bacteriol.* **37:**465–468.

82. **Li, J., H. Ochman, E. A. Groisman, E. F. Boyd, F. Solomon, K. Nelson, and R. K. Selander.** 1995. Relationship between evolutionary rate and cellular location among the Inv/Spa invasion proteins of *Salmonella enterica*. *Proc. Natl. Acad. Sci. USA* **92:**7252–7256.

83. **Maurelli, A. T., R. E. Fernandez, C. A. Bloch, C. K. Rode, and A. Fasano.** 1998. "Black holes" and bacterial pathogenicity: a large genomic deletion that enhances the virulence of Shigella spp. and enteroinvasive *Escherichia coli*. *Proc. Natl. Acad. Sci. USA* **95:**3943–3948.

84. **Maynard Smith, J., N. H. Smith, M. O'Rourke, and B. G. Spratt.** 1993. How clonal

are bacteria *Proc. Natl. Acad. Sci. USA* **90:** 4384–4388.

85. **McClelland, M., K. E. Sanderson, J. Spieth, S. W. Clifton, P. Latreille, L. Courtney, S. Porwollik, J. Ali, M. Dante, F. Y. Du, S. F. Hou, D. Layman, S. Leonard, C. Nguyen, K. Scott, A. Holmes, N. Grewal, E. Mulvaney, E. Ryan, H. Sun, L. Florea, W. Miller, T. Stoneking, M. Nhan, R. Waterston, and R. K. Wilson.** 2001. Complete genome sequence of *Salmonella enterica* serovar Typhimurium LT2. *Nature* **413:**852–856.

86. **McDaniel, T. K., K. G. Jarvis, M. S. Donnenberg, and J. B. Kaper.** 1995. A genetic locus of enterocyte effacement conserved among diverse enterobacterial pathogens. *Proc. Natl. Acad. Sci. USA* **92:**1664–1668.

87. **Milkman, R.** 1996. Recombinational exchange among clonal populations, p. 2663–2684. *In* F. C. Neidhardt, R. Curtiss III, J. L. Ingraham, E. C. C. Lin, K. B. Low, B. Magasanik, W. S. Reznikoff, M. Riley, M. Schaechter, and H. E. Umbarger (ed.), *Escherichia coli and Salmonella typhimurium: Cellular and Molecular Biology,* 2nd ed., vol. 2. ASM Press, Washington, D.C.

88. **Mills, D. M., V. Bajaj, and C. A. Lee.** 1995. A 40-kb chromosomal fragment encoding *Salmonella typhimurium* invasion genes is absent from the corresponding region of the *Escherichia coli* K-12 chromosome. *Mol. Microbiol.* **15:**749–759.

89. **Mirold, S., K. Ehrbar, A. Weissmuller, R. Prager, H. Tschape, H. Russman, and W. D. Hardt.** 2001. *Salmonella* host cell invasion emerged by acquisition of a mosaic of separate genetic elements, including pathogenicity island 1 (SPI1), SPI5, and *sopE2*. *J. Bacteriol.* **183:** 2348–2358.

90. **Morona, R., C. Daniels, and L. Van Den Bosch.** 2003. Genetic modulation of *Shigella flexneri* 2a lipopolysaccharide O antigen modal chain length reveals that it has been optimized for virulence. *Microbiology* **149:**925–939.

91. **Nataro, J. P., and J. B. Kaper.** 1998. Diarrheagenic *Escherichia coli*. *Clin. Microbiol. Rev.* **11:**142–201.

92. **Nelson, K., and R. K. Selander.** 1994. Intergenic transfer and recombination of the 6-phosphogluconate dehydrogenase gene (*gnd*) in enteric bacteria. *Proc. Natl. Acad. Sci. USA* **91:**10227–10231.

93. **Nelson, K., T. S. Whittam, and R. K. Selander.** 1991. Nucleotide polymorphism and evolution in the glyceraldehyde-3-phosphate dehydrogenase gene (*gapA*) in natural populations of *Salmonella* and *Escherichia coli. Proc. Natl. Acad. Sci. USA* **88:**6667–6671.

94. **Noller, A. C., M. C. McEllistrem, O. C. Stine, J. G. Morris, Jr., D. J. Boxrud, B. Dixon, and L. H. Harrison.** 2003. Multilocus sequence typing reveals a lack of diversity among *Escherichia coli* O157:H7 isolates that are distinct by pulsed-field gel electrophoresis. *J. Clin. Microbiol.* **41:** 675–679.

95. **Ochman, H., and E. A. Groisman.** 1996. Distribution of pathogenicity islands in *Salmonella* spp. *Infect. Immun.* **64:**5410–5412.

96. **Ochman, H., and R. K. Selander.** 1984. Standard reference strains of *Escherichia coli* from natural populations. *J. Bacteriol.* **157:**690–693.

97. **Ochman, H., T. S. Whittam, D. A. Caugant, and R. K. Selander.** 1983. Enzyme polymorphism and genetic population structure in *Escherichia coli* and *Shigella. J. Gen. Microbiol.* **129:**2715–2726.

98. **Parkhill, J., G. Dougan, K. D. James, N. R. Thomson, D. Pickard, J. Wain, C. Churcher, K. L. Mungall, S. D. Bentley, M. T. Holden, M. Sebaihia, S. Baker, D. Basham, K. Brooks, T. Chillingworth, P. Connerton, A. Cronin, P. Davis, R. M. Davies, L. Dowd, N. White, J. Farrar, T. Feltwell, N. Hamlin, A. Haque, T. T. Hien, S. Holroyd, K. Jagels, A. Krogh, T. S. Larsen, S. Leather, S. Moule, P. O'Gaora, C. Parry, M. Quail, K. Rutherford, M. Simmonds, J. Skelton, K. Stevens, S. Whitehead, and B. G. Barrell.** 2001. Complete genome sequence of a multiple drug resistant *Salmonella enterica* serovar Typhi CT18. *Nature* **413:**848–852.

99. **Parkhill, J., B. W. Wren, N. R. Thomson, R. W. Titball, M. T. Holden, M. B. Prentice, M. Sebaihia, K. D. James, C. Churcher, K. L. Mungall, S. Baker, D. Basham, S. D. Bentley, K. Brooks, A. M. Cerdeno-Tarraga, T. Chillingworth, A. Cronin, R. M. Davies, P. Davis, G. Dougan, T. Feltwell, N. Hamlin, S. Holroyd, K. Jagels, A. V. Karlyshev, S. Leather, S. Moule, P. C. Oyston, M. Quail, K. Rutherford, M. Simmonds, J. Skelton, K. Stevens, S. Whitehead, and B. G. Barrell.** 2001. Genome sequence of *Yersinia pestis,* the causative agent of plague. *Nature* **413:**523–527.

100. **Perna, T. P., G. I. Plunkett III, V. Burland, B. Mau, J. D. Glasner, D. J. Rose, G. F. Mayhew, P. S. Evans, J. Gregor, H. A. Kirkpatrick, G. Posfai, J. Hackett, S. Klink, A. Boutin, Y. Shao, L. Miller, E. J. Grotbeck, N. W. Davis, A. Lim, E. T. Dimalanta, K. D. Potamousis, J. Apodaca, T. S. Anantharaman, J. Lin, G. Yen, D. C. Schwartz, R. A. Welch, and F. R. Blattner.** 2001. Genome sequence of enterohaemorrhagic *Escherichia coli* O157:H7. *Nature* **409:**529–533.

101. **Popoff, M. Y.** 2001. *Antigenic Formulas of the Salmonella Serovars,* 8th ed. WHO Collaborating Centre for Reference and Research on *Salmonella,* Institut Pasteur, Paris, France.

102. **Porwollik, S., E. F. Boyd, C. Choy, P. Cheng, L. Florea, E. Proctor, and M. McClelland.** 2004. Characterization of *Salmonella enterica* subspecies I genovars by use of microarrays. *J. Bacteriol.* **186:**5883–5898.

103. **Porwollik, S., R. M. Wong, and M. McClelland.** 2002. Evolutionary genomics of *Salmonella:* gene acquisitions revealed by microarray analysis. *Proc. Natl. Acad. Sci. USA* **99:**8956–8961.

104. **Pupo, G. M., D. K. R. Karaolis, R. Lan, and P. R. Reeves.** 1997. Evolutionary relationships among pathogenic and nonpathogenic *Escherichia coli* strains inferred from multilocus enzyme electrophoresis and *mdh* sequence studies. *Infect. Immun.* **65:**2685–2692.

105. **Pupo, G. M., R. Lan, and P. R. Reeves.** 2000. Multiple independent origins of Shigella clones of *Escherichia coli* and convergent evolution of many of their characteristics. *Proc. Natl. Acad. Sci. USA* **97:**10567–10572.

106. **Pupo, G. M., R. Lan, P. R. Reeves, and P. Baverstock.** 2000. Population genetics of *Escherichia coli* in a natural population of native Australian rats. *Environ. Microbiol.* **2:**594–610.

107. **Rabsch, W., H. L. Andrews, R. A. Kingsley, R. Prager, H. Tschape, L. G. Adams, and A. J. Baumler.** 2002. *Salmonella enterica* serotype Typhimurium and its host-adapted variants. *Infect. Immun.* **70:**2249–2255.

108. **Rakin, A., S. Schubert, C. Pelludat, D. Brem, and J. Heesemann.** 1999. The high-pathogenicity island of *Yersiniae*, p. 77–89. *In* J. B. Kaper and J. Hacker (ed.), *Pathogenicity Islands and Other Mobile Virulence Elements.* ASM Press, Washington, D.C.

109. **Ratiner, Y. A.** 1998. New flagellin-specifying genes in some *Escherichia coli* strains. *J. Bacteriol.* **180:**979–984.

110. **Reeves, M. W., G. M. Evins, A. A. Heiba, B. D. Plikaytis, and J. J. Farmer III.** 1989. Clonal nature of *Salmonella typhi* and its genetic relatedness to other salmonellae as shown by multilocus enzyme electrophoresis, and proposal of *Salmonella bongori. J. Clin. Microbiol.* **27:**313–320.

111. **Reeves, P. R.** 1992. Variation in O antigens, niche specific selection and bacterial populations. *FEMS Microbiol. Lett.* **100:**509–516.

112. **Reid, S. D., C. J. Herbelin, A. C. Bumnaugh, R. K. Selander, and T. S. Whittam.** 2000. Parallel evolution of virulence in pathogenic *Escherichia coli. Nature* **406:**64–67.

113. **Revell, P. A., and V. L. Miller.** 2001. *Yersinia* virulence: more than a plasmid. *FEMS Microbiol. Lett.* **205:**159–164.

114. **Riley, L. W., R. S. Remis, S. D. Helgerson, H. B. McGee, J. G. Wells, B. R. Davis, R. J.** Hebert, E. S. Olcott, L. M. Johnson, N. T. Hargrett, P. A. Blake, and M. L. Cohen. 1983. Hemorrhagic colitis associated with a rare *Escherichia coli* serotype. *N. Engl. J. Med.* **308:**681–685.

115. **Riley, M., and K. E. Sanderson.** 1990. Comparative genetics of *Escherichia coli* and *Salmonella typhimurium*, p. 85–95. *In* K. Drlica and M. Riley (ed.), *The Bacterial Chromosome.* American Society for Microbiology, Washington D.C.

116. **Rolland, K., N. Lambert-Zechovsky, B. Picard, and E. Denamur.** 1998. *Shigella* and enteroinvasive *Escherichia coli* strains are derived from distinct ancestral strains of *E. coli. Microbiology* **144:**2667–2672.

117. **Samuel, G., J.-P. Hogbin, L. Wang, and P. R. Reeves.** 2004. Relationships of the *Escherichia coli* O157, O111, and O55 O-antigen gene clusters with those of *Salmonella enterica* and *Citrobacter freundii*, which express identical O antigens. *J. Bacteriol.* **186:**6536–6543.

118. **Schubert, S., A. Rakin, H. Karch, E. Carniel, and J. Heesemann.** 1998. Prevalence of the "high-pathogenicity island" of *Yersinia* species among *Escherichia coli* strains that are pathogenic to humans. *Infect. Immun.* **66:**480–485.

119. **Selander, R. K., P. Beltran, and N. H. Smith.** 1991. Evolutionary genetics of *Salmonella*, p. 25–27. *In* R. K. Selander, A. G. Clark, and T. S. Whittam (ed.), *Evolution at the Molecular Level.* Sinauer Associates, Sunderland, Mass.

120. **Selander, R. K., P. Beltran, N. H. Smith, R. M. Barker, P. B. Crichton, D. C. Old, J. M. Musser, and T. S. Whittam.** 1990. Genetic population structure, clonal phylogeny and pathogenicity of *Salmonella paratyphi* B. *Infect. Immun.* **58:**1891–1901.

121. **Selander, R. K., P. Beltran, N. H. Smith, H. Reiner, F. A. Rubin, D. J. Kopecko, K. Ferris, B. T. Tall, A. Cravioto, and J. M. Musser.** 1990. Evolutionary genetic relationships of clones of *Salmonella* serovars that cause human typhoid and other enteric fevers. *Infect. Immun.* **58:**2262–2275.

122. **Selander, R. K., D. A. Caugant, and T. S. Whittam.** 1987. Genetic structure and variation in natural populations of *Escherichia coli*, p. 1625–1648. *In* F. C. Neidhardt, J. L. Ingraham, B. Magasanik, M. Schaechter, and H. E. Umbarger (ed.), Escherichia coli *and* Salmonella typhimurium: *Cellular and Molecular Biology*, vol. 2. American Society for Microbiology, Washington, D.C.

123. **Selander, R. K., J. Li, and K. Nelson.** 1996. Evolutionary genetics of *Salmonella enterica*, p. 2691–2707. *In* F. C. Neidhardt, R. Curtiss III, J. L. Ingraham, E. C. C. Lin, K. B. Low, B. Magasanik,

W. S. Reznikoff, M. Riley, M. Schaechter, and H.
E. Umbarger (ed.), Escherichia coli and
Salmonella typhimurium: Cellular and Molecular
Biology, 2nd ed., vol. 2. American Society for
Microbiology, Washington, D.C.

124. **Selander, R. K., and N. H. Smith.** 1990.
Molecular population genetics of Salmonella. Rev.
Med. Microbiol. **1:**219–228.

125. **Shaikh, N., and P. I. Tarr.** 2003. Escherichia coli
O157:H7 Shiga toxin-encoding bacteriophages:
integrations, excisions, truncations, and evolutionary implications. J. Bacteriol. **185:**3596–3605.

126. **Skurnik, M., and L. Zhang.** 1996. Molecular
genetics   and   biochemistry   of   Yersinia
lipopolysaccharide. APMIS **104:**849–872.

127. **Smith, D. G., S. W. Naylor, and D. L. Gally.**
2002. Consequences of EHEC colonisation in
humans and cattle. Int. J. Med. Microbiol. **292:**
169–183.

128. **Souza, V., M. Rocha, A. Valera, and L. E.
Eguiarte.** 1999. Genetic structure of natural
populations of Escherichia coli in wild hosts on different continents. Appl. Environ. Microbiol. **65:**
3373–3385.

129. **Spratt, B. G., and M. C. Maiden.** 1999.
Bacterial population genetics, evolution and
epidemiology. Philos. Trans. R. Soc. Lond. B **354:**
701–710.

130. **Stolzfus, A., J. Leslie, and R. Milkman.** 1988.
Molecular evolution of the Escherichia coli chromosome. I. Analysis of structure and variation in a
previously uncharacterised region between trp
and tonB. Genetics **120:**345–358.

131. **Sulakvelidze, A.** 2000. Yersiniae other than Y.
enterocolitica, Y. pseudotuberculosis, and Y. pestis: the
ignored species. Microbes Infect. **2:**497–513.

132. **Tarr, P. I.** 1995. Escherichia coli O157:H7: clinical, diagnostic, and epidemiological aspects of
human infection. Clin. Infect. Dis. **20:**1–8.

133. **Tarr, P. I., L. M. Schoening, Y. L. Yea, T. R.
Ward, S. Jelacic, and T. S. Whittam.** 2000.
Acquisition of the rfb-gnd cluster in evolution of
Escherichia coli O55 and O157. J. Bacteriol.
182:6183–6191.

134. **Tsubokura, M., and S. Aleksi.** 1995. A simplified antigenic scheme for serotyping of Yersinia
pseudotuberculosis: phenotypic characterization of
reference strains and preparation of O and H factor sera. Contrib. Microbiol. Immunol. **13:**99–105.

135. **Venkatesan, M. M., M. B. Goldberg, D. J.
Rose, E. J. Grotbeck, V. Burland, and F. R.
Blattner.** 2001. Complete DNA sequence and
analysis of the large virulence plasmid of Shigella
flexneri. Infect. Immun. **69:**3271–3285.

136. **Wang, L., D. Rothemund, H. Curd, and P. R.
Reeves.** 2003. Species-wide variation in the
Escherichia coli flagellin (H antigen) gene. J.
Bacteriol. **185:**2936–2943.

137. **Wauters, G., S. Aleksi, J. Charlier, and G.
Schulze.** 1991. Somatic and flagellar antigens of
Yersinia enterocolitica and related species.
Contrib. Microbiol. Immunol. **12:**239–243.

138. **Wei, J., M. B. Goldberg, V. Burland, M. M.
Venkatesan, W. Deng, G. Fournier, G. F.
Mayhew, G. Plunkett III, D. J. Rose, A.
Darling, B. Mau, N. T. Perna, S. M. Payne, L.
J. Runyen-Janecky, S. Zhou, D. C. Schwartz,
and F. R. Blattner.** 2003. Complete genome
sequence and comparative genomics of Shigella
flexneri serotype 2a strain 2457T. Infect. Immun.
71:2775–2786.

139. **Welch, R. A., V. Burland, G. Plunkett III, P.
Redford, P. Roesch, D. Rasko, E. L. Buckles,
S. R. Liou, A. Boutin, J. Hackett, D. Stroud,
G. F. Mayhew, D. J. Rose, S. Zhou, D. C.
Schwartz, N. T. Perna, H. L. Mobley, M. S.
Donnenberg, and F. R. Blattner.** 2002.
Extensive mosaic structure revealed by the com-
plete genome sequence of uropathogenic
Escherichia coli. Proc. Natl. Acad. Sci. USA **99:**
17020–17024.

140. **Whittam, T. S.** 1995. Genetic population struc-
ture and pathogenicity in enteric bacteria,
p. 217–245. In S. Baumberg, J. P. W. Young,
E. M. H. Wellington, and J. R. Saunders (ed.),
Population Genetics of Bacteria (Symposium 52).
Cambridge University Press, Cambridge, United
Kingdom.

141. **Whittam, T. S., and S. E. Ake.** 1993. Genetic
polymorphisms and recombination in natural
populations of Escherichia coli, p. 223–245. In N.
Takahata and A. G. Clark (ed.), Mechanisms of
Molecular Evolution. Japan Scientific Societies
Press, Tokyo, Japan.

142. **Wildschutte, H., D. M. Wolfe, A. Tarnewitz,
and J. G. Lawrence.** 2004. Protozoan predation,
diversifying selection, and the evolution of antigenic diversity in Salmonella. Proc. Natl. Acad. Sci.
USA **101:**10644–10649.

143. **Wolf, M. K.** 1997. Occurrence, distribution, and
associations of O and H serogroups, colonization
factor antigens, and toxins of enterotoxigenic
Escherichia coli. Clin. Microbiol. Rev. **10:**569–584.

144. **Wong, K. K., M. McClelland, L. C. Stillwell,
E. C. Sisk, S. J. Thurston, and J. D. Saffer.**
1998. Identification and sequence analysis of a
27-kilobase chromosomal fragment containing a
Salmonella pathogenicity island located at 92
minutes on the chromosome map of Salmonella
enterica serovar typhimurium LT2. Infect. Immun.
66:3365–3371.

145. **Wood, M. W., M. A. Jones, P. R. Watson, S.
Hedges, T. S. Wallis, and E. E. Galyov.** 1998.
Identification of a pathogenicity island required
for Salmonella enteropathogenicity. Mol. Microbiol.
29:883–891.

MYCOBACTERIAL EVOLUTION: INSIGHTS FROM GENOMICS AND POPULATION GENETICS

Alexander S. Pym and Peter M. Small

16

It is difficult to convey the magnitude of the public health consequence of tuberculosis. Despite a coordinated global effort to control it with antibiotics and a vaccine, *Mycobacterium tuberculosis* infects approximately one-third of the world's population and kills one person every 15 seconds (45). Part of its success is due to the complex nature of its transmission and pathogenesis. *M. tuberculosis* is an obligate human pathogen that is transmitted by aerosol from patients with pulmonary tuberculosis. Following infection via the lungs, the majority of individuals mount T-cell-mediated immunity that can effectively constrain the growth of *M. tuberculosis*. Critically, this immune response is usually only capable of containing the infection and rarely sterilizes the lungs. This allows the bacteria to establish what is known as a latent infection, the exact physiological and anatomical nature of which is unknown. Most latent infections are thought to be perpetual, though in at least 5% of cases (10% per year in the presence of human immunodeficiency virus coinfection), the apparently dormant bacteria can exploit lapses in host immunity to multiply and establish overt disease. This results

in enormous bacterial pulmonary loads and the consequent reinitiation of aerosol transmission and infection of new cases. Thus, although *M. tuberculosis* is highly pathogenic, with the capacity to cause severe pulmonary disease required for transmission, it can also exist in a quasi-commensal state with its host, permitting the establishment of a large reservoir of dormantly infected individuals. This has ensured its persistence within human populations and makes the global eradication of tuberculosis a daunting task. The delicate balance that *M. tuberculosis* has established with its host suggests that the evolution of this pathogen has been a complex and extended process.

Until recently, the evolution of tuberculosis remained largely in the realms of speculation. However, the genomics revolution has had the same dramatic effect on the study of *M. tuberculosis* as it has had on the study of other bacterial pathogens. The complete genome sequence of a strain of *M. tuberculosis* was first published in 1998 (33), and since then the genome sequence of a second isolate (49) has been completed, as well as the sequences of two other pathogenic mycobacteria, *Mycobacterium bovis* (54) and *Mycobacterium leprae* (34), the bacteria responsible for bovine tuberculosis and the human disease leprosy. This has stimulated the field of mycobacterial genetics and is finally providing

Alexander S. Pym, Medical Research Council of South Africa, 491 Ridge Road, P.O. Box 70380, Overport 4067, Durban, South Africa. *Peter M. Small,* Global Health Program, P.O. Box 23350, Seattle, WA 98102.

Evolution of Microbial Pathogens, Edited by H. S. Seifert and V. J. DiRita, © 2006 ASM Press, Washington, D.C.

some concrete insights into the molecular evolution of tuberculosis. As with other organisms, the generation of genetic data has greatly outstripped their interpretation. This promises to continue with the completion and comparison of other mycobacterial genomes. We have therefore structured this chapter around the different genetic approaches that are providing insights into the evolution of *M. tuberculosis* and have specifically emphasized important new findings emerging from recent studies of population genetics.

EVOLUTION OF THE GENUS *MYCOBACTERIUM*

One of the first attempts at mycobacterial systematics was proposed by Timpe and Runyon in 1954 (144). They divided the genus into four large groups based on pigmentation and growth rates. This seminal work not only formed the basis for a system of classification for the phenotypic identification of mycobacteria still in use today (146) but also highlighted an association between growth rate and pathogenicity. Dividing the mycobacteria into two groups based on the ability to form clearly visible colonies in more or less than 7 days revealed that, among the obligate or opportunistic mycobacterial pathogens, slow growers outnumbered fast growers by over 4 to 1 (160). Subsequent molecular analyses of the mycobacteria showed that the division between slow and fast growers is phylogenetically coherent (122, 135, 146), and also established that the slow-growing bacteria are closely related (Fig. 1). In addition, with the exception of *M. simiae,* the slow growers all have a particular 16S rRNA secondary structure in the form of a short insertion in helix 18, confirming that they represent a distinct lineage, well resolved from the fast-growing species (135, 146). Importantly, from an evolutionary perspective, these studies reveal a slow-growing lineage divergent from the more diversely branched fast-growing species, demonstrating that fast growth was the ancestral phenotype.

A second striking observation from mycobacterial phylogenetics is that, among the slow growers, the three obligate pathogens affecting humans—*M. tuberculosis, M. leprae,* and *M. ulcerans*—are grouped together (Fig. 1). Furthermore, these species are branched with the *M. avium* complex, which includes the important veterinary pathogens *M. paratuberculosis* and *M. avium,* as well as the most common opportunistic mycobacterial pathogen affecting AIDS patients. Although genes required for mycobacterial pathogenesis could have evolved in a single species, with subsequent dissemination through horizontal transfer, a more plausible explanation is that the existing pathogens diverged from a common pathogenic ancestor, to exploit different hosts and niches. In support of this is the fact that at least *M. marinum* and *M. avium* share with *M. tuberculosis* the same strategy for survival within macrophages, which is considered critical for pathogenicity (5, 32, 138, 165). Following phagocytosis, each of these species effectively inhibits acidification and phagosome-lysosome fusion, enabling them to grow and prosper within the phagosome. Although the precise mycobacterial genes required for modulating phagosomal maturation have not yet been fully defined (155, 158), a recent analysis of the intramacrophage transcriptome of *M. avium* found that many of the genes up-regulated were orthologous to *M. tuberculosis* factors implicated in virulence and intracellular survival (67). Taken together, this information suggests that many of the key virulence determinants of *M. tuberculosis* are present in other mycobacterial pathogens. Further phenotypic studies are now required to determine which of the newly identified mycobacteria (146) can also survive within macrophages.

The convincing association of pathogenicity and slow growth poses several interesting questions. Was the development of slow growth an essential element in the evolution of pathogenic mycobacteria or simply an epiphenomenon? Under what selective pressure was the transition from fast-growing environmental bacteria to slow-growing intracellular pathogen made? And what were the genomic changes that accompanied such a transition? These intriguing questions remain unanswered, but it

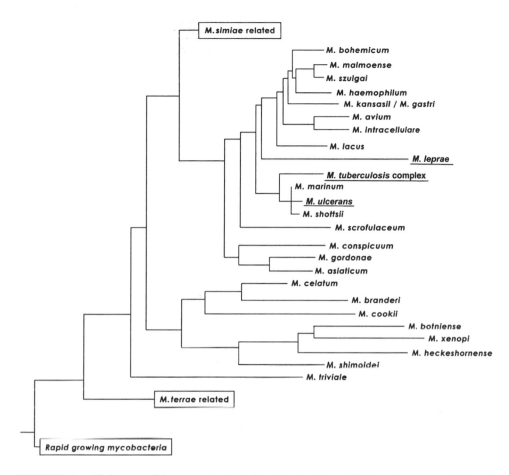

FIGURE 1 Phylogeny of slow-growing *Mycobacterium* based on 16S rRNA sequences (adapted from reference 146). Phylogenetic distances are not precise. Species that are underlined correspond to the obligate human pathogens. The *Mycobacterium tuberculosis* complex corresponds to *M. tuberculosis, M. microti, M. africanum, M. bovis, M. caprae,* and *M. canettii,* which have identical 16S rRNA sequences.

is tempting to speculate that a slowing of growth rate could have been important for colonizing cells. By growing slowly, the intracellular burden of bacteria is lower, perhaps enabling host cells to tolerate intracellular organisms longer. Surprisingly little is known about how *M. tuberculosis* regulates its growth rate. It has been proposed that, because *M. tuberculosis* possesses only a single *rrn* operon, ribosomal production is restricted and as a consequence protein biosynthesis and growth as well. However, some fast-growing mycobacteria also contain only a single copy of the *rrn* operon, suggesting that regulation of rRNA transcrip-

tion or other mechanisms exist (90), such as autocrine growth factors (98). The environment under which these complex regulatory pathways and mechanisms of intracellular survival evolved is also unknown. Evidence that *M. avium* can survive and replicate within the waterborne amoebae (31, 92) raises the possibility that colonization of free-living unicellular organisms was an essential step in the evolution of mycobacterial virulence, as has been suggested for other pathogens (63).

A more complete understanding of the evolution of pathogenic mycobacteria will ultimately require definition of the genomic

TABLE 1 Sizes of complete or nearly complete mycobacterial genome sequences

Organism	Genome size (Mb)	Growth rate[a]	Human pathogen[b]
Streptomyces coelicolor	8.7	F	N
Streptomyces avermitilis	9.0	F	N
Mycobacterium smegmatis	7.0[c]	F	N
Mycobacterium marinum	6.6	S	Y
Mycobacterium ulcerans	5.7[c]	S	Y
Mycobacterium avium	5.4	S	O
Mycobacterium paratuberculosis	4.7	S	?
Mycobacterium tuberculosis	4.4	S	Y
Mycobacterium bovis	4.4	S	Y
Mycobacterium bovis BCG	4.3	S	Vaccine
Mycobacterium leprae	3.3	S	Y

[a] F, fast; S, slow.

[b] O, opportunistic pathogen; Y, yes; N, no. *Mycobacterium paratuberculosis* is the agent responsible for John's disease of cattle but has also been tenuously linked with Crohn's disease of humans.

[c] Sizes are from unfinished or unpublished projects and therefore may not be precise.

changes that accompanied the transition to a pathogenic lifestyle. Fortunately, the genomes of a diverse variety of species are complete or on the verge of completion (Table 1). A comparison of these genomes (currently unavailable) will allow the definition of the set of genes required for each of the different niches occupied by the individual pathogens. It will be of particular interest to determine whether there are genes unique to *M. tuberculosis* relative to the other closely related species. These genes are likely to code for key determinants of virulence, which enable *M. tuberculosis* to exploit the human host so successfully.

One conspicuous theme to emerge from these sequencing projects is the small genome size of the obligate pathogenic mycobacteria (*M. leprae* and *M. tuberculosis*) relative to *M. smegmatis* (23), a fast-growing environmental species (Table 1). *M. tuberculosis*, for example, has a genome close to 4.5 Mb in size compared to approximately 7 Mb for *M. smegmatis* and 7.8 Mb for *Streptomyces coelicolor* (8), a soil-dwelling bacteria from the same taxonomic order *(Actinomycetales)*. This confirms that the obligate pathogens have undergone a complex and lengthy evolutionary divergence from the fast-growing species.

Pronounced genome downsizing has also occurred in endosymbionts and obligate intracellular bacteria (3, 55, 127, 136). This is attrib-

uted to the combination of genetic isolation and the loss of genes expendable for an intracellular existence (105). It seems likely that a similar but less dramatic process may have occurred with the mycobacterial pathogens, during the adoption of their more specialized niches. Pertinently, though, the genome of *M. tuberculosis* is well maintained, with greater than 90% utilization of its potential coding capacity and scarcity of pseudogenes (33) indicating that extensive genome degradation has not accompanied genome downsizing. This is in contrast to the genomes of some obligate intracellular parasites, such as *Rickettsia prowazekii* (3) and *M. leprae* (34), in which gene inactivation has outstripped gene deletion. In the case of *M. leprae*, only 49.5% of the genome represents protein-coding sequences, with a further 27% corresponding to recognizable pseudogenes.

VIRULENCE GENES OF *M. TUBERCULOSIS*

It is only within the last decade that we have gained any insight into the molecular basis of virulence for *M. tuberculosis*. This came about following the rapid development of classical molecular techniques for genetically manipulating *M. tuberculosis* (111) in conjunction with the whole genome sequence (33), and the rediscovery of animal models of tuberculosis. Recently, there has been a sharp increase in the

TABLE 2 Selected experimentally defined virulence factors of *M. tuberculosis*[a]

Category	Gene name	Protein function	Reference(s)
Cell wall			
Protein	erp	Exported repetitive protein	9
Lipid synthesis	pks 12	Polyketide synthase	129
	pcaA	Mycolic acid cyclopropane synthesis	56
	ppsABCDE	Phenolphthiocerol synthesis	26, 38
	ms17, pks10	Dimycocerosyl phthiocerol synthesis	128
Lipid transport	mmpL7	Transmembrane transport protein	26, 38
Cell-cell interaction	hbhA	Heparin-binding hemagglutinin adhesin	113
	pknG	Protein kinase	158
Metabolism	glnAl	Glutamine synthesis	148
	icl	Isocitrate lyase	89
	narGHJI	Nitrate reductase	161
DNA repair and replication	dnaE2	DNA polymerase	15
Protein secretion	secA2	Accessory secretion factor	17
	esat6	Early secreted antigen	116, 159
Resistance to oxidative stress	katG	Catalase-peroxidase	81, 118, 163
Cation transport	mgtC	Putative magnesium transporter	24
Gene regulation	furA	Transcriptional regulator	117
	phoP	Two-component regulatory system	112
	senX3/regX3	Two-component regulatory system	109
	mprA	Two-component regulatory system	167
	sigH	Sigma factor	75
	rpoV	Sigma factor	36
	sigF	Sigma factor	30

[a]The genes were included if adequate experimental data using well-characterized mutants, mostly single gene knockouts, were available showing attenuation in an animal model of tuberculosis. Some of the listed studies used *M. bovis* or *M. bovis* BCG. Auxotrophic mutants, essential genes, and genes of unknown function have been ignored. Other genetic determinants of virulence have been proposed on the basis of growth impairment in macrophages, though this is considered a less rigorous test of virulence.

number of genes associated with virulence, pathogenicity, and intracellular survival. In the case of *M. tuberculosis,* a virulence determinant has come to be defined as a gene that, if inactivated, leads to a reduction in growth rate, persistence, or lethality in an animal model (usually mice). These genes can be divided into several broad categories as illustrated in Table 2. These categories include genes involved in responses to environmental stress, cell wall structure, lipid metabolism, transcriptional regulators, and signaling pathways, as well as a long list of genes with unknown function.

However, as with other organisms, there are methodological as well as semantic problems with defining virulence factors. These studies do not distinguish between genes that are required for optimal viability of mycobacteria and those that are unique and essential for the

virulence of pathogenic species such as *M. tuberculosis.* Thus, many of the "virulence determinants" that have been described in *M. tuberculosis* are also present in the nonpathogenic *M. smegmatis* (121). This paradox is particularly evident for genes involved in structural components of the cell wall. The complex cell wall of *M. tuberculosis* is a hallmark of all mycobacteria that provides protection against environmental stresses, and therefore it is hardly surprising that many of the genes involved in its synthesis and integrity are highly conserved among the mycobacterial species and implicated in virulence (6). These genes are therefore not virulence determinants in an evolutionary sense, as they are not the genetic substrate that has allowed *M. tuberculosis* to become virulent and colonize a new niche. In fact, it is likely that the classical concept of "virulence" factors may not be entirely applicable to *M. tuberculosis*. A more productive model for understanding this organism may be to consider the bacteria and host as involved in a complex dialogue, with each modulating the other. Elucidating the molecules that mediate this dialogue would be extremely informative, but may require fundamentally novel approaches that simultaneously incorporate key aspects of both host and pathogen.

HORIZONTAL GENE TRANSFER AND MOBILE GENETIC ELEMENTS OF *M. TUBERCULOSIS*

The acquisition of novel genes by horizontal transfer has been instrumental in the evolution of many bacterial pathogens (104, 105). In this model of evolution, a nonpathogenic environmental bacterium laterally acquires specific genes (or pathogenicity islands) from another species, which confer traits required for pathogenicity and exploitation of a host. The archetypes of this model (described elsewhere in this book) are the closely related pathogenic *Escherichia coli*, *Shigella*, and *Salmonella* species. The genomes of these species are mosaics, each with a highly similar core of genes corresponding to those obtained vertically from their common ancestor, interspersed with laterally acquired genes (frequently identified on the basis of their aberrant G+C content or codon usage). Phages, plasmids, and transposons have all been identified as efficient vehicles for the horizontal transfer of virulence genes between bacterial species.

In contrast to the preeminence of horizontal transfer in the molecular evolution of *E. coli* and other pathogens, there is as yet little evidence that lateral gene flow has played a dominant role in the recent evolution of *M. tuberculosis* pathogenicity. Analysis of three complete genome sequences of *M. tuberculosis* complex organisms (33, 49, 54) has so far failed to identify genomic islands that deviated significantly from the overall 65% G+C content of the genomes or have abnormal codon usage. A genomic region apparently with low G+C content has been reported in *M. avium* (145), but the same base pair aberrations are not conserved in the orthologous coding sequences of *M. tuberculosis*. One notable exception to the constant genome G+C content is the large PE-PGRS gene family (33). These 60+ genes encode proteins of unknown function, which are characterized by numerous glycine-alanine repeats. Their G+C content of over 70% is most likely a reflection of this probable structural motif (4), rather than a sign of lateral gene transfer.

Plasmids have been isolated from various mycobacterial species, and some have been successfully adapted to create efficient tools for genetically modifying *M. tuberculosis*, which is naturally plasmid free. However, a plasmid-borne virulence factor has been identified for one mycobacterium. It was recently shown that the polyketide synthases required to produce the macrolide toxin of *M. ulcerans* are encoded on a 174-kb plasmid (137). This toxin, mycolactone, is cytotoxic and immunosuppressive and causes the severe necrosis associated with the skin ulceration characteristic of infection by *M. ulcerans*.

Although there is a lack of pathogenicity islands and plasmids, 3.4% of the *M. tuberculosis* genome is composed of mobile genetic elements. Analysis of the *M. tuberculosis* H37Rv complete genome identified 56 loci with homology to insertion sequences (ISs) (33, 60) from eight distinct IS families. Thirty of these were copies of six different ISs, with IS*6110* (16 copies) and IS*1081* (6 copies) being the only high-copy-number elements. Bioinformatics showed that some of these had been previously described, but also identified 30 other loci that included members of seven different IS families. Many of these elements appeared to be defective, but at least two were highly similiar to sequences identified in two other species, *M. intracellulare* and another high-G+C-content nocardiform, *Rhodococcus opacus*, raising the possibility of genetic exchange between these diverse actinomycetes. It appears that IS*6110* is the only highly variable IS in *M. tuberculosis* and can occur in over 25 copies per genome. This variability is potentially of phenotypic importance because IS*6110* insertion sites are often within coding sequences leading to gene inactivation. Homologous recombination between adjacently inserted elements can also lead to deletion of intervening DNA (22, 66, 150, 154).

The intimate association of phages and bacterial virulence genes (157) has focused attention on the two prophagelike elements, phiRv1 and phiRv2, detected in the genome of *M. tuberculosis* H37Rv (33, 64). Each encodes several phagelike proteins, but neither possesses a complete set of genes capable of independently generating an intact infectious particle. However, phiRv1 is integrated at a different site in the *M. tuberculosis* CDC1551 genome, and has been shown to have a functional integration/excision system, indicating it is mobile and not a defunct prophage (11). The eight nonphagelike proteins in phiRv1 are small and of unknown function, and two of these are pseudogenes in the CDC1551 copy of phiRv1, giving few clues to their function or whether they confer a selective advantage to their hosts. Both prophages can be lost/acquired independently (65) and are variably present in clinical isolates of *M. tuberculosis* (21, 147), with phiRv1 frequently so, suggesting that neither is essential. Furthermore, loss of phages has been associated with transmission (147). The specific effects of these phages on mycobacterial physiology need to be further elucidated, but to date, neither appears to be of significant importance for virulence.

Phages do not appear to have contributed to the specialization of *M. tuberculosis,* but they may have played a role in the diversification of mycobacteria. Genome comparisons of 10 mycobacteriophages, isolated from various environmental sources, have revealed an extraordinary genetic diversity (110). Approximately 50% of the average 600 coding sequences per genome were found to be unique, unrelated to genes from phages and other sequenced organisms. Among the coding sequences, not matching other phage sequences, were homologues to genes in a wide variety of organisms. The overall architecture of the phage genomes was complex, reflecting multiple episodes of gene acquisition by illegitimate recombination. The combination of extreme genome plasticity and diversity suggests that mycobacterial phages could have acted as conduits for gene transfer between different species, a process that may have benefited the environmental ancestors of *M. tuberculosis.* Interestingly, traces of ancient horizontal transfer events have been detected in the genome of *M. tuberculosis* (52, 76). Some of these are attributed to the movement of eukaryotic genes, possibly reflecting a prolonged association between a mycobacterium and a eukaryotic host, although they could have been passed via an intermediary species. Others point to the acquisition of bacterial genes as has been proposed for elements of the fatty acid biosynthetic pathway (76), in which the environmental α-proteobacteria are heavily implicated. More extensive phylogenomic analyses are needed to ascertain the extent of lateral gene transfer in the shaping of the ancestral genome of *M. tuberculosis.*

POPULATION GENETICS OF *M. TUBERCULOSIS*

Single Nucleotide Polymorphisms

One of the most significant genetic observations with relevance to understanding the evolution of *M. tuberculosis* has been the lack of single nucleotide polymorphisms (SNPs) detected among clinical isolates of *M. tuberculosis*. Musser and coworkers, who were using DNA sequencing to identify chromosomal mutations associated with drug resistance, first observed this low rate of SNPs (72, 134). Compiling data from 26 structural genes, they amassed 2 Mb of sequences from a large collection of *M. tuberculosis* strains. Within this large data set, they were only able to identify 32 polymorphisms that were not associated with drug resistance, 30 of which were synonymous. From this they computed a synonymous substitution rate (number of synonymous substitutions per synonymous site) of less than 1.2×10^{-4}. In a subsequent study, they found a virtual absence of sequence variability in 24 further genes known to encode targets for host immunity, showing that this low rate of SNPs was present in a broader range of genes (99).

The lack of SNPs in clinical isolates of *M. tuberculosis* has been confirmed by comparing the complete genome sequences of two *M. tuberculosis* strains (10, 49, 68): H37Rv (33), a strain from the United States maintained in laboratories since its isolation in 1905, and CDC1551, a more recent outbreak strain also from the United States (49, 149). Whole-genome alignment of the two *M. tuberculosis* strains revealed only 1,075 SNPs between the two 4.4-Mb genomes (49). Approximately 85% of these mutations occurred in coding regions, and comparison of 3,535 genes orthologous to both genomes translated into a synonymous mutation rate of 3.6×10^{-4} (49). Although higher than the estimates of Musser and colleagues, as would be expected for an analysis that includes nonstructural genes, this is still 2 orders of magnitude less than rates derived from complete genome comparisons or multi-locus sequencing of other bacteria such as *E. coli, Helicobacter pylori,* and *Neisseria menigitidis* (70, 139).

The lack of sequence diversity detected in these studies has been taken as evidence that *M. tuberculosis* has undergone clonal expansion after recently emerging from a tight bottleneck. It has been suggested that this followed a recent speciation or subspeciation event (134). A similar scenario has been evoked to explain the low sequence diversity found among isolates of *Yersinia pestis* (1). Using a rate of synonymous substitution per year derived from nucleotide comparisons between *E. coli* and *Salmonella enterica* serovar Typhimurium and the 120- to 160-million-year estimate for speciation between these two bacteria (107, 126), this bottleneck is predicted to have occurred only 15,000 to 20,000 years ago (72), or 33,500 to 36,400 years (68) using the higher synonymous mutation levels computed from whole-genome comparisons. Although a similar synonymous substitution rate per site per year has been established for other organisms, there are well-recognized limitations to assuming a universal substitution rate for all bacteria (102). These include the influences of differing generation times, mutation rates, and population sizes, which are discussed in the following paragraphs.

Although the number of generations per year for *M. tuberculosis* in natural populations is unknown, it is likely to be less than the 300 estimated for populations of *E. coli* (106, 107), first because *M. tuberculosis* has an intrinsically slow generation time (at least 12 h in vitro or in experimental infections) but also because of the phenomenon of latency. The exact physiological and metabolic state of the tubercle bacilli that permits them to remain "dormant" for decades in their hosts is unknown but is widely believed to be a nonreplicative or rarely replicative state (84), effectively reducing the generation time. If mutations accumulate principally during replicative cycles and tuberculosis is maintained in populations through lengthy periods of latency, followed by a short burst of reactivation and transmission, then this extended generation time would influence the rate at which substitutions occur.

The frequency of mutations conferring resistance to antibiotics can be used to compare mutation rates. Early studies showed that, at least for the reference strain *M. tuberculosis* H37Rv, the number of drug-resistant mutants per bacterium per generation ranged from 10^{-7} to 10^{-10} for various antimycobacterial agents (40, 41), perhaps reflecting differences in the genetic targets for each drug. The mechanism of resistance to rifampin is the same in many bacteria, namely, mutations in a restricted region of the highly conserved *rpoB* gene, allowing direct comparison of mutation rates between species. And more recent studies, using selection for rifampin resistance, have reported mutation rates per generation similar to those in other bacteria (13, 15, 162).

However, the in vitro mutation rate may not be a true reflection of what is actually occurring during human infection. The exact physiological state of persistent bacilli in the latent part of the *M. tuberculosis* life cycle is often compared to the classical stationary phase of other bacteria. Hypermutability has been reported during stationary phase for the fast-growing *M. smegmatis* (73), though this has yet to be verified for slow-growing mycobacteria. This raises the possibility that so-called adaptive or stationary-phase mutation (50) could be a significant source of genetic diversity during latency. Intriguingly, analysis of the H37Rv genome suggests that *M. tuberculosis* is lacking some of the proteins involved in strand-specific mismatch repair (MMR) (94). In other bacteria, such a defect is associated with a "mutator" phenotype (higher rates of spontaneous mutation and recombination) (37) and has been identified in wild populations of pathogens (79, 108). Although the lack of an MMR could be compensated for during DNA replication by other fidelity systems (95), it is conceivable that its absence may contribute to enhanced adaptive mutation. Other aspects of DNA replication and repair appear to be specific for *M. tuberculosis*. In a recent study (15), it was demonstrated that mutation levels of *M. tuberculosis* can be enhanced by DNA-damaging agents, including H_2O_2. The genetic basis of this inducible mutagenesis was found to be different from that observed in *E. coli*. Up-regulation of a *dnaE2*, a second and error-prone copy of the replicative DNA polymerase *dnaE1*, was elegantly shown to be the sole effector. Moreover, *dnaE2* was induced during mouse infection and was required for maximal virulence. This strongly suggests that DnaE2 could enhance mutagenesis in response to the insult of reactive oxygen and nitrogen species generated by the immune system, and may even be a mechanism for producing mutants with an enhanced capacity to survive within the host. In summary, assumptions based on crude in vitro mutation rates for *M. tuberculosis* are unlikely to be accurate.

The substitution is affected not only by the mutation rate, but also by the rate at which randomly occurring mutations become fixed within a population. This process of genetic drift is accelerated in small populations of organisms. The population size of *M. tuberculosis* has not been formally estimated but is usually assumed to be large (72, 134) because one-third of the world's population is reported to be latently infected with *M. tuberculosis* (45).

However, this is based on high rates of reactivity to skin tests with *M. tuberculosis* antigens and could be an overestimate, since environmental mycobacteria can give false-positive results. In addition, less than 10% of these latently infected individuals will ever develop disease, and a significant proportion of these presumed reactivators will have actually acquired tuberculosis from another source. Moreover, the effective population size will be smaller still, because transmission between humans corresponds to a tight transmission bottleneck, as the infective dose for tuberculosis is thought to be only several bacteria. This situation is reminiscent of endosymbionts, whose vertical transmission through cytoplasmic inheritance results in a small effective population size and accelerated rates of sequence evolution (96, 164). In combination with the lack of horizontal transfer, this results in the accumulation of mildly deleterious mutations, manifesting as an increase in nonsynonymous mutations. A similar low ratio of synonymous to nonsynonymous substitutions (1.6, in contrast to 12.3 for *E. coli*) (70) observed in *M. tuberculosis* (49, 134) might also be a reflection of population size, though there are other plausible explanations.

Inadequate sampling is another factor that could influence the accuracy of any assessment of genetic diversity within a population. In the original study of Sreevatsan et al. (134), results were compiled from 842 strains originally isolated from impressively diverse global sources. This suggests their finding of limited polymorphisms among contemporary *M. tuberculosis* strains is accurate. However, recent reports of human *M. canettii* infections (91, 114) hint at a greater genetic diversity. *M. canettii* was first identified in 1969 because of a distinctive smooth colony morphology, has only been isolated from humans, and appears to causes a disease indistinguishable from classical tuberculosis. Subsequent analysis of this and subsequent isolates from cases of human tuberculosis demonstrate that, while it shares an identical 16S rRNA sequence and many phenotypic characteristics with other members of the *M. tuberculosis* complex, it appears to be genetically apart, with a unique direct repeat sequence, polymorphisms in structural genes, and a low copy number of IS*1081* (21, 39, 58, 150, 152). Of particular note is the *recA* sequence of *M. canetti,* which is reported to have 22 substitutions relative to the H37Rv sequence, 18 of which occur in this gene's intein (152). Recently, phylogenies based on large sequence polymorphisms (LSPs) or SNPs have confirmed that *M. canettii* is deeply branched from the other *M. tuberculosis* complex members (21, 62).

Further genetic analysis of *M. canettii* strains is still required to quantify exactly how divergent these isolates are, but their existence calls into question a recent speciation event for *M. tuberculosis.* An alternate explanation is the presence of an ancient human tuberculosis pathogen, with the restricted diversity of classical *M. tuberculosis* strains that are responsible for the current tuberculosis pandemic representing a more recent clonal expansion. Unlike distant events on the evolutionary timescale, small changes in timing can radically alter our perceptions of the ecological changes that might have accounted for recent changes in population structure. For example, if the clonal expansion of modern tuberculosis strains occurred closer to 100,000 years ago, it would coincide with the global dispersal of humans, as opposed to 10,000 years and the growth of human populations associated with urbanization. Further work on mutation rates, generation times, and population size is required to accurately date the time of this expansion. This would help to elucidate whether the emergence of a dominant *M. tuberculosis* clone was due to bacterial factors that conferred a selective advantage, or simply the colonization of expanding human populations by a slowly evolving pathogen.

Large Sequence Polymorphisms

The completion of genome sequences allied to microarray technology has enabled investigators to calibrate genetic diversity in terms of LSPs. This approach allows genomes to be compared in terms of gene content and is providing novel insights into bacterial evolution (47, 71, 78, 103). In essence, genomic DNA

from a test isolate is hybridized to a microarray representing the entire gene content of a reference strain, or preferably multiple strains. On the basis of the intensity of hybridization signals from the microarray, the presence or absence of each gene in the test isolate is determined. The absence of any gene is preferably then confirmed using a secondary method, usually PCR. These types of studies have established that, in certain bacteria such as *H. pylori* (124) and *Staphylococus aureus* (48), over 20% of genes are variably distributed among strains.

Given the lack of SNPs within populations of *M. tuberculosis* (134), it was of particular interest to determine if LSPs or other sources of genetic variability are important in *M. tuberculosis.* An initial study of 16 clinical isolates of *M. tuberculosis* showed that there was indeed variability at the level of gene content, with only one strain having no deletions relative to the reference strain H37Rv represented on the high-density oligoarray (74). In total, these deletions were predicted to interrupt 93 coding sequences, equivalent to approximately 2.3% of the annotated H37Rv genome (27). This study paradigm has now been extended to 100 *M. tuberculosis* strains isolated in San Francisco over a 12-year period (147). Each strain was selected on the basis of a unique IS*6110* restriction fragment length polymorphism pattern to ensure that the diversity of the 2,500+ strain collection was adequately sampled. Specifically, this extended data set allows cases of tuberculosis due to transmission in San Francisco to be distinguished from cases contracted outside the city (130). San Francisco is at the center of a large cosmopolitan conurbation, and the imported isolates therefore reflect the diverse origins of the immigrant populations of this city, enabling a vicarious sampling of global *M. tuberculosis* populations (14). Analysis of the sequences absent from these 100 strains revealed a higher level of diversity than in the previous study, as would be anticipated from a larger sample, with at least 5.5% of coding sequences being variably distributed among the strains. This is likely to be a conservative estimate as the array used in the study was unable to perform in certain areas of the genome rich in repetitive sequences, including the polymorphic GC-rich repetitive sequence (PGRS) gene family. It is difficult to make direct comparisons with other bacteria as the process by which strains are selected, the number of strains that are analyzed, the resolution of the microarray used, and the diligence with which putative deletions are confirmed will all influence interpretation. Nevertheless, the number of variable genes appears to be significantly lower than reported for other pathogens (43, 48, 124). This limited variation in gene loss among the 100 test isolates is in keeping with the low levels of SNPs seen in other global collections (134), confirming the genetic homogeneity of circulating *M. tuberculosis* strains.

A total of 68 different LSPs were detected among the 100 isolates, ranging in size from 189 to 11,985 bp. These were predicted to disrupt from 0 to 50 (median of 19) coding sequences per strain. Unlike the majority of SNPs, LSPs are more likely to involve a loss of function and are therefore likely to have phenotypic consequences. In principle, LSPs could enhance strain fitness, reduce fitness, or be neutral for the strain. Most of the 224 genes predicted to have been deleted and disrupted by the 68 mutations have not been studied experimentally, and therefore the consequences of the majority of LSPs are unclear. LSPs occurred only in a single isolate in most cases, with few occurring in multiple strains. Although this frequency distribution could reflect the rarity of LSPs, predictions of the mutation-selection balance are consistent with deletions on average being associated with a slight loss of fitness (147). Other LSPs, though, might lead to a selective advantage under certain circumstances. An example of this is the loss of *katG,* which encodes a catalase-peroxidase required both for the activation of the prodrug isoniazid and for protection against reactive oxygen species (168). This deletion confers a selective advantage during antimycobacterial therapy, as the loss of KatG results in isoniazid resistance due to failure of drug activation, but also renders the strain vulnerable to oxidative damage

and therefore a loss of fitness in the absence of isoniazid (69, 81, 117, 123, 163).

Microarray studies of other pathogens have identified hypervariable loci often coinciding with defined pathogenicity islands or virulence gene-bearing mobile elements, such as the PA and PZ regions of *H. pylori* (2, 124). The evolutionary history of these regions is complex, involving horizontal gene transfer, ongoing bouts of recombination, and gene shuffling (48). No comparable loci were detected among the 100 strains. However, in eight cases LSPs were found to involve overlapping regions. In some cases these aggregations of deletions are due to the intrinsic plasticity of the sequences themselves. Examples of these are the DR (150) and *plcD* (22, 66) regions that are known to be preferential sites for the insertion of IS*6110.* This makes them susceptible to homologous recombination between adjacently situated ISs, leading to the deletion of the intra-element sequence (22). With the other aggregations, there are no obvious sequence anomalies that could explain why these loci are prone to deletion. For example, two strains had unique deletions both involving *ephA* (147), and strains of *M. bovis* are also known to have a distinct deletion in this region (Fig. 2) (7, 59). The independent loss of *ephA,* predicted to encode an epoxide hydrolase, in three different clones suggests this may be a neutral or even advantageous mutation in terms of strain fitness. Similarly, two overlapping LSPs interrupted *lppA,* which encodes a lipoprotein. Six other putative lipoproteins (*lpqS, lprP, lppC, lppN, lppB,* and *lpqH*) were among the variable genes. Lipoproteins are known to be important antigens of *M. tuberculosis,* and therefore their high rate of deletion could be driven by the selective pressures of the immune system. Ultimately, the influence of specific mutations needs to be tested experimentally. Larger scale studies using population-based molecular epidemiology are also needed to examine how individual LSPs affect strain fitness in humans.

A comparison of the two complete genome sequences of *M. tuberculosis* confirmed the limited extent of LSPs found in the population-

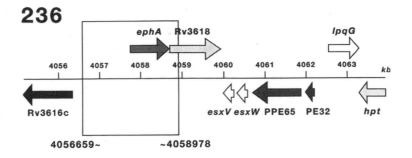

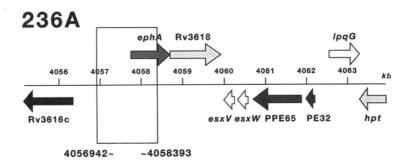

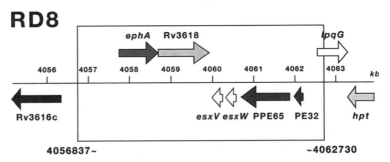

FIGURE 2 Large sequence polymorphisms in the epoxide hydrolase locus of three *M. tuberculosis* complex strains. The large rectangular boxes correspond to the DNA fragment absent from each strain, with the precise H37Rv genome coordinates marking the extent of each deletion. Deletions 236 and 236A were detected in strains isolated from San Francisco, and RD8 was originally detected in *M. bovis* BCG strains (7, 59). The distinct end points for each polymorphism indicate that these genomic deletions have occurred independently. The annotation is according to the H37Rv sequence (27): Rv 3618, function unknown; *ephA*, epoxide hydrolase; *esxV* and *esxW*, members of the early secretory antigen family; PPE65 and PE32, members of two large gene families of unknown function; *lpqG*, lipoprotein; and *hpt*, involved in purine salvage.

based study (10, 49). Only 51 insertions of greater than 10 bp (26 in H37Rv and 35 in CDC1551) were detected in coding regions of the two genomes, corresponding to 25 complete coding sequences. However, 35 of these occurred in the large PPE and PE-PGRS gene families (33), which correspond to almost 10% of the genome. Both families encode for proteins comprising a conserved amino-terminal domain, some of which have a carboxy terminus characterized by variable numbers of family-specific repetitive motifs. The sequence diversity is largely due to variation in the number of carboxy-terminal repeats and has been successfully used for strain typing (77). Only the PGRS family has been studied in any depth, and some of the proteins have been found to be immunogenic and localized to the cell wall, as well as implicated in pathogenesis (4, 18, 26, 42, 119). Their precise function is unknown, but it has been hypothesized that they are a source of antigenic variation, which may allow *M. tuberculosis* to manipulate or evade the immune response (33). Although this may not be the principal cellular function of the PGRS proteins, it is a plausible explanation of how variability is generated and maintained over an extensive part of an otherwise highly conserved genome. It will be interesting to determine if similar sequence diversity also exists in the PGRS genes of other mycobacteria (115) not subject to the selective pressure of an immune system.

Population Structure

Despite the limited genetic diversity detected in clinical isolates, it is of interest to elucidate more finely the population structure of *M. tuberculosis*. Studies of other bacterial pathogens have shown that population structures can vary from clonality to a virtual panmictic state (83, 131). Determining the relative contributions of de novo mutation and recombination for generating genetic diversity is important for understanding the ongoing evolution of *M. tuberculosis*.

The deletional analysis of 100 San Francisco clinical isolates described above provided a useful data set for probing population structure (65). Because the use of a high-density array in combination with specific software can accurately predict the margins of putative deletions (74, 125), the junction sequences could be easily sequenced to provide a specific "start-stop" genomic coordinate for each LSP. Comparison of these deletion end points revealed that 27 of the 68 LSPs were in more than one strain. The conservation of the coordinates, the absence of

flanking repetitive DNA, and their frequent truncation of conserved coding sequences strongly suggested that these genomic deletions represent unique event polymorphisms (21, 23, 65), mutations that do not occur independently in multiple individuals. In addition, in the absence of lateral gene transfer, they are irreversible. They are therefore ideal for establishing phylogenies. Strikingly maximum parsimony tree constructions revealed that 65 out of 68 of these deletions mapped onto a single tree, with only 3 deletions displaying contradiction. Of the three incongruent LSPs, two were prophages and one was flanked by IS6110, all mobile genetic elements capable of independent excision. The impressive congruency of the individual deletion phylogenies confirms that the LSPs detected by this microarray approach are indeed due to loss of DNA rather than lateral gene flow into the reference strain H37Rv. It also suggests that recombination, at least between large sequences, is not evident in the analyzed strains, and supports the widespread view that tuberculosis is a clonal infection.

This clonal structure recently has been shown for a different population of *M. tuberculosis* strains (141). One of the prerequisites for recombination in an obligate pathogen is the presence of a mixed infection of at least two genetically distinct strains. The contemporaneous isolation of two distinct clones from a single patient has been reported (16, 29, 166), and a recent study suggests this may be more common than previously thought (53). However, it is possible that in areas of high transmission, such as those occurring in communities with a high prevalence of human immunodeficiency virus infection, the opportunities for mixed infections arise more frequently. This was the rationale for Supply et al. (141) to search for linkage disequilibrium between genetic markers in 209 isolates of *M. tuberculosis* collected over a 6-year period from an urban South African community. They used mycobacterial interspersed repetitive units, which are human microsatellitelike loci amenable to variable number of tandem repeat type of analysis (88, 140). Twelve of these loci, which are hypervariable in their number of repeats and are scattered around the genome, exhibited highly significant linkage disequilibrium, suggesting that, even in this high-incidence community, recombination between *M. tuberculosis* clones was exceedingly rare.

Further studies, using different genetic markers and populations, are obviously required to confirm that the clonal nature of *M. tuberculosis* seen in these collections of isolates is an accurate reflection of global populations, particularly as limited genetic diversity can hinder the detection of recombination. Nevertheless, the results of these two studies suggest that de novo mutation, and not recombination, is the predominant mechanism for the ongoing genetic diversification of *M. tuberculosis*. This has important implications for predicting how *M. tuberculosis* might evolve in response to human interventions, such as drug therapy and vaccination.

Clonal Families

The genetic homogeneity of *M. tuberculosis* initially proved a challenge for molecular epidemiologists. However, a series of techniques with sufficient discriminatory power have now been developed that can be used in combination to differentiate individual strains (77). These tools have been successfully employed to elucidate the transmission dynamics of *M. tuberculosis* in a wide variety of settings (25). As the number of molecular epidemiological studies has increased, researchers are starting to focus on more fundamental questions relevant to the evolution of tuberculosis, in particular whether there are families of closely related strains, and whether these clonal groupings have particular phenotypic properties. Most of the studies have concentrated on the W or Beijing family of strains. This family was initially identified by a distinctive and easily recognizable spoligotype (153), a molecular epidemiological technique exploiting variation in the direct repeat region (61, 150), and was subsequently shown, using a variety of other molecular markers, to represent a group of closely related strains (12). Beijing family strains are highly prevalent in China,

Russia, and some other East Asian countries (57). They have also been reported in surveys from other continents, including the United States and Africa (151). The ecological abundance of Beijing strains has been taken as evidence of an emerging hypervirulent clonal family (12, 57). Although there are some studies describing unique phenotypic properties of Beijing strains (80, 85, 86, 120), there are no convincing longitudinal data showing expansion within a defined population (57).

The identification of other strain families has been hampered by the limitations of existing molecular markers. Recent reports, though, point to other dominant clones in different human populations (44, 100, 101, 133, 151). This suggests a more global phylogeographical structure for *M. tuberculosis*, in which segregated human populations have been colonized by specific clones. Evidence for this comes from a study in San Francisco (65). Because of the comprehensive nature of the sampling (130), it can be established with some certainty which cases have reactivated infections, and if this occurs in immigrants, reasonably inferred that the infecting strain of *M. tuberculosis* has been acquired in their country of origin. By mapping place of birth of proven cases of reactivation tuberculosis onto the phylogeny of the isolate, it is therefore possible to test agnostically for phylogeographical structure. This revealed a strong correlation between phylogenetic clade and three broad geographical regions (Fig. 3), suggesting a stable association of genetically differentiated strains with specific host populations. These associations probably reflect the historical or prehistorical dissemination of *M. tuberculosis* associated with human migrations, as has been established for *H. pylori* populations (46). Resolving the geographical structure of *M. tuberculosis* on a more global scale could reveal where and when this pathogen emerged. If there are genuine biological differences between these strains, as has been stated in the older literature (93), this information may be of practical significance for patient management or vaccine design.

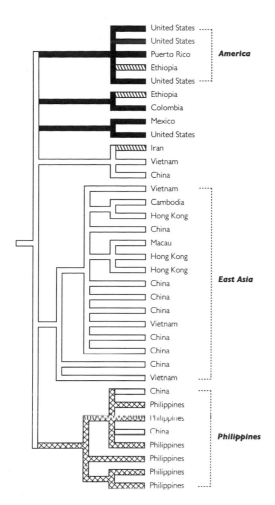

United States
United States
Puerto Rico   **America**
Ethiopia
United States
Ethiopia
Colombia
Mexico
United States
Iran
Vietnam
China
Vietnam
Cambodia
Hong Kong
China
Macau
Hong Kong
Hong Kong   **East Asia**
China
China
China
Vietnam
China
China
China
Vietnam
China
Philippines
Philippines
China
Philippines   **Philippines**
Philippines
Philippines
Philippines

FIGURE 3 Phylogeographical structure of reactivating *M. tuberculosis* strains in San Francisco. The phylogeny was constructed by maximum parsimony using large sequence polymorphisms detected by microarray analysis. The place of birth of the source case for each strain is shown on the right. White, crossed, black, and lined shadings have been superimposed, corresponding to East Asia, the Philippines, the Americas, or other places of birth, to reveal distinct geographical clades.

EVOLUTION OF THE *M. TUBERCULOSIS* COMPLEX

M. tuberculosis is in fact a single member of a group of subspecies known as the *M. tuberculosis* complex, all with identical 16S rRNA sequences. The members of this complex can be distinguished using a variety of phenotypic assays and have been traditionally thought of as discrete subspecies. This classification was based on the historical importance of distinguishing between *M. tuberculosis* and *M. bovis* when, prior to pasteurization, the latter was responsible for large numbers of childhood cases of tuberculosis due to the contamination of milk with bovine tuberculosis. Subsequently, the other members of the complex (*M. microti* and *M. africanum*) were identified because of phenotypic characteristics intermediate to *M. tuberculosis* and *M. bovis*. *M. bovis* appears to have a much broader host range than *M. tuberculosis*, and has been isolated from species as diverse as seals, badgers, llamas, captive primates, possums, and deer (35, 142, 143). In contrast, *M. tuberculosis* is responsible for over 95% of human tuberculosis cases and is only sporadically isolated from animal species. Whereas *M. africanum* is a human pathogen, apparently geographically restricted to parts of Africa (51, 156), *M. microti* is a pathogen of voles, a small mammalian species (19, 28). This led to the seemingly logical assumption that *M. tuberculosis* evolved directly from the promiscuous pathogen *M. bovis* to occupy the more specialized niche of humans, with the domestication of animals providing a convenient ecological change to account for this adaptation (134).

Recent comparative genomic studies have called into question this simple zoonotic model of evolution for *M. tuberculosis*. Following the completion of the *M. tuberculosis* genome sequence, various groups used whole-genome DNA hybridization experiments to determine the chromosomal gene content of *Mycobacterium bovis* BCG (7, 20, 59, 82, 125). These studies were attempting to define the genetic basis of attenuation that occurred during the serial passage of the virulent *M. bovis* progenitor strain that resulted in the live tuberculosis vaccine BCG. Eleven of the genomic deletions or regions of difference (RDs) detected in the BCG strains analyzed, ranging in size from 1 to over 12 kb, were subsequently found to occur in classical strains of *M. bovis* (7, 21, 59, 97). This immediately challenged the assumption that *M. bovis* was the direct progenitor of *M. tuberculosis* as the human pathogen appeared to have the larger genome (23).

The completion of an *M. bovis* genome sequence has confirmed these RDs and importantly also established that there were no genes or genomic regions unique to *M. bovis*. The RDs have normal base pair composition, and their borders frequently interrupt coding sequences. The junction of RD9, for example, truncates *cobL,* a gene encoding a precorrin methyltransferase that is highly conserved in diverse bacteria (23). Taken together, this information confirms that the *M. bovis-M. tuberculosis* RDs are deletions in the *M. bovis* genome and that the animal pathogen does have the smaller genome. There has also been further loss of coding capacity in *M. bovis* in the form of 31 pseudogenes. The balance of the gene losses is reflected in the 3,951 total annotated coding sequences in the *M. bovis* (54) genome compared to 3,995 in *M. tuberculosis* H37Rv (27).

The corollary of the genome shrinkage of *M. bovis* is that its apparent broader host range must be due to gene loss or inactivation rather than the acquisition of specific virulence factors. Mutations leading to loss of function but increased pathogenicity have been identified in other bacteria (132), such as the loss of lysine decarboxylase from *Shigella flexneri* as a result of a genomic deletion, which leads to metabolic changes that increase enterotoxin production and virulence (87). Among the disrupted *M. bovis* genes, it is not known which produce functional losses that are phenotypically important. Decreased antigenic burden (*esx* family members), alteration in cell wall lipids *(pks6),* loss of transporters *(mntH, mmpL1, mmpL6),* global regulatory changes *(pknD),* and metabolic shifts *(glpK, ugpA)* are all possibilities (54). The rabbit model of infection, in which *M. bovis* is more pathogenic than *M. tuberculosis,* provides a suitable experimental system for formally testing the role of gene loss in mycobacterial virulence.

Further reconstruction of the evolutionary history of *M. bovis* was obtained by using the RDs to resolve the phylogenetic relationships of the phenotypically intermediary members of the complex. Brosch et al. were able to construct a rooted phylogeny using the distribution of the *M. bovis* deletions within a large collection of strains representing the entire *M. tuberculosis* complex (21). This revealed a direct lineage from *M. tuberculosis,* via *M. africanum* and *M. microti*–like transitional strains, to the *M. bovis* group. This has subsequently been substantiated using a battery of SNPs (62).

Strictly speaking, these results merely show that *M. tuberculosis* is genomically closer than *M. bovis* to the common complex ancestor and do not reveal what was the host preference of this ancestor. However, *M. bovis* could be an example of a reverse zoonosis given that the progenitor of the animal pathogens *M. microti* and *M. bovis* was an *M. africanum*-like strain that to date is considered an exclusively human pathogen. Although the global movement of cattle during the last century contributed to the dissemination of *M. bovis,* it is probable that a more ancient dispersal of an animal-adapted clone must have occurred to account for the occurrence of *M. tuberculosis* complex members in wild animal populations as diverse as Scottish voles, Argentinean seals, and South African hydraxes (21).

CONCLUDING REMARKS

In terms of cumulative mortality and morbidity, *M. tuberculosis* is the most successful pathogen in the history of mankind. The disease burden has driven an immense effort to understand it from a medical and public health perspective. Indeed, its clinical manifestations, treatment, and epidemiology are understood in considerable detail. The success of *M. tuberculosis* is undoubtedly a consequence of a finely tuned dialogue that has evolved over this time period between pathogen and host. Until recently, however, there was little formal effort to understand *M. tuberculosis* from an evolutionary perspective. Recent advances in genomics now make it possible to explore the evolution of *M. tuberculosis.* Because this organism has such a unique lifestyle, these lessons may provide fundamental insights into the nature and consequences of genetic variability among pathogenic bacteria. Furthermore, it is our ultimate hope that this insight will contribute to the development of practical interventions to address the immense global burden.

CHAPTER SUMMARY

- *Mycobacterium tuberculosis*, the causative agent of tuberculosis, is a highly successful and mortal pathogen infecting one-third of the world's population.
- Within the large genus *Mycobacterium*, the obligate and opportunistic pathogens are closely related and share common determinants of virulence.
- Mutation rather than horizontal gene transfer has driven the recent evolution of *Mycobacterium tuberculosis* and its adaptation to the human host.
- Limited genetic diversity among contemporary strains suggests that *M. tuberculosis* has undergone a recent clonal expansion.
- *M. tuberculosis* exhibits a strong phylogeographical population structure. The existence of dominant clones within human populations raises the possibility of pathogen-host coevolution.
- The *M. tuberculosis* complex subspecies, with their diverse host range, may have evolved from a progenitor human pathogen.

ACKNOWLEDGMENTS

We acknowledge the contributions and helpful comments of Anthony Tsolaki and Aaron Hirsch.

This work was in part supported by National Institute of Allergy and Infectious Diseases grant AI 34238. A.S.P. was in receipt of a Fellowship from the Wellcome Trust.

REFERENCES

1. Achtman, M., K. Zurth, G. Morelli, G. Torrea, A. Guiyoule, and E. Carniel. 1999. *Yersinia pestis*, the cause of plague, is a recently emerged clone of *Yersinia pseudotuberculosis*. *Proc. Natl. Acad. Sci. USA* **96:**14043–14048.
2. Alm, R. A., L. S. Ling, D. T. Moir, B. L. King, E. D. Brown, P. C. Doig, D. R. Smith, B. Noonan, B. C. Guild, B. L. deJonge, G. Carmel, P. J. Tummino, A. Caruso, M. Uria-Nickelsen,

D. M. Mills, C. Ives, R. Gibson, D. Merberg, S. D. Mills, Q. Jiang, D. E. Taylor, G. F. Vovis, and T. J. Trust. 1999. Genomic-sequence comparison of two unrelated isolates of the human gastric pathogen *Helicobacter pylori*. *Nature* **397:**176–180.
3. Andersson, S. G., A. Zomorodipour, J. O. Andersson, T. Sicheritz-Ponten, U. C. Alsmark, R. M. Podowski, A. K. Naslund, A. S. Eriksson, H. H. Winkler, and C. G. Kurland. 1998. The genome sequence of *Rickettsia prowazekii* and the origin of mitochondria. *Nature* **396:**133–140.
4. Banu, S., N. Honore, B. Saint-Joanis, D. Philpott, M. C. Prevost, and S. T. Cole. 2002. Are the PE-PGRS proteins of *Mycobacterium tuberculosis* variable surface antigens? *Mol. Microbiol.* **44:**9–19.
5. Barker, L. P., K. M. George, S. Falkow, and P. L. Small. 1997. Differential trafficking of live and dead *Mycobacterium marinum* organisms in macrophages. *Infect. Immun.* **65:**1497–1504.
6. Barry, C. E., III. 2001. Interpreting cell wall 'virulence factors' of *Mycobacterium tuberculosis*. *Trends Microbiol.* **9:**237–241.
7. Behr, M. A., M. A. Wilson, W. P. Gill, H. Salamon, G. K. Schoolnik, S. Rane, and P. M. Small. 1999. Comparative genomics of BCG vaccines by whole-genome DNA microarray. *Science* **284:**1520–1523.
8. Bentley, S. D., K. F. Chater, A. M. Cerdeno-Tarraga, G. L. Challis, N. R. Thomson, K. D. James, D. E. Harris, M. A. Quail, H. Kieser, D. Harper, A. Bateman, S. Brown, G. Chandra, C. W. Chen, M. Collins, A. Cronin, A. Fraser, A. Goble, J. Hidalgo, T. Hornsby, S. Howarth, C. H. Huang, T. Kieser, L. Larke, L. Murphy, K. Oliver, S. O'Neil, E. Rabbinowitsch, M. A. Rajandream, K. Rutherford, S. Rutter, K. Seeger, D. Saunders, S. Sharp, R. Squares, S. Squares, K. Taylor, T. Warren, A. Wietzorrek, J. Woodward, B. G. Barrell, J. Parkhill, and D. A. Hopwood. 2002. Complete genome sequence of the model actinomycete *Streptomyces coelicolor* A3(2). *Nature* **417:**141–147.
9. Berthet, F. X., M. Lagranderie, P. Gounon, C. Laurent-Winter, D. Ensergueix, P. Chavarot, F. Thouron, E. Maranghi, V. Pelicic, D. Portnoi, G. Marchal, and B. Gicquel. 1998. Attenuation of virulence by disruption of the *Mycobacterium tuberculosis erp* gene. *Science* **282:**759–762.
10. Betts, J. C., P. Dodson, S. Quan, A. P. Lewis, P. J. Thomas, K. Duncan, and R. A. McAdam. 2000. Comparison of the proteome of *Mycobacterium tuberculosis* strain H37Rv with clinical isolate CDC 1551. *Microbiology* **146**(Pt. 12): 3205–3216.
11. Bibb, L. A., and G. F. Hatfull. 2002. Integration

and excision of the *Mycobacterium tuberculosis* prophage-like element, phiRv1. *Mol. Microbiol.* **45:**1515–1526.

12. **Bifani, P. J., B. Mathema, N. E. Kurepina, and B. N. Kreiswirth.** 2002. Global dissemination of the *Mycobacterium tuberculosis* W-Beijing family strains. *Trends Microbiol.* **10:**45–52.

13. **Billington, O. J., T. D. McHugh, and S. H. Gillespie.** 1999. Physiological cost of rifampin resistance induced in vitro in *Mycobacterium tuberculosis. Antimicrob. Agents Chemother.* **43:**1866–1869.

14. **Borgdorff, M. W., M. A. Behr, N. J. Nagelkerke, P. C. Hopewell, and P. M. Small.** 2000. Transmission of tuberculosis in San Francisco and its association with immigration and ethnicity. *Int. J. Tuberc. Lung Dis.* **4:**287–294.

15. **Boshoff, H. I., M. B. Reed, C. E. Barry III, and V. Mizrahi.** 2003. DnaE2 polymerase contributes to in vivo survival and the emergence of drug resistance in *Mycobacterium tuberculosis. Cell* **113:**183–193.

16. **Braden, C. R., G. P. Morlock, C. L. Woodley, K. R. Johnson, A. C. Colombel, M. D. Cave, Z. Yang, S. E. Valway, I. M. Onorato, and J. T. Crawford.** 2001. Simultaneous infection with multiple strains of *Mycobacterium tuberculosis. Clin. Infect. Dis.* **33:**e42–e47.

17. **Braunstein, M., B. J. Espinosa, J. Chan, J. T. Belisle, and R. W. Jacobs, Jr.** 2003. SecA2 functions in the secretion of superoxide dismutase A and in the virulence of *Mycobacterium tuberculosis. Mol. Microbiol.* **48:**453–464.

18. **Brennan, M. J., G. Delogu, Y. Chen, S. Bardarov, J. Kriakov, M. Alavi, and W. R. Jacobs, Jr.** 2001. Evidence that mycobacterial PE-PGRS proteins are cell surface constituents that influence interactions with other cells. *Infect. Immun.* **69:**7326–7333.

19. **Brodin, P., K. Eiglmeier, M. Marmiesse, A. Billault, T. Garnier, S. Niemann, S. T. Cole, and R. Brosch.** 2002. Bacterial artificial chromosome-based comparative genomic analysis identifies *Mycobacterium microti* as a natural ESAT-6 deletion mutant. *Infect. Immun.* **70:**5568–5578.

20. **Brosch, R., S. V. Gordon, A. Billault, T. Garnier, K. Eiglmeier, C. Soravito, B. G. Barrell, and S. T. Cole.** 1998. Use of a *Mycobacterium tuberculosis* H37Rv bacterial artificial chromosome library for genome mapping, sequencing, and comparative genomics. *Infect. Immun.* **66:**2221–2229.

21. **Brosch, R., S. V. Gordon, M. Marmiesse, P. Brodin, C. Buchrieser, K. Eiglmeier, T. Garnier, C. Gutierrez, G. Hewinson, K. Kremer, L. M. Parsons, A. S. Pym, S. Samper, D. van Soolingen, and S. T. Cole.** 2002. A new evolutionary scenario for the *Mycobacterium tuberculosis* complex. *Proc. Natl. Acad. Sci. USA* **99:**3684–3689.

22. **Brosch, R., W. J. Philipp, E. Stavropoulos, M. J. Colston, S. T. Cole, and S. V. Gordon.** 1999. Genomic analysis reveals variation between *Mycobacterium tuberculosis* H37Rv and the attenuated *M. tuberculosis* H37Ra strain. *Infect. Immun.* **67:**5768–5774.

23. **Brosch, R., A. S. Pym, S. V. Gordon, and S. T. Cole.** 2001. The evolution of mycobacterial pathogenicity: clues from comparative genomics. *Trends Microbiol.* **9:**452–458.

24. **Buchmeier, N., A. Blanc-Potard, S. Ehrt, D. Piddington, L. Riley, and E. A. Groisman.** 2000. A parallel intraphagosomal survival strategy shared by *Mycobacterium tuberculosis* and *Salmonella enterica. Mol. Microbiol.* **35:**1375–1382.

25. **Burgos, M. V., and A. S. Pym.** 2002. Molecular epidemiology of tuberculosis. *Eur. Respir. J. Suppl.* **36:**54s–65s.

26. **Camacho, L. R., D. Ensergueix, E. Perez, B. Gicquel, and C. Guilhot.** 1999. Identification of a virulence gene cluster of *Mycobacterium tuberculosis* by signature-tagged transposon mutagenesis. *Mol. Microbiol.* **34:**257–267.

27. **Camus, J. C., M. J. Pryor, C. Medigue, and S. T. Cole.** 2002. Re-annotation of the genome sequence of *Mycobacterium tuberculosis* H37Rv. *Microbiology* **148:**2967–2973.

28. **Cavanagh, R., M. Begon, M. Bennett, T. Ergon, I. M. Graham, P. E. De Haas, C. A. Hart, M. Koedam, K. Kremer, X. Lambin, P. Roholl, and D. van Soolingen.** 2002. *Mycobacterium microti* infection (vole tuberculosis) in wild rodent populations. *J. Clin. Microbiol.* **40:**3281–3285.

29. **Chaves, F., F. Dronda, M. Alonso-Sanz, and A. R. Noriega.** 1999. Evidence of exogenous reinfection and mixed infection with more than one strain of *Mycobacterium tuberculosis* among Spanish HIV-infected inmates. *AIDS* **13:**615–620.

30. **Chen, P., R. E. Ruiz, Q. Li, R. F. Silver, and W. R. Bishai.** 2000. Construction and characterization of a *Mycobacterium tuberculosis* mutant lacking the alternate sigma factor gene, sigF. *Infect. Immun.* **68:**5575–5580.

31. **Cirillo, J. D., S. Falkow, L. S. Tompkins, and L. E. Bermudez.** 1997. Interaction of *Mycobacterium avium* with environmental amoebae enhances virulence. *Infect. Immun.* **65:**3759–3767.

32. **Clemens, D. L., and M. A. Horwitz.** 1995. Characterization of the *Mycobacterium tuberculosis* phagosome and evidence that phagosomal maturation is inhibited. *J. Exp. Med.* **181:**257–270.

33. **Cole, S. T., R. Brosch, J. Parkhill, T. Garnier, C. Churcher, D. Harris, S. V. Gordon, K.**

Eiglmeier, S. Gas, C. E. Barry III, F. Tekaia, K. Badcock, D. Basham, D. Brown, T. Chillingworth, R. Connor, R. Davies, K. Devlin, T. Feltwell, S. Gentles, N. Hamlin, S. Holroyd, T. Hornsby, K. Jagels, A. Krogh, A. McLean, S. Moule, L. Murphy, K. Oliver, J. Osborne, M. A. Quail, M.-A. Rajandream, J. Rogers, S. Rutter, K. Seeger, J. Skelton, R. Squares, S. Squares, J. E. Sulston, K. Taylor, S. Whitehead, and B. G. Barrell. 1998. Deciphering the biology of *Mycobacterium tuberculosis* from the complete genome sequence. *Nature* **393**:537–544.

34. Cole, S. T., K. Eiglmeier, J. Parkhill, K. D. James, N. R. Thomson, P. R. Wheeler, N. Honore, T. Garnier, C. Churcher, D. Harris, K. Mungall, D. Basham, D. Brown, T. Chillingworth, R. Connor, R. M. Davies, K. Devlin, S. Duthoy, T. Feltwell, A. Fraser, N. Hamlin, S. Holroyd, T. Hornsby, K. Jagels, C. Lacroix, J. Maclean, S. Moule, L. Murphy, K. Oliver, M. A. Quail, M. A. Rajandream, K. M. Rutherford, S. Rutter, K. Seeger, S. Simon, M. Simmonds, J. Skelton, R. Squares, S. Squares, K. Stevens, K. Taylor, S. Whitehead, J. R. Woodward, and B. G. Barrell. 2001. Massive gene decay in the leprosy bacillus. *Nature* **409**:1007–1011.

35. Coleman, J. D., and M. M. Cooke. 2001. *Mycobacterium bovis* infection in wildlife in New Zealand. *Tuberculosis* (Edinburgh) **81**:191–202.

36. Collins, D. M., R. P. Kawakami, G. W. de Lisle, L. Pascopella, B. R. Bloom, and W. R. Jacobs. 1995. Mutation of the principal sigma factor causes loss of virulence in a strain of the *Mycobacterium tuberculosis* complex. *Proc. Natl. Acad. Sci. USA* **92**:8036–8040.

37. Cox, E. C. 1976. Bacterial mutator genes and the control of spontaneous mutation. *Annu. Rev. Genet.* **10**:135–156.

38. Cox, J. S., B. Chen, M. McNeil, and W. R. Jacobs, Jr. 1999. Complex lipid determines tissue-specific replication of *Mycobacterium tuberculosis* in mice. *Nature* **402**:79–83.

39. Daffe, M., M. McNeil, and P. J. Brennan. 1991. Novel type-specific lipooligosaccharides from *Mycobacterium tuberculosis*. *Biochemistry* **30**:378–388.

40. David, H., and C. M. Newman. 1971. Some observations on the genetics of isoniazid resistance in the tubercle bacilli. *Am. Rev. Respir. Dis.* **104**:508–515.

41. David, H. L. 1970. Probability distribution of drug-resistant mutants in unselected populations of *Mycobacterium tuberculosis*. *Appl. Microbiol.* **20**:810–814.

42. Delogu, G., and M. J. Brennan. 2001. Comparative immune response to PE and PE-PGRS

antigens of *Mycobacterium tuberculosis*. *Infect. Immun.* **69**:5606–5611.

43. Dorrell, N., J. A. Mangan, K. G. Laing, J. Hinds, D. Linton, H. Al-Ghusein, B. G. Barrell, J. Parkhill, N. G. Stoker, A. V. Karlyshev, P. D. Butcher, and B. W. Wren. 2001. Whole genome comparison of *Campylobacter jejuni* human isolates using a low-cost microarray reveals extensive genetic diversity. *Genome Res.* **11**:1706–1715.

44. Douglas, J. T., L. Qian, J. C. Montoya, J. M. Musser, J. D. van Embden, D. van Soolingen, and K. Kremer. 2003. Characterization of the Manila family of *Mycobacterium tuberculosis*. *J. Clin. Microbiol.* **41**:2723–2726.

45. Dye, C., S. Scheele, P. Dolin, V. Pathania, and M. C. Raviglione. 1999. Consensus statement. Global burden of tuberculosis: estimated incidence, prevalence, and mortality by country. WHO Global Surveillance and Monitoring Project. *JAMA* **282**:677–686.

46. Falush, D., T. Wirth, B. Linz, J. K. Pritchard, M. Stephens, M. Kidd, M. J. Blaser, D. Y. Graham, S. Vacher, G. I. Perez-Perez, Y. Yamaoka, F. Megraud, K. Otto, U. Reichard, E. Katzowitsch, X. Wang, M. Achtman, and S. Suerbaum. 2003. Traces of human migrations in *Helicobacter pylori* populations. *Science* **299**:1582–1585.

47. Fitzgerald, J. R., and J. M. Musser. 2001. Evolutionary genomics of pathogenic bacteria. *Trends Microbiol.* **9**:547–553.

48. Fitzgerald, J. R., D. E. Sturdevant, S. M. Mackie, S. R. Gill, and J. M. Musser. 2001. Evolutionary genomics of *Staphylococcus aureus*: insights into the origin of methicillin-resistant strains and the toxic shock syndrome epidemic. *Proc. Natl. Acad. Sci. USA* **98**:8821–8826.

49. Fleischmann, R. D., D. Alland, J. A. Eisen, L. Carpenter, O. White, J. Peterson, R. DeBoy, R. Dodson, M. Gwinn, D. Haft, E. Hickey, J. F. Kolonay, W. C. Nelson, L. A. Umayam, M. Ermolaeva, S. L. Salzberg, A. Delcher, T. Utterback, J. Weidman, H. Khouri, J. Gill, A. Mikula, W. Bishai, W. R. Jacobs, Jr., J. C. Venter, and C. M. Fraser. 2002. Whole-genome comparison of *Mycobacterium tuberculosis* clinical and laboratory strains. *J. Bacteriol.* **184**:5479–5490.

50. Foster, P. L. 1999. Mechanisms of stationary phase mutation: a decade of adaptive mutation. *Annu. Rev. Genet.* **33**:57–88.

51. Frothingham, R., P. L. Strickland, G. Bretzel, S. Ramaswamy, J. M. Musser, and D. L. Williams. 1999. Phenotypic and genotypic characterization of *Mycobacterium africanum* isolates from West Africa. *J. Clin. Microbiol.* **37**:1921–1926.

52. Gamieldien, J., A. Ptitsyn, and W. Hide. 2002.

Eukaryotic genes in *Mycobacterium tuberculosis* could have a role in pathogenesis and immunomodulation. *Trends Genet.* **18:**5–8.

53. **Garcia de Viedma, D., M. Marin, M. J. Ruiz Serrano, L. Alcala, and E. Bouza.** 2003. Polyclonal and compartmentalized infection by *Mycobacterium tuberculosis* in patients with both respiratory and extrarespiratory involvement. *J. Infect. Dis.* **187:**695–699.

54. **Garnier, T., K. Eiglmeier, J. C. Camus, N. Medina, H. Mansoor, M. Pryor, S. Duthoy, S. Grondin, C. Lacroix, C. Monsempe, S. Simon, B. Harris, R. Atkin, J. Doggett, R. Mayes, L. Keating, P. R. Wheeler, J. Parkhill, B. G. Barrell, S. T. Cole, S. V. Gordon, and R. G. Hewinson.** 2003. The complete genome sequence of *Mycobacterium bovis*. *Proc. Natl. Acad. Sci. USA* **100:**7877–7882.

55. **Gil, R., B. Sabater-Munoz, A. Latorre, F. J. Silva, and A. Moya.** 2002. Extreme genome reduction in *Buchnera* spp.: toward the minimal genome needed for symbiotic life. *Proc. Natl. Acad. Sci. USA* **99:**4454–4458.

56. **Glickman, M. S., J. S. Cox, and W. R. Jacobs, Jr.** 2000. A novel mycolic acid cyclopropane synthetase is required for coding, persistence, and virulence of *Mycobacterium tuberculosis*. *Mol. Cell* **5:**717–727.

57. **Glynn, J. R., J. Whiteley, P. J. Bifani, K. Kremer, and D. van Soolingen.** 2002. Worldwide occurrence of Beijing/W strains of *Mycobacterium tuberculosis*: a systematic review. *Emerg. Infect. Dis.* **8:**843–849.

58. **Goh, K. S., E. Legrand, C. Sola, and N. Rastogi.** 2001. Rapid differentiation of *"Mycobacterium canettii"* from other *Mycobacterium tuberculosis* complex organisms by PCR-restriction analysis of the *hsp65* gene. *J. Clin. Microbiol.* **39:**3705–3708.

59. **Gordon, S. V., R. Brosch, A. Billault, T. Garnier, K. Eiglmeier, and S. T. Cole.** 1999. Identification of variable regions in the genomes of tubercle bacilli using bacterial artificial chromosome arrays. *Mol. Microbiol.* **32:**643–655.

60. **Gordon, S. V., B. Heym, J. Parkhill, B. Barrell, and S. T. Cole.** 1999. New insertion sequences and a novel repeated sequence in the genome of *Mycobacterium tuberculosis* H37Rv. *Microbiology* **145**(Pt. 4):881–892.

61. **Groenen, P. M., A. E. Bunschoten, D. van Soolingen, and J. D. van Embden.** 1993. Nature of DNA polymorphism in the direct repeat cluster of *Mycobacterium tuberculosis;* application for strain differentiation by a novel typing method. *Mol. Microbiol.* **10:**1057–1065.

62. **Gutacker, M. M., J. C. Smoot, C. A. Migliaccio, S. M. Ricklefs, S. Hua, D. V. Cousins, E. A. Graviss, E. Shashkina, B. N. Kreiswirth, and J. M. Musser.** 2002. Genome-wide analysis of synonymous single nucleotide polymorphisms in *Mycobacterium tuberculosis* complex organisms. Resolution of genetic relationships among closely related microbial strains. *Genetics* **162:**1533–1543.

63. **Harb, O. S., L. Y. Gao, and Y. Abu Kwaik.** 2000. From protozoa to mammalian cells: a new paradigm in the life cycle of intracellular bacterial pathogens. *Environ. Microbiol.* **2:**251–265.

64. **Hendrix, R. W., M. C. Smith, R. N. Burns, M. E. Ford, and G. F. Hatfull.** 1999. Evolutionary relationships among diverse bacteriophages and prophages: all the world's a phage. *Proc. Natl. Acad. Sci. USA* **96:**2192–2197.

65. **Hirsh, A. E., A. G. Tsolaki, K. DeRiemer, M. W. Feldman, and P. M. Small.** 2004. Stable association between strains of *Mycobacterium tuberculosis* and their human host populations. *Proc. Natl. Acad. Sci. USA* **101:**4871–4876.

66. **Ho, T. B., B. D. Robertson, G. M. Taylor, R. J. Shaw, and D. B. Young.** 2000. Comparison of *Mycobacterium tuberculosis* genomes reveals frequent deletions in a 20 kb variable region in clinical isolates. *Yeast* **17:**272–282.

67. **Hou, J. Y., J. E. Graham, and J. E. Clark-Curtiss.** 2002. *Mycobacterium avium* genes expressed during growth in human macrophages detected by selective capture of transcribed sequences (SCOTS). *Infect. Immun.* **70:**3714–3726.

68. **Hughes, A. L., R. Friedman, and M. Murray.** 2002. Genome wide pattern of synonymous nucleotide substitution in two complete genomes of *Mycobacterium tuberculosis*. *Emerg. Infect. Dis* **8:**1342–1346.

69. **Johnsson, K., and P. G. Schultz.** 1994. Mechanistic studies of the oxidation of isoniazid by the catalase peroxidase from *Mycobacterium tuberculosis*. *J. Am. Chem. Soc.* **116:**7425–7426.

70. **Jordan, I. K., I. B. Rogozin, Y. I. Wolf, and E. V. Koonin.** 2002. Microevolutionary genomics of bacteria. *Theor. Popul. Biol.* **61:**435–447.

71. **Joyce, E. A., K. Chan, N. R. Salama, and S. Falkow.** 2002. Redefining bacterial populations: a post-genomic reformation. *Nat. Rev. Genet.* **3:**462–473.

72. **Kapur, V., T. S. Whittam, and J. M. Musser.** 1994. Is *Mycobacterium tuberculosis* 15,000 years old? *J. Infect. Dis.* **170:**1348–1349.

73. **Karunakaran, P., and J. Davies.** 2000. Genetic antagonism and hypermutability in *Mycobacterium smegmatis*. *J. Bacteriol.* **182:**3331–3335.

74. **Kato-Maeda, M., J. T. Rhee, T. R. Gingeras, H. Salamon, J. Drenkow, N. Smittipat, and P. M. Small.** 2001. Comparing genomes within the species *Mycobacterium tuberculosis*. *Genome Res.* **11:**547–554.

75. **Kaushal, D., B. G. Schroeder, S. Tyagi, T.**

Yoshimatsu, C. Scott, C. Ko, L. Carpenter, J. Mehrotra, Y. C. Manabe, R. D. Fleischmann, and W. R. Bishai. 2002. Reduced immuno-pathology and mortality despite tissue persistence in a *Mycobacterium tuberculosis* mutant lacking alternative sigma factor, SigH. *Proc. Natl. Acad. Sci. USA* **99:**8330–8335.

76. **Kinsella, R. J., D. A. Fitzpatrick, C. J. Creevey, and J. O. McInerney.** 2003. Fatty acid biosynthesis in *Mycobacterium tuberculosis:* lateral gene transfer, adaptive evolution, and gene duplication. *Proc. Natl. Acad. Sci. USA* **100:**10320–10325.

77. **Kremer, K., D. van Soolingen, R. Frothingham, W. H. Haas, P. W. Hermans, C. Martin, P. Palittapongarnpim, B. B. Plikaytis, L. W. Riley, M. A. Yakrus, J. M. Musser, and J. D. van Embden.** 1999. Comparison of methods based on different molecular epidemiological markers for typing of *Mycobacterium tuberculosis* complex strains: interlaboratory study of discriminatory power and reproducibility. *J. Clin. Microbiol.* **37:**2607–2618.

78. **Lawrence, J. G., and H. Ochman.** 1998. Molecular archaeology of the *Escherichia coli* genome. *Proc. Natl. Acad. Sci. USA* **95:**9413–9417.

79. **LeClerc, J. E., B. Li, W. L. Payne, and T. A. Cebula.** 1996. High mutation frequencies among *Escherichia coli* and *Salmonella* pathogens. *Science* **274:**1208–1211.

80. **Li, Q., C. C. Whalen, J. M. Albert, R. Larkin, L. Zukowski, M. D. Cave, and R. F. Silver.** 2002. Differences in rate and variability of intracellular growth of a panel of *Mycobacterium tuberculosis* clinical isolates within a human monocyte model. *Infect. Immun.* **70:**6489–6493.

81. **Li, Z., C. Kelley, F. Collins, D. Rouse, and S. Morris.** 1998. Expression of *katG* in *Mycobacterium tuberculosis* is associated with its growth and persistence in mice and guinea pigs. *J. Infect. Dis.* **177:**1030–1035.

82. **Mahairas, G. G., P. J. Sabo, M. J. Hickey, D. C. Singh, and C. K. Stover.** 1996. Molecular analysis of genetic differences between *Mycobacterium bovis* BCG and virulent *M. bovis. J. Bacteriol.* **178:**1274–1282.

83. **Maiden, M. C., J. A. Bygraves, E. Feil, G. Morelli, J. E. Russell, R. Urwin, Q. Zhang, J. Zhou, K. Zurth, D. A. Caugant, I. M. Feavers, M. Achtman, and B. G. Spratt.** 1998. Multilocus sequence typing: a portable approach to the identification of clones within populations of pathogenic microorganisms. *Proc. Natl. Acad. Sci. USA* **95:**3140–3145.

84. **Manabe, Y. C., and W. R. Bishai.** 2000. Latent Mycobacterium tuberculosis—persistence, patience, and winning by waiting. *Nat. Med.* **6:**1327–1329.

85. **Manca, C., L. Tsenova, C. E. Barry III, A.** Bergtold, S. Freeman, P. A. Haslett, J. M. Musser, V. H. Freedman, and G. Kaplan. 1999. *Mycobacterium tuberculosis* CDC1551 induces a more vigorous host response in vivo and in vitro, but is not more virulent than other clinical isolates. *J. Immunol.* **162:**6740–6746.

86. **Manca, C., L. Tsenova, A. Bergtold, S. Freeman, M. Tovey, J. M. Musser, C. E. Barry III, V. H. Freedman, and G. Kaplan.** 2001. Virulence of a *Mycobacterium tuberculosis* clinical isolate in mice is determined by failure to induce Th1 type immunity and is associated with induction of IFN-alpha/beta. *Proc. Natl. Acad. Sci. USA* **98:**5752–5757.

87. **Maurelli, A. T., R. E. Fernandez, C. A. Bloch, C. K. Rode, and A. Fasano.** 1998. "Black holes" and bacterial pathogenicity: a large genomic deletion that enhances the virulence of *Shigella* spp. and enteroinvasive *Escherichia coli. Proc. Natl. Acad. Sci. USA* **95:**3943–3948.

88. **Mazars, E., S. Lesjean, A. L. Banuls, M. Gilbert, V. Vincent, B. Gicquel, M. Tibayrenc, C. Locht, and P. Supply.** 2001. High-resolution minisatellite-based typing as a portable approach to global analysis of *Mycobacterium tuberculosis* molecular epidemiology. *Proc. Natl. Acad. Sci. USA* **98:**1901–1906.

89. **McKinney, J. D., K. Honer zu Bentrup, E. J. Munoz-Elias, A. Miczak, B. Chen, W. T. Chan, D. Swenson, J. C. Sacchettini, W. R. Jacobs, Jr., and D. G. Russell.** 2000. Persistence of *Mycobacterium tuberculosis* in macrophages and mice requires the glyoxylate shunt enzyme isocitrate lyase. *Nature* **406:**735–738.

90. **Menendez, M. C., M. J. Garcia, M. C. Navarro, J. A. Gonzalez-y-Merchand, S. Rivera-Gutierrez, L. Garcia-Sanchez, and R. A. Cox.** 2002. Characterization of an rRNA operon (rrnB) of *Mycobacterium fortuitum* and other mycobacterial species: implications for the classification of mycobacteria. *J. Bacteriol.* **184:**1078–1088.

91. **Miltgen, J., M. Morillon, J. L. Koeck, A. Varnerot, J. F. Briant, G. Nguyen, D. Verrot, D. Bonnet, and V. Vincent.** 2002. Two cases of pulmonary tuberculosis caused by *Mycobacterium tuberculosis* subsp canetti. *Emerg. Infect. Dis.* **8:**1350–1352.

92. **Miltner, E. C., and L. E. Bermudez.** 2000. *Mycobacterium avium* grown in *Acanthamoeba castellanii* is protected from the effects of antimicrobials. *Antimicrob. Agents Chemother.* **44:**1990–1994.

93. **Mitchison, D. A., J. G. Wallace, A. L. Bhatia, J. B. Selkon, T. V. Subbaiah, and M. C. Lancaster.** 1960. A comparison of the virulence in Guinea-pigs of South Indian and British tubercle bacilli. *Tubercle* **41:**1–22.

94. **Mizrahi, V., and S. J. Andersen.** 1998. DNA

repair in *Mycobacterium tuberculosis*. What have we learnt from the genome sequence? *Mol. Microbiol.* **29**:1331–1339.

95. **Mizrahi, V., S. S. Dawes, and H. Rubin.** 2000. DNA replication, p. 159–172. In G. F. Hatfull and W. R. Jacobs (ed.), *Molecular Genetics of Mycobacteria.* ASM Press, Washington, D.C.

96. **Moran, N. A.** 1996. Accelerated evolution and Muller's rachet in endosymbiotic bacteria. *Proc. Natl. Acad. Sci. USA* **93**:2873–2878.

97. **Mostowy, S., D. Cousins, J. Brinkman, A. Aranaz, and M. A. Behr.** 2002. Genomic deletions suggest a phylogeny for the *Mycobacterium tuberculosis* complex. *J. Infect. Dis.* **186**:74–80.

98. **Mukamolova, G. V., O. A. Turapov, D. I. Young, A. S. Kaprelyants, D. B. Kell, and M. Young.** 2002. A family of autocrine growth factors in *Mycobacterium tuberculosis*. *Mol. Microbiol.* **46**:623–635.

99. **Musser, J. M., A. Amin, and S. Ramaswamy.** 2000. Negligible genetic diversity of *Mycobacterium tuberculosis* host immune system protein targets: evidence of limited selective pressure. *Genetics* **155**:7–16.

100. **Nguyen, D., P. Brassard, J. Westley, L. Thibert, M. Proulx, K. Henry, K. Schwartzman, D. Menzies, and M. A. Behr.** 2003. Widespread pyrazinamide-resistant *Mycobacterium tuberculosis* family in a low-incidence setting. *J. Clin. Microbiol.* **41**:2878–2883.

101. **Niobe-Eyangoh, S. N., C. Kuaban, P. Sorlin, P. Cunin, J. Thonnon, C. Sola, N. Rastogi, V. Vincent, and M. C. Gutierrez.** 2003. Genetic biodiversity of *Mycobacterium tuberculosis* complex strains from patients with pulmonary tuberculosis in Cameroon. *J. Clin. Microbiol.* **41**:2547–2553.

102. **Ochman, H., S. Elwyn, and N. A. Moran.** 1999. Calibrating bacterial evolution. *Proc. Natl. Acad. Sci. USA* **96**:12638–12643.

103. **Ochman, H., and I. B. Jones.** 2000. Evolutionary dynamics of full genome content in Escherichia coli. *EMBO J.* **19**:6637–6643.

104. **Ochman, H., J. G. Lawrence, and E. A. Groisman.** 2000. Lateral gene transfer and the nature of bacterial innovation. *Nature* **405**:299–304.

105. **Ochman, H., and N. A. Moran.** 2001. Genes lost and genes found: evolution of bacterial pathogenesis and symbiosis. *Science* **292**:1096–1099.

106. **Ochman, H., and A. C. Wilson.** 1987. Evolution in bacteria: evidence for a universal substitution rate in cellular genomes. *J. Mol. Evol.* **26**:74–86.

107. **Ochman, H., and A. C. Wilson.** 1987. Evolutionary history of enteric bacteria, p. 1649–1654. In F. C. Neidhardt, J. L. Ingraham, K. B. Low, B. Magasanik, M. Shaechter, and H. E. Umbarger (ed.), Escherichia coli *and* Salmonella typhimurium: *Molecular and Cellular Aspects,* vol. 2. American Society for Microbiology, Washington, D.C.

108. **Oliver, A., R. Canton, P. Campo, F. Baquero, and J. Blazquez.** 2000. High frequency of hypermutable *Pseudomonas aeruginosa* in cystic fibrosis lung infection. *Science* **288**:1251–1254.

109. **Parish, T., D. A. Smith, G. Roberts, J. Betts, and N. G. Stoker.** 2003. The senX3-regX3 two-component regulatory system of *Mycobacterium tuberculosis* is required for virulence. *Microbiology* **149**:1423–1435.

110. **Pedulla, M. L., M. E. Ford, J. M. Houtz, T. Karthikeyan, C. Wadsworth, J. A. Lewis, D. Jacobs-Sera, J. Falbo, J. Gross, N. R. Pannunzio, W. Brucker, V. Kumar, J. Kandasamy, L. Keenan, S. Bardarov, J. Kriakov, J. G. Lawrence, W. R. Jacobs, Jr., R. W. Hendrix, and G. F. Hatfull.** 2003. Origins of highly mosaic mycobacteriophage genomes. *Cell* **113**:171–182.

111. **Pelicic, V., J. M. Reyrat, and B. Gicquel.** 1998. Genetic advances for studying *Mycobacterium tuberculosis* pathogenicity. *Mol. Microbiol.* **28**:413–420.

112. **Perez, E., S. Samper, Y. Bordas, C. Guilhot, B. Gicquel, and C. Martin.** 2001. An essential role for phoP in *Mycobacterium tuberculosis* virulence. *Mol. Microbiol.* **41**:179–187.

113. **Pethe, K., S. Alonso, F. Biet, G. Delogu, M. J. Brennan, C. Locht, and F. D. Menozzi.** 2001. The heparin-binding haemagglutinin of *M. tuberculosis* is required for extrapulmonary dissemination. *Nature* **412**:190–194.

114. **Pfyffer, G. E., R. Auckenthaler, J. D. van Embden, and D. van Soolingen.** 1998. *Mycobacterium canettii*, the smooth variant of *M. tuberculosis*, isolated from a Swiss patient exposed in Africa. *Emerg. Infect. Dis.* **4**:631–634.

115. **Poulet, S., and S. T. Cole.** 1995. Characterization of the highly abundant polymorphic GC-rich-repetitive sequence (PGRS) present in *Mycobacterium tuberculosis*. *Arch. Microbiol.* **163**:87–95.

116. **Pym, A. S., P. Brodin, R. Brosch, M. Huerre, and S. T. Cole.** 2002. Loss of RD1 contributed to the attenuation of the live tuberculosis vaccines *Mycobacterium bovis* BCG and *Mycobacterium microti*. *Mol. Microbiol.* **46**:709–717.

117. **Pym, A. S., P. Domenech, N. Honore, J. Song, V. Deretic, and S. T. Cole.** 2001. Regulation of catalase-peroxidase (KatG) expression, isoniazid sensitivity and virulence by furA of *Mycobacterium tuberculosis*. *Mol. Microbiol.* **40**:879–889.

118. **Pym, A. S., B. Saint-Joanis, and S. T. Cole.** 2002. Effect of *katG* mutations on the virulence of *Mycobacterium tuberculosis* and the implication for transmission in humans. *Infect. Immun.* **70:** 4955–4960.

119. **Ramakrishnan, L., N. A. Federspiel, and S. Falkow.** 2000. Granuloma-specific expression of Mycobacterium virulence proteins from the glycine-rich PE-PGRS family. *Science* **288:** 1436–1439.

120. **Reed, M. B., P. Domenech, C. Manca, H. Su, A. K. Barczak, B. N. Kreiswirth, G. Kaplan, and C. E. Barry III.** 2004. A glycolipid of hypervirulent tuberculosis strains that inhibits the innate immune response. *Nature* **431:**84–87.

121. **Reyrat, J. M., and D. Kahn.** 2001. Mycobacterium smegmatis: an absurd model for tuberculosis? *Trends Microbiol.* **9:**472–474.

122. **Rogall, T., J. Wolters, T. Flohr, and E. C. Bottger.** 1990. Towards a phylogeny and definition of species at the molecular level within the genus *Mycobacterium. Int. J. Syst. Bacteriol.* **40:** 323–330.

123. **Saint-Joanis, B., H. Souchon, M. Wilming, K. Johnsson, P. M. Alzari, and S. T. Cole.** 1999. Use of site-directed mutagenesis to probe the structure, function and isoniazid activation of the catalase/peroxidase, KatG, from *Mycobacterium tuberculosis. Biochem. J.* **338:**753–760.

124. **Salama, N., K. Guillemin, T. K. McDaniel, G. Sherlock, L. Tompkins, and S. Falkow.** 2000. A whole-genome microarray reveals genetic diversity among *Helicobacter pylori* strains. *Proc. Natl. Acad. Sci. USA* **97:**14668–14673.

125. **Salamon, H., M. Kato-Maeda, P. M. Small, J. Drenkow, and T. R. Gingeras.** 2000. Detection of deleted genomic DNA using a semiautomated computational analysis of GeneChip data. *Genome Res.* **10:**2044–2054.

126. **Sharp, P. M.** 1991. Determinants of DNA sequence divergence between *Escherichia coli* and *Salmonella typhimurium:* codon usage, map position and concerted evolution. *J. Mol. Evol.* **33:**23–33.

127. **Shigenobu, S., H. Watanabe, M. Hattori, Y. Sakaki, and H. Ishikawa.** 2000. Genome sequence of the endocellular bacterial symbiont of aphids *Buchnera* sp. APS. *Nature* **407:**81–86.

128. **Sirakova, T. D., V. S. Dubey, M. H. Cynamon, and P. E. Kolattukudy.** 2003. Attenuation of *Mycobacterium tuberculosis* by disruption of a *mas*-like gene or a chalcone synthase-like gene, which causes deficiency in dimycocerosyl phthiocerol synthesis. *J. Bacteriol.* **185:**2999–3008.

129. **Sirakova, T. D., V. S. Dubey, H. J. Kim, M. H. Cynamon, and P. E. Kolattukudy.** 2003. The largest open reading frame (pks12) in the *Mycobacterium tuberculosis* genome is involved in pathogenesis and dimycocerosyl phthiocerol synthesis. *Infect. Immun.* **71:**3794–3801.

130. **Small, P. M., P. C. Hopewell, S. P. Singh, A. Paz, J. Parsonnet, D. C. Ruston, G. F. Schecter, C. L. Daley, and G. K. Schoolnik.** 1994. The epidemiology of tuberculosis in San Francisco. A population-based study using conventional and molecular methods. *N. Engl. J. Med.* **330:**1703–1709.

131. **Smith, J. M., N. H. Smith, M. O'Rourke, and B. G. Spratt.** 1993. How clonal are bacteria? *Proc. Natl. Acad. Sci. USA* **90:**4384–4388.

132. **Sokurenko, E. V., D. L. Hasty, and D. E. Dykhuizen.** 1999. Pathoadaptive mutations: gene loss and variation in bacterial pathogens. *Trends Microbiol.* **7:**191–195.

133. **Sola, C., I. Filliol, E. Legrand, S. Lesjean, C. Locht, P. Supply, and N. Rastogi.** 2003. Genotyping of the *Mycobacterium tuberculosis* complex using MIRUs: association with VNTR and spoligotyping for molecular epidemiology and evolutionary genetics. *Infect. Genet. Evol.* **3:**125–133.

134. **Sreevatsan, S., X. Pan, K. E. Stockbauer, N. D. Connell, B. N. Kreiswirth, T. S. Whittam, and J. M. Musser.** 1997. Restricted structural gene polymorphism in the *Mycobacterium tuberculosis* complex indicates evolutionarily recent global dissemination. *Proc. Natl. Acad. Sci. USA* **94:**9869–9874.

135. **Stahl, D. A., and J. W. Urbance.** 1990. The division between fast- and slow-growing species corresponds to natural relationships among the mycobacteria. *J. Bacteriol.* **172:**116–124.

136. **Stephens, R. S., S. Kalman, C. Lammel, J. Fan, R. Marathe, L. Aravind, W. Mitchell, L. Olinger, R. L. Tatusov, Q. Zhao, E. V. Koonin, and R. W. Davis.** 1998. Genome sequence of an obligate intracellular pathogen of humans: *Chlamydia trachomatis. Science* **282:**754–759.

137. **Stinear, T. P., A. Mve-Obiang, P. L. Small, W. Frigui, M. J. Pryor, R. Brosch, G. A. Jenkin, P. D. Johnson, J. K. Davies, R. E. Lee, S. Adusumilli, T. Garnier, S. F. Haydock, P. F. Leadlay, and S. T. Cole.** 2004. Giant plasmid-encoded polyketide synthases produce the macrolide toxin of *Mycobacterium ulcerans. Proc. Natl. Acad. Sci. USA* **101:**1345–1349.

138. **Sturgill-Koszycki, S., P. H. Schlesinger, P. Chakraborty, P. L. Haddix, H. L. Collins, A. K. Fok, R. D. Allen, S. L. Gluck, J. Heuser, and D. G. Russell.** 1994. Lack of acidification in Mycobacterium phagosomes produced by exclusion of the vesicular proton-ATPase. *Science* **263:**678–681.

139. Suerbaum, S., J. M. Smith, K. Bapumia, G. Morelli, N. H. Smith, E. Kunstmann, I. Dyrek, and M. Achtman. 1998. Free recombination within *Helicobacter pylori*. *Proc. Natl. Acad. Sci. USA* **95**:12619–12624.

140. Supply, P., E. Mazars, S. Lesjean, V. Vincent, B. Gicquel, and C. Locht. 2000. Variable human minisatellite-like regions in the *Mycobacterium tuberculosis* genome. *Mol. Microbiol.* **36**:762–771.

141. Supply, P., R. M. Warren, A. L. Banuls, S. Lesjean, G. D. Van Der Spuy, L. A. Lewis, M. Tibayrenc, P. D. Van Helden, and C. Locht. 2003. Linkage disequilibrium between minisatellite loci supports clonal evolution of *Mycobacterium tuberculosis* in a high tuberculosis incidence area. *Mol. Microbiol.* **47**:529–538.

142. Thoen, C. O., W. D. Richards, and J. L. Jarnagin. 1977. Mycobacteria isolated from exotic animals. *J. Am. Vet. Med. Assoc.* **170**:987–990.

143. Thorel, M. F., C. Karoui, A. Varnerot, C. Fleury, and V. Vincent. 1998. Isolation of *Mycobacterium bovis* from baboons, leopards and a sea-lion. *Vet. Res.* **29**:207–212.

144. Timpe, R. D., and E. H. Runyon. 1954. The relationship of "atypical" acid-fast bacteria to human disease. *Lab. Clin. Med.* **44**:202–209.

145. Tizard, M., T. Bull, D. Millar, T. Doran, H. Martin, N. Sumar, J. Ford, and J. Hermon-Taylor. 1998. A low G+C content genetic island in *Mycobacterium avium* subsp. *paratuberculosis* and *M. avium* subsp. *silvaticum* with homologous genes in *Mycobacterium tuberculosis*. *Microbiology* **144**(Pt. 12):3413–3423.

146. Tortoli, E. 2003. Impact of genotypic studies on mycobacterial taxonomy: the new mycobacteria of the 1990s. *Clin. Microbiol. Rev.* **16**:319–354.

147. Tsolaki, A. G., A. E. Hirsh, K. DeRiemer, J. A. Enciso, M. Z. Wong, M. Hannan, Y. O. Goguet de la Salmoniere, K. Aman, M. Kato-Maeda, and P. M. Small. 2004. Functional and evolutionary genomics of *Mycobacterium tuberculosis*: insights from genomic deletions in 100 strains. *Proc. Natl. Acad. Sci. USA* **101**:4865–4870.

148. Tullius, M. V., G. Harth, and M. A. Horwitz. 2003. Glutamine synthetase GlnA1 is essential for growth of *Mycobacterium tuberculosis* in human THP-1 macrophages and guinea pigs. *Infect. Immun.* **71**:3927–3936.

149. Valway, S. E., M. P. Sanchez, T. F. Shinnick, I. Orme, T. Agerton, D. Hoy, J. S. Jones, H. Westmoreland, and I. M. Onorato. 1998. An outbreak involving extensive transmission of a virulent strain of *Mycobacterium tuberculosis*. *N. Engl. J. Med.* **338**:633–639.

150. van Embden, J. D., T. van Gorkom, K. Kremer, R. Jansen, B. A. van Der Zeijst, and L. M. Schouls. 2000. Genetic variation and evolutionary origin of the direct repeat locus of *Mycobacterium tuberculosis* complex bacteria. *J. Bacteriol.* **182**:2393–2401.

151. van Helden, P. D., R. M. Warren, T. C. Victor, G. van der Spuy, M. Richardson, and E. Hoal-van Helden. 2002. Strain families of *Mycobacterium tuberculosis*. *Trends Microbiol.* **10**:167–168; author reply 168.

152. van Soolingen, D., T. Hoogenboezem, P. E. de Haas, P. W. Hermans, M. A. Koedam, K. S. Teppema, P. J. Brennan, G. S. Besra, F. Portaels, J. Top, L. M. Schouls, and J. D. van Embden. 1997. A novel pathogenic taxon of the *Mycobacterium tuberculosis* complex, Canetti: characterization of an exceptional isolate from Africa. *Int. J. Syst. Bacteriol.* **47**:1236–1245.

153. van Soolingen, D., L. Qian, P. E. de Haas, J. T. Douglas, H. Traore, F. Portaels, H. Z. Qing, D. Enkhsaikan, P. Nymadawa, and J. D. van Embden. 1995. Predominance of a single genotype of *Mycobacterium tuberculosis* in countries of east Asia. *J. Clin. Microbiol.* **33**:3234–3238.

154. Vera-Cabrera, L., M. A. Hernandez-Vera, O. Welsh, W. M. Johnson, and J. Castro-Garza. 2001. Phospholipase region of *Mycobacterium tuberculosis* is a preferential locus for IS6110 transposition. *J. Clin. Microbiol.* **39**:3499–3504.

155. Vergne, I., J. Chua, and V. Deretic. 2003. Tuberculosis toxin blocking phagosome maturation inhibits a novel Ca2+/calmodulin-PI3K hVPS34 cascade. *J. Exp. Med.* **198**:653–659.

156. Viana-Niero, C., C. Gutierrez, C. Sola, I. Filliol, F. Boulahbal, V. Vincent, and N. Rastogi. 2001. Genetic diversity of *Mycobacterium africanum* clinical isolates based on IS6110-restriction fragment length polymorphism analysis, spoligotyping, and variable number of tandem DNA repeats. *J. Clin. Microbiol.* **39**:57–65.

157. Wagner, P. L., and M. K. Waldor. 2002. Bacteriophage control of bacterial virulence. *Infect. Immun.* **70**:3985–3993.

158. Walburger, A., A. Koul, G. Ferrari, L. Nguyen, C. Prescianotto-Baschong, K. Huygen, B. Klebl, C. Thompson, G. Bacher, and J. Pieters. 2004. Protein kinase G from pathogenic mycobacteria promotes survival within macrophages. *Science* **304**:1800–1804.

159. Wards, B. J., G. W. de Lisle, and D. M. Collins. 2000. An esat6 knockout mutant of *Mycobacterium bovis* produced by homologous recombination will contribute to the development of a live tuberculosis vaccine. *Tuber. Lung Dis.* **80**:185–189.

160. **Wayne, L. G.** 1985. The "atypical" mycobacteria; recognition and disease association. *Crit. Rev. Microbiol.* **26:**185–222.

161. **Weber, I., C. Fritz, S. Ruttkowski, A. Kreft, and F. C. Bange.** 2000. Anaerobic nitrate reductase (narGHJI) activity of *Mycobacterium bovis* BCG in vitro and its contribution to virulence in immunodeficient mice. *Mol. Microbiol.* **35:** 1017–1025.

162. **Werngren, J., and S. E. Hoffner.** 2003. Drug-susceptible *Mycobacterium tuberculosis* Beijing genotype does not develop mutation-conferred resistance to rifampin at an elevated rate. *J. Clin. Microbiol.* **41:**1520–1524.

163. **Wilson, T. M., G. de Lisle, and D. M. Collins.** 1995. Effect of *inhA* and *katG* on isoniazid resistance and virulence of *Mycobacterium bovis. Mol. Microbiol.* **15:**1009–1015.

164. **Woolfit, M., and L. Bromham.** 2003. Increased rates of sequence evolution in endosymbiotic bacteria and fungi with small effective population sizes. *Mol. Biol. Evol.* **20:**1545–1555.

165. **Xu, S., A. Cooper, S. Sturgill-Koszycki, T. van Heyningen, D. Chatterjee, I. Orme, P. Allen, and D. G. Russell.** 1994. Intracellular trafficking in *Mycobacterium tuberculosis* and *Mycobacterium avium*-infected macrophages. *J. Immunol.* **153:**2568–2578.

166. **Yeh, R. W., P. C. Hopewell, and C. L. Daley.** 1999. Simultaneous infection with two strains of *Mycobacterium tuberculosis* identified by restriction fragment length polymorphism analysis. *Int. J. Tuberc. Lung Dis.* **3:**537–539.

167. **Zahrt, T. C., and V. Deretic.** 2001. *Mycobacterium tuberculosis* signal transduction system required for persistent infections. *Proc. Natl. Acad. Sci. USA* **98:**12706–12711.

168. **Zhang, Y., B. Heym, B. Allen, D. Young, and S. Cole.** 1992. The catalase-peroxidase gene and isoniazid resistance of *Mycobacterium tuberculosis. Nature* **358:**591–593.

THE EVOLUTION OF HUMAN
FUNGAL PATHOGENS

Judith N. Steenbergen and A. Casadevall

17

Fungi are ubiquitous organisms that serve a critical role in the maintenance of life through the recycling of nutrients by consuming and contributing to the decomposition of organic matter. Additionally, a few fungal species, such as *Candida albicans,* have close relationships with animal hosts and are referred to as commensal fungi. All pathogenic fungi are unicellular organisms. Although serologic and skin reactivity studies suggest that human infection with fungal organisms is common, invasive fungal disease is relatively rare and occurs most commonly in individuals with compromised immune systems, such as patients with AIDS or malignancy (76). For clarity, the term "infection" is used here to mean acquisition of the microbe into the body of the host, and the term "disease" refers to the state when the host-fungus interaction has resulted in sufficient host damage for clinical manifestations to become apparent (21, 23). Furthermore, "pathogenicity" is defined as the ability of a microbe to cause damage to a host, and "virulence" is the relative degree of damage that a microbe can cause to a host (21). Virulence is viewed as a

microbial property that is expressed only in a susceptible host (22).

Of the greater than 100,000 fungal species identified to date, approximately 300 species have pathogenic relationships with animals and plants. Despite this low number, pathogenic fungi can have devastating affects on diverse populations, as exemplified by two recent epidemics: the American chestnut tree blight and the decline in the populations of Australian and Central American frogs (7). First, the Asian chestnut blight fungus, *Cryphonectria parasitica,* caused the extinction of the American chestnut tree from the eastern United States forests (1). This had wide-reaching effects, including the extinction of several insect species that presumably depended on the trees for survival. A second example is the decline in the amphibian populations of both Queensland, Australia, and Central America caused by a cutaneous Chytridiomycosis infection (7). This fungus was isolated from ill and dead frogs from the two distinct regions. DNA analysis revealed that the isolated fungi were highly similar (7). Both the chestnut tree blight and the amphibian deaths exemplify the wide-reaching effects that fungal diseases can have on various kingdoms and the populations that depend on them.

Fungal pathogens of plants have been extensively studied because of their economic

Judith N. Steenbergen, Department of Microbiology and Immunology, Albert Einstein College of Medicine, Bronx, NY 10461. *A. Casadevall,* Departments of Microbiology and Immunology and of Medicine, Albert Einstein College of Medicine, Bronx, NY 10461.

Evolution of Microbial Pathogens, Edited by H. S. Seifert and V. J. DiRita, © 2006 ASM Press, Washington, D.C.

importance. Given the myriad of fungus-host interactions in the biota, the subject of evolution of fungal pathogens is immense and cannot be done justice in one chapter. Hence, in this chapter we have chosen to focus primarily on the subset of human pathogenic fungi. Even among this relatively small subset of organisms, there is extensive variation in phylogenetic ancestry, pathogenic strategies, ecology, prevalence, and outcome of infection. Hence, generalizations about the evolution of fungal virulence are difficult, but some common themes can be identified.

Fungi are classified into several phylogenetic groups, including *Chytridiomycetes, Zygomycetes,* both filamentous and yeast forms of *Ascomycetes,* and *Basidiomycetes* (68). Fungal pathogenicity is not associated with all the fungal phyla; the majority of plant and animal mycoses are caused by the *Ascomycetes, Basidiomycetes,* and *Zygomycetes* groups (68). The phylogenetic division of fungi that contains the largest number of human pathogenic species is the *Ascomycetes,* which includes *Blastomyces dermatitidis, Histoplasma capsulatum,* and *Saccharomyces cerevisiae* (68). In addition, both *Candida* spp. and *Pneumocystis jiroveci* (formerly *carinii*) have been categorized into the ascomycetes-like group since they share certain characteristics of the true ascomycetes (68).

THE INCIDENCE OF FUNGUS-RELATED DISEASES

Globally, less than 0.0001% of the fungal species identified have been shown to cause disease in humans (104). Furthermore, fungi did not emerge as major human pathogens until the late 20th century. Although endemic fungal infections undoubtedly occurred prior to the 20th century, the major fungal diseases (e.g., cryptococcosis, aspergillosis, blastomycosis, histoplasmosis) were not described until the late 1800s and early 1900s since they occurred at relatively low frequencies in human populations comprised predominantly of immunocompetent hosts. However, in the mid-20th century, medical progress resulted in the introduction of antibiotics, steroid therapies,

chemotherapy for malignancies, indwelling catheters, and new surgical procedures. Each of these advancements was associated with an increased risk for the acquisition of fungal disease. By the late 20th century, fungal diseases had become a major medical problem. For example, by 1988 almost 40% of all deaths from nosocomial infectious diseases were due to fungi (113). Another major development responsible for an increased incidence of fungal diseases was the AIDS epidemic. Advanced human immunodeficiency virus (HIV) infection is associated with a markedly enhanced susceptibility to fungal disease. Therefore, the prevalence of certain types of mycotic diseases increased rapidly with the progression of the AIDS epidemic (76). For example, the prevalence of mucocutaneous candidiasis, aspergillosis, cryptococcosis, and histoplasmosis in selected populations with advanced HIV disease was 90%, 4%, 5 to 10%, and 20%, respectively (33, 75). The high fatality linked to AIDS-associated fungal disease increases the importance of these statistics. For instance, 80% of AIDS patients with aspergillosis will succumb to the disease (75). The advent of highly active antiretroviral therapy in the mid-1990s significantly diminished the prevalence of fungal disease in patients with AIDS in resource-rich countries (53). However, in the resource-poor countries of Africa and Southeast Asia, cryptococcosis remains rampant among patients with AIDS.

The increased incidence of fungal disease has stimulated interest in the field of medical mycology. The problem of fungal diseases is complicated by unsatisfactory treatment options. Relatively few drugs are available for the treatment of fungal infections. The most effective antifungal drug is amphotericin B, which was introduced in the late 1950s and has a high incidence of side effects. Recently, newer drugs have become available in the form of the azoles and pneumocandins, which have fewer serious adverse effects. One of the central problems in antifungal drug development contributing to the dearth of new agents is that animals and fungi are each other's closest relatives; consequently, it is more difficult to identify differences in biochemical pathways that can be exploited in drug development (34).

THE EPIDEMIOLOGY OF FUNGAL DISEASES

Since fungal diseases are generally not transmitted from person to person, their prevalence in a population is usually a function of the immunological state of the host and the type of exposure. The absence of contagiousness combined with their primary occurrence in well-defined populations has reduced the interest in fungal diseases by public health authorities, and few are reportable to health authorities. Consequently, it is difficult to obtain hard data on the incidence and prevalence of fungal diseases in human populations. For most fungal pathogens, the prevalence of disease among immunocompetent humans is remarkably low. For example, the prevalence of cryptococcosis in the United States prior to the AIDS epidemic was estimated at 1 to 2 cases per million (46). In contrast, by the 1990s the prevalence of cryptococcosis in several cities in the United States approached 1 case per 100,000, reflecting the large number of patients with HIV infection in the population (54). The low frequency of disease among immunocompetent individuals is in sharp contrast to the incidence of infection, which can approach 100% of the population. For example, in New York City the prevalence of *Cryptococcus neoformans* infection as measured by the presence of antibody is greater than 90% (48). Similarly, skin testing of military recruits using an *H. capsulatum* antigen preparation demonstrated that histoplasmosis was a common infection that is generally controlled by normal immune functions (35). It is now known that, in certain areas near the Ohio and Mississippi river valleys, the prevalence of *H. capsulatum* infection is as high as 90%, yet the prevalence of histoplasmosis is low (116). The discordance between a very high prevalence of infection, as measured by immunological criteria, and a very low prevalence of disease illustrates the fact that most fungal pathogens are organisms that tend to have relatively low virulence for human hosts with intact immune systems.

The prevalence of fungal infection and disease in immunocompetent hosts can rise rapidly as a result of special circumstances that increase the magnitude of the inoculum delivered at the time of exposure. Outbreaks of histoplasmosis have occurred following community events in which contaminated trees are removed, leading to airborne release of infectious particles (52). Epidemics of coccidioidomycosis have followed seismic events that disturb soils contaminated with *Coccidioides immitis* (96). For example, the 1994 outbreak of coccidioidomycosis in Ventura County followed a sizeable earthquake that is thought to have aerosolized *C. immitis* arthrospores (96). In fact, analysis of the prevalence of coccidioidomycosis in central California over several decades suggests that increases in cases were related to the duration of droughts rather than the emergence of new pathogenic clones (40). *Aspergillus fumigatus,* often considered a nosocomial infection, may be inappropriately labeled as such since aspergillosis outbreaks are often associated with hospital construction (55). Construction activities are presumed to aerosolize *A. fumigatus* spores, providing large inocula that overwhelm the meager defenses of immunocompromised individuals (55). This is a clear example in which the combination of an immunocompromised population and environmental changes leads to increased disease. There is currently an ongoing outbreak of cryptococcosis caused by *C. neoformans* var. *gattii* on Vancouver Island (58). This event is remarkable because infections due to variety *gattii* were previously limited primarily to tropical and subtropical regions (69). The cause of the Vancouver outbreak is unknown, but there is speculation that recent global climate changes may have altered local weather. Weather changes could make the environment more permissive for *C. neoformans* var. *gattii,* consequently increasing the frequency and the magnitude of exposure to this organism.

In contrast to other animal species, such as insects and amphibians, mammals are more resistant as a species to invasive fungal disease. The higher mammalian body temperatures undoubtedly contribute to protection against fungi by creating a nonpermissive environment for the growth of many species of fungi. However, higher temperature is not the sole explanation since there is a gradient of fungal susceptibility in mammals. For example, koala bears are particularly susceptible to disseminated cryptococcosis in part due to increased exposure (66, 67). Among mammals, humans appear to be highly resistant to fungal diseases. The prevalence of fungal disease in the human population is usually a function of two factors: the immunological state of the individuals and the size of the fungal inoculum during exposure. Conditions that result in impaired immunological function are invariably associated with an increase in the prevalence of fungal disease. On the other hand, the reports of histoplasmosis after tree-cutting activities and coccidioidomycosis after earthquakes suggest that exposures with sufficiently large inoculums can overcome the intrinsic high resistance of humans and lead to disease.

FUNGAL DISEASE TAXONOMY

Insects are the only group of organisms whose variety is speculated to be greater than that of fungi (50). Within this vast fungal kingdom, the *Zygomycota, Ascomycota,* and *Basidiomycota* contain pathogenic species (50). These pathogenic fungal species are dispersed throughout the three phyla. The large *Ascomycota* phylum contains medically important fungi in only 9 of the total 46 orders (50). Phylogenetic trees have historically been based on morphological characteristics (68). However, advances in molecular biology have allowed a greater understanding of pathogenic and nonpathogenic fungi. With the advent of DNA typing methods, it is now possible to distinguish individual pathogenic strains within a species and the evolutionary relationships between various species (105, 106).

Some of the closest relatives of the medically important fungal pathogens are nonpathogenic

strains (10, 11). Using DNA fingerprinting, karyotype analysis, and various sequencing techniques, it was established that pathogenic and nonpathogenic fungal species are often phylogenetic neighbors (Figs. 1 and 2). For example, rRNA gene sequencing has shown that the nonpathogenic *Chrysosporium parvum* is more closely related to *B. dermatitidis* than either is to *H. capsulatum* (10, 11). Also, rRNA sequencing determined that the closest relative of the pathogenic fungus *C. immitis* is the nonpathogenic *Uncinocarpus reesii* (11). The phylogenetic interspersal of nonpathogenic and pathogenic fungi is a general theme in mycology, which implies that the potential for human pathogenicity among fungi has arisen independently several times in evolutionary history (10, 11).

SOME COMMON THEMES IN FUNGAL PATHOGENESIS

The major fungal pathogens constitute a diverse group of organisms (Table 1). Despite their genetic differences, certain themes emerge when one considers fungal diseases as a group. As noted previously, infections with fungi appear to be extremely common, but disease is rare and often manifests itself in hosts with impaired immune function (76). In immunocompetent hosts, the initial infection is either asymptomatic or a self-limited illness (76). For the endemic fungal infections—histoplasmosis, coccidioidomycosis, blastomycosis, aspergillosis, paracoccidioidomycosis, and cryptococcosis—infection is presumably acquired by inhalation of fungal particles that produces localized lung damage or pneumonia. This pneumonia tends to resolve spontaneously, but each of these organisms is capable of establishing a latent infection by surviving in granulomas, often inside macrophages (59). If the individual becomes immunosuppressed at a later time in life, the fungus can reactivate with local disease and/or dissemination (59). Without treatment, most disseminated fungal infections are invariably lethal (59). However, fungal disease often takes a chronic and pro-

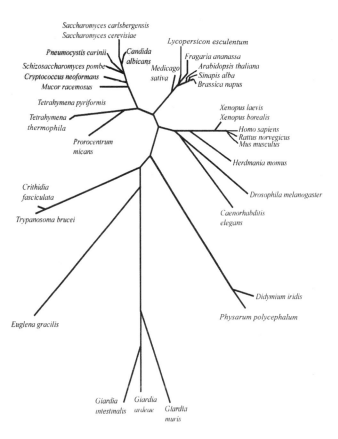

FIGURE 1 Fitch-Margoliash distance tree based on 23S-like rRNA sequences (adapted from reference 38). The phylogenetic tree demonstrates the taxonomic location of fungi within the kingdoms.

gressive course that kills the host slowly. Hence, it was common in the preantibiotic era for systemic fungal infections to progress gradually from minimal symptoms to death over the course of many months. Therapy tends to require prolonged administration of antifungal drugs for resolution of infection. Although disease can often be controlled, many systemic fungal diseases are not curable with antifungal therapy in the setting of immune impairment. Hence, patients with advanced HIV disease complicated by systemic fungal diseases such as aspergillosis, cryptococcosis, coccidioidomycosis or histoplasmosis usually require lifelong therapy. In recent years, the advent of highly active antiretroviral therapy has produced a remarkable reduction in AIDS-related systemic fungal disease because of immune reconstitution (53). Paradoxically, some individuals with

chronic fungal disease controlled on maintenance antifungal therapy have developed worsening of disease as their immunological status has improved (72). Presumably, these individuals retain large amounts of fungal cells and antigens in their tissues that can elicit strong inflammatory responses in the setting of a competent immune system (72). The increased prevalence of invasive fungal disease in patients with advanced HIV disease combined with occasional cases of immune-reconstitution syndromes illustrate the contribution of the host immune system to both susceptibility and disease.

A remarkable aspect of many invasive fungal diseases is that males are more likely to be affected than females (3, 20). For example, the ratio of cases of cryptococcosis in men to cases in women is up to 10:1 in certain studies (20).

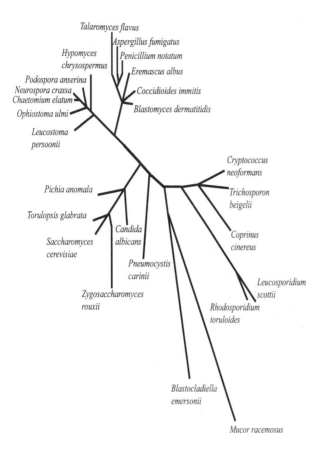

FIGURE 2 Fitch-Margoliash distance tree based on 16S-like rRNA sequences (adapted from reference 38). The phylogenetic tree demonstrates the interspersal of pathogenic and nonpathogenic fungi.

Paracoccidioidomycosis is another example of a fungal disease with an excess of cases in males, with a male-to-female ratio ranging from 13:1 to 78:1 (2). Although this phenomenon is not well understood, it has been hypothesized that it reflects the hormonal milieu of the host. Ovariectomized female mice given testosterone were unable to control *Paracoccidioides brasiliensis* infection, while normal female mice are resistant to disease progression (3). Similarly, castrated male mice given 17β-estradiol were able to restrict initial *P. brasiliensis* growth (3). The enhanced susceptibility of males highlights the critical role played by the host in the manifestation of fungal virulence.

MAJOR TYPES OF FUNGAL PATHOGENS

Fungal pathogens can be divided into two main categories: the commensal and the saprophytic fungi. A commensal fungus is an organism that colonizes a host without damaging the host (22). *C. albicans* is the primary fungal commensal organism in humans; however, this organism has pathogenic potential in normal individuals, as demonstrated by candidal vaginitis. Most cases of *Candida* vaginitis occur when the endogenous bacterial flora is disrupted, suggesting that commensal bacteria reduce the pathogenic potential of *C. albicans* (74). Although *C. albicans* is a free-living organism that does not need a host for propagation, it is intimately associated with humans. It is primarily found in specific niches such as the mouth, gastrointestinal tract, and vagina (74). With the exception of *Candida* spp. and *Malassezia furfur*, all other pathogenic fungi discussed here are saprophytic. In contrast to commensals, a saprophytic fungus is one that ordinarily feeds and grows in dead or decaying matter. Person-to-person transmission of pathogenic saprophytic fungal infections is exceedingly rare. Therefore,

TABLE 1 Fungal pathogens, disease, and virulence

Microbe	Disease(s)	Host susceptibility	Ecologic niche	Virulence determinants	General reference
Aspergillus spp.	Aspergillosis, fungal sinusitis	Neutropenia	Decaying vegetation, soils	Melanin, proteases, toxic products	71
Blastomyces dermatitidis	Blastomycosis	Uncertain	Soils, decaying vegetation	Adhesins	63
Candida spp.	Thrush, vaginal candidiasis, invasive candidiasis	Neutropenia, AIDS, steroid therapy	Skin, vagina, oral mucosa, gastrointestinal flora	Adhesins, proteases, hyphal formation, phenotypic switching	56
Cryptococcus neoformans	Cryptococcosis	T-cell defects, AIDS, steroid therapy	Soils, avian excreta, eucalyptus trees	Capsule, melanin, laccase, phospholipase, mating type	87
Coccidioides immitis	Coccidioidomycosis	T-cell defects, AIDS, pregnancy	Soils	Uncertain	59
Histoplasma capsulatum	Histoplasmosis	T-cell defects, AIDS	Soils, decaying vegetation	Uncertain	119
Malassezia furfur	Pityriasis versicolor	None associated	Skin	Immunomodulation?	5
Paracoccidioides brasiliensis	*Paracoccidioides brasiliensis*	Alcohol use, malnutrition, AIDS	Soils	Melanin?, dimorphism?	9
Sporothrix schenckii	Sporotrichosis	None known for cutaneous disease, AIDS for disseminated infection	Plants	Melanin?	59

infections with saprophytic fungi are generally acquired from the environment, and humans are considered terminal hosts. One possible exception to this generalization is the fungus *P. jiroveci,* which has not been found in the environment, cannot be easily grown in vitro, and may be acquired by human-to-human transmission (81). Currently, the ecology and epidemiology of *P. jiroveci* are sufficiently uncertain that one cannot reliably classify it as a commensal or saprophytic fungus. Hence, we will not consider *P. jiroveci* further in this chapter; interested readers are referred to authoritative reviews (18, 81). The pathogenic saprophytic fungi are described in Table 1.

GENERALIST VERSUS SPECIALIST PATHOGENS

Pathogens can be classified as generalists or specialists depending on their host range (120). A generalist pathogen is one that infects and

causes disease in more than one host, while an ecological specialist is a pathogen that infects and causes disease in only one host (120). It has been hypothesized that evolution occurs faster in smaller niches, and therefore a specialist was thought to have an evolutionary advantage because it could specifically coevolve with its host (120). However, the majority of pathogens are generalists. This finding indicates that there are evolutionary benefits for a pathogen to be a generalist (120). Human fungal pathogens tend to be promiscuous with regard to potential hosts, such that greater than 60% of human pathogens are capable of infecting more than one host species (107). This multihost phenomenon is even more notable in domestic animals, in which more than 80% of fungal pathogens cause disease in more than one host species (28). Generalism depends on both the ability of the pathogen to infect multiple host species and transmissibility of the pathogen among multiple hosts (120). Pathogens transmitted by direct contact are less likely to be generalists since they are presumably not well adapted to survival in the environment. This could in turn explain why the saprophytic opportunistic fungal pathogens are all generalists, as defined by their ability to infect various mammalian species (120).

Most pathogenic fungi are excellent examples of generalist pathogens. For instance, a typical paracoccidioidomycosis granuloma containing fungal cells was found in a lung section of an armadillo, indicating that armadillos not only are carriers of *P. brasiliensis* but also can become infected, with significant host damage (109). In fact, *Sporothrix schenckii, H. capsulatum,* and *C. immitis* can also infect armadillos, and each of these fungi has been found in other mammals, including dogs, badgers, and horses (6, 37, 85).

MICROEVOLUTION VERSUS MACROEVOLUTION

The evolution of virulence is a complex subject because virulence is a microbial property that is expressed only in a susceptible host. Hence, the subject of microbial virulence is difficult to consider independently of the host. The majority of the remainder of this chapter will focus on broad areas of the macroevolution of fungal pathogenesis, but first a brief explanation of microevolution and its relevance to fungal pathogenesis and drug resistance is warranted.

Microevolution occurs in a matter of days or weeks and can be responsible for the development of new strains and variants of a species (78). The ability of an organism to undergo microevolution is believed to be a vital characteristic for survival (78). Phase variation and differential gene expression are mechanisms by which a pathogen can change its virulence, specificity, or ability to be detected by the host's immune system (78). Microevolution can be a result of both epigenetic and genetic changes. Inheritable information that is not encoded on the DNA sequence is called "epigenetic." Two different well-studied patterns of epigenetic

inheritance in fungi are DNA methylation and chromatin folding. Inheritance of DNA methylation sites has been demonstrated in *S. cerevisiae* (8, 65). DNA methylation is a mechanism by which extra information can be added to the DNA that is not encoded in the sequence. This methylation is destroyed during DNA replication; however, DNA methylation is potentially inheritable based on the specific palindromic sequences surrounding the methylation sites (62). Chromatin tertiary structure is also an important epigenetic element and is responsible for the differential expression of various genes. *S. cerevisiae* methylation of histone H3 is an example that incorporates both chromatin structure and methylation as important aspects of genetic expression (80).

In fungi, the two important genetic changes that result in microevolution are genetic rearrangements and point mutations. Recently, however, it was proposed by J. D. Walton that fungi might use horizontal gene transfer as a means to exchange gene clusters encoding secondary metabolite information that could confer an evolutionary advantage (112). Since there are at this time no tangible data to confirm this hypothesis, we will limit our discussion to examples of genetic rearrangements and point mutations in the microevolution of fungi.

Treatment of patients with candidiasis using fluconazole has been associated with the emergence of resistant strains. Resistance can be gained through various point mutations that can affect the fluconazole efflux transporters or alter the ergosterol biosynthetic pathway (42, 114). Furthermore, constitutive overexpression of the target gene can result in enhanced enzyme activity (114). White et al. analyzed serial *C. albicans* isolates from a single AIDS patient and demonstrated that prolonged use of fluconozole selected for resistant mutants (114). Resistance increased gradually through the sum of multiple random mutations, with the final result being highly resistant isolates (114). This result was similar to those of previous studies using DNA fingerprinting analysis that showed a single *Candida* strain was generally responsible for recurrent vaginitis in patients (74, 99). Throughout treatment and the length of the study, it was evident that various minor genetic changes occurred that resulted in the survival of more fit pathogens, and each of these pathogens developed its own combination of fluconozole-resistant mechanisms (74, 92).

Experimental evolutionary studies of *C. albicans* and *S. cerevisiae* populations exposed to antifungal agents in vitro have shown that point mutations and other changes can occur very rapidly (30, 74). Growth of these fungal species in the presence of antifungal agents resulted in the emergence of resistant populations whose replication potential was not affected as measured by colony growth under certain conditions that included various amounts of drug (30, 74). In fact, the emergence of drug resistance resulting from a particular mechanism in a population was random and led to the establishment of only one predominant type of drug-resistant mechanism (30, 74). These experiments indicate that strains can evolve rapidly under selective pressure and suggest that the same phenomena may apply to circumstances such as those found in the human host, where the immune system can be expected to exert major selective influences on the fungal population.

Similar strain variation was seen with *C. neoformans* exposed to laboratory conditions. Analysis of an American Type Culture Collection strain maintained in independent laboratories under various conditions revealed that the various isolates differed in virulence, karyotype, and such phenotypic characteristics as protease and melanin production (43). Presumably, differences in the laboratory conditions in which these isolates were maintained resulted in different selective pressures. This led to the emergence in variants with significant phenotypic and karyotypic differences (43). Again, this provides a powerful example of the capacity of fungi to rapidly change when confronted with different selective pressures.

Another evolutionary development for *Candida* spp. is alternative codon usage, whereby

Candida spp. translate a codon that is normally specific for leucine (e.g., CUG) to serine (94). It was determined through reconstructive studies in *S. cerevisiae* that ambiguous translation provides a selective advantage to *Candida* strains (93). Ambiguous CUG codon usage induces the expression of a specific subset of genes involved in a stress response, which may contribute to the ability of *Candida* spp. to establish themselves in their hosts (93). This was the first instance in which it was shown that codon ambiguity is driven by selection, thus implicating it as an important force in the evolution of a species (93).

MACROEVOLUTION

Macroevolution can be described as evolutionary changes at the level of species and above. Therefore, macroevolution in terms of speciation has led to the development of multiple pathogenic fungal species (4). To develop an understanding of the complex and diverse pathogenesis of the different fungi, it is important to account for the fact that fungal pathogenicity for mammals has evolved independently several times (10, 11). Therefore, there is no unifying theory on how fungi developed the ability to cause disease. Throughout the rest of this chapter, we will propose different hypotheses and supporting data on the evolution and development of fungal pathogenesis

Population Structure, Evolution, and Virulence

Many human pathogenic fungi have the capacity to reproduce sexually or clonally. Sexual reproduction results in a recombining population structure in which all the individuals are genetically different as a result of gene recombination and reassortment. Clonal reproduction results in a clonal population structure in which the individuals are each related to a common ancestor and diverge by the accumulation of mutation, gene gain and loss, duplication, etc. Since virulence is a microbial characteristic that is expressed in a susceptible host, it is dependent on the genetic composition of the particular strain. Hence, knowing the population structure of a fungal pathogen is important for understanding its genetic potential for virulence and the mechanisms available to the species for evolution. Since most fungi can reproduce clonally and sexually, fungal population structures can be clonal, recombining, or mixed, wherein some fraction of the population is clonally related and the remainder has sexual origins. In the past decade, the availability of DNA typing has allowed investigators to discriminate among species, subspecies, and individuals within a species. This has stimulated intensive investigation into the population structure of different fungi that continues to the present. The most comprehensive review in this area was written by Taylor and collaborators in 1999 and remains the major authoritative work in the field (105).

For both *C. neoformans* and *H. capsulatum,* mating has been demonstrated in the laboratory between **a** and α strains. Studies using isoenzyme electrophoresis, restriction fragment length polymorphisms, and random amplified polymorphic DNA analysis have each provided strong evidence for a clonal population structure in *C. neoformans* (12, 25, 44, 77). Also arguing for a predominantly clonal population structure is the fact that the overwhelming majority of *C. neoformans* isolates in the environment are mating type α. However, the fact that some strains can be induced to mate in the laboratory suggests that the ability for sexual reproduction is not a vestigial characteristic, since it is unlikely that such a complicated process would have been maintained in evolutionary history unless it was used. In fact, molecular studies have also provided evidence for recombination in *C. neoformans.* Hybrid genotypes of *C. neoformans* have now been described for serotype AD, suggesting origin from crosses between serotypes A and D (121). Furthermore, an analysis of *C. neoformans* URA5 sequence data returned a large number of most parsimonious trees, a result that argues against a strictly clonal mode of reproduction (105). Hence, these results suggest that the population structure for *C. neoformans* is predominantly clonal with a recombining subset.

For *H. capsulatum,* early studies of mitochondrial DNA and rRNA restriction fragment length polymorphisms revealed that most isolates could be assigned to three groups (110). A recent study of *H. capsulatum* isolates from Indianapolis, Indiana, using biallelic molecular markers revealed that every isolate had a distinct genotype and concluded that the population structure from this site was recombining (19). In contrast to *C. neoformans* and *H. capsulatum,* sexual reproduction has not been demonstrated for *C. albicans, A. fumigatus,* or *C. immitis.* For *C. albicans,* molecular evidence indicates that the population structure is predominantly clonal, but there is also evidence for recombination (41, 49). For *A. fumigatus,* current evidence suggests that the population structure is clonal (reviewed in reference 105). For *C. immitis,* molecular studies have provided evidence for cryptic species, populations that are genetically isolated, and evidence for recombination in certain populations (17, 64, 105).

Emergence of Virulence among Commensal Human Fungal Pathogens

When considering the emergence of virulence among commensal human fungi, we will focus on two species, *C. albicans* and *M. furfur,* which illustrate the mechanisms by which normally harmless microbes can cause disease. The sheer number of symptomatic infections caused by *C. albicans* makes it a major human pathogen. As mentioned previously, *C. albicans* is normally a commensal inhabitant of the skin and gastrointestinal tract that can cause disease in three different settings: (i) immature or impaired host immune function, (ii) breach of the integument and mucosal barriers, and (iii) disruption of the ecology of the normal human microbial flora by antibiotic therapy. There is evidence that *Candida* spp. carried asymptomatically in different anatomical locations are, in some individuals, genetically different, suggesting that different ecological niches in the human body select for individual types of strains (98).

Various genetic studies have shown that *Candida* spp. reproduce clonally, though several reports suggest that sexual reproduction may occur in specific circumstances. Sexual reproduction is a significant way to increase the allelic variation in a population, thereby increasing the potential for maximum fitness in an environment. Therefore, a specific mechanism by which *Candida* spp. may have evolved pathogenic strategies is through sexual inheritance of virulence genes. However, there is no current research to support this notion.

Because *Candida*-related disease is often inversely proportional to host immunological status, this organism is generally considered an opportunistic pathogen (97). Hence, the emergence of virulence in *C. albicans* is intimately associated with alterations to host variables. Infection (e.g., acquisition of the organism) occurs shortly after birth, usually originates from the mother, and most commonly results in the establishment of a commensal state that is maintained for the life of the host (97). However, the initial acquisition of *C. albicans* can result in a neonatal symptomatic infection, possibly as a result of an immature immune system. Hence, *C. albicans* is a significant cause of mycotic disease in the neonatal period of life and is a major pathogen for premature infants. The insertion of intravascular catheters and surgical procedures breach the skin and provide access for *C. albicans* to deeper tissues. Chemotherapy that disrupts the mucosal barrier and produces neutropenia is a major risk factor for invasive candidiasis. Broad-spectrum antimicrobial drugs are associated with an increased risk for candidiasis as a result of depletion of the normal bacterial flora, creating a niche for the proliferation of *Candida*. However, it is important to note that certain host factors may influence the pathogenic potential of *C. albicans*. In this regard, estrogen receptors have been described in *C. albicans* that could conceivably explain the observation that vaginal candidiasis is more frequent during certain states of the menstrual cycle (36, 83).

Genetic analysis of commensal and patho-genic *C. albicans* strains isolated from a single geographical locale revealed that they could be grouped together in a major cluster (57). The commensal and pathogenic strains of *C. albicans* were genetically indistinguishable. The *C. albicans* strains were divided into major and minor groups using DNA fingerprinting. Since pathogenic and commensal organisms were intertwined, it was determined that pathogenic and commensal *C. albicans* are clonal in origin (57). This result is fully consistent with the view that candidiasis is caused by organisms that are commensal in ordinary circumstances. Similarly, analysis of *C. albicans* strains using a moderately repetitive sequence probe revealed that isolates from women with *Candida* vaginitis were not genetically distinguishable from commensal isolates from women in the same geographical locale (95). Candidal vulvovaginitis is an often recurrent disease that affects otherwise immunologically competent women. The pathogenesis of recurrent vaginitis is poorly understood, but molecular studies have shed some light into the ecology of *Candida* in the vaginal tract. Analysis of serial isolates from 18 women with recurrent infection revealed that, for each individual, the same *Candida* strain was responsible for sequential infections (74). In approximately 50% of the patients, the recurrent strain exhibited small genetic variations indicating that substrains of the initial infecting strain were responsible for recurrent vaginitis (74). Furthermore, for many women *C. albicans* could also be recovered from their sexual partners, and that strain was identical or closely related to the "pathogenic" strain recovered from the vaginitis episode (95). These results indicate great complexity in the ecology and pathogenesis of this disease, with the occurrence of genetic changes combined with maintenance of reservoirs in male partners.

Candida colonizes various mammals, and it is speculated that each mammalian species is colonized by a specific species or subspecies of *Candida* (29). Opportunistic infections have been reported in marine mammals, domestic mammals, and wild mammals. Since this chapter is primarily concerned with human pathogens, we will not expound, though we do note that *Candida* has evolved a complex relationship with a range of mammals.

Historically, the majority of *Candida* infections were caused by *C. albicans.* However, in recent years candidiasis caused by non-*C. albicans* species has increased. The fact that clinically significant infections caused by *C. tropicalis, C. parapsilisis, C. krusei,* and *C. glabrata* are more prevalent is of significant concern since their prognosis and treatment are often different from *C. albicans* (84). The incidence of candidiasis caused by *C. albicans* in hospitalized patients decreased from 60 to 47% over a 3.5-year period commensurate with an increase in clinically significant infections by other *Candida* spp. (84). This significant change is thought to be caused by the introduction of antifungal agents, a major concern since the non-*C. albicans* species are generally resistant to fluconazole (84). Also contributing to the changing epidemiology of candidiasis is an increase in the numbers of immunocompromised individuals who are on preventative antifungal therapies. Hence, the combination of changing hosts and selection pressure from antifungal drug use is believed to have altered the epidemiology of candidiasis to reduce the prevalence of infections due to *C. albicans* while increasing those due to non-*C. albicans* spp. This suggests that, when a particular commensal is displaced from its niche, another may occupy its place. This is a clear example of how pharmacotherapy alters the host-pathogen relationship and drives the evolution of pathogenic strains.

Malassezia species are cutaneous commensal fungi that cause a variety of dermatological and systemic infections. In immunocompetent individuals, *Malassezia* has been shown to be involved in dandruff, folliculitis, atopic eczema, and pityriasis versicolor (5). A comprehensive study determined that 100% of the human subjects tested were colonized with *Malassezia* species, and the highest incidence was found on the chest, ear, upper back, forehead, and cheeks (5). In the mid 1990s, the taxonomy of *Malassezia* species began to be unraveled

through sequencing of the large-subunit rRNA (51). These studies determined and named seven *Malassezia* species: *M. furfur, M. slooffise, M. pachydermatis, M. restricta, M. globosa, M. obtuse,* and *M. sympodialis* (51). Specific virulence attributes have not been established for *Malassezia* species, and little is known about the evolutionary history of this fungus. However, since *Malassezia* has not been found in the environment, it is possible that the fungus has specifically evolved with humans.

Malassezia systemic infections caused by catheterization can be severe and often affect premature neonates (5). A noteworthy aspect of the pathogenesis of invasive *Malassezia* infections is their association with the use of intravenous lipid therapy. This fungus has a nutritional requirement for certain lipids that are only found in the skin, and ordinarily cannot cause invasive disease because internal tissues are a nutritionally nonpermissive environment (5). In patients receiving intravenous lipid therapy, the administration of the lipids removes this nutritional restriction, allowing the fungus to replicate in internal tissues and cause disease. For tissue-invasive *Malassezia,* discontinuing the lipid infusion can be therapeutic, as it removes the nutritional support required for growth in internal organs (5). The pathogenesis of invasive *Malassezia* infections provides a dramatic example of how a medical procedure can increase the virulence of a fungal organism for a host and illustrates the intimate relationship between host and pathogen in the evolution of fungal virulence.

Emergence of Virulence among Saprophytic Human Pathogens

Serial laboratory passage can attenuate virulence of saprophytic fungal pathogens, as has been demonstrated for *H. capsulatum, P. brasiliensis, C. neoformans,* and *B. dermatitidis* (13, 14, 45). This attenuation can sometimes be reversed after passage of the fungi through an animal model. Although animal infections with these fungi have occasionally been described, it is unlikely that animal passage is a sufficiently frequent event to maintain the virulence of the fungal population in its natural ecological niche. This is particularly apparent when one considers that many of these fungi maintain virulence though they are found in soils inches below the surface. Given that virulence is a complex trait, it would appear that it requires strong selective pressures for maintenance in the environment. Experiments in *B. dermatitidis, H. capsulatum,* and *C. neoformans* have demonstrated that fungal cells isolated from the environment can cause disease in experimental animals (70, 100, 122). Also, these saprophytic fungal pathogens have a range of specific virulence factors required for infection of humans, including capsule, melanin synthesis, adhesions, inhibition of phagolysosomal fusion, and many others (59). Therefore, it seems paradoxical that saprophytic fungi are pathogenic when isolated from the environment since they do not require mammalian infection for their life cycle.

Alternatively to animal passage, ecological factors may be responsible for selecting and maintaining virulence in saprophytic fungi. One possibility is that virulence is a by-product of strategies selected in the environment for survival against other microorganisms. In this regard, soils are highly complex communities that include fungi, bacteria, ciliates, and amoeboid organisms. Three decades ago, Bulmer and collaborators showed that certain amoebae were predators for *C. neoformans* (16, 82, 91). Hence, we hypothesized that virulence originated, and was maintained, as a consequence of pressure from other microorganisms (103). Since many of the pathogenic saprophytic fungi invade macrophages, we focused our attention on particular amoeboid predators, which resemble vertebrate phagocytic cells in their ability to ingest fungal cells. Our initial studies focused on the soil amoeba *Acanthamoeba castellanii* (103). This particular amoeba was selected because it was extensively studied as a possible host for the bacterial pathogen *Legionella pneumophila* (88).

A. castellanii is an environmental, soil amoeba that feeds on both bacteria and fungi for nourishment and serves as a host for both bacterial and fungal pathogens (Fig. 3) (88, 111). We demonstrated that phagocytosis of *C. neoformans* resulted in replication of the fungal cells inside amoebae, resulting in amoebae death

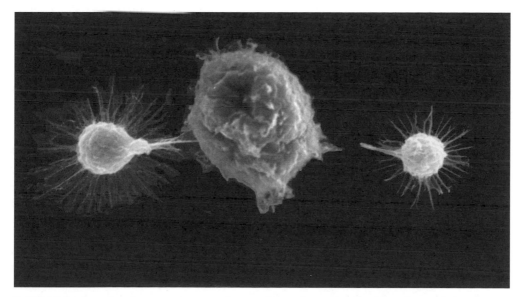

FIGURE 3 Scanning electron microscopy image of *C. neoformans* (small cells) with *Acanthamoeba castellanii* (large cell). This image demonstrates the interactions between the fungal cells and amoeba 30 min postincubation.

(103). Fungal characteristics associated with virulence for mammalian hosts were studied for virulence to amoebae by comparing the outcome of fungus-amoeba interactions using mutants with defined defects (103). Polysaccharide capsule, melanin production, and phospholipase expression were each shown to be important virulence factors in both amoeba and macrophage infection by *C. neoformans* (103). Furthermore, we observed that the intracellular pathogenic strategies of *C. neoformans* for amoebae and macrophages were strikingly similar (103). For both types of host cells, there was accumulation of polysaccharide-filled vesicles in the cytoplasm and disruption of phagosomal membranes. Both immunofluorescence and immunogold transmission electron microscopy demonstrated a cytotoxic buildup of polysaccharide in the amoebae cells (103). This polysaccharide buildup has been associated with macrophage toxicity (39). As mentioned previously, *C. neoformans* has a wide host range, and this study could further explain this phenomenon since it was postulated that the ability to subvert soil amoebae is translated into macrophage survival in a vertebrate host.

Also, using *C. neoformans* as a model yeast, it was demonstrated that passaging the fungal cells through the genetically tractable *Dictyostelium discoideum* amoebae increased the fungal virulence in a mouse model (101). Eighty percent of mice infected with passaged *C. neoformans* cells died within the first 20 days postinfection, while at day 20, only 20% of mice infected with cultured *C. neoformans* cells had died. This experiment strongly suggested that fungal virulence might be maintained in the environment through interactions with soil amoebae (101). Subsequent studies have evaluated the interaction of *A. castellanii* and the soil fungi *B. dermatitis, H. capsulatum,* and *S. schenkii* (102). Like the observations with *C. neoformans,* the interaction of these fungi with *A. castellanii* resulted in the death of amoebae (102). Passage of an avirulent *H. capsulatum* strain through *A. castellanii* resulted in an increase in virulence for mice (102). In addition, small animals such as the worms may also provide strong selective pres-

sures for the emergence and maintenance of traits associated with virulence for mammals (79). These results support the hypothesis that the virulence of certain soil fungi for mammalian hosts is maintained in the environment through the interaction with ecological predators such as *A. castellanii.*

Virulence Factors in the Context of Environmental Survival

For those fungal pathogens that have their niche in the environment, and are free living, it is very unlikely that their virulence factors are the result of a requirement for animal virulence, since their survival is not dependent on any animal host. Among the pathogenic fungi, *C. neoformans* has the best defined virulence factors, and its life cycle is fairly well understood. *C. neoformans* is frequently found in soils contaminated with pigeon excreta and can be recovered from the ground in a state that is virulent for animals. As noted above, we have proposed that virulence for this fungus is a result of selection pressures by amoebae and other environmental predators that confer upon it the ability to survive and cause disease in an animal host (96). According to this hypothesis, virulence factors should have dual function, being selected by environmental pressures yet providing a survival advantage in the animal host. Analysis of *C. neoformans* virulence factors reveals that this is indeed the case, since each has a potentially identifiable role in promoting survival in the environment (Table 2). Although there is insufficient information for the construction of a similar table for the other environmental pathogenic fungi, it is possible that the same applies to them.

CONCLUDING REMARKS

Pathogenic fungi are a diverse group of organisms that became a major health concern in the 20th century due to an increase in the immunocompromised population. These pathogenic fungi are ubiquitous, and most are found associated with soil and decomposing matter. Through taxonomy studies, it was determined that virulence has evolved several times inde-

TABLE 2 *C. neoformans* virulence factors and their possible role in the environment

Virulence factor	Function in virulence	Potential function in environment	Reference(s)
Capsule	Antiphagocytic for macrophages	Antiphagocytic for amoeba	15, 103
	Required for intracellular survival	Required for survival against amoeba predators	39, 103
	Immunomodulator	Delays desiccation	86, 108
Melanin synthesis	Protects against free radicals	Enhances survival in amoebae	24, 103
	Immunomodulator	Protects against heavy metals	47, 60
	Fe acquisition?	Fe acquisition?	61
		Protects against temperature extremes	90
		Resistance against enzymatic degradation	89
Phospholipase	Intracellular replication	Nutritional role?	31
Proteases	Host tissue damage?	Nutritional role?	26, 27
Laccase	Melanin synthesis	Melanin synthesis	73, 117
	Interference with oxidative burst	Wood degradation	118
Urease	Uncertain	Uncertain	32
Matα	Haploid fruiting leading to basidiospore formation	Uncertain	115

pendently, therefore indicating that fungal virulence significantly benefits environmental fungi. Though the specific mechanisms of evolution and development of virulence factors have not been elucidated, there are clear data implicating soil amoebae as a natural predator that may maintain virulence in the fungal habitat. Given increasing interest in this area, we anticipate that future studies will shed additional light on the evolution of fungal pathogenesis.

CHAPTER SUMMARY

- The incidence of fungal diseases in humans is increasing.
- The major pathogenic fungi have different phylogenetic lineages.
- Most pathogenic fungi are nonspecific pathogens capable of causing disease in many different hosts.
- A high basal metabolic temperature in mammals provides defense against many fungal species.
- Virulence in pathogenic fungi may arise from selection pressures exerted by other microbes such as amoebae.

REFERENCES

1. **Anagnostakis, S. L.** 2004. Chestnut blight: the classical problem of an introduced pathogen. *Mycologia* **79**:23–37.
2. **Aristizabal, B. H., K. V. Clemons, A. M. Cock, A. Restrepo, and D. A. Stevens.** 2002. Experimental *Paracoccidioides brasiliensis* infection in mice: influence of the hormonal status of the host on tissue responses. *Med. Mycol.* **40**:169–178.
3. **Aristizabal, B. H., K. V. Clemons, D. A. Stevens, and A. Restrepo.** 1998. Morphological transition of *Paracoccidioides brasiliensis* conidia to yeast cells: in vivo inhibition in females. *Infect. Immun.* **66**:5587–5591.
4. **Arnold, S. J., M. E. Pfrender, and A. G. Jones.** 2001. The adaptive landscape as a conceptual bridge between micro- and macroevolution. *Genetica* **112–113**:9–32.
5. **Ashbee, H. R., and E. G. Evans.** 2002. Immunology of diseases associated with Malassezia species. *Clin. Microbiol. Rev.* **15**:21–57.
6. **Bauder, B., A. Kubber-Heiss, T. Steineck, E. S. Kuttin, and L. Kaufman.** 2000. Granulomatous skin lesions due to histoplasmosis in a badger *(Meles meles)* in Austria. *Med. Mycol.* **38**:249–253.
7. **Berger, L., R. Speare, P. Daszak, D. E. Green, A. A. Cunningham, C. L. Goggin, R. Slocombe, M. A. Ragan, A. D. Hyatt, K. R. McDonald, H. B. Hines, K. R. Lips, G. Marantelli, and H. Parkes.** 1998. Chytridiomycosis causes amphibian mortality associated with population declines in the

rain forests of Australia and Central America. *Proc. Natl. Acad. Sci. USA* **95**:9031–9036.

8. **Bernstein, B. E., E. L. Humphrey, R. L. Erlich, R. Schneider, P. Bouman, J. S. Liu, T. Kouzarides, and S. L. Schreiber.** 2002. Methylation of histone H3 Lys 4 in coding regions of active genes. *Proc. Natl. Acad. Sci. USA* **99:** 8695–8700.

9. **Borges-Walmsley, M. I., D. Chen, X. Shu, and A. R. Walmsley.** 2002. The pathobiology of Paracoccidioides brasiliensis. *Trends Microbiol.* **10:**80–87.

10. **Bowman, B. H., J. W. Taylor, and T. J. White.** 1992. Molecular evolution of the fungi: human pathogens. *Mol. Biol. Evol.* **9:**893–904.

11. **Bowman, B. H., T. J. White, and J. W. Taylor.** 1996. Human pathogenic fungi and their close nonpathogenic relatives. *Mol. Phylogenet. Evol.* **6:**89–96.

12. **Brandt, M., L. C. Hutwagner, L. A. Klug, W. S. Baughman, D. Rimland, E. A. Graviss, R. J. Hamill, C. Thomas, P. G. Pappas, A. L. Reingold, and R. W. Pinner.** 1996. Molecular subtype distribution of *Cryptococcus neoformans* in four areas of the United States. *J. Clin. Microbiol.* **34:**912–917.

13. **Brass, C., C. M. Volkmann, D. E. Philpott, H. P. Klein, C. J. Halde, and D. A. Stevens.** 1982. Spontaneous mutant of *Blastomyces dermatitidis* attenuated in virulence for mice. *Sabouraudia* **20:**145–158.

14. **Brummer, E., A. Restrepo, L. H. Hanson, and D. A. Stevens.** 1990. Virulence of *Paracoccidiodes brasiliensis:* the influence of in vitro passage and storage. *Mycopathologia* **109:**13–17.

15. **Buchanan, K. L., and J. W. Murphy.** 1998. What makes *Cryptococcus neoformans* a pathogen? *Emerg. Infect. Dis.* **4:**71–83.

16. **Bunting, L. A., J. B. Neilson, and G. S. Bulmer.** 1979. *Cryptococcus neoformans:* gastronomic delight of a soil ameba. *Sabouraudia* **17:**225–232.

17. **Burt, A., B. M. Dechairo, G. L. Koenig, D. A. Carter, T. J. White, and J. W. Taylor.** 1997. Molecular markers reveal differentiation among isolates of *Coccidioides immitis* from California, Arizona and Texas. *Mol. Ecol.* **6:**781–786.

18. **Cailliez, J. C., N. Seguy, C. M. Denis, E. M. Aliouat, E. Mazars, L. Polonelli, D. Camus, and E. Dei-Cas.** 1996. Pneumocystis carinii: an atypical fungal micro-organism. *J. Med. Vet. Mycol.* **34:**227–239.

19. **Carter, D. A., A. Burt, J. W. Taylor, G. L. Koenig, and T. J. White.** 1996. Clinical isolates of *Histoplasma capsulatum* from Indianapolis, Indiana, have a recombining population structure. *J. Clin. Microbiol.* **34:**2577–2584.

20. **Casadevall, A., and J. R. Perfect.** 1998. *Cryptococcus neoformans.* American Society for Microbiology, Washington, D.C.

21. **Casadevall, A., and L. Pirofski.** 1999. Host-pathogen interactions: redefining the basic concepts of virulence and pathogenicity. *Infect. Immun.* **67:**3703–3713.

22. **Casadevall, A., and L. Pirofski.** 2001. Host-pathogen interactions: the attributes of virulence. *J. Infect. Dis.* **184:**337–344.

23. **Casadevall, A., and L. Pirofski.** 2000. Host-pathogen interactions: the basic concepts of microbial commensalism, colonization, infection, and disease. *Infect. Immun.* **68:**6511–6518.

24. **Casadevall, A., A. L. Rosas, and J. D. Nosanchuk.** 2000. Melanin and virulence in *Cryptococcus neoformans. Curr. Opin. Microbiol.* **3:**354–358.

25. **Chen, F., B. P. Currie, L.-C. Chen, S. G. Spitzer, E. D. Spitzer, and A. Casadevall.** 1995. Genetic relatedness of *Cryptococcus neoformans* clinical isolates grouped with the repetitive DNA probe CNRE-1. *J. Clin. Microbiol.* **33:**2818–1822.

26. **Chen, L.-C., E. Blank, and A. Casadevall.** 1996. Extracellular proteinase activity of *Cryptococcus neoformans. Clin. Diagn. Lab. Immunol.* **3:**570–574.

27. **Chen, L.-C., and A. Casadevall.** 1999. Variants of a *Cryptococcus neoformans* strain elicit different inflammatory responses in mice. *Clin. Diagn. Lab. Immunol.* **6:**266–268.

28. **Cleaveland, S., M. K. Laurenson, and L. H. Taylor.** 2001. Diseases of humans and their domestic mammals: pathogen characteristics, host range and the risk of emergence. *Philos. Trans. R. Soc. Lond B Biol. Sci.* **356:**991–999.

29. **Connole, M. D., H. Yamaguchi, D. Elad, A. Hasegawa, E. Segal, and J. M. Torres-Rodriguez.** 2000. Natural pathogens of laboratory animals and their effects on research. *Med. Mycol.* **38**(Suppl. 1):59–65.

30. **Cowen, L. E., A. Nantel, M. S. Whiteway, D. Y. Thomas, D. C. Tessier, L. M. Kohn, and J. B. Anderson.** 2002. Population genomics of drug resistance in *Candida albicans. Proc. Natl. Acad. Sci. USA* **99:**9284–9289.

31. **Cox, G. M., H. C. McDade, S. C. Chen, S. C. Tucker, M. Gottfredsson, L. C. Wright, T. C. Sorrell, S. D. Leidich, A. Casadevall, M. A. Ghannoum, and J. R. Perfect.** 2001. Extracellular phospholipase activity is a virulence factor for Cryptococcus neoformans. *Mol. Microbiol.* **39:**166–175.

32. **Cox, G. M., J. Mukherjee, G. T. Cole, A. Casadevall, and J. R. Perfect.** 2000. Urease as a virulence factor in experimental cryptococcosis. *Infect. Immun.* **68:**443–448.

33. **Currie, B. P., and A. Casadevall.** 1994. Estimation of the prevalence of cryptococcal infection among HIV infected individuals in New York City. *Clin. Infect. Dis.* **19:**1029–1033.

34. **DiDomenico, B.** 1999. Novel antifungal drugs. *Curr. Opin. Microbiol.* **2:**509–515.

35. **Edwards, L. B., F. A. Acquaviva, V. T. Livesay, F. W. Cross, and C. E. Palmer.** 1969. An atlas of sensitivity to tuberculin, PPD-B, and histoplasmin in the United States. *Am. Rev. Respir. Dis.* **99**(Suppl.)**:**132.

36. **Eschenbach, D. A., S. S. Thwin, D. L. Patton, T. M. Hooton, A. E. Stapleton, K. Agnew, C. Winter, A. Meier, and W. E. Stamm.** 2000. Influence of the normal menstrual cycle on vaginal tissue, discharge, and microflora. *Clin. Infect. Dis.* **30:**901–907.

37. **Etana, D.** 1999. Isolates of fungi from symptomatic carthorses in Awassa, Ethiopia. *Zentralbl. Veterinarmed. B* **46:**443–451.

38. **Fan, M., B. P. Currie, R. R. Gutell, M. A. Ragan, and A. Casadevall.** 1994. The 16S-like, 5.8S, and 23S-like rRNAs of the two varieties of *Cryptococcus neoformans:* sequence, secondary structure, phylogenetic analysis, and restriction fragment polymorphisms. *J. Med. Vet. Mycol.* **32:**163–180.

39. **Feldmesser, M., Y. Kress, P. Novikoff, and A. Casadevall.** 2000. *Cryptococcus neoformans* is a facultative intracellular pathogen in murine pulmonary infection. *Infect. Immun.* **68:**4225–4237.

40. **Fisher, M. C., G. L. Koenig, T. J. White, and J. W. Taylor.** 2000. Pathogenic clones versus environmentally driven population increase: analysis of an epidemic of the human fungal pathogen *Coccidioides immitis. J. Clin. Microbiol.* **38:**807–813.

41. **Forche, A., G. Schonian, Y. Graser, R. Vilgalys, and T. G. Mitchell.** 1999. Genetic structure of typical and atypical populations of Candida albicans from Africa. *Fungal Genet. Biol.* **28:**107–125.

42. **Franz, R., S. L. Kelly, D. C. Lamb, D. E. Kelly, M. Ruhnke, and J. Morschhauser.** 1998. Multiple molecular mechanisms contribute to a stepwise development of fluconazole resistance in clinical *Candida albicans* strains. *Antimicrob. Agents Chemother.* **42:**3065–3072.

43. **Franzot, S. P., B. C. Fries, W. Cleare, and A. Casadevall.** 1998. Genetic relationship between *Cryptococcus neoformans* var. *neoformans* strains of serotypes A and D. *J. Clin. Microbiol.* **36:**2200–2204.

44. **Franzot, S. P., J. S. Hamdan, B. P. Currie, and A. Casadevall.** 1997. Molecular epidemiology of *Cryptococcus neoformans* in Brazil and the United States: evidence for both local genetic differences and a global clonal population structure. *J. Clin. Microbiol.* **35:**2243–2251.

45. **Franzot, S. P., J. Mukherjee, R. Cherniak, L. Chen, J. S. Hamdan, and A. Casadevall.** 1998. Microevolution of a standard strain of *Cryptococcus neoformans* resulting in differences in virulence and other phenotypes. *Infect. Immun.* **66:**89–97.

46. **Friedman, G. D.** 1983. The rarity of cryptococcosis in Northern California: the 10-year experience of a large defined population. *Am. J. Epidemiol.* **117:**230–234.

47. **Garcia-Rivera, J., and A. Casadevall.** 2001. Melanization of Cryptococcus neoformans reduces the susceptibility to the antimicrobial effects of silver nitrate. *Med. Mycol.* **39:**353–357.

48. **Goldman, D. L., H. Khine, J. Abadi, D. J. Lindenberg, L. Pirofski, R. Niang, and A. Casadevall.** 2001. Serologic evidence for Cryptococcus infection in early childhood. *Pediatrics* 107, E66.

49. **Graser, Y., M. Volovsek, J. Arrington, G. Schonian, W. Presber, T. G. Mitchell, and R. Vilgalys.** 1996. Molecular markers reveal that population structure of the human pathogen *Candida albicans* exhibits both clonality and recombination. *Proc. Natl. Acad. Sci. USA* **93:**12473–12477.

50. **Guarro, J., J. Gene, and A. M. Stchigel.** 1999. Developments in fungal taxonomy. *Clin. Microbiol. Rev.* **12:**454–500.

51. **Guillot, J., and E. Gueho.** 1995. The diversity of *Malassezia* yeasts confirmed by rRNA sequence and nuclear DNA comparisons. *Antonie Leeuwenhoek* **67:**297–314.

52. **Gustafson, T. L., L. Kaufman, R. Weeks, L. Ajello, R. H. Hutcheson, Jr., S. L. Wiener, D. W. Lambe, Jr., T. A. Sayvetz, and W. Schaffner.** 1981. Outbreak of acute pulmonary histoplasmosis in members of a wagon train. *Am. J. Med.* **71:**759–765.

53. **Haddad, N. E., and W. G. Powderly.** 2001. The changing face of mycoses in patients with HIV/AIDS. *AIDS Read.* **11:**365–368.

54. **Hajjeh, R. A., L. A. Conn, D. S. Stephens, W. Baughman, R. Hamill, E. Graviss, P. G. Pappas, C. Thomas, A. Reingold, G. Rothrock, L. C. Hutwagner, A. Schuchat, M. E. Brandt, and R. W. Pinner.** 1999. Cryptococcosis: population-based multistate active surveillance and risk factors in human immunodeficiency virus-infected persons. Cryptococcal Active Surveillance Group. *J. Infect. Dis.* **179:**449–454.

55. **Hajjeh, R. A., and D. W. Warnock.** 2001. Counterpoint: invasive aspergillosis and the environment—rethinking our approach to prevention. *Clin. Infect. Dis.* **33:**1549–1552.

56. **Haynes, K.** 2001. Virulence in Candida species. *Trends Microbiol.* **9**:591–596.

57. **Hellstein, J., H. Vawter-Hugart, P. Fotos, J. Schmid, and D. R. Soll.** 1993. Genetic similarity and phenotypic diversity of commensal and pathogenic strains of *Candida albicans* isolated from the oral cavity. *J. Clin. Microbiol.* **31**:3190–3199.

58. **Hoang, L. M., J. A. Maguire, P. Doyle, M. Fyfe, and D. L. Roscoe.** 2004. *Cryptococcus neoformans* infections at Vancouver Hospital and Health Sciences Centre (1997–2002): epidemiology, microbiology and histopathology. *J. Med. Microbiol.* **53**:935–940.

59. **Hogan, L. H., S. M. Levitz, and B. S. Klein.** 1996. Virulence factors of medically important fungi. *Clin. Microbiol. Rev.* **9**:469–488.

60. **Huffnagle, G. B., G.-H. Chen, J. L. Curtis, R. A. McDonald, R. M. Strieter, and G. B. Toews.** 1995. Down-regulation of the afferent phase of T cell-mediated pulmonary inflammation and immunity by a high melanin-producing strain of *Cryptococcus neoformans.* *J. Immunol.* **155**:3507–3516.

61. **Jacobson, E. S., and J. D. Hong.** 1997. Redox buffering by melanin and Fe(II) in *Cryptococcus neoformans.* *J. Bacteriol.* **179**:5340–5346.

62. **Jeltsch, A.** 2002. Beyond Watson and Crick: DNA methylation and molecular enzymology of DNA methyltransferases. *Chembiochem* **3**:274–293.

63. **Klein, B. S.** 2000. Molecular basis of pathogenicity in *Blastomyces dermatitidis:* the importance of adhesion. *Curr. Opin. Microbiol.* **3**:339–343.

64. **Koufopanou, V., A. Burt, and J. W. Taylor.** 1997. Concordance of gene genealogies reveals reproductive isolation in the pathogenic fungus Coccidioides immitis. *Proc. Natl. Acad. Sci. USA* **94**:5478–5482.

65. **Kouzarides, T.** 2002. Histone methylation in transcriptional control. *Curr. Opin. Genet. Dev.* **12**:198–209.

66. **Krockenberger, M. B., P. J. Canfield, and R. Malik.** 2002. *Cryptococcus neoformans* in the koala *(Phascolarctos cinereus):* colonization by C n. var. gattii and investigation of environmental sources. *Med. Mycol.* **40**:263–272.

67. **Krockenberger, M. B., P. J. Canfield, and R. Malik.** 2003. *Cryptococcus neoformans* var. *gattii* in the koala *(Phascolarctos cinereus):* a review of 43 cases of cryptococcosis. *Med. Mycol.* **41**:225–234.

68. **Kwon-Chung, K. J.** 1994. Phylogenetic spectrum of fungi that are pathogenic to humans. *Clin. Infect. Dis.* **19**(Suppl. 1):S1–S7.

69. **Kwon-Chung, K. J., and J. E. Bennett.** 1984. High prevalence of *Cryptococcus neoformans* var. *gattii* in tropical and subtropical regions. *Zbl. Bakt. Hyg. A* **257**:213–218.

70. **Kwon-Chung, K. J., B. L. Wickes, L. Stockman, G. D. Roberts, D. Ellis, and D. H. Howard.** 1992. Virulence, serotype, and molecular characteristics of environmental strains of *Cryptococcus neoformans* var. *gattii.* *Infect. Immun.* **60**:1869–1874.

71. **Latge, J. P.** 1999. *Aspergillus fumigatus* and aspergillosis. *Clin. Microbiol. Rev.* **12**:310–350.

72. **Legendre, U., M. Battegay, I. Nuttli, P. Dalquen, and P. Nuesch.** 2002. Simultaneous occurrence of 2 HIV-related immune reconstitution diseases after initiation of highly active antiretroviral therapy. *Scand. J. Infect. Dis.* **33**:388–389.

73. **Liu, L., R. P. Tewari, and P. R. Williamson.** 1999. Laccase protects *Cryptococcus neoformans* from antifungal activity of alveolar macrophages. *Infect. Immun.* **67**:6034–6039.

74. **Lockhart, S. R., B. D. Reed, C. L. Pierson, and D. R. Soll.** 1996. Most frequent scenario for recurrent *Candida* vaginitis is strain maintenance with "substrain shuffling": demonstration by sequential DNA fingerprinting with probes Ca3, C1, and CARE2. *J. Clin. Microbiol.* **34**:767–777.

75. **Marques, S. A., A. M. Robles, A. M. Tortorano, M. A. Tuculet, R. Negroni, and R. P. Mendes.** 2000. Mycoses associated with AIDS in the Third World. *Med. Mycol.* **38**(Suppl. 1):269–279.

76. **McNeil, M. M., S. L. Nash, R. A. Hajjeh, M. A. Phelan, L. A. Conn, B. D. Plikaytis, and D. W. Warnock.** 2001. Trends in mortality due to invasive mycotic diseases in the United States, 1980–1997. *Clin. Infect. Dis.* **33**:641–647.

77. **Meyer, W., K. Marszewska, M. Amirmostofian, R. P. Igreja, C. Hardtke, K. Methling, M. A. Viviani, A. Chindamporn, S. Sukroongreung, M. A. John, D. H. Ellis, and T. C. Sorrell.** 1999. Molecular typing of global isolates of Cryptococcus neoformans var. neoformans by polymerase chain reaction fingerprinting and randomly amplified polymorphic DNA—a pilot study to standardize techniques on which to base a detailed epidemiological survey. *Electrophoresis* **20**:1790–1799.

78. **Morschhauser, J., G. Kohler, W. Ziebuhr, G. Blum-Oehler, U. Dobrindt, and J. Hacker.** 2000. Evolution of microbial pathogens. *Philos. Trans. R. Soc. Lond B Biol. Sci.* **355**:695–704.

79. **Mylonakis, E., F. M. Ausubel, J. R. Perfect, J. Heitman, and S. B. Calderwood.** 2002. Killing of *Caenorhabditis elegans* by *Cryptococcus neoformans* as a model of yeast pathogenesis. *Proc. Natl. Acad. Sci. USA* **99**:15675–15680.

80. **Nagy, P. L., J. Griesenbeck, R. D. Kornberg, and M. L. Cleary.** 2002. A trithorax-group complex purified from *Saccharomyces cerevisiae* is required for methylation of histone H3. *Proc. Natl. Acad. Sci. USA* **99**:90–94.

81. Nakamura, Y., and M. Wada. 1998. Molecular pathobiology and antigenic variation of *Pneumocystis carinii*. *Adv. Parasitol.* **41**:63–107.

82. Neilson, J. B., R. A. Fromtling, and G. S. Bulmer. 1981. Pseudohyphal forms of *Cryptococcus neoformans:* decreased survival in vivo. *Mycopathologia* **73**:57–59.

83. Nelson, A. L. 1997. The impact of contraceptive methods on the onset of symptomatic vulvovaginal candidiasis within the menstrual cycle. *Am. J. Obstet. Gynecol.* **176**:1376–1380.

84. Nguyen, M. H., J. E. Peacock, Jr., A. J. Morris, D. C. Tanner, M. L. Nguyen, D. R. Snydman, M. M. Wagener, M. G. Rinaldi, and V. L. Yu. 1996. The changing face of candidemia: emergence of non-Candida albicans species and antifungal resistance. *Am. J. Med.* **100**:617–623.

85. Ono, M. A., A. P. Bracarense, H. S. Morais, S. M. Trapp, D. R. Belitardo, and Z. P. Camargo. 2001. Canine paracoccidioidomycosis: a seroepidemiologic study. *Med. Mycol.* **39**:277–282.

86. Ophir, T., and D. L. Gutnick. 1994. A role for exopolysaccharides in the protection of microorganisms from desiccation. *Appl. Environ. Microbiol.* **60**:740–745.

87. Rodrigues, M. L., C. S. Alviano, and L. R. Travassos. 1999. Pathogenicity of *Cryptococcus neoformans:* virulence factors and immunological mechanisms. *Microbes Infect.* **1**:293–301.

88. Rodriguez-Zaragoza, S. 1994. Ecology of free-living amoebae. *Crit. Rev. Microbiol.* **20**:225–241.

89. Rosas, A. L., and A. Casadevall. 2001. Melanin decreases the susceptibility of Cryptococcus neoformans to enzymatic degradation. *Mycopathologia* **151**:53–56.

90. Rosas, A. L., and A. Casadevall. 1997. Melanization affects susceptibility of *Cryptococcus neoformans* to heat and cold. *FEMS Microbiol. Lett.* **153**:265–272.

91. Ruiz, A., J. B. Neilson, and G. S. Bulmer. 1982. Control of *Cryptococcus neoformans* in nature by biotic factors. *Sabouraudia* **20**:21–29.

92. Sanglard, D., F. Ischer, L. Koymans, and J. Bille. 1998. Amino acid substitutions in the cytochrome P-450 lanosterol 14alpha-demethylase (CYP51A1) from azole-resistant *Candida albicans* clinical isolates contribute to resistance to azole antifungal agents. *Antimicrob. Agents Chemother.* **42**:241–253.

93. Santos, M. A., C. Cheesman, V. Costa, P. Moradas-Ferreira, and M. F. Tuite. 1999. Selective advantages created by codon ambiguity allowed for the evolution of an alternative genetic code in *Candida* spp. *Mol. Microbiol.* **31**:937–947.

94. Santos, M. A., and M. F. Tuite. 1995. The CUG codon is decoded in vivo as serine and not leucine in *Candida albicans*. *Nucleic Acids Res.* **23**:1481–1486.

95. Schmid, J., M. Rotman, B. Reed, C. L. Pierson, and D. R. Soll. 1993. Genetic similarity of *Candida albicans* strains from vaginitis patients and their partners. *J. Clin. Microbiol.* **31**:39–46.

96. Schneider, E., R. A. Hajjeh, R. A. Spiegel, R. W. Jibson, E. L. Harp, G. A. Marshall, R. A. Gunn, M. M. McNeil, R. W. Pinner, R. C. Baron, R. C. Burger, L. C. Hutwagner, C. Crump, L. Kaufman, S. E. Reef, G. M. Feldman, D. Pappagianis, and S. B. Werner. 1997. A coccidioidomycosis outbreak following the Northridge, Calif, earthquake. *JAMA* **277**:904–908.

97. Soll, D. R. 2002. *Candida* commensalism and virulence: the evolution of phenotypic plasticity. *Acta Trop.* **81**:101–110.

98. Soll, D. R., R. Galask, J. Schmid, C. Hanna, K. Mac, and B. Morrow. 1991. Genetic dissimilarity of commensal strains of *Candida* spp. carried in different anatomical locations of the same healthy women. *J. Clin. Microbiol.* **29**:1702–1710.

99. Soll, D. R., C. J. Langtimm, J. McDowell, J. Hicks, and R. Galask. 1987. High-frequency switching in *Candida* strains isolated from vaginitis patients. *J. Clin. Microbiol.* **25**:1611–1622.

100. Spitzer, E. D., B. A. Lasker, S. J. Travis, G. S. Kobayashi, and G. Medoff. 1989. Use of mitochondrial and ribosomal DNA polymorphisms to classify clinical and soil isolates of *Histoplasma capsulatum*. *Infect. Immun.* **57**:1409–1412.

101. Steenbergen, J. N., J. D. Nosanchuk, S. D. Malliaris, and A. Casadevall. 2003. *Cryptococcus neoformans* virulence is enhanced after intracellular growth in the genetically malleable host *Dictyostelium discoideum*. *Infect. Immun.* **71**:4862–4872.

102. Steenbergen, J. N., J. D. Nosanchuk, S. D. Malliaris, and A. Casadevall. 2004. Interaction of *Blastomyces dermatitidis, Sporothrix schenckii,* and *Histoplasma capsulatum* with *Acanthamoeba castellanii*. *Infect. Immun.* **72**:3478–3488.

103. Steenbergen, J. N., H. A. Shuman, and A. Casadevall. 2001. *Cryptococcus neoformans* interactions with amoebae suggest an explanation for its virulence and intracellular pathogenic strategy in macrophages. *Proc. Natl. Acad. Sci. USA* **18**:15245–15250.

104. Sternberg, S. 1994. The emerging fungal threat. *Science* **266**:1632–1634.

105. Taylor, J. W., D. M. Geiser, A. Burt, and V. Koufopanou. 1999. The evolutionary biology and population genetics underlying fungal strain typing. *Clin. Microbiol. Rev.* **12**:126–146.

106. **Taylor, J. W., D. J. Jacobson, S. Kroken, T. Kasuga, D. M. Geiser, D. S. Hibbett, and M. C. Fisher.** 2000. Phylogenetic species recognition and species concepts in fungi. *Fungal Genet. Biol.* **31:**21–32.

107. **Taylor, L. H., S. M. Latham, and M. E. Woolhouse.** 2001. Risk factors for human disease emergence. *Philos. Trans. R. Soc. Lond B Biol. Sci.* **356:**983–989.

108. **Vecchiarelli, A.** 2000. Immunoregulation by capsular components of *Cryptococcus neoformans. Med. Mycol.* **38:**407–417.

109. **Vergara, M. L., and R. Martinez.** 1998. Role of the armadillo *Dasypus novemcinctus* in the epidemiology of paracoccidioidomycosis. *Mycopathologia* **144:**131–133.

110. **Vincent, R. D., R. Goewert, W. E. Goldman, G. S. Kobayashi, A. M. Lambowitz, and G. Medoff.** 1986. Classification of *Histoplasma capsulatum* isolates by restriction fragment polymorphisms. *J. Bacteriol.* **165:**813–818.

111. **Visvesvara, G. S., and W. Balamuth.** 1975. Comparative studies on related free-living and pathogenic amebae with special reference to *Acanthamoeba. J. Protozool.* **22:**245–256.

112. **Walton, J. D.** 2000. Horizontal gene transfer and the evolution of secondary metabolite gene clusters in fungi: an hypothesis. *Fungal Genet. Biol.* **30:**167–171.

113. **Wey, S. B., M. Mori, M. A. Pfaller, R. F. Woolson, and R. P. Wenzel.** 1988. Hospital-acquired candidemia. The attributable mortality and excess length of stay. *Arch. Intern. Med.* **148:**2642–2645.

114. **White, T. C., K. A. Marr, and R. A. Bowden.** 1998. Clinical, cellular, and molecular factors that contribute to antifungal drug resistance. *Clin. Microbiol. Rev.* **11:**382–402.

115. **Wickes, B. L., M. E. Mayorga, U. Edman, and J. C. Edman.** 1996. Dimorphism and haploid fruiting in *Cryptococcus neoformans:* association with the alpha-mating type. *Proc. Natl. Acad. Sci. USA* **95:**7327–7331.

116. **Williams, B., M. Fojtasek, P. Connolly-Stringfield, and J. Wheat.** 1994. Diagnosis of histoplasmosis by antigen detection during an outbreak in Indianapolis, Ind. *Arch. Pathol. Lab. Med.* **118:**1205–208.

117. **Williamson, P. R.** 1994. Biochemical and molecular characterization of the diphenol oxidase of *Cryptococcus neoformans:* identification as a laccase. *J. Bacteriol.* **176:**656–664.

118. **Williamson, P. R.** 1997. Laccase and melanin in the pathogenesis of Cryptococcus neoformans. *Front. Biosci.* **2:**e99–e107.

119. **Woods, J. P.** 2002. *Histoplasma capsulatum* molecular genetics, pathogenesis, and responsiveness to its environment. *Fungal Genet. Biol.* **35:**81–97.

120. **Woolhouse, M. E., L. H. Taylor, and D. T. Haydon.** 2001. Population biology of multihost pathogens. *Science* **292:**1109–1112.

121. **Xu, J., R. Vilgalys, and T. G. Mitchell.** 2000. Multiple gene genealogies reveal recent dispersion and hybridization in the human pathogenic fungus Cryptococcus neoformans. *Mol. Ecol.* **9:**1471–1481.

122. **Yates-Siilata, K. E., D. M. Sander, and E. J. Keath.** 1995. Genetic diversity in clinical isolates of the dimorphic fungus *Blastomyces dermatitidis* detected by a PCR-based random amplified polymorphic DNA assay. *J. Clin. Microbiol.* **33:**2171–2175.

INDEX